MRS of the Brain and Neurological Disorders

Supervisors

Akihiro Igata, M. D.

Aichi Comprehensive Health Science Center, President

Tetsuhiko Asakura, M. D.

Kagoshima University, Neurosurgery, Professor Emeritus

Editor & Contributor

Toshiro Fujimoto, M. D.

Yokakai Foundation, President

I.A.M.T

Tokyo Japan

CRC Press

Boca Raton London New York Washington, D.C.

2000

Authorised Translation from Japanese language edition
published by
Terada International Inc./Institute of Advanced Medical Technology, Tokyo
Dr. Koji Terada
Shimoochiai 3-15-20 Shinjukuku Tokyo
Tel :03-3951-9806 Fax :03-5996-7016
E-mail :kterada@t3. rim. or. jp

Akihiro Igata MD., Chief Director, National Sanatorium Chubu Hospital
Tetsuhiko Asakura MD., Emeritus Prof., Kagoshima University
Toshiro Fujimoto MD., President, Yokakai Foundation

Originally published by
Terada International Inc./Institute of Advanced Medical Technology,

Under the Co-publishing Agreement between CRC and
Terada International Inc./Institute of Advanced Medical Technology,

Library of Congress Catalogue-in-Publication Data
Catalogue record is available from the Library of Congress.

Contributors

Supervised by

Akihiro Igata, M.D. (*Aichi Comprehensive Health Science Center, President*)
Tetsuhiko Asakura, M.D. (*Kagoshima University, Neurosurgery, Professor Emeritus*)

Edited by

Toshiro Fujimoto, M.D. (*Yokakai Foundation, President*)

Contributors

Tohru Yamamoto, Ph.D. (*Hokkaido University, College of Medical Technology, Assistant professor*)
Norio Iriguchi, Ph.D. (*Asahi Chemical Industry Co., Ltd.*)
Toshiyuki Miyazaki, Ph.D. (*Asahi Chemical Industry Co., Ltd.*)
Masahiro Sasahira, M.D. (*Obara Hospital, Neurosurgery*)
Kousaku Terada, M.D. (*Imakyure Hospital, Neurosurgery*)
Katsumi Nakamura, M.D. (*Yokakai Foundation, Neurosurgery Center, Director*)
Yasuhiko Utatsu, M.D. (*Kagoshima University, Neurology*)
Toshihiko Nakano (*Yokakai Foundation, South Japan Neuroscience Center, Biochemistry*)
Toshiro Fujimoto, M.D. (*Yokakai Foundation, Psychiatry, President*)

Collaborators

Siemens-Asahi Medical Technologies Ltd.

Akira Iwasaki (*Asahi Chemical Industry Co., Ltd.*)
Yasuhiro Ueshima (*Asahi Chemical Industry Co., Ltd.*)
Koji Ohga (*Asahi Chemical Industry Co., Ltd.*)
Osamu Takizawa (*Siemens-Asahi Medical Technologies Ltd.*)
Junichi Takeda (*Noguchi Institute*)
Hideo Toyoshima (*Asahi Chemical Industry Co., Ltd.*)
Toshio Naoi (*Asahi Chemical Industry Co., Ltd.*)
Jun Hasegawa (deceased) (*Asahi Chemical Industry Co., Ltd.*)
Koichi Hikida (*Asahi Chemical Industry Co., Ltd.*)
Takeshi Maki (*Representative President, Asahi-Kasei Joho System Co., Ltd.*)
Satoshi Yamai (*Asahi Chemical Industry Co., Ltd.*)
Yasuhiro Wada (*Siemens-Asahi Medical Technologies Ltd.*)

Neurosurgery

Koichi Uchimura (*Kagoshima University, Neurosurgery*)
Takao Kisanuki (*Yokakai Foundation, Fujimoto Hospital*)
Shinichi Kodama (*Yokakai Foundation, Fujimoto Hospital, Chief of Neurosurgery*)
Masaru Shimohonji (*Akune City Hospital, Chief of Neurosurgery*)
Wataru Hirakawa (*Kagoshima University, Neurosurgery*)
Katsuro Mamizuka (*Kagoshima Prefectural Ohshima Hospital*)
Nobuhide Moriya (*Kagoshima Prefectural Ohshima Hospital, Chief of Neurosurgery*)
Kazutaka Yatsushiro (*Yokakai Foundation, Fujimoto Hospital, Chief of the Gamma Knife Center*)

Psychiatry

Tsunehisa Uchida (*Yokakai Foundation, Director of Daigo Hospital*)
Masahiro Uchida (*Yokakai Foundation, Fujimoto Hospital*)
Tetsuya Takano (*Yokakai Foundation, Fujimoto Hospital, Chief of Psychiatry*)
Kouzo Takeuchi (*Yokakai Foundation, Fujimoto Hospital, Chief of Psychiatry*)
Masakiyo Nakashima (*Yokakai Foundation, Fujimoto Hospital*)
Takashi Nonaka (*Yokakai Foundation, Fujimoto Hospital*)
Tsuyoshi Fukuzako (*Kagoshima University, Psychiatry*)
Yoshiro Hokazono (*Chief Director of Hokazono Clinic*)
Hiroshi Yamaguchi (*Kurume University, Psychiatry*)
Kouichiro Yamada (*Kagoshima University, Psychiatry*)

Neurology

Koutaro Izumi (*Kagoshima University, Neurology*)
Nobuko Kawahigashi (*Kagoshima University, Neurology*)

Hirokazu Toyama (*Yokakai Foundation, Fujimoto Hospital*)

Masahiro Nagai (*Yokakai Foundation, Fujimoto Hospital, Chief of Neurology*)

Radiological Technician (Yokakai Foundation, Fujimoto Hospital)

Shinji Arimura

Seiji Obara

Noboru Kameda

Atsushi Koudabashi

Yutaka Nakano

Akihiro Hamada

Tetsuro Matsumoto (*Chief of Radiological Technology*)

Photography

Toshiaki Kawasaki

Secretary (Yokakai Foundation, Fujimoto Hospital)

Satomi Matsuyama

Mayumi Yamauchi

Preface

Today, nuclear magnetic resonance spectroscopy (MRS) stands as a unique tool for providing noninvasive access and measurements of important endogenous metabolically active compounds throughout the body, including the brain. The spatial distribution of key energy metabolites, such as adenosine triphosphate (ATP), phosphorylated and unphosphorylated creatine, lactate, glucose, glycogen and fatty acid energy reserves, and compounds associated with neuronal function including glutamate, glutamine, γ-aminobutyric acid (GABA), and N-acetylaspartate, a putative neuronal marker, are all currently observable via phosphorus (^{31}P), hydrogen (^{1}H), and carbon (^{13}C) MRS. All this, at a spatial resolution ranging from less than 1 ml to over 30 ml on now-standard clinical magnetic resonance imaging (MRI) systems operating at fields of 1.5 Tesla and higher. In addition to measuring the static levels of these compounds, dynamic measurements of metabolic flux and response to stimuli are observable by monitoring reactants and products by MRS. Intracellular pH can be monitored through measurements of the ^{31}P MRS chemical shift of inorganic phosphate. Thus, to the extent that these substances and parameters play key roles in brain function, the advent of spatially localized MRS opens a potential flood-gate of rich information about normal and disease processes involving these substances. MRS is a fundamentally new method of probing brain function!

New tools present new opportunities for research and the clinic, and the obvious questions are : Can the technique be used to solve current scientific questions, and can it be applied directly in the clinic to help with diagnosis or patient management? There are new responsibilities of validation as well : do the measurements accurately reflect what they are supposed to, and how do they compare with what is known from conventional methods? *MRS of the Brain and Neurological Disorders* endeavours to address some of these questions in exciting areas of clinical brain MRS by illustration of an extensive series of case studies that includes brain tumors, infarction, arteriovenous malformations, hemorrhage, epilepsy, and psychiatric disorders. Drs. Toshiro Fujimoto, and Koji Terada and their collaborators have assembled an impressive work that demonstrates both the potential and diversity of clinical MRS of the brain today.

In the early 1980s such texts could not be conceived. It has been the advent, firstly of whole-body magnets with sufficiently large apertures to accommodate the body, with homogeneity and magnetic field of sufficient fidelity and strength to perform MRS and, secondly, of methods that permit localization of the MRS signal to the human brain that have afforded us with this opportunity. The noninvasive measurement by MRS of metabolism and compounds linked to neuronal function in stroke, dementias, epilepsy, tumors, psychiatric disorders and the like visited in the pages herein cannot help but shed some light on these disorders. Often the results seem unexpected, but that's what makes things interesting, yes?

Paul A. Bottomley, Ph. D.
Baltimore, Maryland USA
July 1999

Words of Recommendation

Teruo Nagai
Professor Emeritus, Gunma University
Executive Director, Japan Radioisotope Association

The Science Council of Japan regards "science of the brain and problems of the mind" as one of the most important scientific research subjects in Japan to be approached toward the 21st century. Our time is truly the "era of the brain."

The brain is the organ in which functional differentiation among regions is most advanced. It is, moreover, one of the tissues of the body that exhibits very high levels of metabolism. Therefore, physiologic and biochemical information concerning the kinetics and metabolism of substances as well as anatomical and morphological information must be evaluated for clarification of normal functions of the brain and clinical diagnosis.

Among techniques of diagnostic imaging, X-ray CT and MRI capture primarily anatomical and morphological information, and PET, SPECT, EEG, MEG (magnetoencephalography) by SQUID (superconducting quantum interference device), fMRI (functional MRI), and MRS (MR spectroscopy) collect primarily physiologic and biochemical information.

It has already been some time since the introduction of MRI to daily medical practice, and MRA (MR angiography) is no longer a novelty. MR medicine seems to have entered a stage of maturation, but we have as yet to see the development of MRI and MRS, and the establishment of their clinical usefulness.

MRI is a method to represent the density distribution of a substance that emits strong NMR signals, usually from the hydrogen nucleus (^{1}H, i. e., proton) in tissue as two-dimensional images.

MRS is a method to represent the quantity, metabolic processes, and changes with time of a specific metabolite which, however, has a low signal intensity (compounds present in the tissue such as ^{1}H, ^{31}P, and ^{23}Na or those administered as stable radiolabeled compounds such as ^{2}D, ^{13}C, and ^{19}F) at a particular site of a tissue as spectra.

Although there is no positional information in the spectrum per se, metabolic information can be represented by two-dimensional chemical shift imaging.

The publication of this volume, written by Dr. Toshiro Fujimoto, as the first systematic textbook of MRS in Japan, is truly a timely event and is good news to many Japanese doctors who aspire to learn brain science and MR medicine.

The author, Dr. Fujimoto, specialized in psychiatric medicine after his graduation from the University of Tokyo Faculty of Medicine in 1969 and studied traditional psychiatry with Professor André Buge and pediatric psychiatry with Professor Didier-Jacques Duché at l'Hôpital de la Salpêtrière in Paris. After returning to Japan, he became engaged in clinical practice at Yokakai Fujimoto Hospital, founded by his father, and has put the psychiatry that he learned in France into practice.

Recently, under the guidance of former professor Haruo Akimoto of the University of Tokyo, he has performed MRI and MRS in about 1,200 patients with brain disorders including brain tumors, cerebral infarction, cerebral arteriovenous malformation, Moya Moya disease, and cerebral hemorrhage using Japan's only 2T superconductive MRI system (Siemens-Asahi 2T). Concerned with neurological functional abnormalities, in particular, he has obtained novel findings of profound interest in psychoses such as schizophrenia, depression, epilepsy, dementia, and alcoholism, which have remained largely unexplored by MR imaging.

The ^{1}H and ^{31}P spectra presented in this volume are all excellent, and they are considered to indicate the potential of MRS and the direction of its future development.

The activities of Dr. Fujimoto in the field of MR medicine are truly impressive. His frequent appearances at academic conferences as well as the publication of a number of papers in Japanese and English, and books that he co-authored have contributed to the present nation-wide renown of Fujimoto Hospital.

Publication of a book, whose contents surpass works of representative universities of this country, by a hospital at the forefront of clinical service is at once a matter of wonder and a splendid achievement that suggests how front-line clinical hospitals can and should operate in the future.

One of the greatest objectives of brain research today is to approach the association between the metabolism of substances in the brain and mental activities, i. e. "science of the brain and problems of the mind." In this sense, this volume, *MRS of the Brain and Neurological Disorders*, is expected to serve as a bridge that carries us from natural science primarily concerned with substances to human science centered around the mind.

A Message of Congratulation on the Publication of *MRS of the Brain and Neurological Disorders*

Haruo Akimoto
Professor Emeritus, Kanazawa University
Former Professor, University of Tokyo

MRS of the Brain and Neurological Disorders, authored and edited by my respected friend, Dr. Toshiro Fujimoto, has been completed and is now ready to be published. Dr. Fujimoto is one of the few pioneers in the field of MRS who quickly directed attention to its possible contribution to the research of psychiatric and neurological disorders, and he has aggressively carried out research using an MRS system that he developed in conjunction with Siemens-Asahi. In this volume published by Dr. Fujimoto and his co-workers, accomplishments of MRS studies in Japan to date are compiled. The appearance of this book should be greatly appreciated for the development of psychiatry and neurology.

As described in detail in the first part, "Basic Principles of MRS", MRS is a technique to represent metabolic products in the body as a spectrum on the basis of the principles of magnetic resonance. MRS is advantageous in that it allows direct *in vivo* identification and detection of metabolic products, and is an epoch-making examination for the diagnosis and prognosis of brain disorders as well as investigation of their etiology. Presently, MRS can detect spectra of nuclei such as ^{31}P, ^{1}H, ^{7}Li, ^{13}C, ^{19}F, and ^{23}Na, but ^{31}P MRS and ^{1}H MRS are used most widely. In this book, also, the results of investigations primarily using these two modalities are discussed.

^{31}P MRS is a method to detect signals from phospholipids such as phosphomonoester (PME) and phosphodiester (PDE), high-energy compounds such as adenosine triphosphate (ATP) and creatine phosphate (PCr), and inorganic phosphate (Pi).

In the second part, "Clinical Applications", the results of MRS studies concerning psychiatric disorders such as schizophrenia, mood disorders, and alcoholism as well as neurological disorders such as brain tumors, cerebral infarction, cerebral hemorrhage, cerebral arteriovenous malformation, dementia, and epilepsy are described on the basis of abundant data, and I found them quite informative.

As a psychiatrist, I take the greatest interest in the studies of schizophrenia by Dr. Fujimoto and his co-workers. An English report of such a study was published in Acta Psychiatrica in 1992, and it is regarded as the first attempt to study schizophrenia by MRS along with the reports of American researchers J. W. Pettegrew (1989) and J. A. Stanley (1991). ^{1}H MRS provides information about metabolic products such as *N*-acetylaspartate (NAA), creatine plus creatine phosphate (Cr), choline containing compounds (Cho), glutamic acid and glutamine, inositol, γ-aminobutyric acid (GABA), and lactic acid in various regions of the brain. By this method, Dr. Fujimoto and his co-workers (1996) demonstrated that there are areas of low NAA levels other than the epileptogenic foci in the brain of patients with temporal lobe epilepsy and that their location is associated with clinical symptoms and the course of the disease.

I sincerely hope that MRS, which is still unfamiliar in Japan, attracts more attention from many research and clinical institutions, investigators, and practitioners with the publication of this volume and makes a great contribution to research as well as the diagnosis and treatment of psychiatric and neurological disorders.

Preface to the First Edition

The presentation by Professor Paul A. Bottomley entitled "Technical Feasibility of Clinical ^{1}H Imaging and ^{31}P Spectroscopy" at the Third Annual Meeting of the Society of Magnetic Resonance in Medicine (SMRM) held in New York in 1984 was extremely enlightening. The presentation, in which the expression "compatibility of imaging and spectroscopy technology" was used because the term MRS (magnetic resonance spectroscopy) was not in general use, was exceedingly original and fresh. Being able to obtain the spectrum of metabolites directly and non-invasively from a particular area of the brain was a welcome advancement to researchers of the brain. The editor and co-authors of this book have since been absorbed in MRS and are deeply engaged in its research. Although considerable time seems to have elapsed, it is actually only 15 years since the 1984 SMRM. Since then the development of MRS has progressed at a dazzling pace.

In this book, the results of examination and diagnosis using a 2 Tesla MRS system installed at Yokakai Foundation, Fujimoto Hospital in Miyakonojo, Miyazaki Prefecture, Japan in 1988 are compiled to demonstrate the usefulness of MRS in the diagnosis of brain and neurological disorders. This book is characterized by the fact that 85 cases ranging from neurological disorders to psychiatric disorders have been accumulated by clinical application of a single MRS instrument. The MR spectrum shows magnetic field dependence or instrument dependence, but comparisons among cases are possible because imaging conditions including the pulse sequences are equalized as much as possible. The spectra presented here were obtained primarily by ^{31}P chemical shift imaging supplemented by images obtained by the ^{1}H single voxel method. The MRS system used was first developed jointly as the Asahi Super 200 by Asahi Medical and the editor's group, and the ^{31}P chemical shift imaging method developed for the said MRS system was used. This is another characteristic of this book. The Asahi Super 200 was later remodeled into the Siemens-Asahi 2 Tesla. The efforts that were put into the development of this new instrument are described in further detail in the Introduction.

Chapter 1 of Part I, Background and Theoretical Basis, is about the history of MRS and the process of evolution of the MRS equipment to its present form, with research trends of physics, chemistry, and medicine in Western Europe and the United States presented in tabular form. In connection with the chronological table, references in the early to middle period in the history of MRS are listed for those who wish to study MRS in greater depth. Dr. Tohru Yamamoto, Dr. Toshiyuki Miyazaki and Dr. Norio Iriguchi, who authored Chapter 2, Basic Principles of MRS, were involved in the development of this system, including the baseline correction method and the quadrature type ^{31}P head coil, during the period of Asahi Chemical Industry. In their chapter, which is written on the basis of their experience and expertise accumulated over many years of devotion to the development of MRS, the most important parts of MRS are explained clearly and in an expert manner. In Chapter 3, and ^{1}H MRS, part of the notes taken by the editor and the authors during the study to understand the ^{31}P and ^{1}H spectra are summarized. The theory of magnetic resonance is profound, and biochemical investigation of the brain by MRS is on its way to being established. Unfortunately, a simple explanation is difficult. We hope that readers find this chapter helpful when they prepare their own notebooks. In

Chapter 4, MRS of Healthy Individuals, the spectra used as controls, which are indispensable for comparison with abnormal spectra, are presented. The ^{31}P spectra and ^{1}H spectra were obtained by the chemical shift imaging method and single voxel method, respectively. The clear differences between these control ^{31}P and ^{1}H spectra and the abnormal spectra shown in Part II, Clinical Applications, serves as persuasive evidence of the reliability of the MRS apparatus referred to in this book.

Part II is a Clinical Applications. In Chapter 5, Dr. Masahiro Sasahira demonstrates a number of cases of brain tumors, ^{31}P spectra, metabolite images and contour maps of tumors including pituitary tumor, meningioma, neurinoma, epidermoid, astrocytoma, glioblastoma, oligodendroglioma, metastatic brain tumor, chondrosarcoma, and mucocele are presented. ^{31}P MRS clearly visualized metabolic abnormalities in these diseases, and the ^{31}P spectra illustrated the process of curing the lesions by radiotherapy and chemotherapy. In Chapter 6, Dr. Kousaku Terada presents a collection of data on cerebral infarction. Changes in compounds such as inorganic orthophosphate (Pi), phosphocreatine (PCr), and ATP from acute cerebral infarction to old infarction are captured clearly by ^{31}P MRS. Changes in the intracellular pH in the infarcted area are also detected, indicating the specificity and usefulness of ^{31}P MRS for disturbance of high-energy phosphate metabolism in cerebral infarction. In Chapter 7, Dr. Kousaku Terada deals with arteriovenous malformation (AVM) and Moya Moya disease. Here, increases in Pi were noted in the region of AVM by ^{31}P MRS. In Chapter 8 presented by Kousaku Terada, intracerebral hemorrhage, changes in the ^{31}P spectrum from the acute stage of cerebral hemorrhage are followed up serially, and increases in Pi at the site of the hematoma are particularly noted. Chapter 9 shows ^{31}P MRS of dementia including dementia of Alzheimer's type, Pick's disease, multi-infarct dementia, and Binswanger's disease. Whether the ^{31}P spectrum shows characteristic changes or not in dementia of Alzheimer type remains controversial, but our cases exhibited changes in phosphomonoesters (PME) and phosphodiesters (PDE), indicating abnormalities in phospholipids. These abnormalities in phospholipids may change according to the stage of dementia. Chapter 10 is concerned with neurological disorders such as multiple sclerosis, leukodystrophy, and Huntington's disease. The usefulness of MRS in these disorders is demonstrated. In Chapter 11, Epilepsy, the results of ^{31}P MRS and ^{1}H MRS are presented. By ^{1}H MRS, neuronal loss or dysfunction in an area including the epileptogenic focus are detected as a reduction in *N*-acetylaspartate (NAA). By ^{31}P chemical shift imaging, on the other hand, abnormalities in the metabolism of high-energy phosphates or abnormalities in their distribution have been detected. In Chapter 12, Psychiatric Disorders, the results of ^{31}P MRS and ^{1}H MRS in conditions such as schizophrenia, bipolar disorders, and alcoholism are shown. In the ^{31}P spectrum, abnormalities in phospholipids or metabolism of high-energy phosphates are occasionally detected. In the ^{1}H spectrum, neuronal loss or dysfunction may be disclosed. Although further evaluation with the examination of more patients is needed, these findings suggest that the detection of metabolic abnormalities of the brain in patients with psychiatric disorders is possible at the clinical level, and that MRS plays an important role in the evaluation of treatment and research.

Currently, MRS is undergoing remarkable improvements, and the MRS system referred to in this book is now obsolete. However, the experience of using this instrument ensured the realization of our expectations for MRS and confirmed our belief that treatment and research of brain and neurological disorders will make rapid progress with further improvements in MRS. Publication of this book has become possible through the efforts of Dr. Koji Terada, Representative of the Institute of Advanced Medical Technology, and we would like to express our whole-hearted appreciation. We have an intense feeling that we have some tie with him, since Dr. Koji Terada was also impressed by Professor Bottomley's presentation at SMRM in 1984. Finally, we would like to close by expressing our deep gratitude to Dr. Paul A. Bottomley, Dr. Haruo Akimoto and Dr. Teruo Nagai, who kindly contributed the Preface and Words of Recommendation to this book in addition to warm encouragement for our undertaking.

March 15, 1999

Tetsuhiko Asakura
Akihiro Igata
Toshiro Fujimoto

Reference

Bottomley, P. A.; Edelstein, W. A.; Leue, W. M. et al. Technical feasibility of clinical ^{1}H imaging and ^{31}P spectroscopy. *In Program and Book of Abstracts: Third Annual Meeting of the Society of Magnetic Resonance in Medicine, New York: USA: SMRM* ; 1984: 68–69.

CONTENTS

Pulse Sequence

The following pulse sequences were used :

^{31}P MRS

Two dimensional ^{31}P chemical shift imaging (2D ^{31}P CSI)

Time of repetition	: TR=2,000 ms
Time of delay	: TD=1.72 ms
Matrix size	: 8×8
Acquisition	: 12
Voxel size	: $3\times3\times4$ cm^3, $1.5\times1.5\times4$ cm^3

^{1}H MRS

^{1}H single voxel method

PRESS (point-resolved spectroscopy)

Time of repetition	: TR=1,500 ms
Time of echo	: TE=135, 270 ms
Acquisition	: 700
Voxel size	: $3\times3\times3$ cm^3

STEAM (stimulated echo acquisition mode)

Time of repetition	: TR=2,000 ms
Time of echo	: TE=60 ms
Acquisition	: 400
Voxel size	: $2.5\times2.5\times2.5$ cm^3

Informed Consent

The examinations of MRI and MRS were performed with the informed consent of patients and their families.

Introduction

Toshiro Fujimoto

All the MRS (magnetic resonance spectroscopy) data in this book were obtained using the 2 Tesla superconductive magnet system of Siemens-Asahi Meditech Co. It will delight me if the story of the birth of this equipment, which provided excellent phosphorus-31(^{31}P) chemical shift imaging for the first time in Japan, is a greater source of information for the world, than my mere indulgence in nostalgia. The forerunner of this equipment was the Asahi Super 200 built by the Asahi Chemical Industry Co., Ltd. The Asahi Super 200 was installed at Yokakai Foundation Fujimoto Hospital in 1988. The hospital had owned a 0.1T resistive magnet type Asahi Mark J since 1983 and it had been used by the departments of neurology, neurosurgery, radiology, and psychiatry under the guidance of the then Professors Akihiro Igata and Tetsuhiko Asakura of Kagoshima University and Professor Katsuji Watanabe of Miyazaki Medical College. The prototype of the Mark J was developed at the University of Aberdeen and showed excellent performance in the measurement of water proton T_1. However, as ^{31}P spectroscopy began to attract attention, particularly in the United States, MR systems all around the world shifted to superconducting magnet types. I was studying changes in water proton T_1 in the brain of patients with psychiatric brain disorders,[1-3] and ^{31}P MRS was all the more attractive to me in that it allowed direct observation of the ^{31}P spectrum and, particularly, because it provided *in vivo* information concerning high-energy phosphates and phospholipids. ^{31}P MRS had the potential of capturing biochemical changes in the brains of patients with still unexplained psychiatric disorders (such as schizophrenia and dementia). It was my hypothesis that causes of psychiatric disorders are obscure because information concerning the *in vivo* metabolism was missing in postmortem analysis of the brain.

In those days, Asahi Chemical Industry Co., Ltd. was making all-out efforts to develop a 2T Asahi Super 200.[4] Research on nuclei including ^{19}F, ^{13}C, ^{31}P, and ^{1}H and related technology such as chemical shift imaging by SIDAC (spectroscopic imaging by dephasing amplitude changing)[5-7] invented by Dr. Toshiyuki Miyazaki and his coworkers had been advancing considerably, and their achievements had been reported at conferences of the Japanese Society of Magnetic Resonance in Medicine[8-30] and the Society of Magnetic Resonance in Medicine (SMRM),[31,32] the Society for Magnetic Resonance Imaging (SMRI),[33] and the Radiological Society of North America (RSNA)[34-37] in the United States. The presentation by Dr. Jun Hasegawa, at the SMRI conference held in San Antonio, Texas in 1987, on his achievement of presenting *in vivo* ^{13}C chemical shift images of the human forearm for the first time in the world was especially splendid.[38] This study received high esteem and was cited in *Magnetic Resonance Imaging, Basic Principles* by Professor Young published in 1988.[39] The term MRIS (magnetic resonance imaging spectroscopy) was first used by the Asahi Chemical Industry group.[40] I conferred with Mrs. Takeshi Maki, Junichi Takeda, Hideo Toyoshima, and Norio Iriguchi of Asahi Chemical Industry in 1987 and set the goal to "obtain a ^{31}P spectrum from a voxel of $2\times2\times2$ cm^3 in the brain within 20 minutes". The technique of water suppression still had to overcome some problems in those days, and greater expectation was attached to ^{31}P MRS than to ^{1}H MRS. My project was accepted on the condition that the

^{31}P spectroscopy be developed jointly.

An Asahi Super 200 was installed in a special wooden building (Photo) made of non-magnetic materials and stainless steel nails, and no helium recycle system was used. As a result, excellent homogeneity of the magnetic field by the standards of those days could be obtained. The MRS part of the Asahi Super 200 was improved while the instrument was actually in clinical use as MRI. However, it was only at night or during holidays that such modifications could take place, and the technical staff of Asahi Chemical Industry shuttled between the research center at Atsugi and my hospital in Miyakonojo, sometimes working through the night for several days straight. The development of the Asahi Super 200 progressed steadily at a surprising speed. Consequently, I could present a study of ^{31}P spectra of schizophrenia and dementia at the 11th Conference of the Japanese Society of Magnetic Resonance in Medicine held at Japan City Center in Tokyo in March 1988.[41,42] I also submitted chemical shift imagings of cerebral infarction, brain tumors, schizophrenia, and dementia, and presented a basic evaluation of ^{31}P MRS at the 12th conference of the same Society in September.[43-50] To my knowledge, these presentations were the first of their kind in Japan. The development of the Super 200 progressed steadily, and the results were periodically released.[51-75] An issue in those days was spatial localization methods, and the single voxel method had a problem associated with the spatial displacement of the voxel due to the difference in chemically shifted resonances. The technical staff at Asahi Chemical Industry had already tested chemical shift imaging by SIDAC and had confirmed that the displacement error was relatively small by chemical shift imaging. Eventually, Dr. Toshiyuki Miyazaki devised a new method for chemical shift imaging including an epoch-making method for baseline correction.[76]

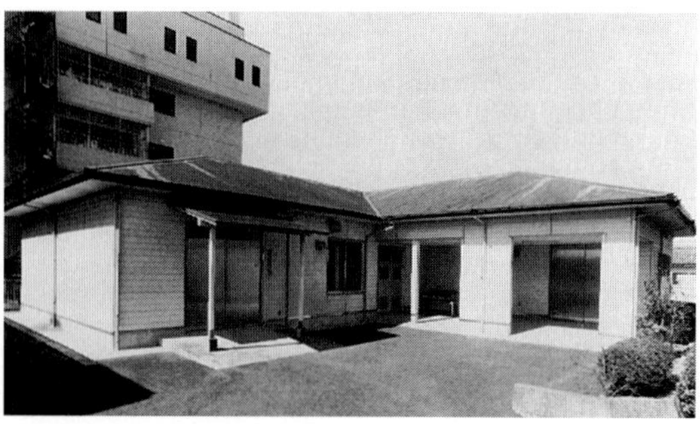

However, the MR section of Asahi Chemical Industry Co., Ltd. was merged with Siemens, and my dream of putting up the flag of the rising sun of medicine in the United States with the Asahi Super 200 was broken. In 1990, the Asahi Super 200 underwent almost total remodeling and, after major changes except for the magnet, it reappeared as a Siemens-Asahi 2 Tesla. As for the name, the fact that the system came to be called simply a Siemens-Asahi 2 Tesla without the name of Magnetom illustrated the pride of Siemens. Since it was regarded as a new MRI system, the medical insurance coverage, which was achieved after so much waiting, was removed, and everything had to be started again. However, this technological fusion between Japan and Germany has resulted in remarkable improvements in the performance of the Siemens-Asahi 2 Tesla. The goal was changed to "obtaining the ^{31}P spectrum from a voxel of $3\times 3\times 4$ cm^3 in the brain as a chemical shift image within 27 minutes" and was quickly attained and claimed as a major success. Since 1991, the results of application of MRS to cerebrovascular disorders, brain tumors, epilepsy, dementia, and psychiatric brain disorders, using Miyazaki's method for baseline correction, have been successively published in Japan and abroad.[77-90] Using the ^{31}P chemical shift imaging function of this system, I discovered abnormalities in membrane phospholipids and the metabolism of high-energy phosphates in the basal ganglia, temporal lobe, and the frontoparietal region in schizophrenic patients. A report of these discoveries was contributed to the Acta Psychiatrica Scandinavica in 1992 and was immediately accepted.[91] One year before this report, Professor Jay W. Pettegrew of the University of Pittsburgh reported abnormalities in the ^{31}P spectrum in the prefrontal area in schizophrenic patients using a surface coil, but my results were obtained by the chemical shift imaging method for the first time in the field of psychiatry, and my paper was different regarding the area from which the ^{31}P spectrum was obtained, and the discussion about phospholipids. My objective of developing ^{31}P MRS was attained. I was then invited to the MRS Workshop on Psychiatric Disorders held by Dr. Raymond F. Deicken at the Veterans Affairs Medical Center in San Francisco on May 23, 1993. At this workshop, where I presented a study of schizophrenia, Professor Michael W. Weiner said, the "Siemens-Asahi 2 Tesla system is the best," while we were eating cake together. I was deeply moved by his words and thought of the faces of the technical staff of Siemens-Asahi. These words of this great professor were more than a sufficient reward for the strenuous effort and struggle of all those who were involved in this work. The technology of ^{31}P chemical shift imaging developed in conjunction with Asahi Chemical Industry has also been applied to ^{1}H chemical shift imaging and, as is well known, has spread world-wide. I was satisfied with these achievements and was about to retire for some time from studies of MRS. However, through the encouragement of Dr. Haruo Akimoto to continue the work, I have envisioned a new research project and have begun preparations.

From my modest personal experience described above, I consider that the determination of the right goal and close cooperation between manufacturing technicians and physicians are vital for developing instruments of a world-class level. Moreover, technicians should attend international conferences along with physicians, globalize their perspectives, make presentations more frequently, and, thus, try to establish the importance of technicians, which have tended to be placed in the shadow of manufacturers in Japan. The challenge by Asahi Chemical Industry and Siemens-Asahi led by Mr. Maki was an experiment of just such a concept and has resulted in wonderful accomplishments in the sense of international technological contribution,[92] although the concept was so novel that the road to its realization was a rough one. Many people who were involved in the development of the Super 200 remain active today by making use of their valuable experiences. I would like to express my respect and gratitude to Mr. Takeshi Maki and other members of the technical staff of Asahi Chemical Industry and Siemens and wish them further success in their careers. In addition, I am also deeply grateful to Professor Takayuki Tsuji of Tokyo University and members of the Department of Neurosurgery and the Third Department of Internal Medicine, Kagoshima University School of Medicine, and Department of Radiology, Miyazaki Medical College, for their guidance and encouragement, which made such a project possible at a private hospital.

References

1) Fujimoto, T.; Yokoyama, Y.; Fujimoto, A. et al. Study of endogenous psychoses using NMR-CT. *Japanese Journal of Clinical Psychiatry* 13 : 1517-1530 ; 1984. [Japanese]
2) Fujimoto, T.; Nakano, T.; Fujii, M. et al. Changes in proton T1 in dog brains due to the administration of haloperidol. *Magn. Reson. Imaging* 5 : 469-474 ; 1987.
3) Fujimoto, T.; Tsuji, T.; Yokoyama, Y. et al. Study of dementia in the elderly using magnetic resonance (MR). Part I. —Measurement of proton spin lattice relaxation time (T1) using low field magnetic resonance. *Japanese Journal of Psychiatric Treatment* 3 : 897-908 ; 1988. [Japanese]
4) Iriguchi, N.; Iwasaki, A.; Yamamoto, T. et al. Spectroscopy using 2 tesla whole body MRS (First report). *Journal of NMR Medicine* 5 (Suppl) : 108 ; 1985. [Japanese]
5) Miyazaki, T.; Yamamoto, T.; Iriguchi, N. et al. Chemical shift imaging using SIDAC (Spectroscopic Imaging by Dephasing Amplitude Changing) method. *Journal of NMR Medicine* 6 (Suppl2) : 125 ; 1986. [Japanese]
6) Miyazaki, T.; Yamamoto, T.; Iriguchi, N. et al.

Spectroscopic imaging by dephasing amplitude changing (SIDAC). *In : Book of Abstracts : Fifth Annual Meeting of the Society of Magnetic Resonance in Medicine, Vol. 3. Montreal, Quebec, Canada : SMRM* ; 1986 : 856–857.

7) Miyazaki, T.; Yamamoto, T.; Iriguchi, N. et al. Chemical shift imaging using SIDAC (Spectroscopic Imaging by Dephasing Amplitude Changing) method (Second report). *Journal of NMR Medicine* 7 (Suppl1) : 105 ; 1987. [Japanese]

8) Manabe, A.; Miyazaki, T.; Toyoshima, H. 0.1-T human fat/water separation by SIDAC. *Magn. Reson. Med.* 5 : 492–501 ; 1987.

9) Iriguchi, N.; Iwasaki, A.; Yamamoto, T. et al. Study of ^{19}F NMR by 2 tesla MRS. *Journal of NMR Medicine* 6 (Suppl1) : 143 ; 1986. [Japanese]

10) Shimizu, M.; Kobayashi, T.; Morimoto, H. et al. Cancer imaging using missile ^{19}F MRI by anti-CEA antibody and 2T superconducting NMRsytem. *Japanese Journal of Magnetic Resonance in Medicine* 7 (Suppl2) : 225 ; 1987. [Japanese]

11) Iriguchi, N.; Iwasaki, A.; Yamamoto, T. et al. In vivo FTPA imaging using 2 tesla MRS. *Journal of NMR Medicine* 7 (Suppl1) : 107 ; 1987. [Japanese]

12) Hasegawa, J.; Iriguchi, N.; Ueshima, Y. et al. Human natural ^{13}C-imaging. *Japanese Journal of Magnetic Resonance in Medicine* 7 (Suppl2) : 224 ; 1987. [Japanese]

13) Yamamoto, T.; Iriguchi, N.; Hasegawa, J. et al. Possibility of ^{13}C brain imaging. *Journal of NMR Medicine* 7 (Suppl1) : 109 ; 1987. [Japanese]

14) Hasegawa, J.; Iriguchi, N.; Iwasaki, A. et al. Human natural ^{13}C-MR imaging. *Journal of NMR Medicine* 7 (Suppl1) : 110 ; 1987. [Japanese]

15) Iriguchi, N.; Hasegawa, J.; Miyazaki, T. et al. P-31 magnetic resonance imaging. *Japanese Journal of Magnetic Resonance in Medicine* 7 (Suppl2) : 228 ; 1987. [Japanese]

16) Yamai, S.; Iriguchi, N.; Yamamoto, T. et al. In vivo real time ^{31}P spectroscopy using 2 tesla whole body system. *Journal of NMR Medicine* 6 (Suppl2) : 232 ; 1986. [Japanese]

17) Yamai, S.; Iriguchi, N.; Yamamoto, T. et al. In vivo real time ^{31}P spectroscopy using 2 tesla whole body system (Second report). *Journal of NMR Medicine* 7 (Suppl1) : 136 ; 1987. [Japanese]

18) Hasegawa, J.; Iwasaki, A.; Iriguchi, N. et al. Bioimaging using ^{1}H gated decoupling method. *Journal of NMR Medicine* 6 (Suppl2) : 123 ; 1986. [Japanese]

19) Ueshima, Y.; Hasegawa, J.; Iriguchi, N. et al. Fundamental study of Tailored solvent suppression pulse. *Journal of NMR Medicine* 6 (Suppl2) : 130 ; 1986. [Japanese]

20) Yamamoto, T.; Yamai, S.; Iriguchi, N. et al. Absolute evaluation of S/N and quantification of limit. *Journal of NMR Medicine* 6 (Suppl2) : 132 ; 1986. [Japanese]

21) Hasegawa, J.; Ueshima, Y.; Iriguchi, N. et al. 2 tesla whole body imaging. *Journal of NMR Medicine* 6 (Suppl2) : 197 ; 1986. [Japanese]

22) Yamamoto, T.; Hikida, K.; Ueshima, Y. et al. Double speed imaging. *Journal of NMR Medicine* 7 (Suppl1) : 96 ; 1987. [Japanese]

23) Hikida, K.; Yamamoto, T.; Ueshima, Y. et al. Enlarged imaging of local region. *Journal of NMR Medicine* 7 (Suppl1) : 101 ; 1987. [Japanese]

24) Hikida, K.; Iriguchi, N.; Yamamoto, T. et al. Study of inclination of static magnetic field using strong magnetic. *Journal of NMR Medicine* 7 (Suppl1) : 102 ; 1987. [Japanese]

25) Ueshima, Y.; Hasegawa, J.; Yamamoto, T. et al. Volume-Selected Spectroscopy using Tailored pulse. *Journal of NMR Medicine* 7 (Suppl1) : 138 ; 1987. [Japanese]

26) Iriguchi, N.; Yamai, S.; Hikida, K. et al. Localized MR spectroscopy using inclination of static magnetic field. *Journal of NMR Medicine* 7 (Suppl1) : 139 ; 1987. [Japanese]

27) Hikida, K.; Iriguchi, N.; Yamamoto, T. et al. Study of inclination of static magnetic field using strong magnetic (Second report). *Japanese Journal of Magnetic Resonance in Medicine* 7 (Suppl2) : 175 ; 1987. [Japanese]

28) Miyazaki, T.; Iriguchi, N.; Ueshima, Y. et al. Speed analyzing imaging of flow. *Japanese Journal of Magnetic Resonance in Medicine* 7 (Suppl2) : 133 ; 1987. [Japanese]

29) Ueshima, Y. Volume-selected spectroscopy. *Japanese Journal of Magnetic Resonance in Medicine* 7 : 3–23 ; 1987. [Japanese]

30) Yamamoto, T. Chemical shift imaging. *Journal of NMR Medicine* 6 : 221–239 ; 1987. [Japanese]

31) Yamamoto, T.; Yamai, S. Iriguchi, N. et al. An estimation scheme for the S/N of coil. *In : Book of Abstracts : Fifth Annual Meeting of the Society of Magnetic Resonance in Medicine, Vol. 1. Montreal, Quebec, Canada : SMRM* ; 1986 : 211.

32) Iriguchi, N.; Iwasaki, A.; Yamamoto, T. et al. In vivo ^{19}F images obtained within minutes. *In : Book of Abstracts : Fifth Annual Meeting of the Society of Magnetic Resonance in Medicine, Vol. 4. Montreal, Quebec, Canada : SMRM* ; 1986 : 1545.

33) Hikida, K.; Iriguchi, N.; Yamamoto, T. et al. Localized MR utilizing a ferromagnetic cylinder. *In : Program and Abstracts : Fifth Annual Meeting of the Society for Magnetic Resonance Imaging, San*

Antonio, Texas : SMRI ; 1987 : 115.

34) Yamai, S.; Iriguchi, N.; Yamamoto, T. et al. Phosphorus-31 real time spectroscopy. *In : 72nd Scientific Assembly and Annual Meeting of the Radiological Society of North America, Chicago : RSNA* ; 1986 : 341.

35) Iriguchi, N.; Miyazaki, T.; Hasegawa, J. et al. F-19 MR imaging in vivo with FTPA. *In : 72nd Scientific Assembly and Annual Meeting of the Radiological Society of North America, Chicago : RSNA* ; 1986 : 315.

36) Iwasaki, A.; Miyazaki, T.; Iriguchi, N. et al. Field inhomogeneity correction system using spectroscopic imaging by dephasing amplitude changing (SIDAC). *In : 72nd Scientific Assembly and Annual Meeting of the Radiological Society of North America, Chicago : RSNA* ; 1986 : 211.

37) Miyazaki, T.; Yamamoto, T.; Iriguchi N. et al. Spectroscopic imaging by dephasing amplitude changing (SIDAC). *In : 72nd Scientific Assembly and Annual Meeting of the Radiological Society of North America, Chicago : RSNA* ; 1986 : 210.

38) Hasegawa, J.; Iriguchi, N.; Ueshima, Y. et al. Natural abundance carbon-13 NMR imaging of the human arm. *In : Program and Abstracts : Fifth Annual Meeting of the Society for Magnetic Resonance Imaging, San Antonio, Texas : SMRI* ; 1987 : 46.

39) Young, S. W. Magnetic Resonance Imaging : Basic principles. New York : Raven Press ; 1988 : p. 209.

40) Iriguchi, N.; Iwasaki, A.; Yamamoto, T. et al. Whole body 2 tesla MRIS. *Journal of NMR Medicine* 6 (Suppl2) : 196 ; 1986. [Japanese]

41) Fujimoto, T.; Nakano, T.; Suemitsu, J. et al. Study of psychoses using 2 Tesla MR. *Japanese Journal of Magnetic Resonance in Medicine* 8 (Suppl1) : 206 ; 1988. [Japanese]

42) Fujii, M.; Uchida, T.; Fujimoto, T. et al. Study of dementia using 2 Tesla MR. *Japanese Journal of Magnetic Resonance in Medicine* 8 (Suppl1) : 207 ; 1988. [Japanese]

43) Uchimura, K.; Sasahira, M.; Fujimoto, T. et al. Human brain ^{31}P-chemical shift imaging — Case study of cerebral infarction with wide lesions —. *Japanese Journal of Magnetic Resonance in Medicine* 8 (Suppl2) : 280 ; 1988. [Japanese]

44) Sasahira, M.; Uchimura, M.; Fujimoto, T. et al. Phosphorous spectroscopic imaging of brain tumors. *Japanese Journal of Magnetic Resonance in Medicine* 8 (Suppl2) : 281 ; 1988. [Japanese]

45) Fujimoto, T.; Tsuji, T.; Nakano, T. et al. Study of schizophrenia and dementia using ^{31}P spectroscopic imaging by dephasing amplitude changing. *Japanese Journal of Magnetic Resonance in Medicine* 8 (Suppl2) : 279 ; 1988. [Japanese]

46) Noguchi, S.; Nakano, T.; Fujimoto, T. et al. Study of muscle phoshorylase kinase deficiency using ^{31}P-MRS and ^{31}P-MRI. *Japanese Journal of Magnetic Resonance in Medicine* 8 (Suppl2) : 217 ; 1988. [Japanese]

47) Okada, A.; Utatsu, Y.; Fujimoto, T. et al. Study of myasthenia gravis using ^{31}P-NMR spectrum. *Japanese Journal of Magnetic Resonance in Medicine* 8 (Suppl1) : 121 ; 1988. [Japanese]

48) Utatsu, Y.; Okada, A.; Fujimoto, T. et al. Study of muscle diseases using SIDAC (Spectroscopic imaging by dephasing amplitude changing) method. *Japanese Journal of Magnetic Resonance in Medicine* 8 (Suppl2) : 201 ; 1988. [Japanese]

49) Tsuji, T.; Fujimoto, T.; Simooki, S. et al. Effects of head muscle of canine to ^{31}P spectra. *Japanese Journal of Magnetic Resonance in Medicine* 8 (Suppl2) : 143 ; 1988. [Japanese]

50) Shimooki, S.; Sakoda, H.; Fujimoto, T. et al. Evaluation of ^{31}P SIDAC (Spectroscopic imaging by dephasing amplitude changing) method by phantom. *Japanese Journal of Magnetic Resonance in Medicine* 8 (Suppl2) : 278 ; 1988. [Japanese]

51) Fujimoto, T.; Noguchi, S.; Nakano, T. et al. Study of Alzheimer's disease using 2 tesla MR. *Jpn. J. Med. Imaging* 7 : 286 ; 1988. [Japanese]

52) Noguchi, S.; Fujimoto, T.; Mitsuyama, Y. New technology for diagnosis of dementia : Study of usefulness of ^{31}P-MRI. *Jpn. J. Med. Imaging* 7 : 286 ; 1988. [Japanese]

53) Okada, A.; Fujimoto, T. ^{1}H-MR and ^{31}P-MR spectroscopy. *Image Technology & Information Display* 20 : 78-81 ; 1988. [Japanese]

54) Fujimoto, T.; Tsuji, T.; Nakano, T. et al. ^{1}H imaging and ^{31}P spectroscopic imaging in Alzheimer's disease. *International Symposium MRI Update* 93 ; 1988.

55) Sasahira, M.; Uchimura, K.; Fujimoto, T. et al. Phosphorus spectroscopic imaging of human brain. *International Symposium MRI Update* 94 ; 1988.

56) Fujimoto, T.; Noguchi, S.; Nakano, T. et al. MRS of Alzheimer's disease with presinile onset. *In : Abstract of the 12th Japanese Society of CNS CT* 116 ; 1989. [Japanese]

57) Noguchi, S.; Fujimoto, T.; Mitsuyama, Y. et al. Study of usefulness of ^{31}P-MRI for diagnosis of dementia ; comparison with IMP-SPECT. *In : Abstract of the 12th Japanese Society of CNS CT* 183 ; 1989. [Japanese]

58) Sasahira, M.; Uchimura, K.; Fujimoto, T. et al. ^{31}P spectroscopic imaging of brain tumors. *Japanese Journal of Magnetic Resonance in Medicine* 9 (Suppl2) : 236 ; 1989. [Japanese]

59) Sasahira, M.; Uchimura, K.; Fujimoto, T. et al. ^{31}P

spectroscopic imaging of brain tumors. *In : Abstract of the 12th Japanese Society of CNS CT* 191 ; 1989. [Japanese]

60) Uchimura, K.; Sasahira, M.; Fujimoto, T. et al. ^{31}P-chemical shift imaging of cerebral infarction and hemorrhage — Study of energy metabolism using SIDAC method. *In : Abstract of the 12th Japanese Society of CNS CT* 185 ; 1989. [Japanese]

61) Okada, A.; Utatsu, Y.; Fujimoto, T. et al. ^{31}P-MRS imaging of cerebral infarction-relation with SPECT and T_1 relaxation time. *In : Abstract of the 12th Japanese Society of CNS CT* 184 ; 1989. [Japanese]

62) Shimooki, S.; Nakano, T.; Fujimoto, T. et al. A quantitative study of chemical shift imaging by using phantom. *Japanese Journal of Magnetic Resonance in Medicine* 9 (Suppl2) : 309 ; 1989. [Japanese]

63) Noguchi, S.; Fujimoto, T. Application of ^{31}P-magnetic resonance imaging to senile dementia of Alzheimer type. *In : Book of Abstracts : Eighth Annual Meeting and Exhibition of the Society of Magnetic Resonance in Medicine, Vol. 2. Amsterdam, The Netherlands : SMRM* ; 1989 : 669.

64) Fujimoto, T.; Nakano, T.; Noguchi, S. et al. Study of dementia of Alzheimer type using ^{31}P chemical shift imaging and ^{31}P-NMR spectroscopy. *Japanese Journal of Psychiatric Treatment* 4 : 1249-1257 ; 1989. [Japanese]

65) Fujimoto, T.; Nakano, T.; Noguchi, S. et al. In-vivo ^{31}P multivoxel spectroscopy in Alzheimer's disease. *Progress in CT* 11 : 435-441 ; 1989. [Japanese]

66) Fujimoto, T.; Sasahira, M.; Okada, A. et al. Clinical application of ^{31}P chemical shift imaging and spectra. *Innervision* 4 : 33-38 ; 1989. [Japanese]

67) Fujimoto, T.; Nakano, T.; Fujii, M. et al. ^{31}P MRS of chronic schizophrenia. *Japanese Journal of Magnetic Resonance in Medicine* 10 (Suppl1) : 249 ; 1990. [Japanese]

68) Fujimoto, T.; Nakano, T.; Arimitsu, K. et al. Phosphorus-31 MR spectroscopy using 2 tesla MRS in epilepsy. *Japanese Journal of Magnetic Resonance in Medicine* 10 (Suppl2) : 191 ; 1990. [Japanese]

69) Fujii, M.; Fujimoto, T.; Nakano, T. et al. Study of aging and ^{31}P NMR spectra. *Japanese Journal of Magnetic Resonance in Medicine* 10 (Suppl1) : 246 ; 1990. [Japanese]

70) Sasahira, M.; Asakura, T.; Uchimura, K. et al. ^{31}P chemical shift imaging of arteriovenous malformations. *Japanese Journal of Magnetic Resonance in Medicine* 10 (Suppl1) : 199 ; 1990. [Japanese]

71) Shimooki, S.; Fujimoto, T.; Nakano, T. et al. ^{31}P spectrum studies on time course of change in brain metabolism after administration of phenobalbital to canines. *Japanese Journal of Magnetic Resonance in Medicine* 10 (Suppl1) : 356 ; 1990. [Japanese]

72) Fujimoto, T.; Nakano, T.; Sasahira, M. et al. MRS of brain disorders. *Clinical Neuroscience* 8 : 86-89 ; 1990. [Japanese]

73) Sasahira, M.; Uchimura, K.; Fujimoto, T. et al. ^{31}P spectroscopic imaging of brain tumors. *Progress in CT* 12 : 59-66 ; 1990. [Japanese]

74) Fujimoto, T.; Terada, K.; Shimohonji, M. et al. Future of MR spectroscopy. *Image Technology & Information Display* 22 : 81-84 ; 1990. [Japanese]

75) Sasahira, M.; Uchimura, K.; Fujimoto, T. et al. Early detection of cerebral infarction by ^{31}P spectroscopic imaging. *Neuroradiology* 32 : 43-46 ; 1990.

76) Miyazaki, T. Automatic baseline correction for ^{31}P-CSI. *Japanese Journal of Magnetic Resonance in Medicine* 12 : 322-327 ; 1992. [Japanese]

77) Fujimoto, T.; Nakano, T.; Noguchi, S. et al. Study of dementia of the Alzheimer type (presenile onset) using in vivo ^{31}P MR chemical shift imaging. *Japanese Journal of Magnetic Resonance in Medicine* 11 (Suppl1) : 192 ; 1991. [Japanese]

78) Fujimoto, T.; Nakano, T.; Noguchi, S. et al. Study of epilepsy using ^{31}P chemical shift imaging. *Japanese Journal of Magnetic Resonance in Medicine* 11 (Suppl1) : 191 ; 1991. [Japanese]

79) Nakamura, K.; Yatsushiro, K.; Asakura, T. et al. A study of epileptogenic foci on ^{31}P-chemical shift imaging. *Japanese Journal of Magnetic Resonance in Medicine* 11 (Suppl2) : 408 ; 1991. [Japanese]

80) Fujimoto, T.; Nakano, T.; Noguchi, S. et al. Study of dementia, epilepsy and schizophrenia using ^{31}P chemical shift imaging. *Japanese Journal of Magnetic Resonance in Medicine* 11 (Suppl2) : 248 ; 1991. [Japanese]

81) Yatsushiro, K.; Kasamo, S.; Sasahira, M. et al. Evaluation by ^{31}P chemical shift imaging of glioma before and after selective intraarterial chemotherapy and radiation therapy. *Japanese Journal of Magnetic Resonance in Medicine* 11 (Suppl2) : 407 ; 1991. [Japanese]

82) Terada, K.; Shimohonji, M.; Kawanishi, A. et al. Energy metabolism in brain tumor, cerebral infarction and intracerebral hemorrhage studied by ^{31}P chemical shift imaging (CSI). *Japanese Journal of Magnetic Resonance in Medicine* 11 (Suppl1) : 190 ; 1991. [Japanese]

83) Sasahira, M.; Asakura, T.; Uchimura, K. et al. Clinical evaluation of cerebral infarction by ^{31}P chemical shift imaging. *Japanese Journal of Magnetic Resonance in Medicine* 11 (Suppl1) : 189 ; 1991. [Japanese]

84) Fujimoto, T.; Nakano, T. Terada, K. et al. Study of dementia, epilepsy and shizophrenia using ^{31}P-CSI.

Japanese Journal of Clinical Medicine 49 : 233–237 ; 1991. [Japanese]

85) Fujimoto, T.; Nakano, T.; Terada, K. et al. Study of phosphorous 31 MR spectroscopy of interictal epileptic patients using 2 Tesla MR. *In : Book of Abstracts : Tenth Annual Scientific Meeting and Exhibition of the Society of Magnetic Resonance in Medicine, Vol. 1 San Francisco, California, USA : SMRM* ; 1991 : 222.

86) Utatsu, Y.; Izumi, K.; Fujimoto, T. et al. Localized proton MRS of the cerebellum in patients with spinocerebellar degeneration. *Japanese Journal of Magnetic Resonance in Medicine* 12 (Suppl1) : 79 ; 1992. [Japanese]

87) Fujimoto, T.; Nakano, T.; Fujii, M. et al. Study of ^{31}P-NMR spectra of chronic schizophrenia using 2T MRS. *Japanese Journal of Magnetic Resonance in Medicine* 12 (Suppl1) : 80 ; 1992. [Japanese]

88) Fujimoto, T.; Nakano, T.; Noguchi, S. et al. Study of dementia of the Alzheimer type (presenile onset) using in vivo ^{31}P NMR chemical shift imaging. *Jpn. J. Psychiatric Treatment* 7 : 531–540 ; 1992. [Japanese]

89) Fujimoto, T.; Nakano, T.; Takano, T. et al. Study of in vivo phosphorus 31 NMR spectra of chronic schizophrenics. *Japanese Journal of Clinical Psychiatry* 21 : 1471–1480 ; 1992. [Japanese]

90) Fujimoto, T.; Nakano, T.; Takano, T. et al. Study of chronic schizophrenia using ^{31}P chemical shift imaging. *In : Book of Abstracts : Eleventh Annual Scientific Meeting of the Society of Magnetic Resonance in Medicine, Vol. 1. Berlin, Germany : SMRM* ; 1992 : 1935.

91) Fujimoto, T.; Nakano, T.; Takano, T. et al. Study of chronic schizophrenics using ^{31}P magnetic resonance chemical shift imaging. *Acta Psychiatr. Scand.* 86 : 455–462 ; 1992.

92) Collaborator of Jun Hasegawa. Works of Jun Hasegawa. 1996. [Japanese]

PART I

BACKGROUND

AND

THEORETICAL BASIS

Chapter 1 History of MRS

Toshiro Fujimoto

1.1 MAGNET AND PHYSICAL BACKGROUND

The history of MRS (magnetic resonance spectroscopy) began with natural magnets. In China more than 3,000 years ago, vehicles called *shinan-sha* (south-pointing cart) were mounted on a figure whose hand pointed south because of the nature of magnets.[1] Natural magnets were also known in ancient Greece in about 600 B.C. In those days, there was a town called Magnesia in Asia Minor, and there was a town by the same name also in Macedonia. Since both towns produced natural magnets, the word "magnet" was coined from the name of the towns.[2] In China, the phrase "magnet invites iron or attracts it" seen in *Roshi Shunju* compiled in the third century B.C. is the first mention of magnetism. In Japan in the sixth year of Wado (713 A.D.) the people of the Ohmi region presented a "magnet" to the Emperor. This incident recorded in Book 6 of *Shoku Nihongi* is the first reference to magnets in Japan. Interestingly, the character 慈石 was used in those days instead of 磁石 to denote the word magnet as in the present time. This character, 慈 *ji* means to give loving care, to be affectionate, and to have mercy as is still used in expressions such as 慈愛 *jiai* (affection), 慈悲 *jihi* (mercy), and 慈雨 *jiu* (beneficial rain). A magnet is called 慈石 *Jishaku*, because a magnet and iron attract each other just as an affectionate mother and her child are attached to each other by the mystic love between them. It may be the Oriental intuition and wisdom that made our ancestors feel mercy, which is the noblest function of the human spirit, in the physical phenomenon of magnetism.

Here, we make a great leap to Europe in the early 20th century, where quantum mechanics and physics were coming into bloom. At that time, physicists were struggling to establish the concept of spin. According to Tomonaga and Segrè, the struggle was as follows.[3,4] It started with the discovery of the Zeeman effect (1896) by the Dutch physicist, Zeeman. He found that a spectral line splits into several lines when a light is placed in a magnetic field. The reason for this splitting of the spectral line was unknown. To explain this phenomenon, Uhlenbeck and Goudsmit of the Netherlands proposed the concept of spinning electrons in 1925. However, as this concept was so unconventional and contradictory to experimental findings, the two investigators lost confidence in their theory after contributing their paper to a journal and even asked the journal to return the manuscript. The manuscript, however, was already in print.[3,4] The concept of spinning electrons was promoted by Kronig, an American physicist in his 20s, about half a year before the paper of Uhlenbeck and Goudsmit. Unfortunately, the idea was refuted by Pauli, who was an influential figure in physics in those days, and publication of Kronig's theory was abandoned. Pauli maintained his opposition to the theory of spinning electrons even after the appearance of Uhlenbeck and Goudsmit paper. Ironically, however, Dirac noted that Pauli's exclusion principle agrees exactly with the concept of spinning electrons with a minor supplementation. Pauli's exclusion principle has since been linked closely to imaging of spin. This concept of spinning was called spin by the Danish physicist Bohr. Around this time, Estermann and

Stern measured the nuclear magnetic moment of the proton (1933), and Rabi published a theoretical paper about nuclear magnetic resonance in a molecular beam. And in 1911, Kamerlingh Onnes discovered the phenomenon of superconductivity.

In such a surge of advancement in natural science, Bloch and Purcell observed nuclear magnetic resonance (NMR) of protons in 1946 and established this method.[5,6] NMR was applied to medicine and has been developed as magnetic resonance imaging (MRI). Since MRS was developed abreast with that of MRI, a review of the history of MRS inevitably requires a mention of MRI.

1.2 MAJOR ACCOMPLISHMENTS CONCERNING MRS AND MRI

1946

- Purcell, Torrey, Pound[5]
  Observation of nuclear magnetic resonance in paraffin containing protons.
- Bloch, Hansen, Packard[6]
  Observation of nuclear magnetic resonance of the proton in water.

1948

- Bloembergen, Purcell, Pound[7]
  Relaxation effects in NMR absorption.

1950

- Hahn[8]
  Spin echoes.
- Dickinson[9]
  ^{19}F NMR.

1951

- Gabillard[10]
  Measurement of T_2 in an inhomogeneous magnetic field, basic research on the gradient magnetic field.
- Arnold, Dharmatti, Packard[11,12]
  Magnetic resonances of protons in ethyl alcohol.

1954

- Carr, Purcell[13]
  Carr–Purcell technique

1957

- Zimmerman, Brittin[14]
  NMR in multiple phase systems (Zimmerman–Brittin model).

1958

- Meiboom, Gill[15]
  CPMG (Carr–Purcell–Meiboom–Gill) technique.

1959

- Singer[16]
  Measurements of the blood flow rates in the mouse tail.

1963

- Daszkiewicz, Hennel, Lubas[17]
  Fast exchange two state model.

1964

- Barnothy[18]
  Biological effects of magnetic fields.

1965

- Bratton, Hopkins, Weinberg[19]
  NMR studies of living muscle.

1968

- Jackson, Langham[20]
  In vivo proton NMR in rats.

1969

- Koenig, Schillinger[21]
  Measurement of T_1 of apotransferrin by NMRD.

1971

- Damadian[22]

Discrimination between malignant and benign tumors in rats based on the measurement of T_1 and T_2.

1972

- Weisman, Bennett, Maxwell[23]
  In vivo detection of cancer of the mouse by NMR.
- Frey, Knispel, Kruuv[24]
  Studies of T_1 in nonmalignant tumors in mice.
- Battocletti, Linehan, Larson[25]
  NMR blood flowmeter for pulsatile flow.
- Hollis, Saryan, Morris[26]
  NMR study of water in Morris hepatomas.
- Damadian[27]
  The possibility of NMR imaging suggested.

1973

- Hounsfield[28]
  X-ray CT.
- Abe[29]
  Magnetic field focusing method.
- Lauterbur[30]
  NMR zeugmatography.
- Moon, Richards[31]
  Determination of intracellular pH by ^{31}P NMR.
- Mansfield, Grannell[32]
  Determination of spatial structures in solids which relies on NMR 'diffraction' effects.

1974

- Fung, McGaughy[33]
  State of water in muscle.
- Hinshaw[34]
  Spin mapping using a moving gradient magnetic field.
- Garroway, Grannell, Mansfield[35]
  The line scan method by selective excitation.
- Hazlewood, Cleveland, Medina[36]
  Relationship between hydration and proton relaxation time in tissues of tumor-bearing and non-tumor-bearing mice.
- Hutchison, Mallard, Goll[37]
  In vivo imaging using proton resonance.
- Hoult, Busby, Gadian[38]
  Observation of tissue metabolism by ^{31}P NMR.

1975

- Kumar, Welti, Ernst[39,40]
  Fourier Zeugmatography (two or three dimensional images).
- Mansfield, Grannell[41]
  Diffraction and microscopy in solids and liquids by NMR.
- Grannell, Mansfield[42]
  In vivo NMR microscopy.
- Llinás, Wüthrich, Schwotzer[43]
  ^{15}N NMR of living cells.

1976

- Mansfield, Maudsley, Baines[44]
  Fast scan proton density imaging.
- Mansfield, Maudsley[45]
  Planar spin imaging.
- Hinshaw[46]
  Image formation by the sensitive-point method.
- Damadian, Minkoff, Goldsmith[47]
  Visualization of a tumor in a live animal by field focusing nuclear magnetic resonance (FONAR).

1977

- Edzes, Samulski[48]
  A cross-relaxation model.
- Mansfield[49]
  Multi-planar image formation (fast imaging) using NMR spin echoes.
- Hinshaw, Bottomley, Holland[50]
  Thin-section image of the wrist can be compared in quality to those produced by X-ray CT.
- Holland, Bottomley, Hinshaw[51]
  ^{19}F MRI.
- Damadian, Goldsmith, Minkoff[52]
  MRI of the live human body by FONAR technique.

1978

- Chance, Nakase, Bond[53]
  In vivo ^{31}P NMR of the brain of mouse.
- Brooker, Hinshaw[54]
  Thin-section images using reconstruction from a set of projections taken from a selected slice of the sample.
- Hinshaw, Andrew, Bottomley[55]
  Cross-sectional image of rabbits by the sensitive line method.
- Mansfield, Pykett, Morris[56]
  Whole body line-scan imaging. Cross-sectional images through the abdomen.
- Bottomley, Andrew[57]
  RF magnetic field penetration, phase shift and power dissipation in biological tissue.

1979

- Hoult[58]
  Rotating frame zeugmatography.
- Hinshaw, Andrew, Bottomley[59]
  In vivo thin section MR images of the fore-arm and hand.
- Brunner, Ernst[60]
  Two-dimensional Fourier MR imaging.
- Gadian, Radda, Richards[61]
  ^{31}P NMR studies of the living body.

1980

- Moore, Holland[62]
  A whole body multiple sensitive point MR imaging system.
- Bendel, Lai, Lauterbur[63]
  ^{31}P spectroscopic zeugmatography.
- Edelstein, Hutchison, Johnson[64]
  Spin warp MR imaging (two-dimensional Fourier imaging) and a whole-body MR apparatus.
- Ackerman, Grove, Wong[65]
  Development of the surface coil.
- Hawkes, Holland, Moore[66]
  Brain tomography by MR. Clinical evaluation of patients with intracranial abnormalities.

1981

- DeLayre, Ingwall, Malloy[67]
  Gated ^{23}Na MR images of an isolated perfused rat heart.
- Smith, F. W.[68]
  Whole body NMR imaging. Examinations of 200 patients.
- Ordidge, Mansfield, Coupland[69]
  Rapid biomedical imaging by high-speed echo-planar imaging technique.
- Bangert, Mansfield, Coupland[70]
  Whole-body tomographic imaging by MR.
- Ross, Radda, Gadian[71]
  Clinical application of ^{31}P MR.
- Lai, Lauterbur[72]
  Three-dimensional image reconstruction by MR zeugmatography.

1982

- Brown, Kincaid, Ugurbil[73]
  Three-dimensional ^{31}P chemical shift imaging.
- Ordidge, Mansfield, Doyle[74]
  Real time movie images by MR.
- Alfidi, Haaga, El Yousef[75]
  A superconducting, whole-body, MR scanner.
- Young, Bailes, Burl[76]
  A whole body MR tomograph.
- Reid, Smith F. W., Hutchison[77]
  Clinical application of MRI and its safety implications.
- Escanye, Canet, Robert[78]
  Translational diffusion model.
- Fullerton, Potter, Dornbluth[79]
  Fast proton diffusion model.
- Gadian[80]
  Applications of NMR to living systems.
- Bottomley[81]
  Localized ^{31}P MRS by the sensitive point method.
- Bottomley, Kogure, Namon[82]
  ^{31}P NMR of the ischemic rat brain using surface coils.

1983

- Hilal, Maudsley, Simon[83]
  In vivo ^{23}Na images in cats.
- Behar, Den Hollander, Stromski[84]
  In vivo ^{1}H NMR of cerebral hypoxia showing changes of the lactate in the rat brain.
- Pykett, Rosen[85]
  In vivo ^{1}H chemical shift imaging.
- Cady, Costello, Dawson[86]
  ^{31}P MRS in newborn infants.
- Bottomley, Hart, Edelstein[87]
  ^{31}P and ^{1}H MRS of the head.
- Maudsley, Hilal, Perman[88]
  Four-dimensional ^{31}P MRS.

1984

- Bottomley, Foster, Darrow[89]
  DRESS (depth-resolved surface-coil spectroscopy).
- Bottomley[90]
  PRESS (point-resolved spectroscopy).
- Bottomley[91-93]
  Usefulness of ^{1}H, ^{31}P and ^{13}C MRS indicated.
- Hope, Costello, Cady[94]
  In vivo ^{31}P MRS in birth-asphyxiated infants.
- Younkin, Delivoria-Papadopoulos, Leonard[95]
  In vivo ^{31}P MRS of neonate brains.
- Dixon[96]
  Proton spectroscopic imaging (Dixon method).
- Sepponen, Sipponen, Tanttu[97]
  Chemical shift imaging of protons (Sepponen method).
- Hilberman, Subramanian, Haselgrove[98]
  In vivo time-resolved brain ^{31}P MRS.

1985

- Petroff, Prichard, Behar[99]
  Determination of intracellular pH.
- Bottomley, Edelstein, Foster[100]
  ^{1}H MRS by the water suppression method.
- Haase, Frahm, Hänicke[101]
  CHESS (chemical shift selective) imaging.
- Frahm, Merboldt, Hänicke[102]
  STEAM (stimulated echo acquisition mode).
- Hilal, Maudsley, Ra[103]
  ^{23}Na imaging of the human head.

1986

- Hasegawa, Iriguchi, Ueshima[104]
  In vivo ^{13}C imaging of the human arm.
- Bottomley, Drayer, Smith[105]
  Chronic adult cerebral infarction studied by ^{31}P MRS.
- Miyazaki, Yamamoto, Iriguchi[106]
  SIDAC (spectroscopic imaging by dephasing amplitude changing) technique.
- Ordidge, Connelly, Lohman[107]
  ISIS (image-selected *in vivo* spectroscopy) technique.

References

1) Ishii, T.; Kawabata, A.; Toyabe, T. Physics of Magnetic. Sogokagaku Publishing, 1980. [Japanese]
2) Asanuma, M. World of N and S : Magnet. Tokai University Publishing, 1977. [Japanese]
3) Tomonaga, S. Spin : The Period of Maturity of Quantum Mechanics. Cyuokoronsya, 1974. [Japanese]
4) Segrè, d. E. From X-rays to Quarks. Milano : Arnoldo Mondadori Editore, 1983.
5) Purcell, E. M.; Torrey, H. C.; Pound, R. V. Resonance absorption by nuclear magnetic moments in a solid. *Phys. Rev.* 69 : 37-38 ; 1946.
6) Bloch, F.; Hansen, W. W.; Packard, M. Nuclear induction. *Phys. Rev.* 69 : 127 ; 1946.
7) Bloembergen, N.; Purcell, E. M.; Pound, R. V. Relaxation effects in nuclear magnetic resonance absorption. *Phys. Rev.* 73 : 679-712 ; 1948.
8) Hahn, E. L. Spin echoes. *Phys. Rev.* 80 : 580-594 ; 1950.
9) Dickinson, W. C. Dependence of the F^{19} nuclear resonance position on chemical compound. *Phys. Rev.* 77 : 736-737 ; 1950.
10) Gabillard, R. Mesure du temps de relaxation T_2 en présence d'une inhomogénéité de champ magnétique supérieure à la largeur de raie. *C. R. Acad. Sci. Paris* 232 : 1551-1553 ; 1951.
11) Arnold, J. T.; Dharmatti, S. S.; Packard, M. E. Chemical effects on nuclear induction signals from organic compounds. *J. Chem. Phys.* 19 : 507 ; 1951.
12) Arnold, J. T. Magnetic resonances of protons in ethyl

alcohol. *Rhys. Rev.* 102 : 136-150 ; 1956.

13) Carr, H. Y.; Purcell, E. M. Effects of diffusion on free precession in nuclear magnetic resonance experiments. *Phys. Rev.* 94 : 630-638 ; 1954.

14) Zimmerman, J. R.; Brittin, W. E. Nuclear magnetic resonance studies in multiple phase systems : Lifetime of a water molecule in an adsorbing phase on silica gel. *J. Phys. Chem.* 61 : 1328-1333 ; 1957.

15) Meiboom, S.; Gill, D. Modified spin-echo method for measuring nuclear relaxation times. *Rev. Sci. Instrum.* 29 : 688-691 ; 1958.

16) Singer, J. R. Blood flow rates by nuclear magnetic resonance measurements. *Science* 130 : 1652-1653 ; 1959.

17) Daszkiewicz, O. K.; Hennel, J. W.; Lubas, B. et al. Proton magnetic relaxation and protein hydration. *Nature* 200 : 1006-1007 ; 1963.

18) Barnothy, J. M. Chapter 1. Introduction. In : M. F. Barnothy (Ed). Biological Effects of Magnetic Fields. New York : Plenum Press, 1964 : pp. 3-24.

19) Bratton, C. B.; Hopkins, A. L.; Weinberg, J. W. Nuclear magnetic resonance studies of living muscle. *Science* 147 : 738-739 ; 1965.

20) Jackson, J. A.; Langham, W. H. Whole-body NMR spectrometer. *Rev. Sci. Instrum.* 39 : 510-513 ; 1968.

21) Koenig, S. H.; Schillinger, W. E. Nuclear magnetic relaxation dispersion in protein solutions. *J. Biol. Chem.* 244 : 3283-3289 ; 1969.

22) Damadian, R. Tumor detection by nuclear magnetic resonance. *Science* 171 : 1151-1153 ; 1971.

23) Weisman, I. D.; Bennett, L. H.; Maxwell, L. R. et al. Recognition of cancer in vivo by nuclear magnetic resonance. *Science* 178 : 1288-1290 ; 1972.

24) Frey, H. E.; Knispel, R. R.; Kruuv, J. et al. Brief communication : Proton spin-lattice relaxation studies of nonmalignant tissues of tumorous mice. *J. Natl. Cancer Inst.* 49 : 903-906 ; 1972.

25) Battocletti, J. H.; Linehan, J. H.; Larson, S. J. et al. Analysis of a nuclear magnetic resonance blood flowmeter for pulsatile flow. *Transactions on Biomedical Engineering* 19 : 403-407 ; 1972.

26) Hollis, D. P.; Saryan, L. A.; Morris, H. P. A nuclear magnetic resonance study of water in two morris hepatomas. *Hopkins Med. J.* 131 : 441-444 ; 1972.

27) Damadian, R. V. Apparatus and method for detecting cancer in tissue. *United States Patent* 3789832 ; 1972.

28) Hounsfield, G. N. Computerized transverse axial scanning (tomography) : Part Ⅰ. Description of system. *Br. J. Radiol.* 46 : 1016-1022 ; 1973.

29) Abe Z. Measurement of information from the internal parts of objects due to application of nuclear magnetic resonance phenomenon. *Public Official Gazett of Patent.* 601-621 ; 1973. [Japanese]

30) Lauterbur, P. C. Stable isotope distributions by NMR zeugmatography. *Proc 1st international conference on stable isofopes in chemistry biolog and medicine.* 255-260 ; 1973.

31) Moon, R. B.; Richards, J. H. Determination of intracellular pH by ^{31}P magnetic resonance. *J. Biol. Chem.* 248 : 7276-7278 ; 1973.

32) Mansfield, P.; Grannell, P. K. NMR 'diffraction' in solids ? *J. Phys. C : Solid State Phys.* 6 : 422-426 ; 1973.

33) Fung, B. M.; McGaughy, T. W. The state of water in muscle as studied by pulsed NMR. *Biochim. Biophys. Acta* 343 : 663-673 ; 1974.

34) Hinshaw, W. S. Spin mapping : The application of moving gradients to NMR. *Physics Letters* 48A : 87-88 ; 1974.

35) Garroway, A. N.; Grannell, P. K.; Mansfield, P. Image formation in NMR by a selective irradiative process. *J. Phys. C : Solid State Phys.* 7 : 457-462 ; 1974.

36) Hazlewood, C. F.; Cleveland, G.; Medina, D. Relationship between hydration and proton nuclear magnetic resonance relaxation times in tissues of tumor-bearing and non-tumor-bearing mice : Implications for cancer detection. *J. Natl. Cancer Inst.* 52 : 1849-1853 ; 1974.

37) Hutchison, J. M. S.; Mallard, J. R.; Goll, C. C. In-vivo imaging of body structures using proton resonance. In : Magnetic resonance and related phenomena, Proceedings of the 18th Ampere Congress, 9-14 September. Vol. 1, P. S. Allen, E. R. Andrew, and C. A. Bates (Eds). Amsterdam : North-Holland, 1974 : 283-284.

38) Hoult, D. I.; Busby, S. J. W.; Gadian, D. G. et al. Observation of tissue metabolites using ^{31}P nuclear magnetic resonance. *Nature* 252 : 285-287 ; 1974.

39) Kumar, A.; Welti, D.; Ernst, R. R. NMR fourier zeugmatography. *J. Magn. Reson.* 18 : 69-83 ; 1975.

40) Kumar, A.; Welti, D.; Ernst, R. R. Imaging of macroscopic objects by NMR fourier zeugmatography. *Naturwissenschaften* 62 : 34 ; 1975.

41) Mansfield, P.; Grannell, P. K. "Diffraction" and microscopy in solids and liquids by NMR. *Phys. Rev. B.* 12 : 3618-3634 ; 1975.

42) Grannell, P. K.; Mansfield, P. Microscopy *in vivo* by nuclear magnetic resonance. *Phys. Med. Biol.* 20 : 477-482 ; 1975.

43) Llinás, M.; Wüthrich, K.; Schwotzer, W. et al. ^{15}N nuclear magnetic resonance of living cells. *Nature* 257 : 817-818 ; 1975.

44) Mansfield, P.; Maudsley, A. A.; Baines, T. Fast scan proton density imaging by NMR. *J. Phys. E : Sci. Instrum.* 9 : 271-278 ; 1976.

45) Mansfield, P.; Maudsley, A. A. Planar spin imaging by

NMR. *J. Phys. C : Solid State Phys*. 9 : 409–412 ; 1976.

46) Hinshaw, W. S. Image formation by nuclear magnetic resonance : The sensitive-point method. *J. Appl. Phys*. 47 : 3709–3721 ; 1976.

47) Damadian, R.; Minkoff, L.; Goldsmith, M. et al. Field focusing nuclear magnetic resonance (FONAR) : Visualization of a tumor in a live animal. *Science* 194 : 1430–1432 ; 1976.

48) Edzes, H. T.; Samulski, E. T. Cross relaxation and spin diffusion in the proton NMR of hydrated collagen. *Nature* 265 : 521–523 ; 1977.

49) Mansfield, P. Multi-planar image formation using NMR spin echoes. *J. Phys. C : Solid State Phys*. 10 : 55–58 ; 1977.

50) Hinshaw, W. S.; Bottomley, P. A.; Holland, G. N. Radiographic thin-section image of the human wrist by nuclear magnetic resonance. *Nature* 270 : 722–723 ; 1977.

51) Holland, G. N.; Bottomley, P. A.; Hinshaw, W. S. ^{19}F magnetic resonance imaging. *J. Magn. Reson*. 28 : 133–136 ; 1977.

52) Damadian, R.; Goldsmith, M.; Minkoff, L. NMR in cancer : XVI. Fonar image of the live human body. *Physiol. Chem. & Phys*. 9 : 97–100 ; 1977.

53) Chance, B.; Nakase, Y.; Bond, M. et al. Detection of ^{31}P nuclear magnetic resonance signals in brain by *in vivo* and freeze-trapped assays. *Proc. Natl. Acad. Sci. USA* 75 : 4925–4929 ; 1978.

54) Brooker, H. R.; Hinshaw, W. S. Thin-section NMR imaging. *J. Magn. Reson*. 30 : 129–131 ; 1978.

55) Hinshaw, W. S.; Andrew, E. R.; Bottomley, P. A. et al. Display of cross sectional anatomy by nuclear magnetic resonance imaging. *Br. J. Radiol*. 51 : 273–280 ; 1978.

56) Mansfield, P.; Pykett, I. L.; Morris, P. G. et al. Human whole body line-scan imaging by NMR. *Br. J. Radiol*. 51 : 921–922 ; 1978.

57) Bottomley, P. A.; Andrew, E. R. RF magnetic field penetration, phase shift and power dissipation in biological tissue : Implications for NMR imaging. *Phys. Med. Biol*. 23 : 630–643 ; 1978.

58) Hoult, D. I. Rotating frame zeugmatography. *J. Magn. Reson*. 33 : 183–197 ; 1979.

59) Hinshaw, W. S.; Andrew, E. R.; Bottomley, P. A. et al. An *in vivo* study of the fore-arm and hand by thin section NMR imaging. *Br. J. Radiol*. 52 : 36–43 ; 1979.

60) Brunner, P. Ernst, R. R. Sensitivity and performance time in NMR imaging. *J. Magn. Reson*. 33 : 83–106 ; 1979.

61) Gadian, D. G.; Radda, G. K.; Richards, R. E. et al. ^{31}P NMR in living tissue : The road from a promising to an important tool in biology. In : Biological Applications of Magnetic Resonance. New York : Academic Press, 1979 : pp. 463–535.

62) Moore, W. S.; Holland, G. N. Experimental considerations in implementing a whole body multiple sensitive point nuclear magnetic resonance imaging system. *Phil. Trans. R. Soc. Lond. B* 289 : 511–518 ; 1980.

63) Bendel, P.; Lai, C-M.; Lauterbur, P. C. ^{31}P spectroscopic zeugmatography of phosphorus metabolites. *J. Magn. Reson*. 38 : 343–356 ; 1980.

64) Edelstein, W. A.; Hutchison, J. M. S.; Johnson, G. et al. Spin warp NMR imaging and applications to human whole-body imaging. *Phy. Med. Biol*. 25 : 751–756 ; 1980.

65) Ackerman, J. J. H.; Grove, T. H.; Wong, G. G. et al. Mapping of metabolites in whole animals by ^{31}P NMR using surface coils. *Nature* 283 : 167–170 ; 1980.

66) Hawkes, R. C.; Holland, G. N.; Moore, W. S. et al. Nuclear magnetic resonance (NMR) tomography of the brain : A preliminary clinical assessment with demonstration of pathology. *J. Comput. Assist. Tomogr*. 4 : 577–586 ; 1980.

67) DeLayre, J. L.; Ingwall, J. S.; Malloy, C. et al. Gated sodium-23 nuclear magnetic resonance images of an isolated perfused working rat heart. *Science* 212 : 935–936 ; 1981.

68) Smith, F. W. Whole body nuclear magnetic resonance imaging. *Radiography* XLVII : 297–300 ; 1981.

69) Ordidge, R. J.; Mansfield, P.; Coupland, R. E. Rapid biomedical imaging by NMR. *Br. J. Radiol*. 54 : 850–855 ; 1981.

70) Bangert, V.; Mansfield, P.; Coupland, R. E. Whole-body tomographic imaging by NMR. *Br. J. Radiol*. 54 : 152–154 ; 1981.

71) Ross, B. D.; Radda, G. K.; Gadian, D. G. et al. Examination of a case of suspected mcardle's syndrome by ^{31}P nuclear magnetic resonance. *N. Engl. J. Med*. 304 : 1338–1343 ; 1981.

72) Lai, C-M.; Lauterbur, P. C. True three-dimensional image reconstruction by nuclear magnetic resonance zeugmatography. *Phys. Med. Biol*. 26 : 851–856 ; 1981.

73) Brown, T. R.; Kincaid, B. M.; Ugurbil, K. NMR chemical shift imaging in three dimensions. *Proc. Natl. Acad. Sci. USA* 79 : 3523–3526 ; 1982.

74) Ordidge, R. J.; Mansfield, P.; Doyle, M. et al. Real time movie images by NMR. *Br. J. Radiol*. 55 : 729–733 ; 1982.

75) Alfidi, R. J.; Haaga, J. R.; El Yousef, S. J. et al. Preliminary experimental results in humans and animals with a superconducting, whole-body, nuclear magnetic resonance scanner. *Radiology* 143 : 175–181 ; 1982.

76) Young, I. R.; Bailes, D. R.; Burl, M. et al. Initial

clinical evaluation of a whole body nuclear magnetic resonance (NMR) tomograph. *J. Comput. Assist. Tomogr*. 6 : 1-18 ; 1982.

77) Reid, A.; Smith, F. W.; Hutchison, J. M. S. Nuclear magnetic resonance imaging and its safety implications: follow-up of 181 patients. *Br. J. Radiol*. 55 : 784-786; 1982.

78) Escanye, J. M.; Canet, D.; Robert, J. Frequency dependence of water proton longitudinal nuclear magnetic relaxation times in mouse tissues at 20℃. *Biochim. Biophys. Acta* 721 : 305-311 ; 1982.

79) Fullerton, G. D.; Potter, J. L.; Dornbluth, N. C. NMR relaxation of protons in tissues and other macromolecular water solutions. *Magn. Reson. Imaging* 1 : 209-228 ; 1982.

80) Gadian, D. G. Nuclear Magnetic Resonance and its Applications to Living Systems. Oxford : Clarendon Press, 1982.

81) Bottomley, P. A. Localized NMR spectroscopy by the sensitive point method. *J. Magn. Reson*. 50 : 335-338 ; 1982.

82) Bottomley, P. A.; Kogure, K.; Namon, R. et al. Cerebral energy metabolism in rats studied by phosphorus nuclear magnetic resonance using surface coils. *Magn. Reson. Imaging* 1 : 81-85 ; 1982.

83) Hilal, S. K.; Maudsley, A. A.; Simon, H. E. et al. In vivo NMR imaging of tissue sodium in the intact cat before and after acute cerebral stroke. *AJNR Am. J. Neuroradiol*. 4 : 245-249 ; 1983.

84) Behar, K. L.; Den Hollander, J. A.; Stromski, M. E. et al. High-resolution ^{1}H nuclear magnetic resonance study of cerebral hypoxia *in vivo*. *Proc. Natl. Acad. Sci. USA* 80 : 4945-4948 ; 1983.

85) Pykett, I. L.; Rosen, B. R. Nuclear magnetic resonance: *In vivo* proton chemical shift imaging. *Radiology* 149: 197-201 ; 1983.

86) Cady, E. B.; Costello, A. M. de L.; Dawson, M. J. et al. Non-invasive investigation of cerebral metabolism in newborn infants by phosphorus nuclear magnetic resonance spectroscopy. *Lancet* 1059-1062 ; 1983.

87) Bottomley, P. A.; Hart, H. R.; Edelstein, W. A. et al. NMR imaging/spectroscopy system to study both anatomy and metabolism. *Lancet* 273-274 ; 1983.

88) Maudsley, A. A.; Hilal, S. K.; Perman, W. H. et al. Spatially resolved high resolution spectroscopy by "four-dimensional" NMR. *J. Magn. Reson*. 51 : 147-152 ; 1983.

89) Bottomley, P. A.; Foster, T. B.; Darrow, R. D. Depth-resolved surface-coil spectroscopy (DRESS) for *in vivo* ^{1}H, ^{31}P, and ^{13}C NMR. *J. Magn. Reson*. 59 : 338-342 ; 1984.

90) Bottomley, P. A. Selective volume method for performing localized NMR spectroscopy. US Patent 4480228 : 1984.

91) Bottomley, P. A. NMR in medicine. *Computerized Radiol*. 8 : 57-77 ; 1984.

92) Bottomley, P. A. NMR : a new perspective on medicine. *New York State Journal of Medicine* 84 : 438-440 ; 1984.

93) Bottomley, P. A.; Hart, Jr., H. R.; Edelstein, W. A. et al. Anatomy and metabolism of the normal human brain studied by magnetic resonance at 1.5 tesla. *Radiology* 150 : 441-446 ; 1984.

94) Hope, P. L.; Costello, A. M. de L.; Cady, E. B. et al. Cerebral energy metabolism studied with phosphorus NMR spectroscopy in normal and birth-asphyxiated infants. *Lancet* 366-369 ; 1984.

95) Younkin, D. P.; Delivoria-Papadopoulos, M.; Leonard, J. C. et al. Unique aspects of human newborn cerebral metabolism evaluated with phosphorus nuclear magnetic resonance spectroscopy. *Ann. Neurol*. 16 : 581-586 ; 1984.

96) Dixon, W. T. Simple proton spectroscopic imaging. *Radiology* 153 : 189-194 ; 1984.

97) Sepponen, R. E.; Sipponen, J. T.; Tanttu, J. I. A method for chemical shift imaging : Demonstration of bone marrow involvement with proton chemical shift imaging. *J. Comput. Assist. Tomogr*. 8 : 585-587 ; 1984.

98) Hilberman, M.; Subramanian, V. H.; Haselgrove, J. et al. *In vivo* time-resolved brain phosphorus nuclear magnetic resonance. *J. Cereb. Blood Flow Metabol*. 4 : 334-342 ; 1984.

99) Petroff, O. A. C.; Prichard, J. W.; Behar, K. L. et al. Cerebral intracellular pH by ^{31}P nuclear magnetic resonance spectroscopy. *Neurology* 35 : 781-788 ; 1985.

100) Bottomley, P. A.; Edelstein, W. A.; Foster, T. H. et al. *In vivo* solvent-suppressed localized hydrogen nuclear magnetic resonance spectroscopy : A window to metabolism ? *Proc. Natl. Acad. Sci. USA* 82 : 2148-2152 ; 1985.

101) Haase, A.; Frahm, J.; Hänicke, W. et al. ^{1}H NMR chemical shift selective (CHESS) imaging. *Phys. Med. Biol*. 30 : 341-344 ; 1985.

102) Frahm, J.; Merboldt, K. D.; Hänicke, W. et al. Stimulated echo imaging. *J. Magn. Reson*. 64 : 81-93 ; 1985.

103) Hilal, S. K.; Maudsley, A. A.; Ra, J. B. et al. In vivo NMR imaging of sodium-23 in the human head. *J. Comput. Assist. Tomogr*. 9 : 1-7 ; 1985.

104) Hasegawa, J.; Iriguchi, N.; Ueshima, Y. et al. Natural abundance carbon-13 NMR imaging of the human arm. *In : Fifth Annual Meeting of the Society for Magnetic Resonance Imaging, San Antonio, Texas : SMRI* ; 1987 : 46.

105) Bottomley, P. A.; Drayer, B. P.; Smith, L. S. Chronic adult cerebral infarction studied by phosphorus NMR spectroscopy. *Radiology* 160 : 763–766 ; 1986.

106) Miyazaki, T.; Yamamoto, T.; Iriguchi, N. et al. Spectroscopic imaging by dephasing amplitude changing (SIDAC). *In : Book of Abstracts : Fifth Annual Meeting of the Society of Magnetic Resonance in Medicine, Montreal, Quebec, Canada : SMRM* ; 1986 : 856–857.

107) Ordidge, R. J.; Connelly, A.; Lohman, J. A. B. Image-selected *in vivo* spectroscopy (ISIS). A new technique for spatially selective NMR spectroscopy. *J. Magn. Reson.* 66 : 283–294 ; 1986.

Chapter 2 Basic Principles of MRS

Tohru Yamamoto, Norio Iriguchi, and Toshiyuki Miyazaki

In this chapter, principles of magnetic resonance spectroscopy (MRS) are described. All data in this volume were obtained and evaluated on those principles. Factors that determine limitations of measurements such as spatial and temporal resolutions are discussed, and primary factors in the performance are explained.

2.1 PRINCIPLES OF MEASUREMENTS

Spectroscopy based on nuclear magnetic resonance (NMR) is used for analysis of molecules. MRS is a method to obtain NMR information concerning biochemical substances such as ATP and lactic acid *in vivo* by collecting magnetic resonance signals from nuclei of biological substances such as ^{31}P and ^{1}H (usually other than water and fat). Therefore, MRS provides molecular-based information such as that concerning biochemical changes in the body, unlike the histomorphological information derived from MRI.

2.1.1 RF coil

Special radio-frequency (RF) coils designed to measure different parts of the body are used to allow the corresponding area to generate magnetic resonance signals and to receive them. In this volume, head MRS using a head volume coil for both transmission and reception was evaluated in a clinical MR system. In this evaluation, a quadrature type head MRI RF coil was used for ^{1}H MRS. However, when MRS is performed using nuclei other than ^{1}H such as ^{31}P, special high-frequency hardware, e.g., a head RF coil for ^{31}P, becomes necessary because of the difference in the resonance frequency. To obtain spectral signals, ^{1}H MR images must be obtained in advance, and the region in which the measurements are made must be targeted. For this reason, there are RF coils that can receive both ^{1}H and ^{31}P signals. In the MRS described in this volume, however, ^{1}H MRI images were obtained using a ^{1}H head RF coil, which was then replaced with a special quadrature type head RF coil for ^{31}P. The use of the head volume coil for ^{31}P improved the detection sensitivity of ^{31}P signals. The patient's head was carefully immobilized to ensure high reproducibility.

2.1.2 Localization

Biochemical activities in the body occur unevenly at the microscopic level, and different tissues, e.g., normal tissue and malignant tumor tissues, exhibit different biochemical activities. Without localization of the area in which magnetic resonance signals are to be collected, a variety of biochemical activities would commingle. Therefore, selection of the region from which signals are collected is one of the keys for successful MRS. Although there are several methods for restricting signal reception, including the use of a surface coil, the three-dimensional localization method, by adding positional information to magnetic resonance signals using a gradient magnetic field similar to that used in MRI, is most often employed in clinical studies. This three-dimensional localization method can be classified into the single-voxel method, in which a single region is excited selectively, and the multivoxel method, in which the magnetic resonance spectra are examined for multiple voxels in a matrix (e.g., 8×8). Fig. 2-1 shows examples of these methods.

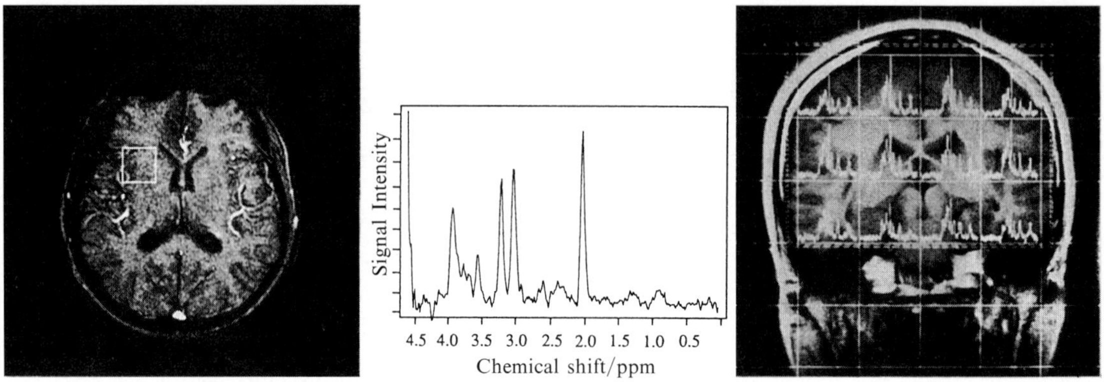

A VOI on a T_1 weighted image. A Spectrum of the VOI.

(1) Single-voxel method. (2) Multivoxel method.

Fig. 2-1 Examples of MRS localization.

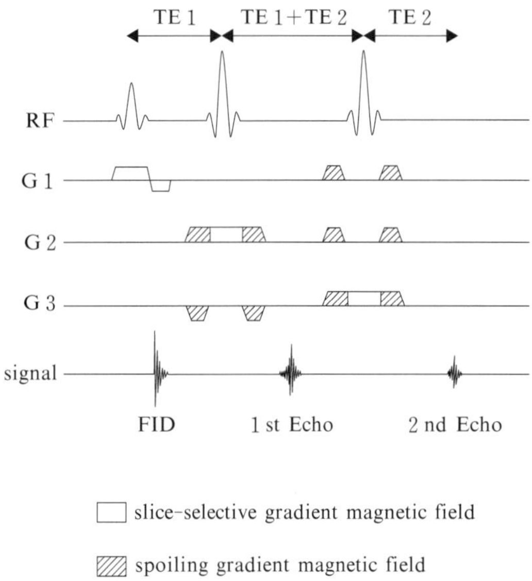

Fig. 2-2 PRESS pulse sequence diagram.

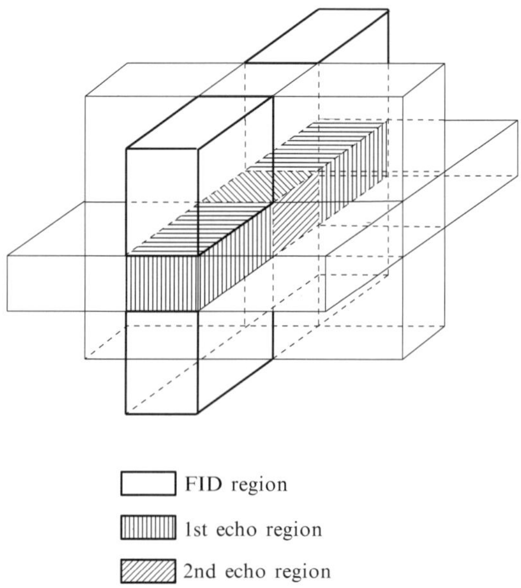

Fig. 2-3 Selected regions of PRESS.

(1) ***Single-voxel method***

PRESS (point-resolved spectroscopy)[1,2]

This method is a technique that makes a specific selected region generate second spin echo signals. Fig. 2-2 shows basic pulse sequence diagram of PRESS. RF pulses in a sequence of 90° -(TE1)-180°-(TE1+TE2)-180°-(TE2)-signal induce two spin echoes. Since the slice-selective gradient magnetic fields corresponding to each RF pulse are different, three perpendicular planes are usually selected. As a result, the part in which the three planes converge becomes the selected region since the second spin echo is generated exclusively in this part. Fig. 2-3 shows the selected regions where magnetic resonance signals are generated according to the gradient magnetic fields. The second spin echo region, in which the selected slices of the three gradient magnetic fields intersect with one another, is the region selected for MRS. Also, the gradient magnetic fields applied before and after the timing of each 180° pulse to cancel the phases of the spins other than those in the selected region are called spoiling gradient magnetic fields. Since the phases of spins in the selected region are

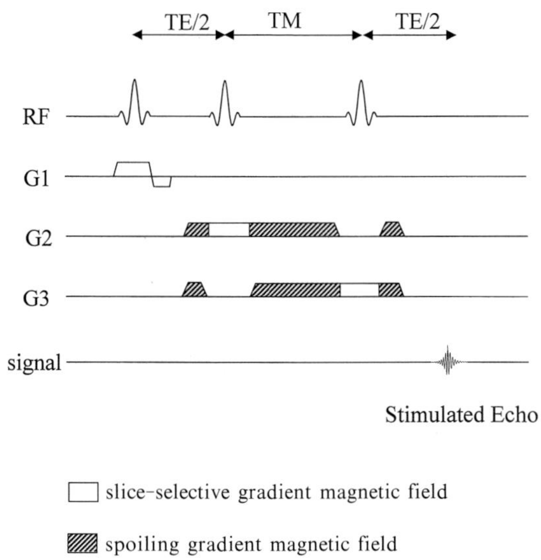

Fig. 2-4 STEAM pulse sequence diagram.

reversed by 180° pulses, the phases of spins induced by spoiling gradient magnetic fields before and after the 180° pulse cancel, and the signal is preserved.

STEAM (stimulated echo-acquisition mode)[3–5]

This technique is used to induce stimulated echo signals[6] exclusively from a given region. Fig. 2-4 shows a basic pulse sequence diagram used in this method. Stimulated echoes are generated by a sequence of 90°-(TE/2)-90°-(TM)-90°-(TE/2)-signals. A stimulated echo is different from a spin echo in that instead of the 180° pulse, it employs two 90° pulses sandwiching the mixing time (TM). Since this TM is independent of TE, it can be made relatively short. Therefore, compared with PRESS, the time from the initial excitation to generation of signal echoes (delay time) can be reduced for measurement of metabolites with short T_2. Although the delay time of STEAM is restricted by factors such as eddy currents described later, measurements on the order of 10 ms can be made.[7]

The stimulated echo is explained qualitatively as follows. The phases of spins induced by the first 90° pulse are distributed isotropically due to T_2 relaxation and spoiling gradient magnetic fields. After the second 90° pulse, half the information of the excited spins is preserved in the direction of B_o (the z axis). Finally, the preserved spin information is transferred to the xy plane by the third 90° pulse, and a stimulated echo is generated after TE/2 similarly to the spin echo. Since only half the information of the induced spin can be obtained, the signal intensity is smaller than in PRESS with a similar delay time. While two 180° pulses are employed in PRESS, the pulses used in STEAM are all 90°. In addition, the region selectivity is higher with 90° pulses. This is a major feature of STEAM. By contrast, the flip angle of the 180° pulses used in PRESS must be carefully adjusted, and RF coils with a homogeneous RF magnetic field are needed, but the flip angle of the 90° pulses used in STEAM need not be so exact.[8] Moreover, in substances having spin-spin coupling such as protons of lactic acid, modulation due to spin-spin coupling can be controlled by adjusting TE or TM. For example, in STEAM with TE=136 ms and TM=30 ms, the Fourier-transformed peak of lactic acid appears negative.

(2) ***Multivoxel method***[9–13]

The single-voxel method provides information only in a single selected region. The multivoxel method is used to simultaneously obtain spectra in multiple regions. In this method, a given field of view (FOV) is divided into several voxels, and the spectrum is examined in each voxel as in Fig. 2-1 (2). In this method, the number of voxels, i.e., the matrix size, is relatively small (e.g., 8×8 or 16×16) compared with MRI, but the method is also called CSI (chemical-shift imaging) because it is a variation of MRI. In MRI, one direction of the space is usually encoded with the frequency using a readout gradient magnetic field. However, a readout gradient magnetic field cannot be used in the multivoxel method, which acquires signals of materials with multiple resonance frequencies, because it causes chemical-shift artifacts. For this reason, after slice-selective excitation, two-dimen-

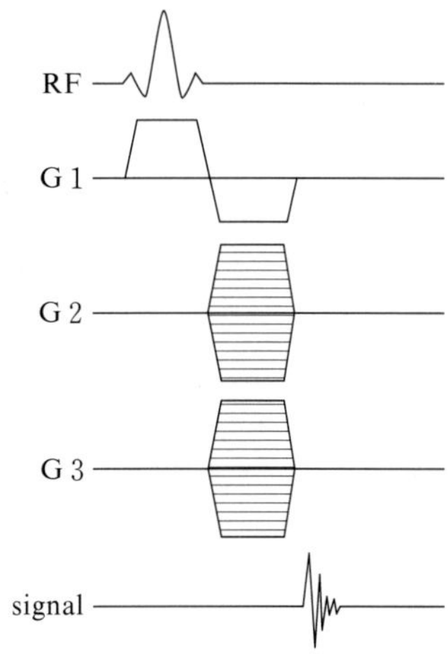

Fig. 2-5 Two-dimensional CSI pulse sequence diagram.

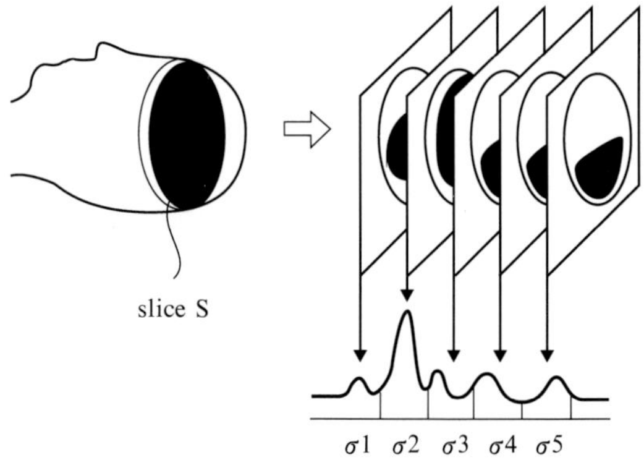

Fig. 2-6 Chemical shift imaging.

sional phase encoding of positional information is made by giving phases to the spins at various positions in two-directional gradient magnetic fields. This method is also called two-dimensional CSI. Its basic pulse sequence diagram is shown in Fig. 2-5. Furthermore, imaging can be done for each chemical shift component in the spectrum obtained from each voxel (chemical-shift imaging [Fig. 2-6]). In the images obtained by this method, the signal intensities of various chemical shifts can be displayed in a mosaic-like pattern because of the sparsity of the matrix density. However, with interpixel interpolation, images such as that shown in Fig. 2-7(1) can be obtained, and a signal intensity contour map can be prepared for each chemical shift as in Fig. 2-7(2). The slice selection thickness of two-dimensional CSI can also be increased, and the position in the direction of slice selection can be encoded by the phase using the gradient magnetic field. This method is called three-dimensional CSI.[14–16] The pulse sequence diagram shown in Fig. 2-5 is an example of those used in the gradient echo method, but the spin echo method can also be used,[17] because only two-dimensional phase encoding in a gradient magnetic field is needed for its application. Moreover, the cerebral parenchyma, for example, can be selected as a volume of interest (VOI) by the single-voxel method, and two-dimensional phase coding can be made in that voxel. Fig. 2-8 shows an example of a pulse sequence diagram used for this purpose. This method is used to suppress fat signals from the surface of the head, especially in ^{1}H MRS of the head.[18,19]

(3) *Comparison of the single-voxel and multivoxel methods*

While the multivoxel method is advantageous, for example, for overall analysis of the distribution of metabolites as shown in Fig. 2-7, localized spectral information cannot be obtained until all encoded data have been acquired, as with MRI. Moreover, data processing is often so time-consuming that measurements with repeated adjustment of the parameters to match the object of measurement is difficult at present. On the other hand, the single-voxel method allows quicker evaluation of the data, thus it is suitable for iterative measurements as in examination of changes in the spectrum with adjustments of parameters such as the repetition time and echo time.[20] Concerning the region selectivity, interference by signals from surrounding portions is smaller in the single-voxel method, particularly STEAM, whereas contamination by signals from surrounding voxels is inevitable in the multivoxel method,

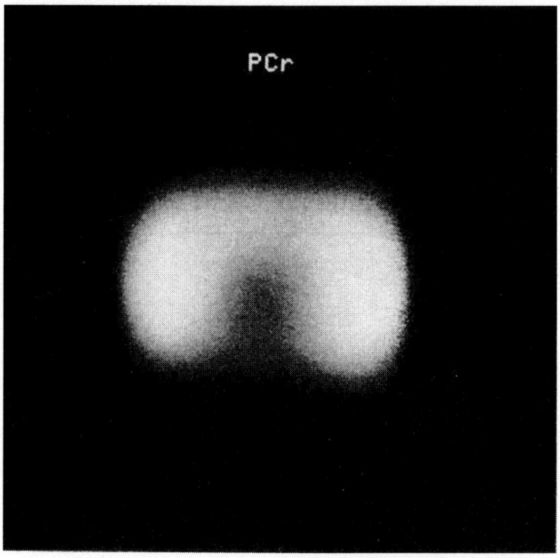

(1) A PCr image after interpixel interpolation.

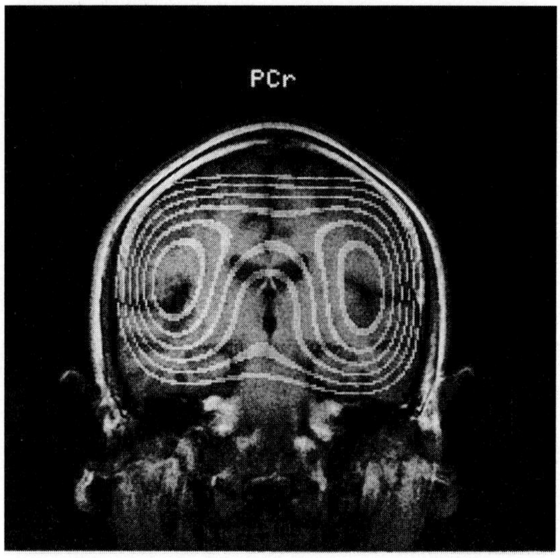

(2) A PCr contour map on a T_1-weighted image.

Fig. 2-7 Two display types of chemical shift imaging.

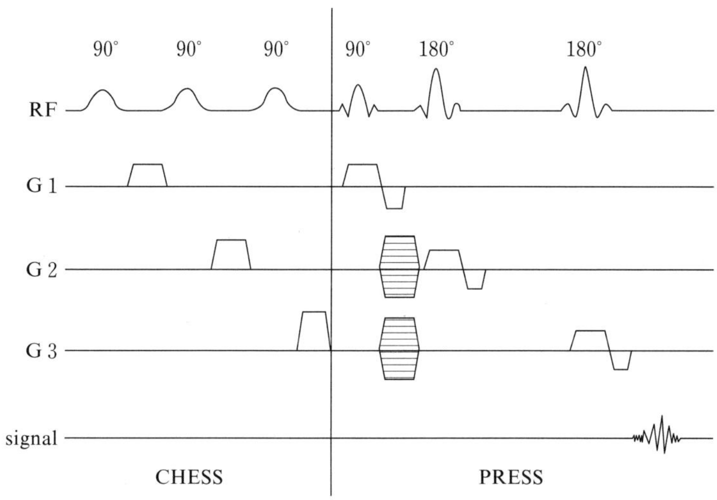

Fig. 2-8 A pulse sequence diagram of two-dimensional CSI with VOI selection by PRESS. CHESS;chemical shift suppression for water suppression (cf. 2.1.3).

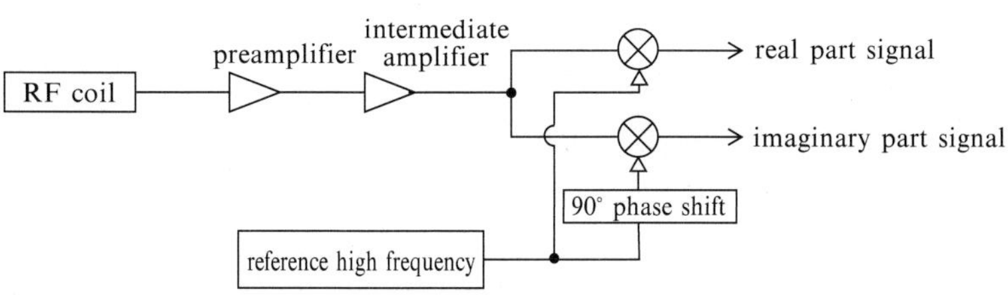

Fig. 2-9 Block diagram of demodulation of high frequency signal.

which theoretically follows the point-spread function.

2.1.3 Water suppression

In ^1H MRS, the amount of ^1H in water is overwhelmingly greater (on the order of 10^3–10^4) than that of metabolites such as NAA and lactic acid. Therefore, magnetic resonance signals from the ^1H in water must be suppressed. CHESS (chemical-shift selective) is a typical method used to achieve this.[21] Fig. 2-8 shows a CSI pulse sequence diagram incorporating water suppression. This suppression sequence is placed prior to the above pulse sequence for localization of nuclei. In this sequence, the suppression RF pulse has the resonance frequency of H_2O, and has a narrow band that does not overlap with the resonance frequency of ^1H of each metabolite. A gradient magnetic field follows the suppression RF pulse to cancel out the directions of spins, i.e., to spoil the phases, of excited ^1H in water.

2.1.4 Reception of signals and RF detection

After radio-frequency signals from various substances, including metabolites with different resonance frequencies according to the differences in the chemical shift, are received with the RF coil, they are amplified by a pre-amplifier and the intermediate amplifier of the receiver, and detected (demodulated) as low-frequency components by two phase-sensitive detectors (PSD) (Fig. 2-9). Detection occurs by picking a lower frequency from the entire frequency by eliminating the reference radio frequency of the apparatus. For example, in a 1.5 T MR apparatus with a standard frequency of 64 MHz, the bandwidth of signals detected is usually 640 Hz or less, because the spectral band of ^1H MRS is about 10 ppm. This conversion to a smaller frequency range allows analogue-digital conversion of signals, and the data can be processed by a computer. Since all frequency signals have complex information with the two components of the amplitude and phase for

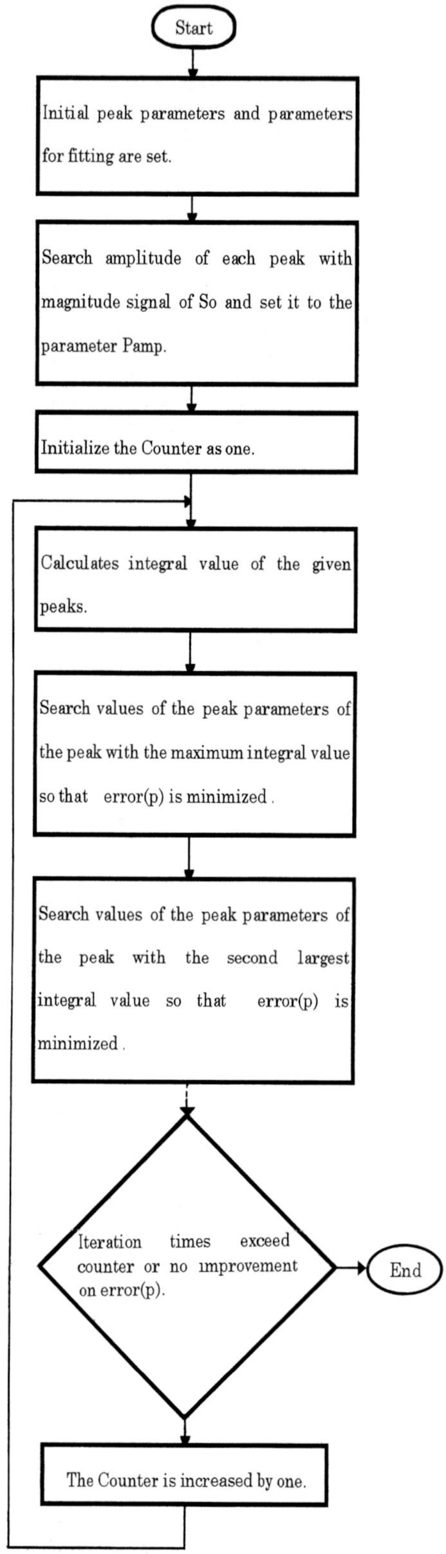

Fig. 2-10 Block diagram of the baseline correction.

each frequency, two kinds of data must be obtained to detect this complex information. For this reason, two components, namely the real signal component with the phase matched with the standard frequency of the system and an imaginary signal component with a phase different by 90°, are collected. Therefore, two spectra, i.e., one real and one imaginary, are obtained by Fourier transformation of each signal component.

2.2 POST-PROCESSING

The spectrum is obtained by post-processing of the real and imaginary parts of the signals after detection. Firstly, automatic baseline correction, one of the key techniques to yield ^{31}P-CSI data, is described. Then, various post-processing techniques are outlined.

2.2.1 Automatic baseline correction for ^{31}P-CSI

(1) ***Baseline correction***

In CSI which provides multi-spectra in a single study, there are two conventional ways to acquire MR signals. One way is to acquire spin echo signals, and the other is to acquire FID (Free Induction Decay) signals. For clinical ^{31}P-CSI, the latter method has the advantage of obtaining a high signal-to-noise ratio for quantitative analysis of the spectra because ATP and PDE have rapid relaxation times compared to the echo time used in the conventional spin echo pulse sequence. In FID data acquisition for ^{31}P-CSI, however, the dead time which is the delay in starting data acquisition due to the application of the slice selection RF pulse and phase encoding gradient pulse prior to data acquisition causes phase distortion after Fourier transformation.

Ordinally, this phase error is removed by the conventional phase correction technique that applies constant and linear order phase (the frequency dependent phase) to the spectrum. After applying the phase correction to the spectrum, the spectrum shows side lobes or "sinc wiggles" on each side of the peak. In this section a totally automated baseline correction technique to remove this baseline distortion is described.[22,23]

(2) ***Theory***

Complete spectrum

Let us define *complete spectrum,* which is obtained under ideal conditions with zero dead time and is also the goal of baseline correction of the observed spectrum.

The time domain signal for the *complete spectrum* is defined as

$$s(t) \equiv \sum_n s_n(t) = \sum_n A_n \times \exp(-a_n t - i\omega_n t) \quad (1)$$

where S_n represents the n-th signal component, A_n represents the amplitude of the n-th signal component, a_n represents the factor for decreasing the n-th signal component, ω_n represents the angular frequency of the n-th signal component, and t represents time. Using Fourier transformation to process $s(t)$, the *complete spectrum* is derived as

$$\begin{aligned} S_c(\omega) &\equiv FT(s(t) \times rect(0, \infty)) \\ &= \sum_n A_n \times (a_n + i\omega)/(a_n^2 + (\omega - \omega_n)^2) \end{aligned} \quad (2)$$

where FT represents Fourier transformation, and the function $rect(\tau_1, \tau_2)$ is a function respective to t defined as

$$\begin{aligned} rect(\tau_1, \tau_2) &= 1 \qquad t = \tau_1 \sim \tau_2 (\tau_1 \leq \tau_2), \\ &= 0 \qquad t \neq \tau_1 \sim \tau_2 \end{aligned}$$

Observed spectrum

Observed signal is defined as

$$\begin{aligned} &s_o(t) \\ &\equiv \sum_n A_n \times \exp(-a_n(t+\Delta t) - i\omega_n(t+\Delta t) + i\phi) \\ &= \sum_n s_n(t) \times \exp(-a_n \Delta t - i\omega_n \Delta t + i\phi) \end{aligned} \quad (3)$$

where Δt represents the dead time, and the observed spectrum after Fourier transformation is as

$$FT(s_o(t) \times rect(0, \infty))$$

$$= \sum_n A_n \times \exp(-a_n \Delta t) \times (a_n + i\omega)/(a_n^2 + (\omega - \omega_n)^2) \times \exp(i\phi - i\omega_n \Delta t) \quad (4)$$

Ordinarily, phase correction is carried out to remove phase distortion, multiplying $\exp(-i\phi + i\omega\Delta t)$ by equation (4), the observed spectrum after phase correction $S_o(\omega)$ is obtained as

$$\begin{aligned} S_o(\omega) &\equiv FT(s_o(t) \times rect(0, \infty)) \times \exp(-i\phi + i\omega\Delta t) \\ &= FT(s_o(t - \Delta t) \times rect(\Delta t, \infty)) \times \exp(-i\phi) \\ &= FT(s(t) \times rect(\Delta t, \infty)) \end{aligned} \quad (5)$$

Baseline correction spectrum

Baseline correction spectrum is a spectrum that compensates for the baseline distortion of $S_o(\omega)$. The *baseline correction spectrum* can be defined as

$$\begin{aligned} S_b(\omega) &\equiv S_c(\omega) - S_o(\omega) \\ &= FT(s(t) \times (rect(0, \infty) - rect(\Delta t, \infty))) \\ &= FT(s(t) \times rect(0, \Delta t)) \end{aligned} \quad (6)$$

Substituting $s(t)$ for equation (1), the *baseline correction spectrum* is derived

$$S_b(\omega) = \int_0^{\Delta t} \sum_n A_n \exp(-a_n t) \exp(i(\omega - \omega_n)t)\, dt \quad (7)$$

and introducing the following assumption

$$\exp(-a_n t) \cong 1 \text{ in the time range } 0 \sim \Delta t \quad (8)$$

the *baseline correction spectrum* is

$$S_b(\omega) \cong \sum_n A_n (\exp(i(\omega - \omega_n)\Delta t) - 1)/i(\omega - \omega_n) \quad (9)$$

Assumption (8) can be accepted in actual ^{31}P-CSI. For example, if a_n is 25 (1/s) at 2T, which corresponds to 1.0 ppm half width of the peak in the frequency domain, and the dead time is 2 ms, $\exp(-a_n t)$ smoothly changes from 1.0 to 0.95 with respect to t=0 to 2 ms.

Taking the real part of equation (9),

$$S_{br}(\omega) \equiv \sum_n A_n \sin(\omega - \omega_n)\Delta t/(\omega - \omega_n) \quad (10)$$

is obtained.

Peak parameters

To estimate the *baseline correction spectrum* with peak related parameters, the following peak parameters are introduced,

$$\begin{aligned} Pamp_n &= A_n / a_n \\ Pwid_n &= a_n \\ Ppos_n &= \omega_n \end{aligned} \quad (11)$$

The real part of the *complete spectrum* $S_{cr}(\omega)$ and the real part of the *baseline correction spectrum* $S_{br}(\omega)$ are represented with peak parameters as

$$S_{cr}(\omega) = \sum_n Pamp_n \times Pwid_n^2/(Pwid_n^2 + (\omega - Ppos_n)^2) \quad (12)$$

$$S_{br}(\omega) = \sum_n Pamp_n \times Pwid_n \sin(\omega - Ppos_n)\Delta t/(\omega - Ppos_n) \quad (13)$$

Equation (13) shows the sum of sinc curves, each with a central frequency and the amplitude of the integral value of each signal component (peak).

Error function to estimate baseline correction spectrum

To estimate values of the peak parameters for baseline correction, an error function of the *baseline correction spectrum* is introduced as

$$error(p) - \int_{-\infty}^{+\infty} (S_{cr}(\omega, p) - (S_{br}(\omega, p) + S_{or}(\omega))^2 dw \quad (14)$$

where p represents peak parameters, $S_{cr}(\omega, p)$ represents a real part of the *complete spectrum*, $S_{br}(\omega, p)$ represents a real part of the *baseline correction spectrum* and $S_{or}(\omega)$ represents a real part of the observed spectrum after Fourier transform. *error* (p) is a summation of the fitting error between the *complete spectrum* calculated with given peak parameters $S_{cr}(\omega, p)$ and the observed spectrum which was baseline corrected using the *baseline correction spectrum* calculated by the given peak parameters $S_{br}(\omega, p)+S_{or}(\omega)$. If the number of peak parameter sets is the same as the number of observed peaks and values of each peak parameter that minimizes the value of this error function can be obtained, the true *baseline correction spectrum* can be calculated, and then the baseline corrected spectrum (the *completed spectrum*) can be obtained.

Estimation scheme of values of peak parameters

In this section, a simple scheme to minimize the error function *error* (p) starting with a set of initial values of peak parameters based on prior knowledge is demonstrated. As equation (13) shows, the *baseline correction spectrum* is the sum of sinc curves, each with a central frequency and the amplitude of the integral value calculated by $Pamp_n \times Pwid_n$ of each signal component (peak). This means the peak with the largest integral value among observed peaks causes the largest baseline distortion. In ^{31}P-CSI MR spectra of the human brain obtained *in vivo*, for example, the dominant peak is PDE and generally a strong baseline distortion is observed around its peak. An algorithm employed in this scheme searches peak parameters of peaks predefined as PME, Pi, PDE, PCr, α-ATP, β-ATP, and γ-ATP changing the values by pre-defined delta values such as the delta peak position and delta amplitude. The search order of the evaluated peaks is determined by integral values calculated by a pre-defined initial condition. Namely, the peak with the largest integral value among the pre-defined peaks is selected first to search for values of the peak parameters which will minimize the value of the error function, and then the peak which has the second largest integral value is selected. After this procedure is applied to all peaks in order, the integral values of the peaks are recalculated again and the search order is reset, then the above sequence is iterated for a pre-defined number of times.

(3) ***Simulation and discussion***

A simulated brain ^{31}P time domain signal which was shifted to the right by 2 msec was used as the observed time domain signal $s(t)$. Different values from the values of the peak parameters used in calculating the simulated signal are set to the peak parameters for the initial condition. To search for the peak parameters value that minimizes the value of *error* (p), the following fitting parameters are used :

Iterations : 4 times

Calculation range : $-30 \sim 20$ ppm (PCr is located at 0 ppm)

Delta position to change the peak position : 0.1 ppm

Amplitude factor to change the peak amplitude : 5% of the peak amplitude

Delta width to change the peak width : 0.2 Hz

In Fig. 2-11 (1), the thin curve shows the real part of the observed spectrum to which phase correction with the first order phase has been applied and the thick curve shows the estimated baseline curve that is $-S_{br}(\omega, p)$. In Fig. 2-11 (2), the thin curve shows the real part of the estimated *complete spectrum* and the thin curve shows the real part of the observed signal that has undergone baseline correction. Comparing the two curves, it is easy to consider that with the technique described above, values of the peak parameters that minimize *error* (p) have been found and baseline correction has been successfully performed.

(4) ***Features of the baseline correction***

The technique for a totally automated baseline correction for ^{31}P-CSI with FID data acquisition has been described and demonstrated. In ^{31}P *in vivo* CSI study, generally it is necessary to process numerous spectra to obtain integral values of the observed peaks to determine metabolite concentrations. As the technique described above can be performed automatically, and the researcher can obtain integral values of the peaks in the processed spectra, which is a one of purposes of postprocessing spectra, the technique is useful for researchers performing quantitative analyses of ^{31}P-CSI study.

2.2.2 Various post-processing techniques

(1) ***Apodization***

After the received MRS radio frequency signals are detected, the signals are usually processed to reduce the noise. Apodization is achieved by multiplying the real and imaginary parts of FID signals detected by a window function such as a Gaussian or exponential function as in Fig. 2-12.[24] This process reduces the noise when the noisy parts of FID signals are strongly attenuated. This results in widening of the half-width of the Fourier transformed spectrum and a reduction of the noise. After apodization, the real and imaginary spectra can be obtained by Fourier transformation of the data of the respective parts. The spectra obtained require correction of the phase for each frequency component.

(2) ***Phase correction***

In the gradient echo method, spins of various components with different resonance frequencies come to be in different phases before magnetic resonance signals are received because of the interval between excitation of the spin and reception of signals (delay time). Complex information with a given amplitude and phase for each frequency appears as a two-dimensional quantity (vector quantity) consisting of the values of the real and imaginary spectra for each frequency in the spectrum obtained. Therefore, differences in the phase among frequencies mean differences in the direction of the vectors, causing differences in the ratio between the values of the real and imaginary spectra among frequencies. Thus, to equalize the direction of the vector at each peak in the spec-

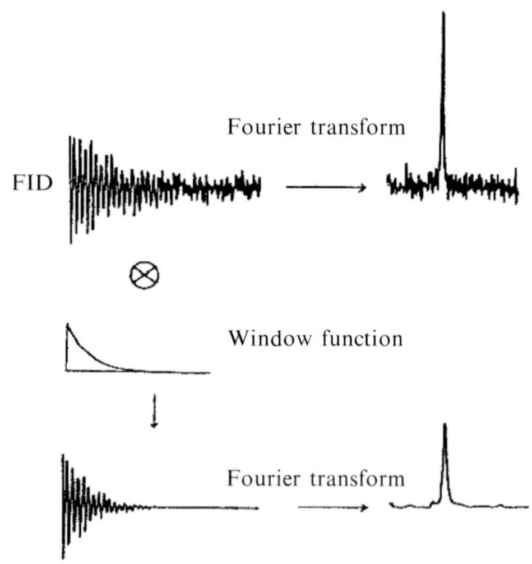

Fig. 2-12 Apodization.

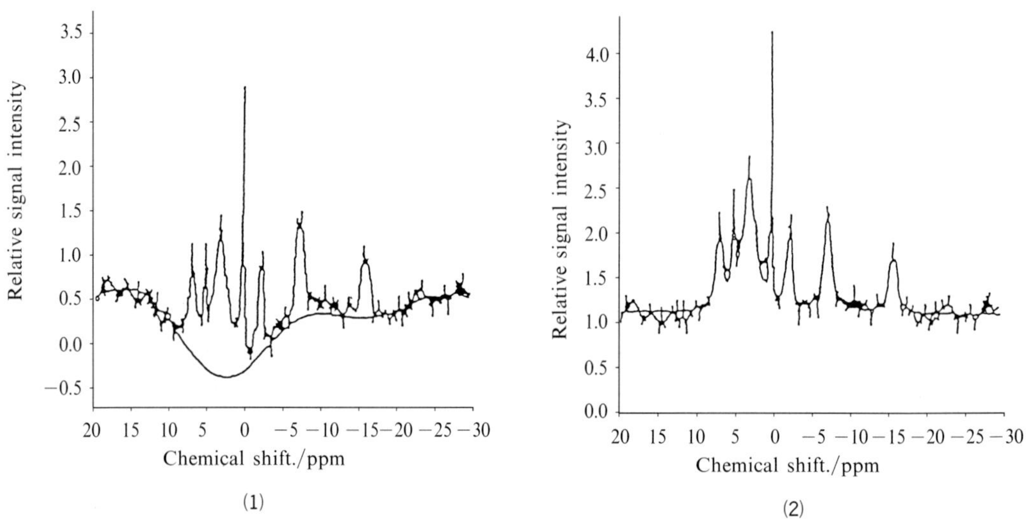

Fig. 2-11 Example of baseline correction.

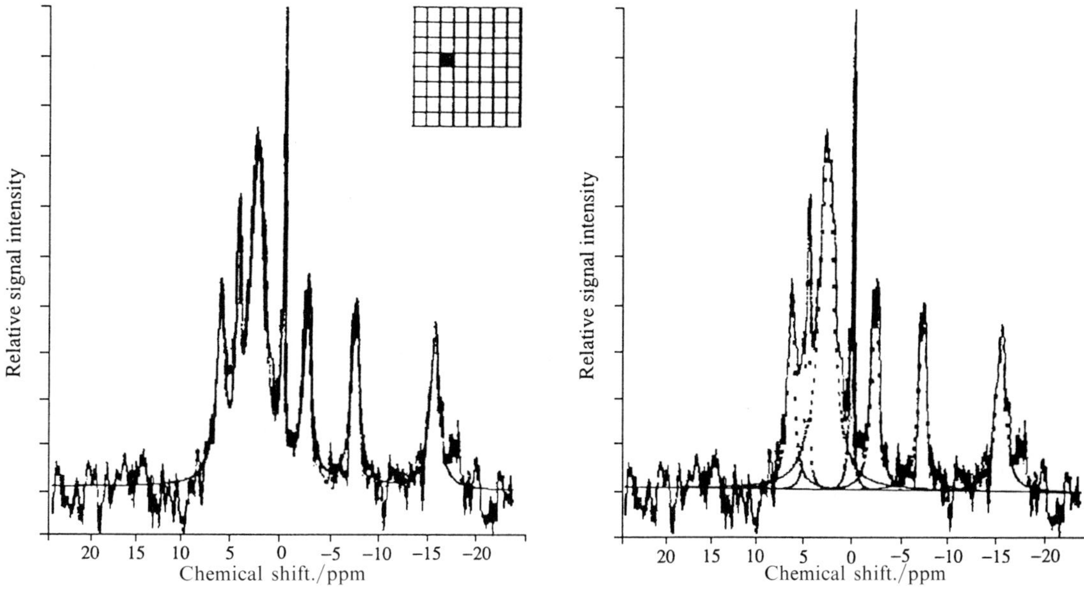

A spectrum after phase and baseline correction.

A spectrum and each separated peak curve.

Fig. 2-13 Separation of spectral peaks by a curve-fitting software.

trum, the phase must be adjusted at each frequency of the spectrum to allow each peak of the real spectrum to be represented with the maximal amplitude. A common procedure for this phase correction consists of constant phase correction followed by linear phase correction.

Constant phase correction

First, in constant phase correction, the phase of the entire spectrum obtained, i.e., the direction of the vector of each frequency component, is increased or decreased simultaneously to maximize and make symmetrical a given peak regarded as a reference in the real spectrum. Other peaks are not maximized by this correction alone.

Linear phase correction

Next, as the phase produced in a given delay time is proportional to the resonance frequency, each peak can be maximized and made symmetrical by correction of the phase proportional to the frequency with a reference peak. This is called linear phase correction. However, the spectrum obtained without baseline correction is arranged along a distorted baseline. Actually, each peak may not be maximized and made symmetrical by constant and linear phase corrections alone. This indicates that phase modulation of a higher order occurs during signal reception. This phenomenon is caused primarily by modulation of the resonance frequency of each spin by the temporal variation of the magnetic field produced by the eddy current caused by the gradient magnetic field (See 2.3.2). This effect of eddy current also appears as a disturbance of the spectral phase in the spin echo method, in which the influence of the delay time on spin phase is normally canceled out by the 180° pulse.

(3) ***Curve fitting***

Signals of components with short T_2 such as those from phospholipids of the cell membrane appear as a spectrum with a large half-width. These components can be isolated by baseline correction and a curve- fitting to separate overlapping peaks of multiple components (Fig. 2-13). Automatic baseline correction in ^{31}P-CSI (See 2.2.1), in particular, is a powerful technique because post-processing must be performed for the spectrum of each of the large number of voxels.

2.3.2 Various limitation factors

(1) ***Spatial resolution***

Limitations in S/N restrict the spatial resolution and make it difficult to obtain good spectra for clinical research. Magnetic resonance signals from metabolites and other substances to be studied by MRS are markedly weaker than signals of water, which is the source of signals used in MRI. Therefore, the voxel size must be considerably greater in MRS than in MRI. In head MRS, the voxel size in ^{31}P MRS with a signal collection time of 15–45 minutes is about 12–27 ml.[14–16,28–32]

(2) ***Spatial contamination***[33,34]

The ^{1}H resonance frequencies of water and lipid are different by about 3.5 ppm so that chemical shift artifacts may arise in MRI. Positional shifts also occur among substances with different resonance frequencies in MRS as long as selective excitation is done using a gradient magnetic field. The positional shift is dependent on the intensity of the gradient magnetic field used. If a selection gradient magnetic field of 4 mT/m is used at a static magnetic field intensity of 2T, for example, the positional shift is about 2.5 mm in ^{1}H MRS, since the chemical shift bandwidth of the subject metabolites is about 5 ppm, and it can be about 15 mm in ^{31}P MRS because the chemical shift bandwidth is about 30 ppm. Therefore, in ^{1}H CSI, in which selection of the VOI (volume of interest) is made, and the single-voxel method, in which three-dimensional region selection is performed using gradient magnetic fields, attention must be paid to the occurrence of a positional shift of the VOI selected for each chemical shift. In the multivoxel method also, positional shift occurs in the slice direction of the selective excitation plane, although no disparity is caused in the phase-encoded position. While an increase of the strength of the gradient magnetic field for selection with the use of wide band RF pulses results in a reduction in such positional shift, the influence of the eddy current, which will be described later, must be taken into consideration. Moreover, as the number of voxels is smaller (16×16 or 8×8) in CSI than in MRI, contamination by signals from neighboring voxels due to the effect of the point-spread function must also be considered in data analysis. Methods to reduce the effect of the point-spread function are also being tested.[35]

(3) ***Temporal resolution***

Since the longitudinal relaxation time varies among metabolites, the spectral pattern differs with the repetition time (TR) of MRS; TR is usually set at 1–3 seconds in consideration of the efficiency of signal collection. When MRS is performed with this TR, the total signal collection time generally becomes 10–30 minutes. However, attempts to improve the temporal resolution at the sacrifice of the spatial resolution are being made and, for example, changes in lactic acid during neural activities in response to photic stimulation are measured by ^{1}H MRS with a temporal resolution of 30 seconds by enlarging the voxel size, which is usually 1–2 ml to 11.2 ml.[36]

(4) ***Delay time***

Since ^{31}P MRS should be able to detect the signals of metabolites with a short T_2 relaxation time such as β-ATP, sequences with a long delay time from the initial excitation to signal collection cannot be used. Therefore, the gradient echo method is used frequently for multivoxel MRS. Also, the image-selected *in vivo* spectroscopy (ISIS)[37] is a useful technique among single-voxel methods. In this volume, CSI is employed as the imaging technique of ^{31}P.

(5) ***Eddy currents***

A gradient magnetic field is accompanied by a fringe magnetic field outside the gradient magnetic field coil. This fringe magnetic field causes eddy currents in metallic parts such as the body of the main magnet, because it changes with time according to the sequence of the gradient magnetic field.

Since the channel of the produced eddy current is influenced by the distribution of electric characteristics of the metallic parts and contact resistance between metals, its control in the manufacturing process of the apparatus is difficult. The magnetic field caused by the eddy current disturbs the behavior of the spin. Moreover, this magnetic field changes with time and often consists of multiple components. This eddy current causes unsatisfactory water suppression or regional selectivity in ^1H MRS, or restrictions of shortening of the echo time, resulting in disturbances of the phase or baseline of the spectrum. Attempts are being made to eliminate the effect of eddy current, e.g., adjustment of the wave form of the gradient magnetic field current and generation of a B_0 magnetic field (spatially homogeneous magnetic field) that compensates for the eddy current magnetic field occurring in response to changes in the gradient magnetic field in a feed-forward manner. The property of disturbance of the spectrum by the eddy current can be estimated by obtaining signals of water from the VOI without water suppression and analyzing them in advance. A method to correct MRS signals obtained for the effect of eddy current by the results of this analysis has been put into practice. Furthermore, by installation of actively shielded gradient magnetic field coils, which prevent the occurrence of a fringe magnetic field from the gradient magnetic field coil, the effect of eddy current is being reduced.[38]

One method to monitor the eddy current is to measure the magnetic field induced by the eddy current using a pick-up coil with an internal diameter of about 2 cm. A gradient magnetic field with a predetermined intensity is applied for about 2 seconds, and the eddy-current magnetic field overlapping the gradient magnetic field generated in the pick-up coil placed in the magnet bore is measured. The eddy-current magnetic field obtained often consists of multiple components with an attenuation time varying from milliseconds to several seconds. However, as the eddy current does not necessarily occur homogeneously in the measurement space, its radical reduction by the use of an actively shielded gradient magnetic field coil is needed.

2.4 FACTORS AFFECTING THE PERFORMANCE

Control and adjustment of various measurement and instrumental parameters are needed to perform optimal MRS under the present conditions using a clinical high-magnetic field MR system. These parameters are classified into controllable and uncontrollable ones by the user. The main controllable parameters are apodization, phase correction, and baseline correction mentioned in 2.2 and the uncontrollable parameters are intrinsic to the system. Important items among them are described below.

2.4.1 Selection of the RF coil

A volume coil for the head is usually used in head MRS because of the homogeneous sensitivity in the brain region. The sensitivity and sensitive region in MRS are matters that must be considered in selection of the RF coil. The sensitivity and the extent of the sensitive region are reciprocal to each other. Since SNR is improved several-fold when the sensitive region is limited by the use of a simple surface coil or a more advanced surface coil in which the phased array technique is employed,[39,40] RF coils custom-designed by each institution are beginning to be used.[41] Designing an RF coil suitable for the target region is the key to such attempts.[27] Also, as surface coils produce inhomogeneous RF magnetic fields, large RF coils for the body are often used in ^1H MRS for transmission to improve the exactness of VOI selection by making the RF magnetic field more homogeneous. Since most clinical MR systems do not have a transmission coil that generates a homogeneous RF magnetic field in ^{31}P MRS, surface coils are used for both transmission and reception. In such cases, additional precautions like the use of the adiabatic pulse,[42] which is an RF pulse technique to improve the uniformity of the flip angle even in inhomogeneous RF magnetic fields, are needed in region selection.

2.4.2 Fat suppression

In the ^1H spectrum, the peak of lactic acid overlaps with that of lipids. In the single-voxel method, especially in PRESS, the signal of lipids is reduced by the use of relatively long echo times because of the short T_2 of the lipid compared with that of lactic acid. The echo time used in this procedure is often 135 ms or 270 ms, in consideration of J modulation by the spin-spin coupling of lactic acid. Additionally, in head ^1H MRS, signals from fat on the surface of the head are stronger than those from other metabolites of measurement, so that fat-signal contamination from voxels of the head surface poses a problem particularly in head CSI. For this reason, the VOI is set in the brain parenchyma by avoiding the head surface, and CSI is performed in this region.[18,19] Actually, prevention of contamination by fat signals is often insufficient simply by determining the VOI in regions other than the head surface because of the effects of the inhomogeneity of the static magnetic field and the RF magnetic field, the eddy current, and various methods to suppress the effects of fat are being attempted. Also, because of improvements in the methods used to suppress signals from tissues outside the cerebral parenchyma, such as fat on the head surface called outer volume suppression (OVS), ^1H CSI is also performed without determination of the VOI that avoids the head surface.[33,34]

2.4.3 Water suppression

In ^1H MRS, water suppression is often done by CHESS.[21] Because narrow band RF pulses are used in this process, the static magnetic field including the area around the target region must be homogeneous. After water suppression, a residual water component is still present in the spectrum obtained. However, software to automatically eliminate the residual water component by the use of a method to analyze the disturbance of the spectrum by the eddy current mentioned above has also become available.

2.4.4 Local shim

The homogeneity of the static magnetic field is particularly important in MRS. Since the static magnetic field is disturbed by the inhomogeneity of the magnetic susceptibility of biological materials, water suppression in ^1H MRS becomes incomplete or the resolution of the spectrum obtained deteriorates. In ^1H MRS, the homogeneity of the static magnetic field in the voxel is preferably 0.05 ppm or less. Usually, global shimming is performed to minimize the half-width of the spectral peak of water protons from the entire head or the selected plane including the target VOI, but inhomogeneity of about 0.1-0.3 ppm remains when the voxel size is $2\times2\times2$ ml in the head.[43] Therefore, the homogeneity of the static magnetic field in VOI is improved primarily by manually adjusting various shim coil currents. There are also automatic local shimming methods,[43,44] and inhomogeneity in the VOI has been reported to be reduced to about one half by a method using the multi-angle projection (MAP) shim.[43]

2.5 PROSPECTS FOR THE FUTURE

Application of techniques of analytical NMR, which has a long history in MRS, is being attempted. For example, measurement of changes in the creatinine kinase rate[45] by saturation-transfer NMR[46] and, although this is still in the stage of animal experiments, methods for acquisition of data concerning neurotransmitters by ^1H-^{15}N MRS[47] are being tested, and pioneer studies aggressively using special hardware and original pulse sequences are being carried out. Also, ^1H MRS, such as ^1H CSI, is being performed using clinical high-magnetic field MR systems and is beginning to be put into practical use for the diagnosis and evaluation of therapeutic effects beyond the research stage. Improvements in operation functions such as simple data processing are essential for this technique to become beneficial for patients, and a marked increase in the productivity of MRS clinical data is desired. Aspects of high- magnetic field MR systems for general clinical use in which improvements in MRS are anticipated are described below.

2.5.1 Improvements in the RF coil technology

To improve SNR, which is the greatest limiting factor in MRS, phased-array surface coils,[39] in which multiple surface coils are combined as shown in Figure. 2-15, are increasingly used.[41,48-50] The phased-array technology is derived from the antenna technology used in devices such as radar designed to change the direction of radiation by arraying multiple antennas and controlling the phase of each antenna. In applying this technology to MR, it is important to sufficiently reduce electromagnetic coupling among the multiple surface coils. This allows reception of independent signals simultaneously by the multiple surface coils and synthesis of images of wide scanning areas through processes including controlling the phases of these signals. Surface coils have inhomogeneous intensities of the RF magnetic field compared with volume coils and are inferior in terms of deep sensitivity, but reasonable sensitivity can be obtained to some depth by the use of surface coils of an appropriate size. Therefore, with the phased-array technology, signals can be collected from a wide area with fair sensitivity through multiple surface coils. For example, when phased-array detectors with surface coils 6-8 cm in diameter are used, the spatial resolution of ^1H MRS in the brain is 0.2-0.4 ml.[41]

2.5.2 Quantification

Quantification of MRS for determination of the absolute concentration of metabolites is being undertaken as the next step of comparison of peaks of the spectrum in relative terms.[51-54] For this purpose, a standard signal that permits conversion of the intensity of the spectrum obtained into the absolute concentration becomes necessary. In ^1H MRS, in particular, there are the internal-standard methods to refer to a material in the body such as the peak of creatine and phosphocreatine[55] and the signal intensity of protons of unsuppressed water[52] and an external-standard method, by which a reference material is determined outside the object of examination. For this quantification, measurements are performed by changing various temporal parameters of MRS, because T_1 and T_2 values must be determined for each peak. Therefore, the single-voxel method is employed more frequently.

References

1) Bottomley, P. A. Selective volume method for performing localized NMR spectroscopy. US patent 4480228. 1984.

2) Bottomley, P. A. Spatial localization in NMR spectroscopy *in vivo*. [Review] *Annals of the New York Academy of Sciences* 508:333-348;1987.

3) Granot, J. Selected volume excitation using stimulated echoes (VEST). Application to spatially localized spectroscopy and imaging. *J. Magn. Reson.* 70 : 488-492 ; 1986.

4) Kimmich, R. ; Hoepfel, D. Volume-selective multipulse spin-echo spectroscopy. *J. Magn. Reson.* 72 : 379-384 ; 1987.

5) Frahm, J. ; Merboldt, K-D. ; Hänicke, W. Localized proton spectroscopy using stimulated echoes. *J. Magn. Reson.* 72 : 502-508 ; 1987.

6) Hahn, E. L. Spin echoes. *Phys. Rev.* 80 : 580-594 ; 1950.

7) Posse, S. ; Schuknecht, B. ; Smith, M. E. et al. Short echo time proton MR spectroscopic imaging. *J. Comput. Assist. Tomogr.* 17 : 1-14 ; 1993.

8) Frahm, J. ; Merboldt, K. D. ; Hänicke, W. et al. Stimulated echo imaging. *J. Magn. Reson.* 64 : 81-93 ; 1985.

9) Brown, T. R. ; Kincaid, B. M. ; Ugurbil, K. NMR chemical shift imaging in three dimensions. *Proc. Natl. Acad. Sci. USA* 79 : 3523-3526 ; 1982.

10) Maudsley, A. A. ; Hilal, S. K. ; Perman, W. H. et al. Spatially resolved high resolution spectroscopy by

"four-dimensional" NMR. *J. Magn. Reson.* 51 : 147-152 ; 1983.

11) Mareci, T. H. ; Brooker, H. R. High-resolution magnetic resonance spectra from a sensitive region defined with pulsed field gradients. *J. Magn. Reson.* 57 : 157-163 ; 1984.

12) Maudsley, A. A. ; Hilal, S. K. ; Simon, H. E. et al. *In vivo* MR spectroscopic imaging with P-31. *Radiology* 153 : 745-750 ; 1984.

13) Yamamoto, T. Chemical shift imaging. *Jpn. J. NMR Med.* 6 : 221-239 ; 1987. [Japanese]

14) Coutts, G. A. ; Bryant, D. J. ; Collins, A. G. et al. ^{31}P magnetic resonance spectroscopy of the normal human brain : approaches using four dimensional chemical shift imaging and phase mapping techniques. *NMR Biomed.* 1 : 190-197 ; 1989.

15) Vigneron, D. B. ; Nelson, S. J. ; Murphy-Boesch, J. et al. Chemical shift imaging of human brain : axial, sagittal, and coronal P-31 metabolite images. *Radiology* 177 : 643-649 ; 1990.

16) Murphy-Boesch, J. ; Stoyanova, R. ; Srinivasan, R. et al. Proton-decoupled ^{31}P chemical shift imaging of the human brain in normal volunteers. *NMR Biomed.* 6 : 173-180 ; 1993.

17) Maudsley, A. A. ; Twieg, D. B. ; Sappey-Marinier, D. et al. Spin echo ^{31}P spectroscopic imaging in the human brain. *Magn. Reson. Med.* 14 : 415-422 ; 1990.

18) Frahm, J. ; Bruhn, H. ; Gyngell, M. L. et al. Localized high-resolution proton NMR spectroscopy using stimulated echoes : initial applications to human brain *in vivo. Magn. Reson. Med.* 9 : 79-93 ; 1989.

19) Moonen, C. T. W. ; von Kienlin, M. ; van Zijl, P. C. M. et al. Comparison of single-shot localization methods (STEAM and PRESS) for *in vivo* proton NMR spectroscopy. *NMR Biomed.* 2 : 201-208 ; 1989.

20) Naruse, S. Basics of MR Spectroscopy. *In : Naruse, S., ed. Practice of Magnetic Resoncence Spectroscopy. Tokyo : Igakushoin* ; 1995 : 64. [Japanese]

21) Haase, A. ; Frahm, J. ; Hänicke, W. et al. ^{1}H NMR chemical shift selective (CHESS) imaging. *Phys. Med. Biol.* 30 : 341-344 ; 1985.

22) Derby, K. ; Hawryszko, C. ; Tropp, J. et al. Baseline deconvolution, phase correction, and signal quantification in Fourier localized spectroscopic imaging. *Magn. Reson. Med.* 12 : 235-240 ; 1989.

23) Miyazaki, T. Automatic baseline correction for ^{31}P-CSI. *Jpn. J. Magn. Reson. Med.* 12 : 322-327 ; 1992. [Japanese]

24) Gadian, D. G. Spectrometer design and operation. *In : Nuclear magnetic resonance and its applications to living systems. New York : Oxford University Press* ; 1982 : 133-158.

25) Hoult, D. I. ; Lauterbur, P. C. The sensitivity of the zeugmatographic experiment involving human samples. *J. Magn. Reson.* 34 : 425-433 ; 1979.

26) Iriguchi, N. ; Yamai, S. ; Hasegawa, J. The NMR sensitivity achievable with a slotted-tube resonator. MAGMA 1 : 122-125 ; 1993. [Japanese]

27) Yamamoto, T. Optimized design of an RF coil for magnetic resonance with quantitative analysis of a signal-to-noise ratio. *Annu. Rep. College Med. Technol. Hokkaido Univ.* 8 : 157-164 ; 1995. [Japanese]

28) Bottomley, P. A. ; Charles, H. C. ; Roemer, P. B. et al. Human *in vivo* phosphate metabolite imaging with ^{31}P NMR. *Magn. Reson. Med.* 7 : 319-336 ; 1988.

29) Tropp, J. S. ; Sugiura, S. ; Derby, K. A. et al. Characterization of MR spectroscopic imaging of the human head and limb at 2.0 T. *Radiology* 169 : 207-212 ; 1988.

30) Lenkinski, R. E. ; Holland, G. A. ; Allman, T. et al. Integrated MR imaging and spectroscopy with chemical shift imaging of P-31 at 1.5 T : initial clinical experience. *Radiology* 169 : 201-206 ; 1988.

31) Taylor, J. S. ; Vigneron, D. B. ; Murphy-Boesch, J. et al. Free magnesium levels in normal human brain and brain tumors : ^{31}P chemical-shift imaging measurements at 1.5 T. *Proc Natl. Acad. Sci. USA* 88 : 6810-6814 ; 1991.

32) Garcia, P. A. ; Laxer, K. D. ; van der Grond, J. et al. Phosphorus magnetic resonance spectroscopic imaging in patients with frontal lobe epilepsy. *Ann. Neurol.* 35 ; 217-221 ; 1994.

33) Spielman, D. M. ; Pauly, J. M. ; Macovski, A. et al. Lipid-suppressed single- and multisection proton spectroscopic imaging of the human brain. *J. Magn. Reson. Imaging* 2 : 253-262 ; 1992.

34) Duyn, J. H. ; Gillen, J. ; Sobering, G. et al. Multisection proton MR spectroscopic imaging of the brain. *Radiology* 188 : 277-282 ; 1993.

35) Gonen, O. ; Hu, J. ; Stoyanova, R. et al. Hybrid three dimensional (1D-Hadamard, 2D-chemical shift imaging) phosphorus localized spectroscopy of phantom and human brain. *Magn. Reson. Med.* 33 : 300-308 ; 1995.

36) Frahm, J. ; Krüger, G. ; Merboldt, K-D. et al. Dynamic uncoupling and recoupling of perfusion and oxidative metabolism during focal brain activation in man. *Magn. Reson. Med.* 35 : 143-148 ; 1996.

37) Ordidge, R. J. ; Connelly, A. ; Lohman, J. A. B. Image-selected *in vivo* spectroscopy (ISIS). A new technique for spatially selective NMR spectroscopy. *J. Magn. Reson.* 66 : 283-294 ; 1986.

38) Mansfield, P. ; Chapman, B. Active magnetic screening of gradient coils in NMR imaging. *J. Magn. Reson.* 66 : 573-576 ; 1986.

39) Roemer, P. B. ; Edelstein, W. A. ; Hayes, C. E. et al.

The NMR phased array. *Magn. Reson. Med.* 16 : 192-225 ; 1990.

40) Hayes, C. E. ; Roemer, P. B. Noise correlations in data simultaneously acquired from multiple surface coil arrays. *Magn. Reson. Med.* 16 : 181-191 ; 1990.

41) Wald, L. L. ; Moyher, S. E. ; Day, M. R. et al. Proton spectroscopic imaging of the human brain using phased array detectors. *Magn. Reson. Med.* 34 : 440-445 ; 1995.

42) Hendrich, K. ; Garwood, M. ; Merkle, H. et al. Spectroscopic imaging using variable angle excitation from adiabatic plane-rotation pulses. *Magn. Reson. Med.* 19 : 496-501 ; 1991.

43) Manabe, A. Multi-angle projection shim (MAPshim) for localized volumes. *In : Book of proceedings : Third Scientific Meeting and Exhibition of the Society of Magnetic Resonance, Vol. 2. Nice, France : SMR* ; 1995 : 696.

44) Webb, P. ; Macovski, A. Rapid, fully automatic, arbitrary-volume *in vivo* shimming. *Magn. Reson. Med.* 20 : 113-122 ; 1991.

45) Chen, W. ; Adriany, G. ; Zhu, X.-H. et al. Increase of creatine kinase rate in visual cortex of human brain during photic stimulation : an ^{31}P NMR magnetization transfer study. *In : Book of proceedings : Fourth Scientific Meeting and Exhibition of the International Society for Magnetic Resonance in Medicine, Vol. 1. New York, USA : ISMRM* ; 1996 : 293.

46) Gadian, D. G. ; Radda, G. K. ; Brown, T. R. et al. The activity of creatine kinase in frog skeletal muscle studied by saturation-transfer nuclear magnetic resonance. *Biochem. J.* 194 : 215-228 ; 1981.

47) Kanamori, K. ; Ross, B. D. ; Tropp, J. Selective, *in vivo* observation of [5-^{15}N] glutamine amide protons in rat brain by ^{1}H-^{15}N heteronuclear multiple-quantum-coherence transfer NMR. *J. Magn. Reson. Series B* 107 : 107-115 ; 1995.

48) Nicklaus, D. J. Use of multiple receive coils for improved signal-to-noise in large field-of-view chemical shift imaging. *In : Works in progress : Ninth Annual Scientific Meeting and Exhibition of the Society of Magnetic Resonance in Medicine, New York, USA : SMRM* ; 1990 : 1142.

49) Hardy, C. J. ; Bottomley, P. A. ; Rohling, K. W. et al. An NMR phased array for human cardiac ^{31}P spectroscopy. *Magn. Reson. Med.* 28 : 54-64 ; 1992.

50) Tan, G. ; Song, W. ; Jesmanowicz, A. et al. Multi-channel magnetic resonance spectroscopy. *In : Book of proceedings : Twelfth Annual Scientific Meeting of the Society of Magnetic Resonance in Medicine, Vol. 1. New York, USA : SMRM* ; 1993 : 370.

51) Christiansen, P. ; Toft, P. ; Larsson, H. B. W. et al. The concentration of *N*-acetyl aspartate, creatine+phosphocreatine, and choline in different parts of the brain in adulthood and senium. *Magn. Reson. Imaging* 11 : 799-806 ; 1993.

52) Christiansen, P. ; Henriksen, O. ; Stubgaard, M. et al. *In vivo* quantification of brain metabolites by ^{1}H-MRS using water as an internal standard. *Magn. Reson. Imaging* 11 : 107-118 ; 1993.

53) Kreis, R. ; Ernst, T. ; Ross, B. D. Absolute quantitation of water and metabolites in the human brain. II. Metabolite concentrations. *J. Magn. Reson. Series B* 102 : 9-19 ; 1993.

54) Ernst, T. ; Kreis, R. ; Ross, B. D. Absolute quantitation of water and metabolites in the human brain. I. Compartments and water. *J. Magn. Reson. Series B* 102 : 1-8 ; 1993.

55) Frahm, J. ; Bruhn, H. ; Gyngell, M. L. et al. Localized proton NMR spectroscopy in different regions of the human brain *in vivo*. Relaxation times and concentrations of cerebral metabolites. *Magn. Reson. Med.* 11 : 47-63 ; 1989.

Chapter 3 Understanding Spectra of ^{31}P MRS and ^{1}H MRS

Toshiro Fujimoto and Toshihiko Nakano

Magnetic resonance spectroscopy (MRS) provides biochemical information *in vivo*, and its combination with the anatomical and pathological information obtained by MRI opens a new perspective of understanding pathophysiology, course of progression, and the effects of treatment in various diseases. There has been a dramatic increase in the number of clinical investigations employing clinical MRS.[1] In order to interpret signals obtained by MRS, an overview of major parameters of magnetic resonance spectroscopy and the biochemical significance of spectra are explained in this chapter. An outline of basic aspects of MRS and metabolites necessary for understanding ^{31}P and ^{1}H spectra will be provided.

3.1 MAJOR PARAMETERS OF MRS

The major parameters of MRS—chemical shift, spin-spin coupling and relaxation time—are explained, as are the techniques of Nuclear Overhauser Effect (NOE), and proton decoupling.

3.1.1 Chemical shift

The magnetic field experienced by a nucleus is not exactly the same as applied magnetic field B_0, because the small field $B_0\sigma$ at the nucleus is produced by the electron cloud within the molecule.[2] The orientation of the $B_0\sigma$ is parallel to the field B_0 in paramagnetic effect and in the opposite direction to the field B_0 in the diamagnetic effect. The effective magnetic field B_{eff} at the nucleus is expressed as[3]

$$B_{eff} = B_0(1-\sigma)$$

where σ is a shielding constant, and the value of σ is positive in the diamagnetic effect and negative in the paramagnetic effect.

Chemical shift is defined as nuclear shielding divided by applied field, and is measured from the suitable reference compound.[4,5] Chemical shift is defined as

$$\delta = \frac{B_{reference} - B_{sample}}{B_{reference}} \times 10^6 \text{ppm}$$

where $B_{reference}$ and B_{sample} are the resonance field strength for the reference and sample nuclei, respectively, when an external magnetic field is applied.

3.1.2 Spin-spin coupling

Magnetic resonance peaks are often split into multiplets, and the spin-spin coupling is responsible for this splitting. The spin-spin coupling is caused by an interaction between spins which is mediated by bonding electrons.[2] The magnitude of the spin-spin interaction between nuclei is called the spin-spin coupling constant (J), which has the unit of Hz. As shown in Figure 3-1 of the ^{31}P spectrum of ATP, ^{31}P signals of α-and γ-ATP are split into doublets through the coupling to neighboring ^{31}P nucleus of β- ATP, and the signal of β-ATP is split into triplet through coupling to two neighboring ^{31}P nuclei of α-and γ-ATP.

3.1.3 Relaxation mechanisms

Relaxation is a process where the spin energy reverts to equilibrium after perturbation of the spin system caused by the resonance absorption of radiation. Relaxation plays an important role in observing resonance phenomenon. There are two

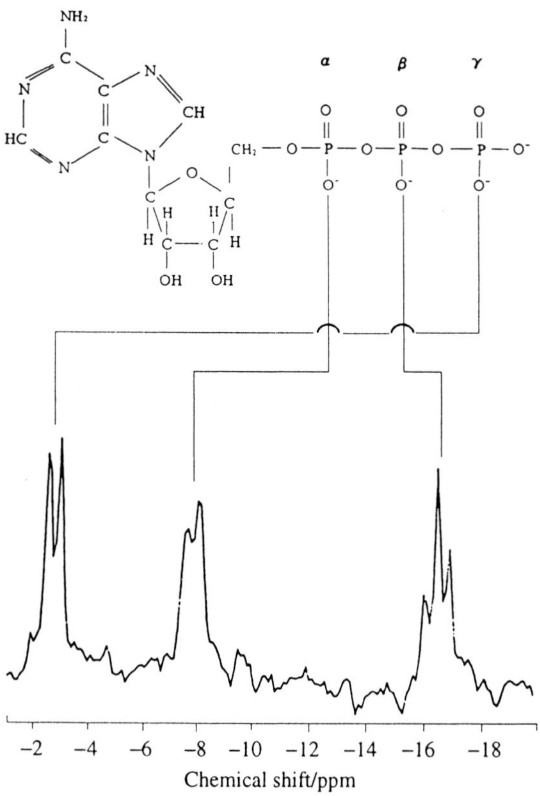

Figure 3-1 Spin-spin coupling of ^{31}P resonance in ATP. The signals from the α-phosphate and γ-phosphate are split into doublets through coupling to the ^{31}P nucleus of the β group, respectively. The β-phosphate signal is split into triplet through coupling to ^{31}P nuclei of α and γ groups.

distinct relaxation processes, spin-lattice (longitudinal) relaxation and spin-spin (transverse) relaxation.[2]

(1) ***Spin-lattice (longitudinal) relaxation***

Spin-lattice relaxation is a process in which the magnetic energy of the nuclear spin system is transferred to "lattice", which refers to the environment surrounding the nucleus.[2] Spin-lattice relaxation is caused by interaction of the interested nucleus with the randomly fluctuating fields due to the thermal motion of magnetic dipoles in the lattice.[3] Spin-lattice relaxation time (T_1) or longitudinal relaxation time is a time constant in this process.

(2) ***Spin-spin (transverse) relaxation***

Spin-spin relaxation is a process based on energy transfer between individual spins, via a flip-flop type mechanism.[6] In the spin-spin relaxation system, no energy is transferred from the nuclei to the lattice. Spin-spin relaxation time or transverse relaxation time (T_2) is a time constant in this process. Measured T_2 value is shorter than true T_2 value because of the inhomogeneity of the magnetic field,[2] and T_2^* is customarily used for showing the measured T_2.

(3) ***Dipole-dipole relaxation mechanism of protons in liquids and variation of T_1 and T_2 with correlation time (τ_c)***

The dominant mechanism of spin relaxation of ^{1}H in liquids is nuclear dipole-dipole interaction. Relaxation time, T_1 and T_2, and line width in MR spectra are associated with the chaotic random motion of molecules in liquids called Brownian motion. This has a time scale, the rotational correlation time (τ_c) defined as the time taken on average for a solute molecule to rotate by one radian or roughly the reciprocal of the rate of tumbling in solution of the relevant piece of the molecule.[7] The spin experiences the fluctuation of the local field due to the random molecular motion of neighbouring magnetic dipoles. The rotational correlation time (τ_c) is influenced by viscosity, temperature, molecular size and molecular shape.[8] The linewidth depends on T_2 and is roughly proportional to the inverse of T_2^*. Variation of T_1 and T_2 of protons with τ_c is shown in Figure 3-2.

3.1.4 Nuclear Overhauser Effect (NOE) and proton decoupling

Nuclear Overhauser Effect (NOE) and proton decoupling are caused by using double resonance techniques where the second radio frequency field is used other than the conventional radio frequency which excites protons from the ground state to the excited state.[9] NOE involves enhancement in the intensity of the resonance signal when

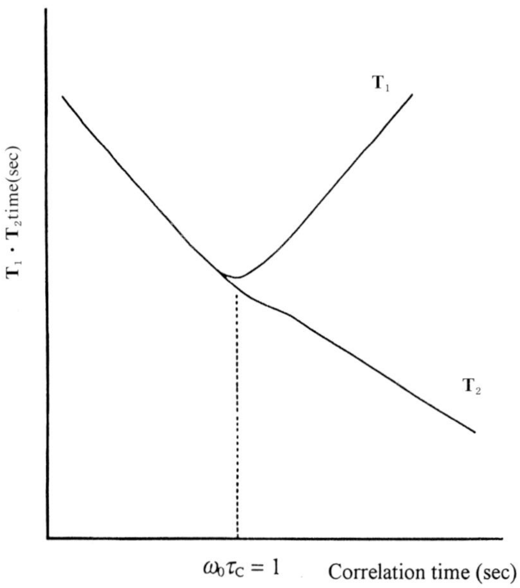

Figure 3-2 Variation of T_1 and T_2 of the protons with τ_c in pure liquid water. When $\omega_0 \tau_c \ll 1$. (ω_0 : spectrometer frequency), T_1 and T_2 are equal. This is the extreme narrowing limit. T_1 passes through a minimum at $\omega_0 \tau_c \fallingdotseq 1$. When $\omega_0 \tau_c \gg 1$, T_1 increases and becomes much longer than T_2. Increased τ_c results in reduced T_2 and increased linewidths.[16]

the electron spin resonance signal from unpaired electrons[10] or the resonance signal from the nuclei coupled to the interested nucleus in the sample are saturated. The NOE causes a significant enhancement of signal intensity in low sensitive nuclei such as ^{13}C. Proton decoupling improves spectral resolution by suppressing the heteronuclear *J* modulation patterns, for which the interaction of ^{1}H-spin with the interested nuclear spin other than ^{1}H nucleus is responsible, because the second radio frequency field causes ^{1}H-spin to disappear.[11] The proton decoupling method applied in ^{31}P MRS at 1.5 T improved spectral resolution substantially and yielded well-resolved ^{31}P resonances of glycerophosphocholine, glycerophosphoethanolamine, and phosphoethanolamine in human brain.[12] The NOE technique was also employed in ^{31}P MRS, and a combination of NOE and chemical shift imaging techniques increased signal-to-noise ratio and allowed shorter examination time to be achieved.[13] It was suggested that sensitivity in ^{31}P spectra, whose coupling protons were decoupled with the broad band proton decoupling technique, is enhanced by NOE.[14] ^{31}P spectra obtained with the proton decoupling technique and with full enhancement by NOE showed well-resolved peaks in the phosphomonoesters (PME) and phosphodiesters (PDE) regions of the human brain.[15] However, the proton decoupling and NOE require continuous irradiation of radio frequency, which may result in excessive heating of tissues. It was reported that in the U. S. A. it is possible to use the proton decoupling technique in ^{31}P MRS studies within the Food and Drug Administration safety guidelines in radio frequency power deposition in human tissue.[11]

3.2 ^{31}P MRS

Clinical ^{31}P MRS shows resonance lines of phosphomonoester (PME), inorganic phosphate (Pi), phosphodiester (PDE), phosphocreatine (PCr), γ-ATP, α-ATP, and β-ATP (Figure 3-3). Peaks of PME and PDE involve information associated with membrane phospholipids and their metabolism. The peaks of PCr, ATP, and Pi provide information concerning high-energy phosphate metabolism. In ^{31}P-MRS, relative values of metabolites, i.e., the ratio of each peak area to the total peak area or the ratios among the peaks, are evaluated. Table 3-1 shows the concentrations of metabolites in the brain and their T_1 and T_2 values.[17–24]

3.2.1 Resonance of PME

The resonance of PME predominantly arises from phosphocholine (PC) and phosphoethanolamine (PE), both of which are the precursors of membrane phospholipids.[25] The peak of PME reflects the anabolic activity of phospholipid metabolism. The level of PME peak is elevated during the development of the brain with neurotic

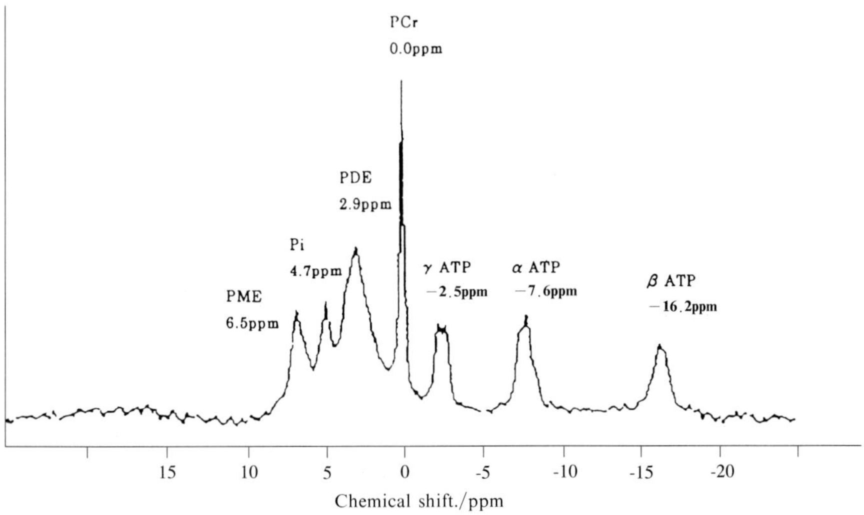

Figure 3-3 ^{31}P spectrum and chemical shift. The chemical shift of each substance is shown and measured with respect to the resonance of phosphocreatine (PCr).

prolifilation.[26] The T_1 value of total PME in the developing brain of normal human beings decreases with age, which was explained by its variable multicomponent nature.[27] This finding may suggest that the phosphoethanolamine (PE) with a long T_1 value dominates in the PME peak of the newborn brain, whereas multiple unresolved resonances with short T_1 values contribute mostly to the PME peak of the adult brain.

3.2.2 Resonance of PDE

The resonance of PDE contains signals of glycerophosphocholine (GPC) and glycerophosphoethanolamine (GPE), both of which are catabolic products of membrane phospholipids.[28] ^{31}P-MRS without off-resonance saturation has broad components centered in the PDE region in *in vivo* brain.[29] This broad resonance of the PDE region was explained by substantial contributions from a fraction of mobile phospholipids,[30] or from the phospholipid bilayer as well as a small contribution from a motionally averaged macromolecule.[31] A large amount of PDE is present in the brain, but little is known about its physiological actions. A study by nuclear magnetic resonance with 4.7T showed that PDE was significantly higher in aged rat brain than in adult controls, suggesting accelerated phospholipid catabolism in aged rat brain.[32]

3.2.3 Phospholipids

More than 60% of total lipids in the brain are phospholipids, and most are contained in membranes. The fundamental structure of the biological membrane is the structure of lipid bilayer, comprised of a complex mixture of phospholipids, glycolipids, and cholesterol.[33] The membrane not only forms the closed boundary of the cell but also plays the important role in regulating information transmission between cells and their environment. As demonstrated by *in vitro* ^{31}P NMR spectroscopy, the phospholipid profile of fresh autopsied human brain extracts showed six main constituents of the biological membrane, namely phosphatidylcholine (lecithin) and phosphatidylethanolamine, phosphatidylserine, phosphatidylinositol, sphingomyelin, and ethanolamine plasmalogen.[34] Phosphatidylcholine was 43.6% in the gray matter and 28.1% in the white matter, and phosphatidylethanolamine 28.1% in the gray matter and 26.8% in the white matter. Precursors of phosphatidylcholine and phosphatidylethanolamine are phos-

Table 3-1 The absolute metabolite concentration, T_1, and T_2 in the brain obtained by ^{31}P MRS.

		PME			Pi			PDE			PCr			γATP			αATP			βATP		
		T_1	T_2	mM	T_1	T_2	mM	T_1	T_2	mM	T_1	T_2	mM	T_1	T_2	mM	T_1	T_2	mM	T_1	T_2	mM
Roth(1989)* [17]		1420		4.0	1450		2.0	1320		11.5	3140		4.9	650			850			800		2.5
Luyten(1989) [18]		2740			1470		2.6	1640			3290		4.3	1360		3.5	970		5.7	1030		3.0
Merboldt(1990) *[19]		4000	70		2500	80	1.0	2000	20		3000	150	5.0	700	30	3.3	700	30	4.0	1000	20	3.3
Bottomley(1992) [20]				3.2			1.4			12.4			4.6									2.8
Jung(1993) [21]															89			84			62	
Lara(1993)* [22]		1700	33	3.0	1400	81	0.7	1300	11	10.9	2700	390	2.7	600	17		1000	28		700	15	2.9
Matson(1993)* [23]				2.3			1.2			7.0			3.1									2.3
Buchli(1994)** [24]	GM			3.1			1.0			10.1			3.1									2.9
	WM			4.3			1.3			14.2			2.9									2.9

All data measured at 1.5T(* :2.0T, ** :2.35T). GM: gray matter WM: white matter
T1, T2 : msec

phocholine (PC) and phosphoethanolamine (PE), respectively (Figure 3-4). Phosphatidylethanolamine is synthesized from CDP-ethanolamine and diacylglycerol (DG). Phosphatidylcholine is synthesized from CDP-choline and diacylglycerol or phosphatidylethanolamine[35]. Anabolic and catabolic pathways of phosphatidylcholine (Figure 3-5) and phosphatidylethanolamine intersect, and biosynthesis of these substances appears to be subject to biochemical feedback and amplification

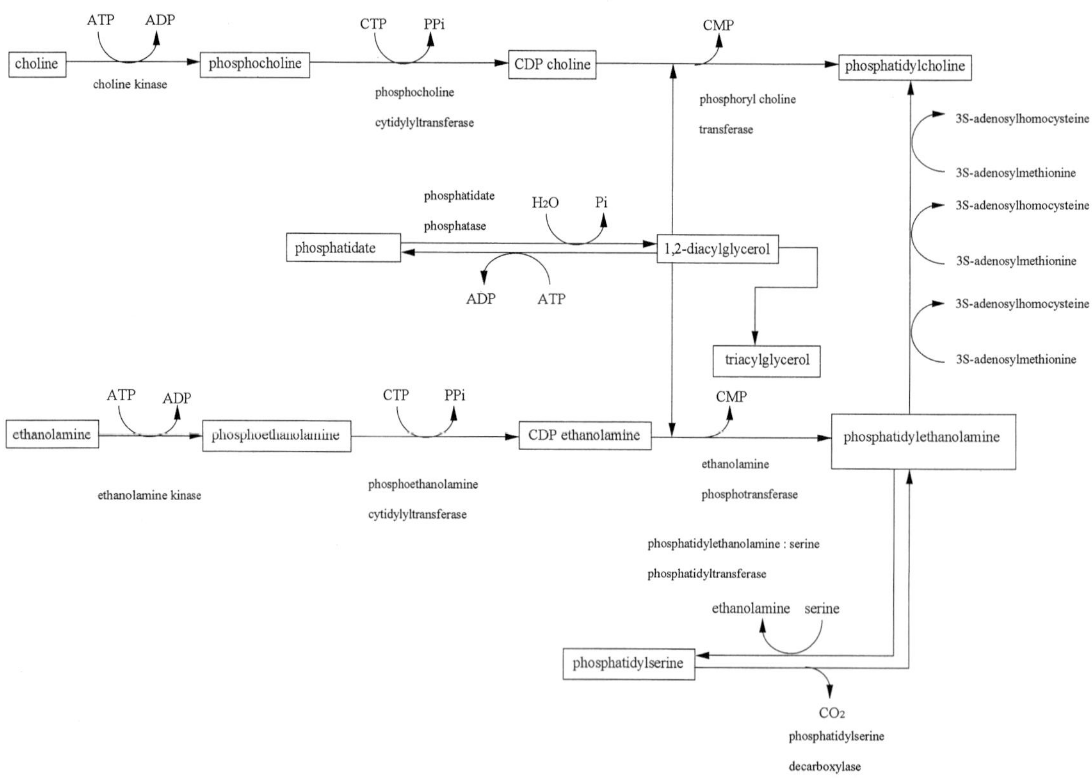

Figure 3-4 Biosynthesis of phosphatidylcholine and phosphatidylethanolamine. Phosphocholine and phosphoethanolamine are precursors used for synthesizing phosphatidylcholine and phosphatidylethanolamine, respectively.

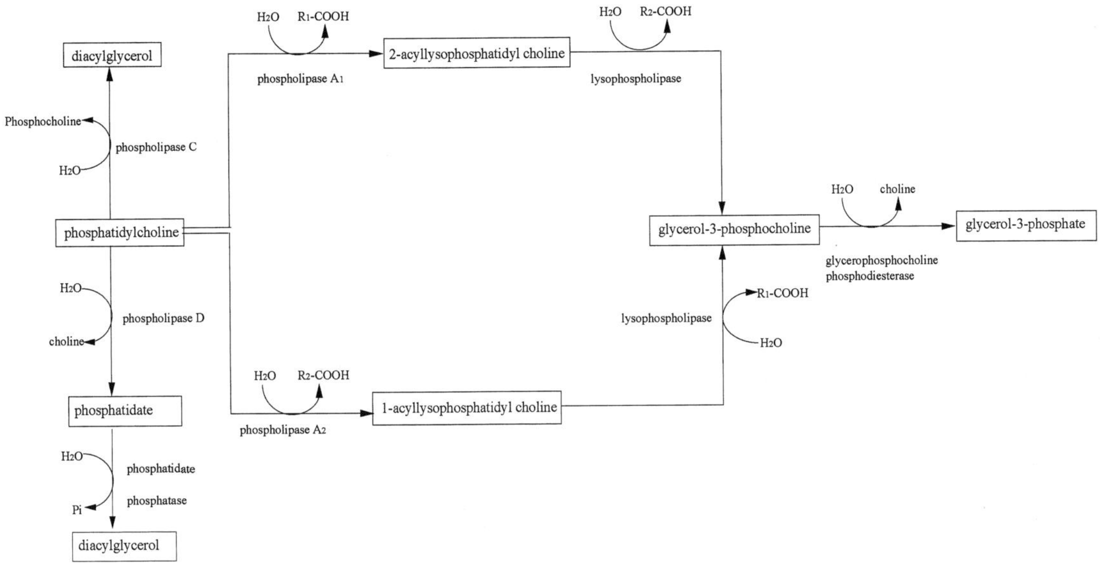

Figure 3-5 Catabolism of phosphatidylcholine.[25,28] Glycerol-3-phosphocholine (glycerophosphcholine) is a catabolic product of phosphatidylcholine, which is formed by the activity of phosphlipases.

through a complicated network.

3.2.4 Resonance of ATP, Pi, and PCr

In ^{31}P-MRS, the peak of γ-ATP contains a small amount of ADP signals. The peak of α-ATP also contains a small amount of ADP signals and nicotinamide adenine dinucleotides (NAD), and the uridine diphosphosugars (galactose, glucose, mannose).[28] The resonance of β-ATP is considered to be the most reliable indicator of tissue ATP level.[36] ATP is the high-energy intermediate that constitutes the most common energy currency in biological systems.[37] Energy obtained from the oxidation of metabolic fuels, such as lipids and carbohydrates, is recovered in the form of ATP with high efficiency in energy conversion.[38] ATP releases a large amount of free energy when hydrolyzed to ADP (adenosine diphosphate) and Pi, or hydrolyzed to AMP (adenosine monophosphate) and pyrophosphate by the cleavage of phosphoanhydride linkage. On the other hand, ATP is synthesized by oxidative phosphorylation in the inner membrane of mitochondria under aerobic condition. ATP is also synthesized in relatively small amounts under anaerobic conditions during the process of glycolysis. This ATP-ADP cycle is the fundamental mode of energy exchange in biologically active systems. The turnover of ATP is very high and its level is stationally maintained.

PCr is considered to be a high-energy reservoir for ATP formation. PCr is formed by the reversible phosphorylation of creatine by ATP as catalyzed by creatine kinase. When the ATP level is relatively high in the resting state, this reaction via creatine kinase proceeds with net synthesis of PCr. When ATP level falls, equilibrium shifts so as to yield net synthesis of ATP through transfer of the activated phosphoryl group from PCr to ADP. The free ADP concentration in the brain is in the order of μM, and it is below the sensitivity of *in vivo* ^{31}P MRS. The reaction mediated by creatine kinase is nearly equilibriated, and ADP concentration can be calculated indirectly by the following equation.[39]

$$[\mathrm{ADP}] = \frac{[\mathrm{C_r}]\,[\mathrm{ATP}]}{[\mathrm{PC_r}]\,[\mathrm{H^+}]}\,\mathrm{K_{ck}}$$

in which Kck is the equilibrium constant.

Cerebral intracellular pH(pHi) can be determined by Petroff's formula[40] from the difference (△) in chemical shift between Pi and PCr.

$$pHi = 6.77 + \log[(\triangle - 3.29)/(5.68 - \triangle)]$$

The free energy of hydrolysis for ATP is usually associated with Mg^{2+} because Mg^{2+} partly binds to the ATP molecule under physiological concentration, and is markedly influenced by pH because hydrolysis of ATP produces H^+ ion.[41] The free magnesium concentration can be calculated from changes in the chemical shift of ATP in binding of Mg^{2+} to ATP and is estimated to be about 0.3 mM in the human brain.[42] PCr/ATP ratio is an indicator of the energetic state of the brain.

3.3 ^{1}H MRS

^{1}H MRS is used to observe resonances of brain metabolites including lactate, *N*-acetylaspartate (NAA) and *N*-acetylaspartylglutamate (NAAG), glutamine (Gln), glutamate (Glu), γ-aminobutyric acid (GABA), creatine and phosphocreatine (Cr), choline containing compounds (Cho), taurine (Tau), and inositol (Ins) (Table 3-2) (Figure 3-6).[43] Generally, three major signals of NAA (2.0ppm), Cr(3.0ppm), and Cho(3.2ppm) can be obtained with high reliability at long-echo time, and relative ratios among these peaks are evaluated. Recently, significant improvements in the quality of ^{1}H MR spectra has allowed quantification of *in vivo* absolute metabolite concentrations. However, quantification of the absolute concentration does have problems such as the overlapping of resonance lines and line broadening due to eddy current, poor field homogeneity, and incomplete water suppression pulse, particularly at short echo times. Table 3-3 shows the concentration of metabolites in the brain and their T_1 and T_2 values obtained by ^{1}H MRS.[44-62]

3.3.1 Resonance of NAA (N-acetylaspartate)

NAA (*N*-acetylaspartate) was found in the central nervous system of vertebrates in high concentration by Tallan et al. in 1956.[63] NAA is the

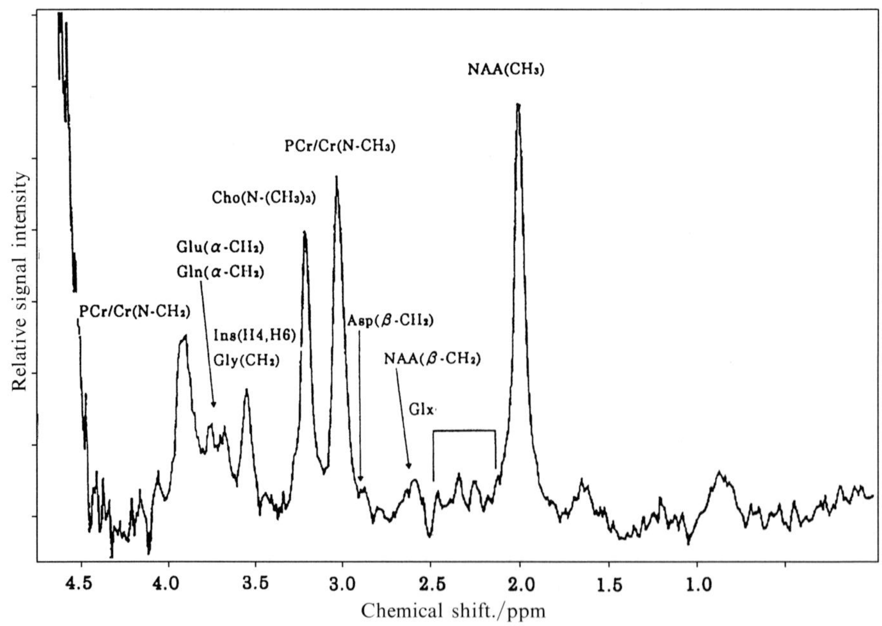

Figure 3-6 ^{1}H spectrum and metabolites.

Table 3-2 Chemical shifts of assigned resonances of brain metabolites obtained by ^{1}H MRS.[43,66]

Metabolite	Abbr.	Proton (s)	Chemical shift (ppm)
Lipids	Lip	CH_3, CH_2	0–2
Valine	Val	CH_3	1.05
Lactate	Lac	CH_3	1.3
Threonine	Thr	γ-CH_3	1.33
Alanine	Ala	β-CH_3	1.48
		α-CH	4.11
Acetate	Ac	CH_3 (C-2)	1.85
γ-Aminobutyrate	GABA	γ-CH_2	2.25
N-Acetyl aspartate	NAA	CH_3	2.0
		β-CH_2	2.6
Glutamate	Glu	β-CH_2	2.1
		γ-CH_2	2.35
		α-CH	3.75
Glutamine	Gln	β-CH_2	2.1
		γ-CH_2	2.45
		α-CH	3.75
Aspartate	Asp	β-CH_2	2.8
Creatine	Cr	N-CH_3	3.0
		N-CH_2	3.9
Phosphocreatine	PCr	N-CH_3	3.0
		N-CH_2	3.9
Cholines	Cho	N-$(CH_3)_3$	3.2
		CH_2 (C-2)	3.52
Taurine	Tau	N-CH_2, S-CH_2	3.3
Inositols	Ins	CH (C-5)	3.29
		CH (C-1 & C-3)	3.54
		CH (C-4 & C-6)	3.63
		CH (C-2)	4.07
Glycine	Gly	α-CH_2	3.5

Table 3-3 The absolute metabolite concentration, T_1, and T_2, in the brain obtained by ^{1}H MRS.

	Lactate			Total NAA			Cr+PCr			Cho			Taurine			Inositol		
	T_1	T_2	mM	T_1	T_2	mM	T_1	T_2	mM	T_1	T_2	mM	T_1	T_2	mM	T_1	T_2	mM
Frahm(1989)[44] occipital	1550	1200		1450	450		1550	240		1150	330		1700	270		900	110	4.9
Hüppi(1991)[45] cerebellum						6.5						1.4			1.8			4.4
Narayana(1991)[46] frontal				1390	320	9.9	1520	240	7.8	1160	270	2.1						
Hennig(1992)[47] parietal					352	8.2		252	5.3		372	1.3						
occipital					329	10.4		251	5.8		331	1.3						
frontal					358	8.4		251	5.6		379	1.5						
cerebellum					383	8.7		274	8.1		307	2.2						
Barker(1993)[48] GM					320	17.2		180	11.6		350	2.0						
WM					430	16.6		210	10.6		360	1.9						
Christiansen(1993a)[49]				1370	299	11.6	1170	190	7.6	1290	270	1.7						
Christiansen(1993b)[50] occipital(a)				1500	344	11.4	1300	220	7.1	1500	360	1.5						
Hänicke(1993)*[51] GM						8.0			6.4			1.1						4.6
WM				1560		7.5	1530		5.5	1150		1.5				1140		3.7
Kreis(1993)[52] GM				1330	399	12.7	1320	204	11.1	1390	401	2.0				1130	279	9.9
WM				1380	483	13.6	1300	209	9.8	1440	325	2.4				1200	197	10.3
Michaelis(1993)[53] GM (parietal)						11.7			8.2			1.4						
WM (parietal)						11.2			6.1			1.8						
Thalamus						11.8			7.5			1.8						
Moats(1994)[54] GM (occipital)(b)				1150	402	9.3	1120	186	8.2	1250	386	1.6				960	157	6.4
WM (occipital)(b)				1160			1080			1030						890		
Toft(1994)[55] striatum (c)					324			216			398						76	
Dezortová(1995)[56]				1450	331	11.8	1550	240	7.2	1150	360	1.6						
Pouwels(1995)*[57] Frontal						7.7			6.0			1.2						4.2
Parietal						8.5			6.4			1.1						4.0
Occipital						9.9			6.5			0.8						3.7
Saunders(1995)[58] GM						15.1			8.2			1.2						
WM						14.5			7.3			2.1						
Pouwels(1998)*[61] GM (frontal)						8.4			6.4			1.4						4.3
WM (frontal)						9.6			5.7			1.8						3.8
GM (parietal)						8.7			6.5			1.1						4.3
WM (parietal)						10.6			5.7			1.7						3.1
GM (occipital)						10.6			6.9			0.9						4.1
WM (occipital)						10.4			5.5			1.6						4.1
Cerebellum						11.0			8.7			2.2						5.8
Thalamus						10.5			6.8			1.8						3.6
Wang(1998)[62] GM (occipital)				1330	399	11.0	1320	204	9.7	1390	401	1.9						
WM (occipital)				1380	483	7.5	1300	209	5.2	1440	325	1.6						

All date measured at 1.5T (*2.0T). GM : gray matter. WM : white matter. T_1 T_2 : msec. (a) : 20-30 years old. (b) : normal elderly. (c) : developing brain.

most abundant next to glutamate in the free amino acid pool of the mammalian brain.[64] NAA is also considered to be a neuronal marker,[65] and its concentration varies with the region of the brain and age. The concentration of NAA *in vitro* is 5.97 mM/kg frozen wet weight of human temporal lobe cortex.[66] The concentration of NAA in adult mammalian brains is higher in the gray matter than in the white matter.[67,68] In the subcellular fractions of the rat brain, NAA is localized in soluble portion of the cell.[69]

The biosynthesis of NAA occurs through the direct acetylation of L-aspartate by L-aspartate-*N*-acetyltransferase (ANAT).[70–72] It was reported that NAA may also be formed from the cleavage of *N*-acetylaspartylglutamate (NAAG) by *N*-acetylated-α-linked acidic dipeptidase.[73] After being synthesized, NAA is exported from the brain mitochondria by dicarboxylic acid translocase to cytoplasm.[74] NAA and other *N*-acylated amino acids are hydrolyzed to the free amino acid and acetate by amidohydrolases (aminoacylases).[75] The function of NAA remains to be clarified, but presumptive functions are as follows.

1) NAA plays an active role in the synthesis of fatty acid during growth and development of the brain. NAA concentration in the rat brain is low at birth but increases rapidly to a mature level within 10–20 days after birth, which is the period of myelination when lipids arc synthesized rapidly.[64] NAA constitutes acetyl transport system for extra-mitochodrial fatty acid synthesis.[76] NAA may also regulate lipogenesis in the brain during the period of myelination.[64] NAA concentration is higher in the gray matter than in the white matter and spinal cord because in the white matter and spinal cord the activity of *N*-acetyl-L-aspartate amidohydrolase II (aminoacylase II) is three times higher than in gray matter.[77]
2) NAA is considered to act as a carbon transport molecule to citrate and to provide cytosolic carbon from intramitocondrial sources.[74]
3) NAA may be a precursor of *N*-acetylaspartylglutamate (NAAG), which may have a regulatory role in neruotransmission.[78]
4) NAA biosynthesis may be related to neuronal protein synthesis. *N*-acylation of aspartate occurs on aspartyl-t-RNA, suggesting that NAA-t-RNA would act as a chain initiator of protein synthesis in neurons.[79]
5) NAA may be a storage form of aspartate, because it neither affects amino acid receptors nor is generally incorporated into peptides.[65]
6) NAA may function as an osmolyte, which involves cerebral osmotic regulation.[80]

Other noteworthy findings include that the NAA level in the ipsilateral striatum reduces after decortication,[81] and that a trans-synaptic decrease in NAA level is caused by acute deafferentation in the central nervous system.[82] Also, NAA concentration is increased by the administration of 5-hydroxytryptophan (5-HTP), as well as certain drugs classified as monoamine oxidase inhibitors, but is reduced by the administration of reserpine and lysergic acid diethylamide (LSD-25).[69] After acute brain injury, a reversible decrease in NAA was observed.[83]

In the brain of healthy rats, the NAA/Cr ratio obtained by *in vivo* MRS is generally considered as a reliable one, because it closely correlates with the NAA/Cr ratio determined by *in vitro* MRS or chromatography.[84] Currently, a reduction of the NAA peak in MRS is considered to reflect the loss or dysfunction of neurons.[85] A defect in metabolism of NAA results in spongy degeneration of the brain (Canavan disease).[86] To clarify whether NAA is a marker for functional and structural integrity of nerurons or not[87] is considered to be an important challenge in the future study of neuropsychiatric disorders.

3.3.2 Resonance of Cr (creatine and phosphocreatine)

The methyl group and methylene group in the creatine and phosphocreatine (Cr) molecule are observed as a single peak in ^{1}H-MRS, respectively. Concentrations of creatine plus phosphocreatine *in vitro* are 7.68 mM/kg frozen wet weight in white matter and 9.63 mM in cortex in post-operative human brain.[66] The ratio of creatine peak to phosphocreatine peak was 2.3:1 in the dog brain.[88]

Cr resonance is considered to be more stable than the peaks of NAA or Cho so that it is occasionally used as a reference. However, it is reduced in the brain of patients with brain tumor or infectious brain masses, and its use as a reference requires caution.[89]

3.3.3 Resonance of Cho (choline containing compounds)

Choline is readily transported through the blood-brain barrier and utilized by the myelinating brain for the biosynthesis of its phospholipids.[90] Choline is a precursor of phosphatidylcholine (Figure 3-4), as well as the metabolite of acetylcholine. Choline itself and its metabolites are present in relatively small amounts, compared to the contents of NAA and Cr.[91] The trimethylamine resonance of choline containing compounds contributes to the resonance at 3.2 ppm and is from glycerophosphocholine (GPC) and phosphocholine (PC) in addition to only a small amount of free choline in the ^{1}H-MRS.[88] The concentrations of GPC and PC in the canine brain were about 1.3 μmol/g wet wt. and 0.5 μmol/g wet wt., respectively. Since GPC and PC are involved in membrane phospholipid metabolism, information associated with phospholipid metabolism can be obtained from the Cho peak (Figures 3-4 and 5). The Cho peak is increased in the fast growing tumor such as the glioma, suggesting a high degree of cell proliferation and probably increased membrane turnover.[92,93] However, interpretation of changes of Cho signals in the brain tumor is difficult, because the other standard compounds are more severely reduced.[89] The Cho peak provides even more useful information when it is evaluated if combined with ^{31}P-MRS technique which yields the peak of PME containing signals of PC, and the peak of PDE containing signals of GPC. The Cho peak was also reported to be increased after 3 hours following oral administration of choline.[94]

3.3.4 Resonance of lactate

Brain lactate is a marker for inadequate oxygen supply to tissues. Lactate concentration in brain tissues increases when oxygen is deficient or energy requirement increases, and when irreversible damage is caused by persistence of pathological conditions. The lactate concentration in normal human brain is below 1 mM.[44,53] *In vivo* detection of the lactate signal is complicated by the overlapping of signals derived from lipids (primarily triglycerides) in the same spectral region. Spectral editing is needed to obtain only the methyl protons signal of lactate.[95,96] The resonance of methyl protons of lactate is split into a doublet at 1.3 ppm because of the three-bond homonuclear coupling between a single methine proton and the three equivalent methyl protons.[97] Measurement of brain lactate concentration showed contradictory results, and all molecules of lactate in tissue do not necessarily contribute to the resonance at 1.3 ppm. A study using cell cultures indicated that the quantity of lactate detected by NMR in long echo time was about 70% of that detected by a biochemical method.[98] Figure 3-7 shows examples of the ^{1}H spectrum of lactate. An elevated pool of brain lactate is observed in epilepsy, stroke, tumor growth, trauma, and other pathological conditions. The lactate level in the human visual cortex was also increased by visual stimulation within the physiological range.[99]

Elevation of lactate concentration is frequently related to acidosis. However, ^{1}H MRS studies of the human brain showed that in certain cases the lactate concentration was increased, accompanying insignificant change or elevation of tissue pH.[100,101] Lactate content was increased after electroshock to the cerebral cortex, but significant change in intracellular pH could not be found. Lactate content was increased in reversible near complete cerebral ischemia and brain tumors, while the tissue pH shifted to alkaline.[101] In interpreting lactate accumulation under different pathophysiological conditions, it should be remembered that lactate accumulation is not necessarily an indicator of tissue acidosis.

3.3.5 Resonance of NAAG (N-acetylaspartylglutamate)

The majority of the NAA signal at 2.0 ppm in ^{1}H-MRS arises from *N*-acetylaspartate (NAA), but includes contributions of other *N*-acetyl moieties such as *N*-acetylaspartylglutamate (NAAG).[47] NAAG is a dipeptide specific to the nervous system,[78] and presents at about 10% of *N*-acetylaspartate (NAA) in the mammalian brain.[102] NAAG is concentrated in neurons and its distribution in the brain is not uniform.[67] Metabolism and function of NAAG remain to be clarified, but NAAG may be synthesized from NAA because NAAG has a structure similar to that of NAA and its concentration is less than 10% of that of NAA.[67] NAAG is hydrolyzed into glutamate (Glu) and NAA by *N*-acetylated-α-linked acidic dipeptidase (NAALADase), a membrane-bound peptidase.[103] The finding that hydrolysis of NAAG elevated the content of extracellular glutamate indicates that glutamate uptake is not tightly coupled with the activity of peptidase; therefore, NAAG is considered to play an important role as a source of glutamate in the synaptic space.[104] NAAG may have a role as the neurotransmitter of the lateral olfactory tract[105] and endogenous neuroexcitants in certain pathways of the hippocampus,[106] and have a function in synaptic communication in the brain.[107,108] After synaptic release, variation in the direct uptake of NAAG as well as extracellular hydrolysis to glutamate may lead to a cascade of receptor- mediated response.[109] NAAG exhibits potent convulsant properties, and its injection into the rat hippocampus causes convulsions similar to that induced by the glutamate receptor agonist, quisqualic acid.[110] Conversely, NAAG has been reported to play a protective role against pentamethylenetetrazol (PTZ) induced seizures.[111] This effect may be explained by the following hypothesis that NAAG has a close relation to a homeostatic mechanism in which excitatory neurotransmission is regulated via control of the availability of glutamate (the excitatory neurotransmitter) at a specific synapse.

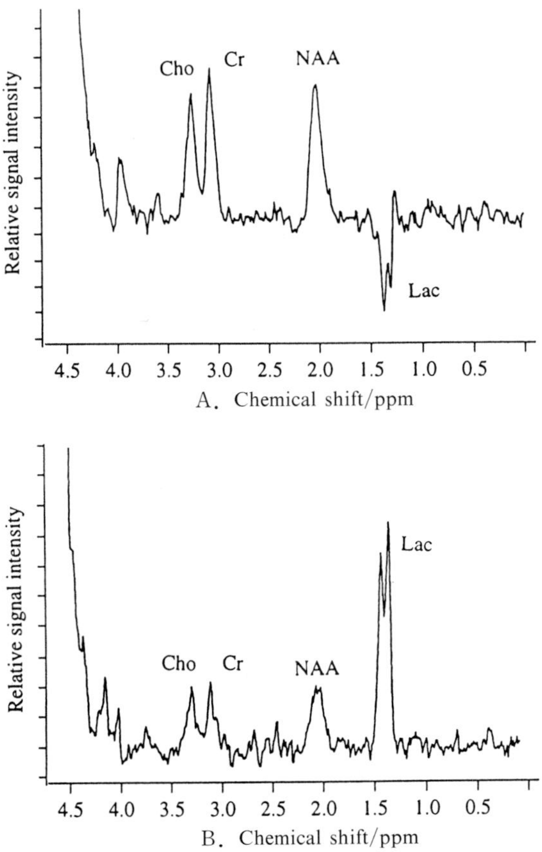

Figure 3-7 Lactate resonance in the lesion of cerebral infarction at 3 days after onset. The methyl proton signal of lactate observed at 135 ms of echo time has a downward direction, while that at 270 ms of echo time has an upward direction.

A. Te=135 ms, Tr=1,500 ms. and voxel size=3×3×3 cm^{3}. (PRESS)

B. Te=270 ms, Tr=1,500 ms. and voxel size=3×3×3 cm^{3}. (PRESS)

3.3.6 Resonance of mI (myo-inositol)

About 70% of the Ins peak at 3.5 ppm is derived from *myo*-inositol, and 15% from *myo*-inositol-monophosphate.[112] In the human brain, the concentration of Ins was estimated to be 4.3 mM in gray matter and 3.1 mM in white matter in the parietal region in ^{1}H MRS.[61]

Functions of *myo*-inositol are unclear, but it is considered to be a storage form of the IP_n messenger system.[112] *Myo*-inositol has a role as a glia-specific marker for *in vivo* MRS studies.[113] *Myo*-inositol functions as an osmotic regulator of the Na^+-*myo*-inositol-cotransporter in the brain.[114,115] According to the inositol depletion hypothesis, lithium strongly blocks the enzyme, *myo*-inositol- 1-monophosphatase and consequently prevents the conversion of inositol monophosphate into *myo*- inositol. However, it has been reported that a decrease in *myo*-inositol content in patients with manic-depressive disease, who are administered lithium, is at present too difficult to detect.[116] *Scyllo*-inositol is observed as a singlet at 3.35 ppm, and its concentration is about 0.43 mM in the gray matter and 0.35 mM in the white matter in the human brain.[117] A common increase of *Myo*- and *scyllo*-Ins was observed in mitochondrial enzyme deficiency and glioma in ^{1}H MRS.[117]

3.3.7 Resonance of Glx (glutamate and glutamine)

The resonance of Glx (glutamate; Glu, and glutamine; Gln) is complicated by the following factors.[118] Glutamate and glutamine have spin systems that are very similar in structure, coupling constants and chemical shifts, and strong coupling between the two β and γ protons exists in both compounds. Resonances of NAA, aspartate, GABA, and Ins also overlap the spectra of Glu and Gln. The MRS with field strength of 4 to 7T is unable to solve the problem of strong coupling for Glu, Gln, and inositol.[119] However, the detection of resonaces of the β-and γ- Glx was improved by using a MRS with 0.5T, because of improved B_0 main-field homogeneity and the collapse of the strongly J-coupled Glx resonances.[120] The glutamate and glutamine concentrations in the cerebral cortex were estimated by ^{1}H MRS to be about 5 mmol/kg wet wt. and about 5.6 mmol/kg wet wt., respectively.[121] In the glutamine/glutamate cycle, glutamate is formed from glutamine by glutaminase in the presynaptic neuron, and the released glutamate from the presynaptic neuron is taken up by astrocytes and converted to glutamine by glutamine synthetase.[122] Glutamate is most abundant in the free amino acid pool and has a role as the most important excitatory neurotransmitter in the central nervous system. Glutamine may be crucial in cerebral function, in detoxification and regulation of neurotransmitter activities.[112] The elevation of glutamine concentration in the brain was observed in hepatic encephalopathy that showed hyperammonemia.[118,122]

3.3.8 Resonance of GABA (γ-aminobutyric acid)

The measurement of cerebral γ-aminobutyric acid (GABA) in ^{1}H MRS is complicated by the overlapping resonances due to other metabolites such as glutamate, glutamine, NAA, creatine, and a macromolecule.[123] Application of spectral editing methods enables the signal of ^{1}H nuclei of GABA to be measured. The GABA concentration in the occipital lobe was estimated to be 1.15 mM, using 4.1T MRS.[123] GABA is the major inhibitory neurotransmitter in the human cortex.[124] GABA is closely related to the metabolism of glutamate, glutamine, and the tricarbonic acid cycle and is formed by decalboxylation of gultamate (Figure 3-8). Although GABA taken back into nerve terminals is recycled, GABA in glia is metabolized to succinic semialdehyde by GABA - T (GABA α-oxoglutarate transaminase).[125] GABA levels were decreased in brain areas in tardive dyskinesia, Huntington's disease, parkinsonism, and idiopathic dyskinesias, and GABA was proposed to play a role in the modulation of extrapyramidal motor

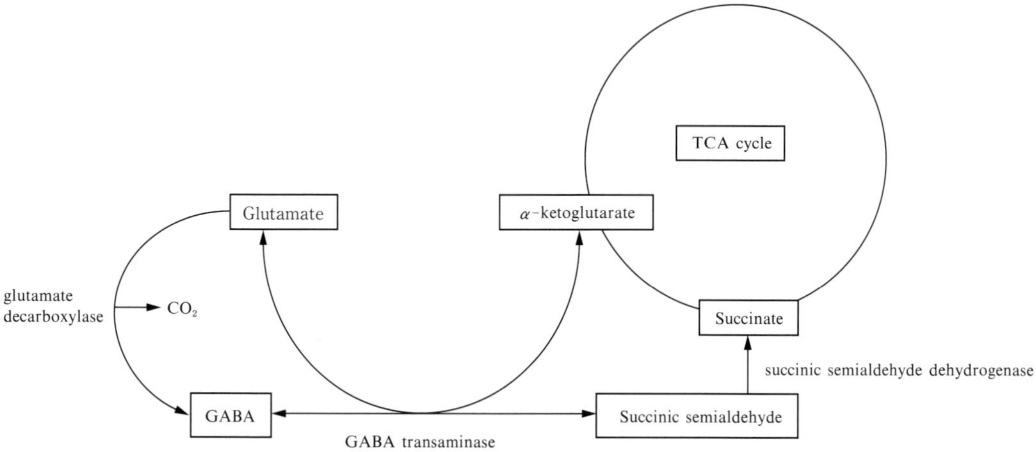

Figure 3-8 Metabolic pathway of GABA.

function.[126] GABA content was also reduced in the brain of schizophrenia.[127] Abnormalities of the GABAergic system are associated with the cause and spread of seizure activity. Inhibitors of GABA-T such as γ-vinyl GABA (vigabatrin), γ-acetylenic GABA and gabacline result in increased concentration of synaptosomal and whole brain GABA, and act as potent anticonvulsants.[128] ^{1}H-edited MRS study demonstrated that GABA level was increased in the occipital lobe of patients treated with vigabatrin (4-amino-hex-5-enoic acid).[129]

References

1) Lenkinski, R. E.; Schnall, M. D. MR spectroscopy and the biochemical basis of neurological disease. In: S. W. Atlas (Ed). Magnetic Resonance Imaging of the Brain and Spine, Second Edition. Philadelphia: Lippincott-Raven Publishers, 1996: pp. 1619-1653.
2) James, T. L. Nuclear Magnetic Resonance in Biochemistry. Principles and Applications. New York: Academic Press, 1975.
3) Gadian, D. G. Nuclear Magnetic Resonance and its Applications to Living Systems. New York: Oxford University Press, 1982.
4) Abraham, R. J.; Fisher, J.; Loftus, P. Introduction to NMR Spectroscopy. Chichester: John Wiley & Sons, 1988.
5) Günther, H. NMR Spectroscopy. Basic Principles, Concepts, and Applications in Chemistry, Second Edition. Chichester: John Wiley & Sons, 1992.
6) Homans, S. W. A Dictionary of Concepts in NMR. Oxford: Clarendon Press, 1989.
7) Sanders, J. K. M.; Hunter, B. K. Modern NMR Spectroscopy. A Guide for Chemists, Second Edition. Oxford: Oxford University Press, 1993.
8) Laszlo, P. NMR of Newly Accessible Nuclei Volume1. Chemical and Biochemical Applications. New York: Academic Press, 1983.
9) Freeman, R. Double resonance. In: D. M. Grant, R. K. Harris (Eds). Encyclopedia of Nuclear Magnetic Resonance Volume 3. Chichester: John Wiley & Sons, 1996: pp. 1740-1749.
10) Freeman, R. A Handbook of Nuclear Magnetic Resonance. Longman Scientific & Technical, 1988.
11) Lamerichs, R. M. J. N.; Luyten, P. R. Proton decoupling during in vivo whole body phosphorus MRS. In: D. M. Grant, R. K. Harris (Eds). Encyclopedia of Nuclear Magnetic Resonance Volume 6. Chichester: John Wiley & Sons, 1996: pp. 3825-3828.
12) Luyten, P. R.; Bruntink, G.; Sloff, F. M. et al. Broadband proton decoupling in human ^{31}P NMR spectroscopy. *NMR Biomed*. 1: 177-183; 1989.
13) Kolem, H.; Miyazaki, T.; Schneider, M. et al. Nuclear Overhauser enhanced localized *in vivo* phosphorus spectroscopy using the CSI technique. *In: Works in Progress: Ninth Annual Scientific Meeting and Exhibition of the Society of Magnetic Resonance in Medicine, New York, USA: SMRM*; 1990: 1331.
14) van Sluis, R.; Payne, G. S.; Leach, M. O. Increased NOE enhancement in ^{1}H decoupled ^{31}P MRS. *Magn. Reson. Med*. 34: 893-897; 1995.
15) Murphy-Boesch, J.; Stoyanova, R.; Srinivasan, R. et al. Proton-decoupled ^{31}P chemical shift imaging of the human brain in normal volunteers. *NMR Biomed*. 6: 173-180; 1993.

16) Akitt, J. W. NMR and Chemistry. An introduction to modern NMR spectroscopy, Third Edition. London: Chapman & Hall, 1992.
17) Roth, K.; Hubesch, B.; Meyerhoff, D. J. et al. Noninvasive quantitation of phosphorus metabolites in human tissue by NMR spectroscopy. *Journal of Magnetic Resonance* 81: 299-311; 1989.
18) Luyten, P. R.; Groen, J. P.; Vermeulen, J. W. A. H. et al. Experimental approaches to image localized human ^{31}P NMR spectroscopy. *Magn. Reson. Med*. 11: 1-21; 1989.
19) Merboldt, K. D.; Chien, D.; Hänicke, W. et al. Localized ^{31}P NMR spectroscopy of the adult human brain *in vivo* using stimulated-echo (STEAM) sequences. *Journal of Magnetic Resonance* 89: 343-361; 1990.
20) Bottomley, P. A.; Cousins, J. P.; Pendrey, D. L. et al. Alzheimer dementia: Quantification of energy metabolism and mobile phosphoesters with P-31 NMR spectroscopy. *Radiology* 183: 695-699; 1992.
21) Jung, W-I.; Widmaier, S.; Bunse, M. et al. ^{31}P transverse relaxation times of ATP in human brain *in vivo*. *Magn. Reson. Med*. 30: 741-743; 1993.
22) Lara, R. S.; Matson, G. B.; Hugg, J. W. et al. Quantitation of in vivo phosphorus metabolites in human brain with magnetic resonance spectroscopic imaging (MRSI). *Magn. Reson. Imaging* 11: 273-278; 1993.
23) Matson, G. B.; Meyerhoff, D. J.; Lawry, T. J. et al. Use of computer simulations for quantitation of ^{31}P ISIS MRS results. *NMR Biomed*. 6: 215-224; 1993.
24) Buchli, R.; Duc, C. O.; Martin, E. et al. Assessment of absolute metabolite concentrations in human tissue by ^{31}P MRS *in vivo*. Part I: Cerebrum, cerebellum, cerebral gray and white matter. *Magn. Reson. Med*. 32: 447-452; 1994.
25) Leach, M.; Le Moyec, L.; Podo, F. Chapter 18, MRS of tumours: Basic Principles. In: J. D. De Certaines, W. M. M. J. Bovée, F. Podo (Eds). Magnetic Resonance Spectroscopy in Biology and Medicine. Oxford: Pergamon Press, 1992: pp. 295-344.
26) Pettegrew, J. W.; Minshew, N. J. Chapter 12, Molecular insights into schizophrenia In: N. C. Andreasen (Ed). Schizophrenia: From Mind to Molecule. Washington, DC: American Psychiatric Press, 1994: pp. 221, 226-228.
27) Gruetter, R.; Fusch, C.; Martin, E. et al. Determination of saturation factors in ^{31}P NMR spectra of the developing human brain. *Magn. Reson. Med*. 29: 7-11; 1993.
28) Pettegrew, J. W. Molecular insights into Alzheimer's disease. *Annals New York Academy of Sciences* 568: 5-28; 1989.
29) McNamara, R.; Arias-Mendoza, F.; Brown, T. R. Investigation of broad resonances in ^{31}P NMR spectra of the human brain *in vivo*. *NMR Biomed*. 7: 237-242; 1994.
30) Cerdan, S.; Subramanian, V. H.; Hilberman, M. et al. ^{31}P NMR detection of mobile dog brain phospholipids. *Magn. Reson. Med*. 3: 432-439; 1986.
31) Murphy, E. J.; Rajagopalan, B.; Brindle, K. M. et al. Phospholipid bilayer contribution to ^{31}P NMR spectra *in vivo*. *Magn. Reson. Med*. 12: 282-289; 1989.
32) Kwee, I. L.; Nakada, T.; Suzuki, N. ^{31}P and 3-fluoro-3-deoxy-$_{D}$-glucose ^{19}F *in vivo* NMR spectroscopy of aged rat brain. *NMR Biomed*. 4: 38-40; 1991.
33) Stryer, L. Biochemistry. Fourth Edition. New York: W. H. Freeman and Company, 1995.
34) Kwee, I. L.; Nakada, T. Phospholipid profile of the human brain: ^{31}P NMR spectroscopic study. *Magn. Reson. Med*. 6: 296-299; 1988.
35) Agranoff, B. E. Chapter 5, Lipids. In: G. J. Siegel, B. W. Agranoff, R. W. Albers, P. B. Molinoff (Eds). Basic Neurochemistry: Molecular, Cellular, and Medical Aspects, Fourth Edition. New York: Raven Press, 1989: pp. 91-107.
36) Bottomley, P. A. Human in vivo NMR spectroscopy in diagnostic medicine: clinical tool or research probe ? *Rodiology* 170: 1-15; 1989.
37) Voet, D.; Voet, J. G. Biochemistry. Second Edition. New York: John Wiley & Sons, 1995.
38) Horton, H. R.; Moran, L. A.; Ochs, R. S. et al. Principles of Biochemistry. Second Edition. Prentice Hall, 1996.
39) Chance, B.; Leigh Jr, J. S.; McLaughlin, A. C. et al. Phosphorus-31 spectroscopy and imaging. In: C. L. Partain, R. R. Price, J. A. Patton, M. V. Kulkarni, A. E. James (Eds). Magnetic Resonance Imaging, Vol. 2. Philadelphia: W. B. Saunders Company, 1988: pp. 1501-1520.
40) Petroff, O. A. C.; Prichard, J. W.; Behar, K. L. et al. Cerebral intracellular pH by ^{31}P nuclear magnetic resonance spectroscopy. *Neurology* 35: 781-788 ; 1985.
41) Williams, G. D.; Smith, M. B. Application of the accurate assessment of intracellular magnesium and pH from the ^{31}P shifts of ATP to cerebral hypoxia-ischemia in neonatal rat. *Magn. Reson. Med*. 33: 853-857; 1995.
42) Halvorson, H. R.; Linde, A. M. Q. V.; Helpern, J. A. et al. Assessment of magnesium concentrations by ^{31}P NMR *in vivo*. *NMR Biomed*. 5: 53-58 ; 1992.
43) Frahm, J.; Bruhn, H.; Gyngell, M. L. et al. Localized high-resolution proton NMR spectroscopy using stimulated echoes: Initial applications to human brain *in vivo*. *Magn. Reson. Med*. 9: 79-93; 1989.

44) Frahm, J.; Bruhn, H.; Gyngell, M. L. et al. Localized proton NMR spectroscopy in different regions of the human brain *in vivo*. Relaxation times and concentrations of cerebral metabolites. *Magn. Reson. Med.* 11: 47–63; 1989.

45) Hüppi, P. S.; Posse, S.; Lazeyras, F. et al. Brain development in preterm and term babies studied with ^{1}H-magnetic resonance spectroscopy using short-echo time STEAM technique. *In: Book of Abstracts: Tenth Annual Scientific Meeting and Exhibition of the Society of Magnetic Resonance in Medicine, Vol. 1. San Francisco, California, USA: SMRM*; 1991: 377.

46) Narayana, P. A.; Johnston, D.; Flamig, D. P. In vivo proton magnetic resonance spectroscopy studies of human brain. *Magn. Reson. Imaging* 9: 303–308; 1991.

47) Hennig, J.; Pfister, H.; Ernst, T. et al. Direct absolute quantification of metabolites in the human brain with *in vivo* localized proton spectroscopy. *NMR Biomed.* 5: 193–199; 1992.

48) Barker, P. B.; Soher, B. J.; Blackband, S. J. et al. Quantitation of proton NMR spectra of the human brain using tissue water as an internal concentration reference. *NMR Biomed.* 6: 89–94; 1993.

49) Christiansen, P.; Henriksen, O.; Stubgaard, M. et al. In vivo quantification of brain metabolites by ^{1}H-MRS using water as an internal standard. *Magn. Reson. Imaging* 11: 107–118; 1993a.

50) Christiansen, P.; Toft, P.; Larsson, H. B. W. et al. The concentration of *N*-acetyl aspartate, creatine+phosphocreatine, and choline in different parts of the brain in adulthood and senium. *Magn. Reson. Imaging* 11: 799–806; 1993b.

51) Hänicke, W.; Michaelis, T.; Merboldt, K. D. et al. On the use of a fully automated data analysis method for *in vivo* MRS. Metabolite concentrations and relaxation times from proton spectra of human brain. *In: Proceedings: Twelfth Annual Scientific Meeting of the Society of Magnetic Resonance in Medicine, Vol. 2. New York, USA: SMRM*; 1993: 977.

52) Kreis, R.; Ernst, T.; Ross, B. D. Absolute quantitation of water and metabolites in the human brain. II. Metabolite concentrations. *Journal of Magnetic Resonance* 102: 9–19; 1993.

53) Michaelis, T.; Merboldt, K-D.; Bruhn, H. et al. Absolute concentrations of metabolites in the adult human brain in vivo: Quantification of localized proton MR spectra. *Radiology* 187: 219–227; 1993.

54) Moats, R. A.; Ernst, T.; Shonk, T. K. et al. Abnormal cerebral metabolite concentrations in patients with probable Alzheimer disease. *Magn. Reson. Med.* 32: 110–115; 1994.

55) Toft, P. B.; Leth, H.; Lou, H. C. et al. Metabolite concentrations in the developing brain estimated with proton MR spectroscopy. *JMRI* 4: 674–680; 1994.

56) Dezortová, M.; Hájek, M.; Hejcmanová, L. The changes of *N*-acetylaspartate and creatine/phosphocreatine concentrations in patients with phenylketonuria. *In: Proceedings: Third Scientific Meeting and Exhibition of the Society of Magnetic Resonance, Vol. 3. Nice, France: SMR*; 1995: 1833.

57) Pouwels, P. J. W.; Hänicke, W.; Frahm, J. On a concentration gradient of cerebral metabolites in human gray matter as determined by quantitative localized proton MRS. *In: Proceedings: Third Scientific Meeting and Exhibition of the Society of Magnetic Resonance, Vol. 3. Nice, France: SMR*; 1995: 1957.

58) Saunders, D. E.; Howe, F. A.; van den Boogaart, A. et al. Ageing of the human adult brain: *In vivo* quantitation of metabolite content with proton magnetic resonance spectroscopy. *In: Proceedings: Third Scientific Meeting and Exhibition of the Society of Magnetic Resonance, Vol. 3. Nice, France: SMR*; 1995: 1804.

59) Hajek M. Quantitative NMR spectroscopy. Comments on methodology of *in vivo* MR spectroscopy in medicine. *Quart. Magn. Res. in Biol. Med.* 2: 165–193; 1995.

60) Henriksen, O. *In vivo* quantitation of metabolite concentrations in the brain by means of proton MRS. *NMR Biomed.* 8: 139–148; 1995.

61) Pouwels, P. J. W.; Frahm, J. Regional metabolite concentrations in human brain as determined by quantitative localized proton MRS. *Magn. Reson. Med.* 39: 53–60; 1998.

62) Wang, Y.; Li, S-J. Differentiation of metabolic concentrations between gray matter and white matter of human brain by *in vivo* ^{1}H magnetic resonance spectroscopy. *Magn. Reson. Med.* 39: 28–33; 1998.

63) Tallan, H. H.; Moore, S.; Stein, W. H. *N*-acetyl-$_{\text{L}}$-aspartic acid in brain. *J. Biol. Chem.* 219: 257–264; 1956.

64) D'Adamo, Jr., A. F.; Yatsu, F. M. Acetate metabolism in the nervous system. *N*-acetyl-$_{\text{L}}$-aspartic acid and the biosynthesis of brain lipids. *J. Neurochem.* 13: 961–965; 1966.

65) Birken, D. L.; Oldendorf, W. H. *N*-acetyl-$_{\text{L}}$-aspartic acid: A literature review of a compound prominent in ^{1}H-NMR spectroscopic studies of brain. *Neurosci. Biobehav. Rev.* 13: 23–31; 1989.

66) Petroff, O. A. C.; Spencer, D. D.; Alger, J. R. et al. High-field proton magnetic resonance spectroscopy of human cerebrum obtained during surgery for epilepsy. *Neurology* 39: 1197–1202; 1989.

67) Miyake, M.; Kakimoto, Y.; Sorimachi, M. A gas

chromatographic method for the determination of *N*-acetyl-L-aspartic acid, *N*-acetyl-α-aspartylglutamic acid and β-citryl-L-glutamic acid and their distributions in the brain and other organs of various species of animals. *J. Neurochem.* 36: 804-810; 1981.

68) Tallan, H. H. Studies on the distribution of *N*-acetyl-L-aspartic acid in brain. *J. Biol. Chem.* 224: 41-45; 1957.

69) McIntosh, J. C.; Cooper, J. R. Studies on the function of *N*-acetyl aspartic acid in brain. *J. Neurochem.* 12: 825-835; 1965.

70) Jacobson, K. B. Studies on the role of *N*-acetylaspartic acid in mammalian brain. *J. Gen. Physiol.* 43: 323-333; 1959.

71) Goldstein, F. B. Biosynthesis of *N*-acetyl-L-aspartic acid. *J. Biol. Chem.* 234: 2702-2706; 1959.

72) Truckenmiller, M. E.; Namboodiri, M. A. A.; Brownstein, M. J. et al. *N*-acetylation of L-aspartate in the nervous system: differential distribution of a specific enzyme. *J. Neurochem.* 45: 1658-1662; 1985.

73) Slusher, B. S.; Robinson, M. B.; Tsai, G. et al. Rat brain *N*-acetylated α-linked acidic dipeptidase activity: Purification and immunologic characterization. *J. Biol. Chem.* 265: 21297-21301; 1990.

74) Patel, T. B.; Clark, J. B. Synthesis of *N*-acetyl-L-aspartate by rat brain mitochondria and its involvement in mitochondrial/cytosolic carbon transport. *Biochem. J.* 184: 539-546; 1979.

75) Goldstein, F. B. Amidohydrolases of brain; enzymatic hydrolysis of *N*-acetyl-L-aspartate and other *N*-acyl-L-amino acids. *J. Neurochem.* 26: 45-49; 1976.

76) D'Adamo, Jr., A. F.; Gidez, L. I.; Yatsu, F. M. Acetyl transport mechanisms. Involvement of N-acetyl aspartic acid in *de novo* fatty acid biosynthesis in the developing rat brain. *Exp. Brain Res.* 5: 267-273; 1968.

77) D'Adamo, Jr., A. F.; Smith, J. C.; Woiler, C. The occurrence of *N*-acetylaspartate amidohydrolase (Aminoacylase II) in the developing rat. *J. Neurochem.* 20: 1275-1278; 1973.

78) Cangro, C. B.; Namboodiri, M. A. A.; Sklar, L. A. et al. Immunohistochemistry and biosynthesis of *N*-acetylaspartylglutamate in spinal sensory ganglia. *J. Neurochem.* 49: 1579-1588; 1987.

79) Clarke, D. D.; Greenfield, S.; Dicker, E. et al. A relationship of *N*-acetylaspartate biosynthesis to neuronal protein synthesis. *J. Neurochem.* 24: 479-485; 1975.

80) Lee, J. H.; Arcinue, E.; Ross, B. D. Brief report: organic osmolytes in the brain of an infant with hypernatremia. *N. Engl. J. Med.* 331: 439-442; 1994.

81) Koller, K. J.; Zaczek, R.; Coyle, J. T. *N*-acetyl-aspartyl-glutamate: regional levels in rat brain and the effects of brain lesions as determined by a new HPLC method. *J. Neurochem.* 43: 1136-1142; 1984.

82) Rango, M.; Spagnoli, D.; Tomei, G. et al. Central nervous system trans-synaptic effects of acute axonal injury: a ^{1}H magnetic resonance spectroscopy study. *Magn. Reson. Med.* 33: 595-600; 1995.

83) De Stefano, N.; Matthews, P. M.; Arnold, D. L. Reversible decreases in *N*-acetylaspartate after acute brain injury. *Magn. Reson. Med.* 34: 721-727; 1995.

84) Burri, R.; Bigler, P.; Straehl, P. et al. Brain development: ^{1}H magnetic resonance spectroscopy of rat brain extracts compared with chromatographic methods. *Neurochem. Res.* 15: 1009-1016; 1990.

85) Koopmans, R. A.; Li, D. K. B.; Zhu, G. et al. Magnetic resonance spectroscopy of multiple sclerosis : in-vivo detection of myelin breakdown products. *Lancet* 341: 631-632; 1993.

86) Matalon, R.; Michals, K.; Sebesta, D. et al. Aspartoacylase deficiency and *N*-acetylaspartic aciduria in patients with canavan disease. *Am. J. Med. Genet.* 29: 463-471; 1988.

87) Tsai, G.; Coyle, J. T. *N*-acetylaspartate in neuropsychiatric disorders. *Prog. Neurobiol.* 46: 531-540; 1995.

88) Barker, P. B.; Breiter, S. N.; Soher, B. J. et al. Quantitative proton spectroscopy of canine brain: *in vivo* and *in vitro* correlations. *Magn. Reson. Med.* 32: 157-163; 1994.

89) Miller, B. L. A review of chemical issues in ^{1}H NMR spectroscopy: *N*-acetyl-L-aspartate, creatine and choline. *NMR Biomed.* 4: 47-52; 1991.

90) Tunggal, B.; Hofmann, K.; Stoffel, W. *In vivo* ^{13}C nuclear magnetic resonance investigations of choline metabolism in rabbit brain. *Magn. Reson. Med.* 13: 90-102; 1990.

91) McIlwain, H.; Bachelard, H. S. Biochemistry and the Central Nervous System. Fifth Edition. Edinburgh: Churchill Livingstone, 1985: pp. 296-297.

92) Gyngell, M. L.; Hoehn-Berlage, M.; Kloiber, O. et al. Localized proton NMR spectroscopy of experimental gliomas in rat brain *in vivo*. *NMR Biomed.* 5: 335-340; 1992.

93) Bruhn, H.; Michaelis, T.; Merboldt, K. D. et al. On the interpretation of proton NMR spectra from brain tumours *in vivo* and *in vitro*. *NMR Biomed.* 5: 253-258; 1992.

94) Stoll, A. L.; Renshaw, P. F.; De Micheli, E. et al. Choline ingestion increases the resonance of choline-containing compounds in human brain: An in vivo proton magnetic resonance study. *Biol. Psychiatry* 37: 170-174; 1995.

95) Hanstock, C. C.; Boisvert, D. P. J.; Bendall, M. R. et al. In vivo assessment of focal brain lactate alterations with NMR proton spectroscopy. *J. Cereb. Blood Flow*

Metab. 8: 208-214; 1988.

96) Hurd, R. E.; Freeman, D. Proton editing and imaging of lactate. *NMR Biomed*. 4: 73-80; 1991.

97) Duyn, J. H.; Frank, J. A.; Moonen, C. T. W. Incorporation of lactate measurement in multi-spin-echo proton spectroscopic imaging. *Magn. Reson. Med*. 33: 101-107; 1995.

98) Kotitschke, K.; Schnackerz, K. D.; Dringen, R. et al. Investigation of the ^{1}H NMR visibility of lactate in different rat and human brain cells. *NMR Biomed*. 7: 349-355; 1994.

99) Prichard, J. W. What the clinician can learn from MRS lactate measurements. *NMR Biomed*. 4: 99-102; 1991.

100) Petroff, O. A. C.; Novotny, E. J.; Avison, M. et al. Cerebral lactate turnover after electroshock: In vivo measurements by ^{1}H/^{13}C magnetic resonance spectroscopy. *J. Cereb. Blood Flow Metab*. 12: 1022-1029; 1992.

101) Paschen, W.; Djuricic, B.; Mies, G. et al. Lactate and pH in the brain: association and dissociation in different pathophysiological states. *J. Neurochem*. 48: 154-159; 1987.

102) Miyake, M.; Morino, H.; Mizobuchi, M. et al. *N*-acetyl-$_{L}$-aspartic acid, *N*-acetyl-α-$_{L}$-aspartyl-$_{L}$-glutamic acid and β-citryl-$_{L}$-glutamic acid in human urine. *Clinica. Chimica. Acta* 120: 119-126; 1982.

103) Meyerhoff, J. L.; Robinson, M. B.; Bixler, M. A. et al. Seizures decrease regional enzymatic hydrolysis of *N*-acetyl-aspartylglutamate in rat brain. *Brain Res*. 505: 130-134; 1989.

104) Cassidy, M.; Neale, J. H. *N*-acetylaspartylglutamate catabolism is achieved by an enzyme on the cell surface of neurons and glia. *Neuropeptides* 24: 271-278; 1993.

105) Ffrench-Mullen, J. M. H.; Koller, K.; Zaczek, R. et al: *N*-acetylaspartylglutamate: Possible role as the neurotransmitter of the lateral olfactory tract. *Proc. Natl. Acad. Sci. USA* 82: 3897-3900; 1985.

106) Bernstein, J.; Fisher, R. S.; Zaczek, R. et al. Dipeptides of glutamate and aspartate may be endogenous neuroexcitants in the rat hippocampal slice. *J. Neurosci*. 5: 1429-1433; 1985.

107) Williamson, L. C.; Eagles, D. A.; Brady, M. J. et al. Localization and synaptic release of *N*-acetylaspartylglutamate in the chick retina and optic tectum. *Eur. J. Neurosci*. 3: 441-451; 1991.

108) Williamson, L. C.; Neale, J. H. Calcium-dependent release of *N*-acetylaspartylglutamate from retinal neurons upon depolarization. *Brain Res*. 475: 151-155; 1988.

109) Cassidy, M.; Neale, J. H. Localization and transport of *N*-acetylaspartylglutamate in cells of whole murine brain in primary culture. *J. Neurochem*. 60: 1631-1638; 1993.

110) Zaczek, R.; Koller, K.; Cotter, R. et al. *N*-acetylaspartylglutamate : An endogenous peptide with high affinity for a brain "glutamate" receptor. *Proc. Natl. Acad. Sci. USA* 80: 1116-1119; 1983.

111) Brancati, A.; D'Arcangelo, P. Effects evoked by pentamethylenetetrazol-induced seizures upon *N*-acetylaspartate and *N*-acetylaspartylglutamate levels in different regions of the rat neuraxis. *Life Sciences* 48: 2229-2232; 1991.

112) Ross, B. D. Biochemical considerations in ^{1}H spectroscopy. Glutamate and glutamine; *myo*-inositol and related metabolites. *NMR Biomed*. 4: 59-63; 1991.

113) Brand A.; Richter-Landsberg, C.; Leibfritz, D. Multinuclear NMR studies on the energy metabolism of glial and neuronal cells. *Dev. Neurosci*. 15: 289-298; 1993.

114) Lien, Y-H. H.; Shapiro, J. I.; Chan, L. Effects of hypernatremia on organic brain osmoles. *J. Clin. Invest*. 85: 1427-1435; 1990.

115) Ibsen, L.; Strange, K. In situ localization and osmotic regulation of the Na^{+}-*myo*-inositol cotransporter in rat brain. *Am. J. Physiol*. 271: 877-885; 1996.

116) Silverstone, P. H.; Hanstock, C. C.; Fabian, J. et al. Chronic lithium does not alter human *myo*-inositol or phosphomonoester concentrations as measured by ^{1}H and ^{31}P MRS. *Biol. Psychiatry* 40: 235-246; 1996.

117) Michaelis, T.; Helms, G.; Merboldt, K-D. et al. Identification of *scyllo*-inositol in proton NMR spectra of human brain *in vivo*. *NMR Biomed*. 6: 105-109; 1993.

118) Kreis, R.; Farrow, N.; Ross, B. D. Localized ^{1}H NMR spectroscopy in patients with chronic hepatic encephalopathy. Analysis of changes in cerebral glutamine, choline and inositols. *NMR Biomed*. 4: 109-116; 1991.

119) Michaelis, T.; Merboldt, K-D.; Hänicke, W. et al. On the identification of cerebral metabolites in localized ^{1}H NMR spectra of human brain *in vivo*. *NMR Biomed*. 4: 90-98; 1991.

120) Prost, R. W.; Mark, L.; Mewissen, M. et al. Detection of glutamate/glutamine resonances by ^{1}H magnetic resonance spectroscopy at 0.5 tesla. *Magn. Reson. Med*. 37: 615-618; 1997.

121) Bovée, W. M. M. J. Quantification of glutamate, glutamine, and other metabolites in *in vivo* proton NMR spectroscopy. *NMR Biomed*. 4: 81-84; 1991.

122) Chamuleau, R. A. F. M. ; Bosman, D. K. ; Bovée, W. M. M. J. et al. What the clinician can learn from MR glutamine/glutamate assays. *NMR Biomed*. 4: 103-108 ; 1991.

123) Hetherington, H. P.; Newcomer, B. R.; Pan, J. W. Measurements of human cerebral GABA at 4.1 T using numerically optimized editing pulses. *Magn.*

Reson. Med. 39: 6-10; 1998.

124) Rothman, D. L.; Petroff, O. A. C.; Behar, K. L. et al. Localized ^{1}H NMR measurements of γ-aminobutyric acid in human brain *in vivo*. *Proc. Natl. Acad. Sci. USA* 90: 5662-5666; 1993.

125) McGeer, P. L.; McGeer, E. G. Chapter 15. Amino acid neurotransmitters. In: G. J. Siegel, B. W. Agranoff, R. W. Albers, P. B. Molinoff (Eds). Basic Neurochemistry : Molecular, Cellular, and Medical Aspects, Fourth Edition. New York: Raven Press, 1989: pp. 311-332.

126) Casey, D. E.; Gerlach, J.; Magelund, G. et al. γ-Acetylenic GABA in tardive dyskinesia. *Arch. Gen. Pschiatry* 37: 1376-1379; 1980.

127) Perry, T. L.; Kish, S. J.; Buchanan, J. et al. γ-aminobutyric-acid deficiency in brain of schizophrenic patients. *Lancet* 3: 237-239; 1979.

128) Behar, K. L.; Boehm, D. Measurement of GABA following GABA-transaminase inhibition by gabaculine: A ^{1}H and ^{31}P NMR spectroscopic study of rat brain *in vivo*. *Magn. Reson. Med*. 31: 660-667; 1994.

129) Petroff, O. A. C.; Rothman, D. L.; Behar, K. L. et al. Initial observations on effect of vigabatrin on in vivo ^{1}H spectroscopic measurements of γ-aminobutyric acid, glutamate, and glutamine in human brain. *Epilepsia* 36: 457-464; 1995.

Chapter 4 MRS of Healthy Individuals

Toshiro Fujimoto

MRS is usually evaluated with regard to the ratio of various peaks. Ideally, the absolute concentration of the target metabolite is desired. However, such quantitative evaluation requires the use of an internal or external standard and determination of the T_1 and T_2 values of each metabolite takes considerable time for the procedure and burdens the subjects. In this volume, therefore, only the ratios among the peaks in the spectrum are evaluated, but sufficiently useful information has been obtained by comparisons of these ratios between patients and healthy controls. In this chapter, relative values of the ^{31}P spectrum obtained by chemical shift imaging (CSI) and the ^{1}H spectrum obtained by the single voxel method in healthy individuals are presented.

4.1 ^{31}P MRS by CSI

4.1.1 Examples of the ^{31}P spectrum of a healthy individual.

^{31}P spectra of voxels 1–10

^{31}P spectra by CSI in a healthy subject (a 54-year-old male) are presented. In Figure 4-1-1, CSI spectra are superimposed on a T_1-weighted image (500/15). In this volume, spectra are obtained primarily in the coronal section because signals with high S/N ratio can be obtained by placing the voxels ($3\times3\times4$ cm^3) in the middle of the brain. Transverse sections of the CSI are used only when they are necessary, because the thickness of the anterior part of the frontal lobe is small, and considerable time is needed for positioning of voxels with 4 cm thick. In Figure 4-1-2, voxels with 4 cm thick are superimposed on a sagittal section of the T_1-weighted image (500/15) to indicate the position of the voxels in the brain. Voxels 1 and 2 correspond to the medial frontal lobe including the parietal lobe, voxels 3 and 6 correspond to the upper temporal lobes including portions of the frontal lobe, voxels 4 and 5 correspond to a region including the basal ganglia, voxels 7 and 10 correspond to the lateral portions of the temporal lobes, and voxels 8 and 9 correspond to a region including mesial portions of the temporal lobes and the brainstem. Spectra of voxels 1–10 indicated in Figure 4-1-1 are shown in Figures 4-1-3 to 4-1-12.

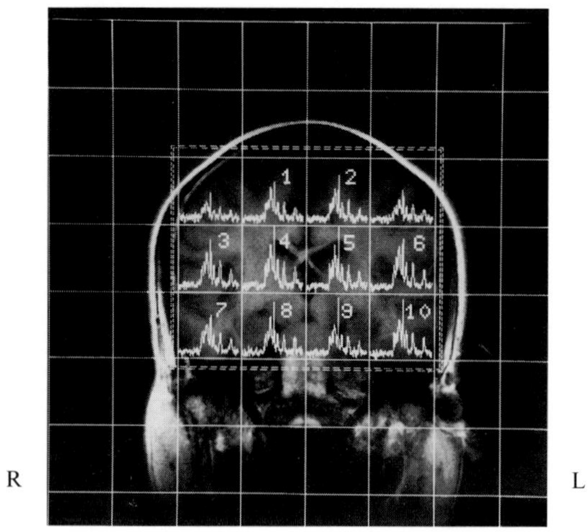

Fig. 4-1-1 ^{31}P CSI with voxels 1 to 10 superimposed on T_1-weighted image (500/15). A voxel size is $3\times3\times4$ cm^3.

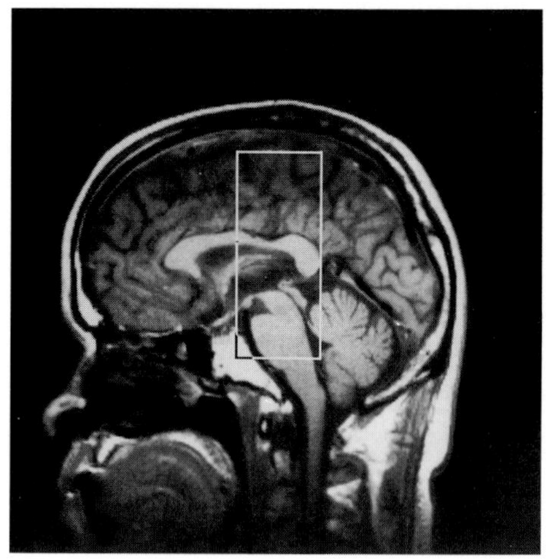

Fig. 4-1-2 Voxels with 4 cm thick are superimposed on a sagittal section of the T_1-weighted image (500/15) to indicate the position of the voxels in the brain.

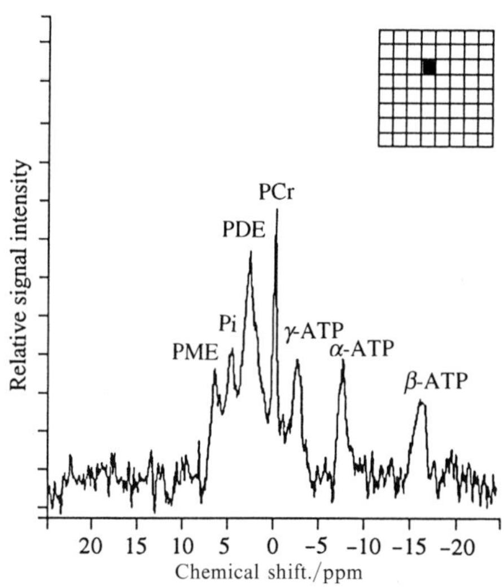

Fig. 4-1-3 ^{31}P spectrum of voxel 1.

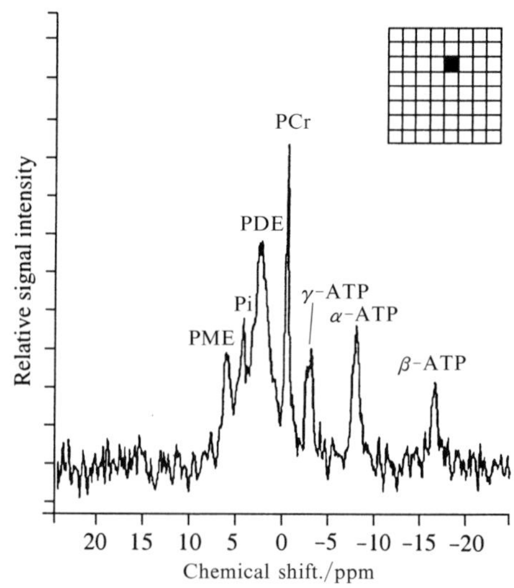

Fig. 4-1-4 ^{31}P spectrum of voxel 2.

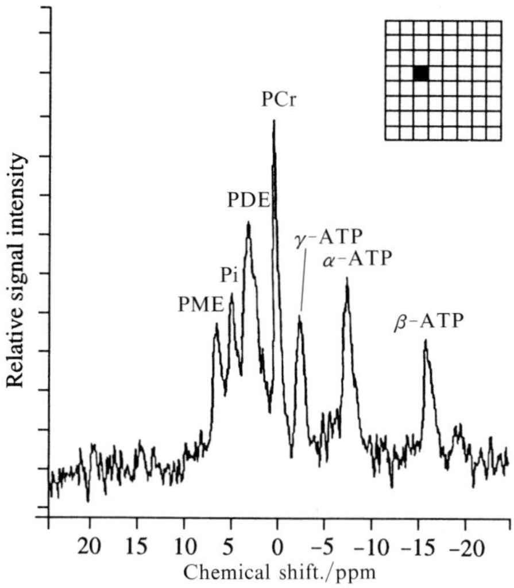

Fig. 4-1-5 ^{31}P spectrum of voxel 3.

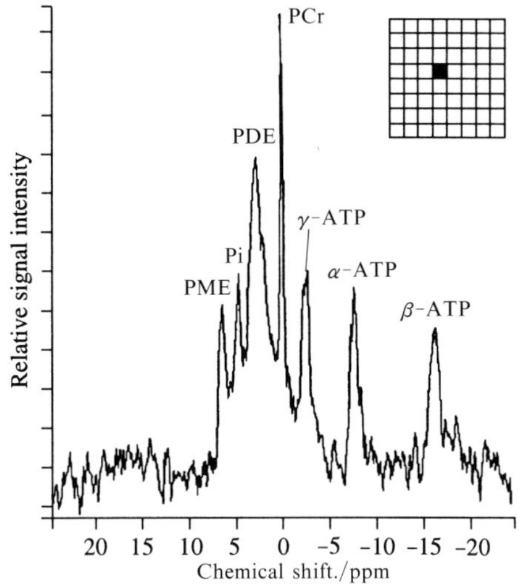

Fig. 4-1-6 ^{31}P spectrum of voxel 4.

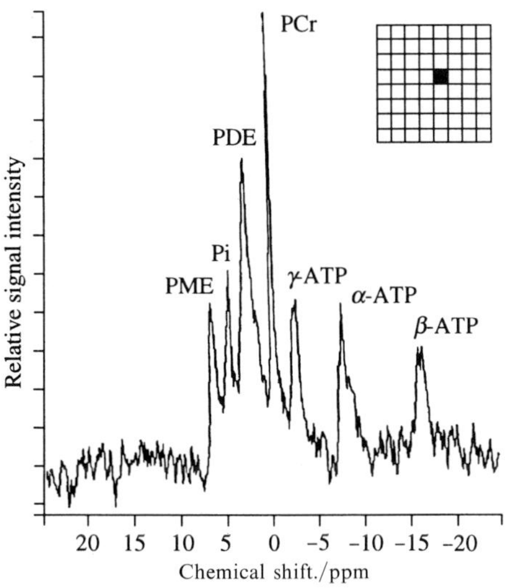

Fig. 4-1-7 ^{31}P spectrum of voxel 5.

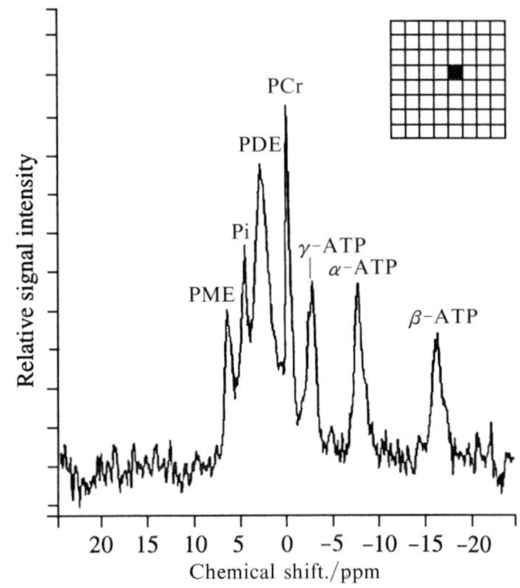

Fig. 4-1-8 ^{31}P spectrum of voxel 6.

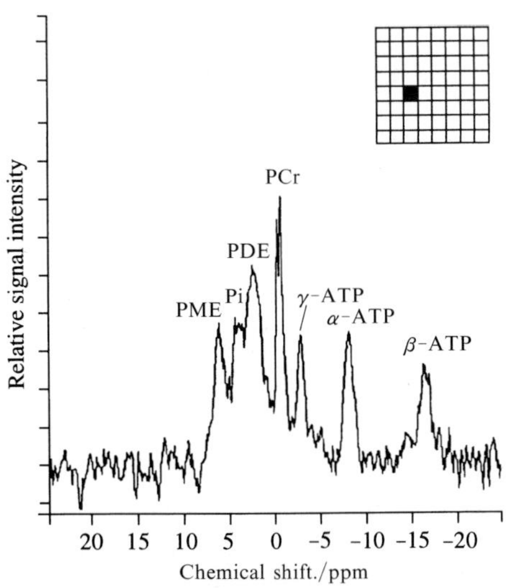

Fig. 4-1-9 ^{31}P spectrum of voxel 7.

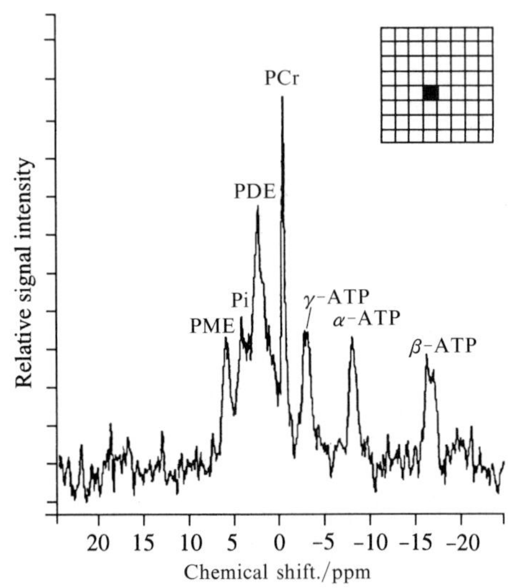

Fig. 4-1-10 ^{31}P spectrum of voxel 8.

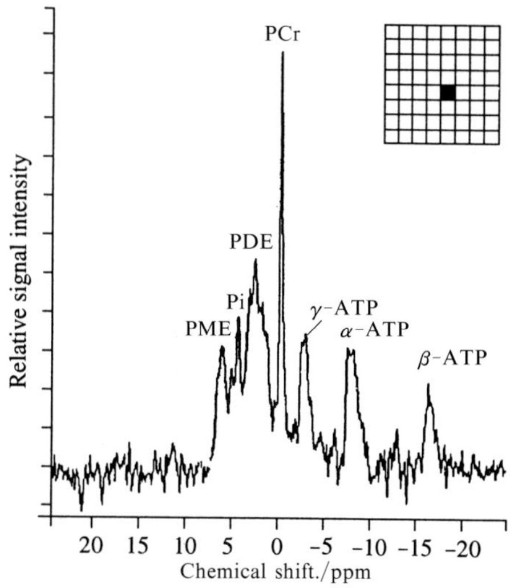

Fig. 4-1-11 ${}^{31}P$ spectrum of voxel 9.

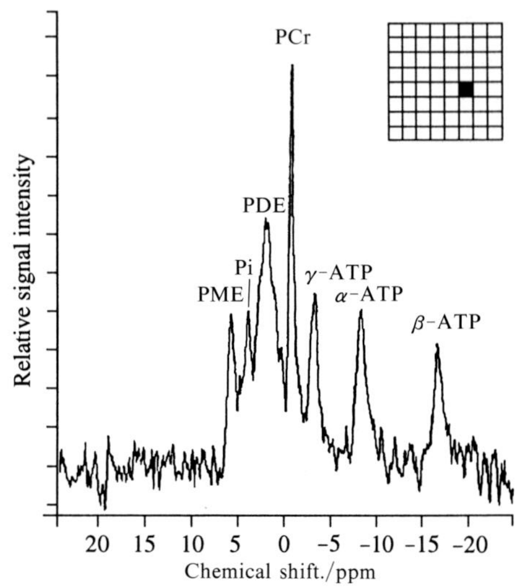

Fig. 4-1-12 ${}^{31}P$ spectrum of voxel 10.

4.1.2 Examples of the ³¹P spectrum in a healthy individual. ³¹P spectra of voxels 11-13 (54 year-old male).

Figure 4-1-13 shows voxels placed in the mesial portions of the temporal lobes by the voxel shift method on the basis of Figure 4-1-1. Figures 4-1-14 and 4-1-16 show ^{31}P spectra of voxels 11 and 13, and Figure 4-1-15 shows a ^{31}P spectrum of voxel 12 covering the brainstem.

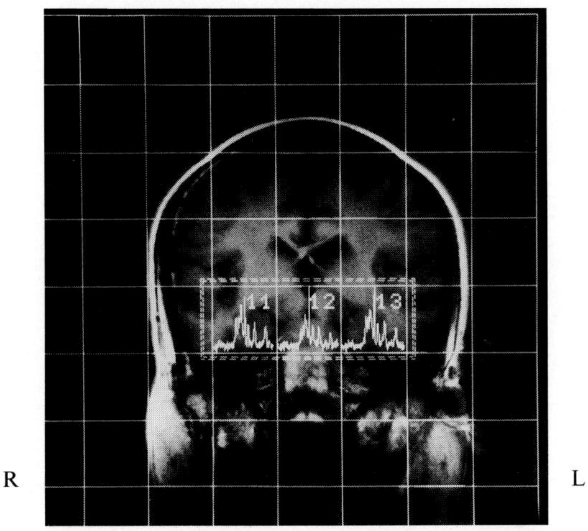

Fig. 4-1-13 ^{31}P CSI with voxels 11 to 13 superimposed on T_1-weighted image. The voxels with size of 3×3×4cm³ are placed in the mesial temporal and brain stem regions.

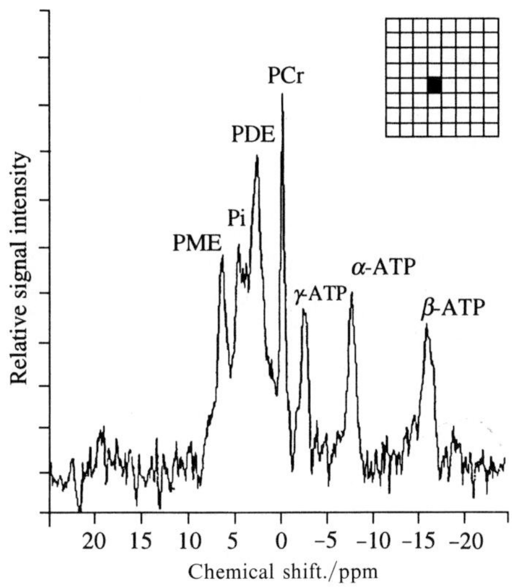

Fig. 4-1-14 ^{31}P spectrum of voxel 11.

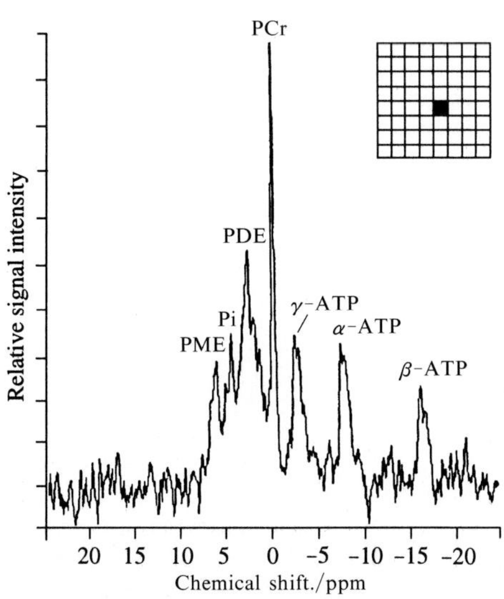

Fig. 4-1-15 ^{31}P spectrum of voxel 12.

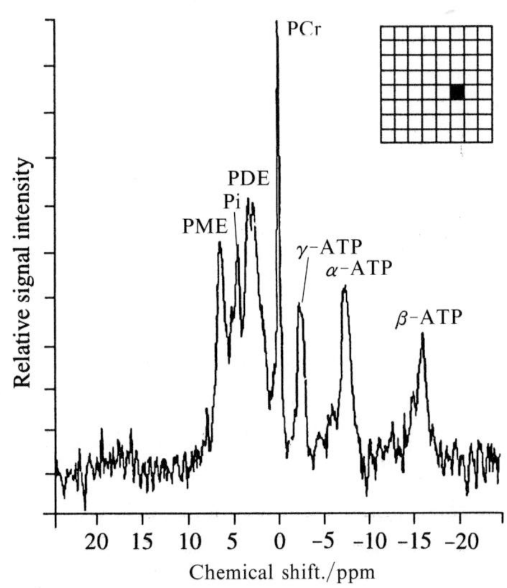

Fig. 4-1-16 ^{31}P spectrum of voxel 13.

4.1.3 Examples of the ^{31}P spectrum in a healthy individual. ^{31}P spectra of voxels 14 and 15 (54 year-old male).

Figures 4-1-17 and 18 show voxels placed in an area that contains the basal ganglia to a maximum degree by the voxel shift method on the basis of Figure 4-1-1, but the voxels also include portions of the lateral ventricles. Figures 4-1-19 and 4-1-20 show ^{31}P spectra of voxels 14 and 15.

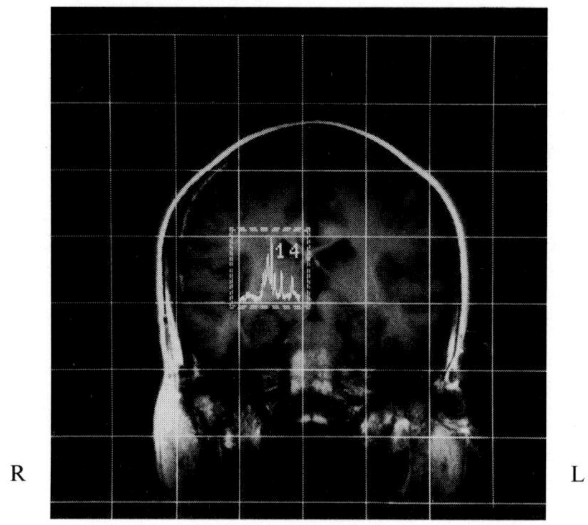

Fig. 4-1-17 ^{31}P CSI with voxel 14 superimposed on T_1-weighted image. The voxel with size of 3×3×4 cm^3 is placed in the right basal ganglia region.

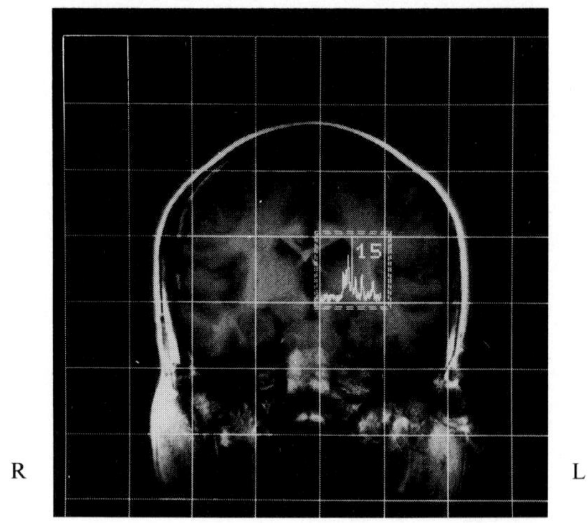

Fig. 4-1-18 ^{31}P CSI with voxel 15 superimposed on T_1-weighted image. The voxel with size of 3×3×4 cm^3 is placed in the left basal ganglia region.

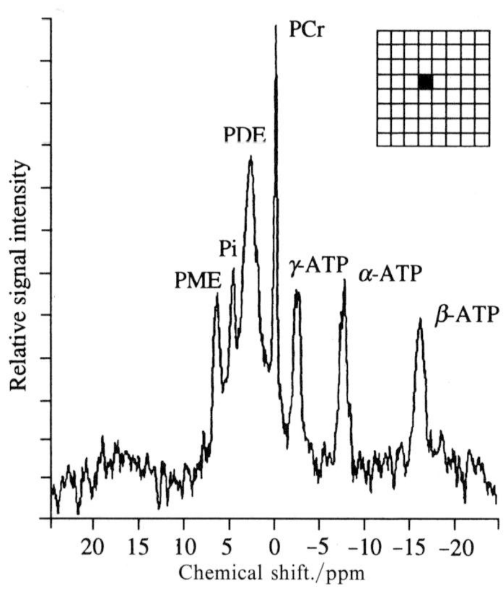

Fig. 4-1-19 ^{31}P spectrum of voxel 14.

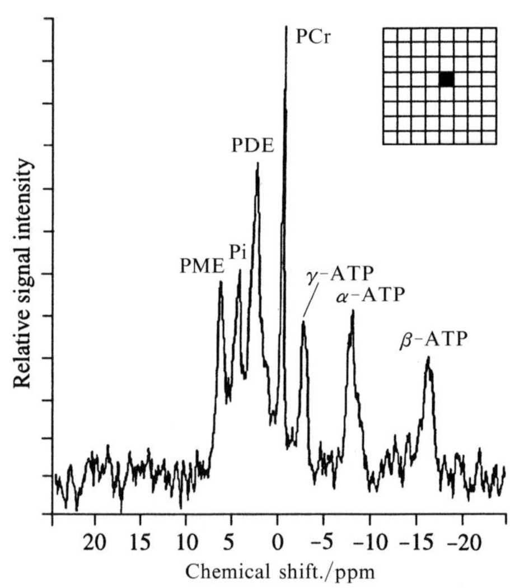

Fig. 4-1-20 ^{31}P spectrum of voxel 15.

4.1.4 Examples of the ^{31}P spectrum in a healthy individual. ^{31}P spectra obtained by averaging over voxels (54 year-old male).

Figures 4-1-21 to 4-1-26 show spectra obtained by averaging over voxels on the basis of Figure 4-1-1. Spectra with high S/N can be obtained by averaging over voxels.

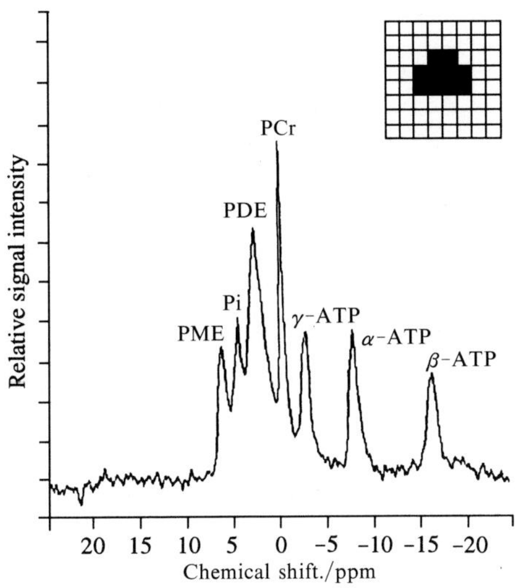

Fig. 4-1-21 ^{31}P spectrum averaging over 10 voxels (from 1 to 10).

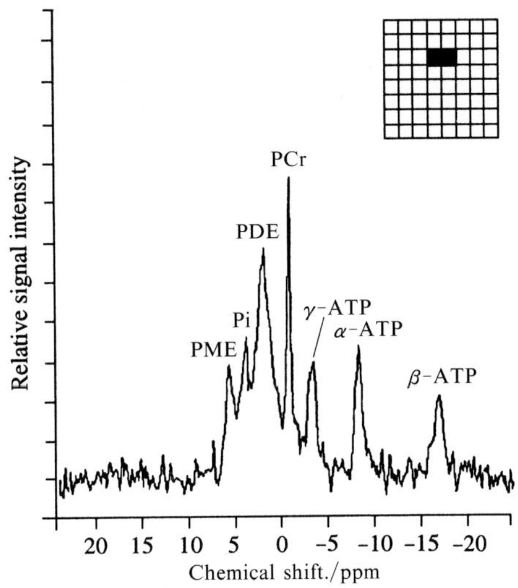

Fig. 4-1-22 ^{31}P spectrum averaging over 2 voxels (1 and 2).

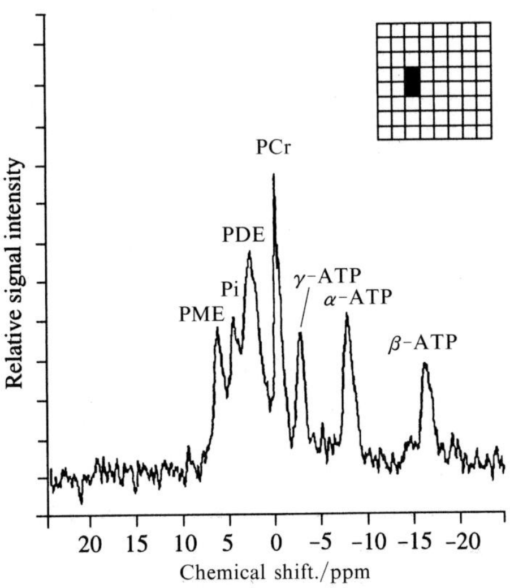

Fig. 4-1-23 ^{31}P spectrum averaging over 2 voxels (3 and 7).

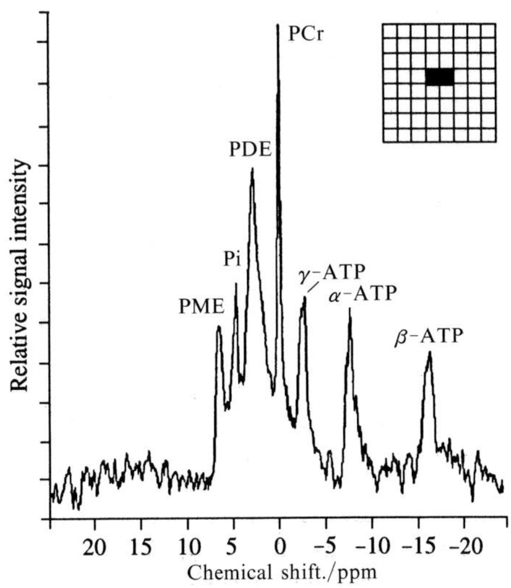

Fig. 4-1-24 ^{31}P spectrum averaging over 2 voxels (4 and 5).

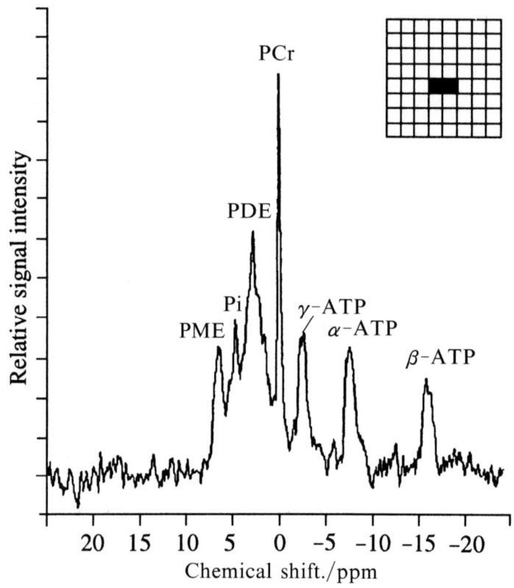

Fig. 4-1-25 ^{31}P spectrum averaging over 2 voxels (8 and 9).

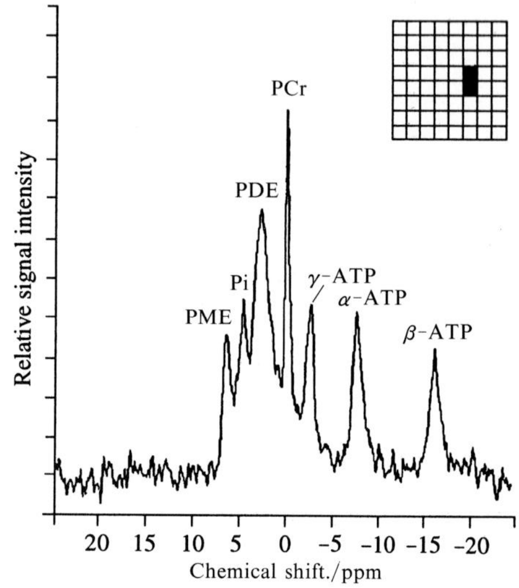

Fig. 4-1-26 ^{31}P spectrum averaging over 2 voxels (6 and 10).

4.1.5 Mean ratios of peaks of the ^{31}P spectrum of healthy individuals

Table 4-1-1 shows the mean percentages of each of the seven peaks of phosphomonoesters (PME), inorganic orthophosphate (Pi), phosphodiesters (PDE), phosphocreatine (PCr), γ-ATP, α-ATP, and β-ATP of the ^{31}P spectrum relative to the total area of the seven peaks in 67 healthy controls (from 20s to 70s). Voxels 1 to 15 correspond to those defined in 4.1.1 to 4.1.3 in a healthy individual. The values of PME/PDE, PCr/Pi, and pHi are also indicated. The pHi was calculated by the Petroff equation.

Table 4-1-1 Percentage of individual peak areas to total observable peak areas of ^{31}P MR spectra from voxel 1 to voxel 15 in control subjects from 20s to 70s.

%PME

		1	2	3	4	5	6	7	8	9	10	11	12	13	14	15
20s (n=5)	MEAN(%)	10.7	11.0	10.3	9.3	9.8	9.7	10.7	10.1	11.1	10.7	9.6	11.2	11.0	9.0	11.0
	SD(%)	(5.4)	(2.9)	(2.3)	(2.7)	(2.8)	(2.0)	(2.4)	(0.6)	(1.1)	(2.2)	(2.4)	(3.7)	(2.8)	(1.3)	(2.9)
30s (n=20)	MEAN(%)	10.6	9.9	10.4	9.8	10.1	9.7	10.2	10.3	10.2	9.7	11.2	10.1	10.1	10.6	10.0
	SD(%)	(2.3)	(1.6)	(1.8)	(1.6)	(2.5)	(2.1)	(2.0)	(2.8)	(2.9)	(2.7)	(2.0)	(2.9)	(2.3)	(2.2)	(2.6)
40s (n=3)	MEAN(%)	9.8	9.0	9.6	10.3	8.6	7.6	9.4	9.9	10.5	9.3	9.9	9.4	9.7	10.5	9.1
	SD(%)	(2.0)	(1.8)	(0.7)	(0.2)	(0.3)	(1.7)	(1.3)	(0.3)	(1.3)	(1.7)	(1.1)	(2.1)	(2.7)	(0.7)	(0.4)
50s (n=16)	MEAN(%)	9.1	10.6	10.8	10.6	10.3	8.9	10.0	10.1	10.7	8.7	10.9	11.3	10.2	11.2	11.4
	SD(%)	(2.7)	(2.7)	(1.6)	(2.6)	(2.8)	(1.1)	(2.1)	(2.2)	(2.7)	(2.2)	(1.8)	(3.7)	(2.2)	(2.5)	(2.3)
60s (n=13)	MEAN(%)	9.2	8.7	9.1	9.3	11.3	8.1	9.8	9.5	9.9	8.4	10.1	9.8	10.1	11.1	11.7
	SD(%)	(2.4)	(2.0)	(2.0)	(2.9)	(3.8)	(1.8)	(2.0)	(2.1)	(2.1)	(2.3)	(2.2)	(2.7)	(1.8)	(4.1)	(3.3)
70s (n=10)	MEAN(%)	12.4	11.4	12.4	9.6	9.0	9.4	11.0	9.9	10.5	10.3	10.9	12.7	12.0	11.5	10.7
	SD(%)	(2.5)	(2.8)	(3.9)	(3.5)	(2.0)	(1.7)	(3.6)	(2.3)	(2.5)	(2.9)	(2.6)	(1.8)	(5.5)	(4.7)	(2.4)

%Pi

		1	2	3	4	5	6	7	8	9	10	11	12	13	14	15
20s (n=5)	MEAN(%)	5.5	6.2	6.2	6.5	4.7	5.0	5.0	5.3	5.6	4.0	4.9	4.3	3.8	6.3	4.3
	SD(%)	(2.7)	(1.7)	(1.0)	(3.5)	(2.0)	(2.4)	(1.5)	(0.8)	(2.4)	(2.0)	(2.2)	(2.1)	(1.7)	(2.6)	(1.4)
30s (n=20)	MEAN(%)	6.1	5.9	6.6	5.2	5.8	5.4	5.8	5.0	5.8	5.3	4.7	4.5	4.9	4.7	5.5
	SD(%)	(1.8)	(1.9)	(1.8)	(1.5)	(2.3)	(1.6)	(1.9)	(1.9)	(1.9)	(2.3)	(1.6)	(2.2)	(1.6)	(1.4)	(1.3)
40s (n=3)	MEAN(%)	5.4	6.0	4.6	4.6	5.3	4.5	6.6	4.6	3.9	4.4	4.9	2.4	5.1	4.3	5.4
	SD(%)	(1.7)	(2.8)	(0.6)	(1.2)	(1.9)	(0.9)	(1.8)	(0.8)	(1.9)	(2.3)	(1.2)	(1.2)	(4.1)	(1.1)	(0.7)
50s (n=16)	MEAN(%)	6.0	5.5	6.5	5.9	6.6	5.2	5.6	4.9	5.6	5.0	4.9	4.6	4.4	5.6	6.5
	SD(%)	(1.8)	(1.7)	(2.2)	(2.6)	(2.5)	(2.8)	(2.1)	(1.1)	(2.4)	(3.0)	(1.8)	(1.3)	(1.5)	(2.9)	(2.2)
60s (n=13)	MEAN(%)	4.9	5.7	5.3	6.4	6.8	5.1	5.6	4.3	5.5	5.1	4.7	4.8	4.9	5.4	6.4
	SD(%)	(2.0)	(3.7)	(1.7)	(2.6)	(3.3)	(2.3)	(2.1)	(2.8)	(2.7)	(2.9)	(1.8)	(2.2)	(1.9)	(2.1)	(2.0)
70s (n=10)	MEAN(%)	5.3	4.4	4.4	4.7	5.9	4.7	4.7	4.6	3.6	4.7	5.1	4.4	4.8	4.8	5.7
	SD(%)	(2.0)	(1.5)	(1.6)	(1.8)	(1.8)	(1.7)	(1.6)	(2.4)	(1.5)	(1.5)	(1.5)	(2.7)	(1.7)	(1.7)	(2.1)

Table 4-1-1 continued.

%PDE

		1	2	3	4	5	6	7	8	9	10	11	12	13	14	15
20s (n=5)	MEAN(%)	39.4	36.0	40.5	39.7	40.6	42.9	39.9	38.9	38.9	38.2	42.0	36.5	41.5	40.3	39.9
	SD(%)	(6.6)	(6.1)	(2.9)	(5.5)	(2.8)	(4.1)	(3.9)	(4.0)	(1.9)	(4.0)	(2.4)	(4.7)	(2.6)	(4.6)	(2.4)
30s (n=20)	MEAN(%)	40.3	39.7	37.2	41.8	39.2	40.6	36.2	39.4	36.2	39.0	39.4	37.2	39.6	40.4	37.8
	SD(%)	(3.5)	(3.1)	(4.6)	(2.6)	(4.2)	(2.7)	(4.4)	(3.5)	(4.2)	(4.3)	(4.2)	(4.4)	(3.4)	(3.4)	(3.5)
40s (n=3)	MEAN(%)	39.7	40.1	39.2	39.6	38.7	41.0	35.5	37.5	34.5	39.7	39.9	36.6	38.8	40.5	36.7
	SD(%)	(3.8)	(5.0)	(3.2)	(3.9)	(5.3)	(3.5)	(1.4)	(3.7)	(1.7)	(3.9)	(1.7)	(1.0)	(2.2)	(0.8)	(4.1)
50s (n=16)	MEAN(%)	41.6	40.7	38.7	35.5	33.3	40.8	35.7	38.6	34.5	39.3	39.0	35.3	39.7	37.5	32.8
	SD(%)	(3.8)	(3.4)	(4.4)	(7.3)	(4.7)	(3.5)	(3.7)	(3.5)	(5.1)	(4.2)	(2.8)	(6.9)	(3.5)	(3.9)	(6.3)
60s (n=13)	MEAN(%)	41.3	41.2	40.6	35.9	33.5	39.1	37.3	36.7	34.0	38.5	40.1	32.6	37.8	36.2	34.1
	SD(%)	(4.8)	(4.8)	(3.7)	(4.4)	(4.7)	(3.9)	(3.6)	(4.4)	(3.7)	(6.1)	(4.3)	(7.1)	(4.1)	(7.0)	(3.9)
70s (n=10)	MEAN(%)	39.5	38.4	40.0	40.9	40.3	41.8	38.8	41.8	41.2	39.3	40.1	39.4	40.8	39.2	40.0
	SD(%)	(6.1)	(4.9)	(3.6)	(5.7)	(4.8)	(1.9)	(3.3)	(3.9)	(3.1)	(3.4)	(3.7)	(4.9)	(3.1)	(7.1)	(6.9)

%PCr

		1	2	3	4	5	6	7	8	9	10	11	12	13	14	15
20s (n=5)	MEAN(%)	9.8	10.2	10.0	10.3	9.8	10.2	11.7	13.4	11.9	11.5	12.1	12.9	10.7	10.6	10.3
	SD(%)	(2.6)	(2.6)	(1.4)	(1.2)	(1.3)	(1.5)	(2.4)	(4.1)	(2.6)	(2.1)	(4.3)	(2.2)	(1.2)	(2.4)	(2.0)
30s (n=20)	MEAN(%)	9.6	9.8	10.8	9.9	10.3	10.1	12.0	11.2	11.5	11.7	10.6	13.8	10.4	10.0	10.4
	SD(%)	(1.3)	(1.2)	(1.5)	(1.3)	(1.6)	(1.3)	(1.8)	(1.4)	(1.5)	(1.5)	(1.0)	(3.2)	(1.2)	(1.4)	(1.8)
40s (n=3)	MEAN(%)	10.7	9.5	9.5	10.3	10.1	12.0	12.3	11.5	12.9	12.8	11.1	12.8	11.5	10.4	11.3
	SD(%)	(0.9)	(1.0)	(1.9)	(1.3)	(0.3)	(1.0)	(1.0)	(1.7)	(1.4)	(1.9)	(0.7)	(1.3)	(1.1)	(1.0)	(0.7)
50s (n=16)	MEAN(%)	9.8	10.3	10.1	11.5	11.4	11.8	12.1	12.5	13.1	12.9	10.5	14.7	11.6	11.3	12.2
	SD(%)	(1.1)	(1.5)	(2.0)	(1.4)	(2.0)	(1.6)	(1.9)	(2.3)	(2.1)	(2.0)	(1.4)	(3.7)	(1.9)	(1.9)	(2.9)
60s (n=13)	MEAN(%)	10.8	11.2	10.6	12.5	12.4	13.0	11.6	14.4	13.4	13.8	11.3	16.1	11.3	13.9	11.2
	SD(%)	(1.5)	(1.3)	(1.7)	(1.9)	(2.5)	(2.5)	(1.1)	(2.1)	(2.1)	(1.4)	(1.3)	(3.9)	(1.0)	(3.4)	(1.3)
70s (n=10)	MEAN(%)	10.1	10.1	11.0	10.3	11.3	11.5	11.9	11.8	12.2	12.0	11.0	11.9	11.3	10.3	11.0
	SD(%)	(1.5)	(1.2)	(1.9)	(1.5)	(1.4)	(1.8)	(1.7)	(1.8)	(1.8)	(1.4)	(1.7)	(2.7)	(1.2)	(2.6)	(1.2)

%γ-ATP

		1	2	3	4	5	6	7	8	9	10	11	12	13	14	15
20s (n=5)	MEAN(%)	9.8	10.8	9.0	10.7	11.0	10.0	10.3	9.6	10.7	10.2	10.0	9.9	9.8	10.3	10.4
	SD(%)	(1.0)	(2.3)	(1.4)	(0.8)	(1.7)	(0.9)	(2.4)	(1.9)	(0.9)	(2.5)	(1.3)	(3.8)	(1.8)	(1.5)	(1.1)
30s (n=20)	MEAN(%)	10.4	10.7	10.5	10.8	11.4	10.7	9.9	10.9	11.6	9.9	10.1	11.6	10.2	10.4	11.2
	SD(%)	(2.4)	(1.7)	(1.5)	(1.2)	(1.9)	(1.4)	(1.8)	(2.2)	(2.3)	(2.3)	(1.3)	(3.2)	(1.5)	(1.6)	(1.8)
40s (n=3)	MEAN(%)	10.4	10.4	10.1	10.9	12.0	10.6	10.1	9.0	11.7	10.2	9.8	10.9	11.6	9.9	12.3
	SD(%)	(1.3)	(2.1)	(0.6)	(0.8)	(0.9)	(2.3)	(0.8)	(0.9)	(1.0)	(1.4)	(0.8)	(1.2)	(1.9)	(0.7)	(0.9)
50s (n=16)	MEAN(%)	10.6	10.0	10.2	11.6	14.4	10.4	10.4	10.9	11.1	10.4	10.0	10.8	10.1	10.3	11.8
	SD(%)	(2.1)	(1.5)	(1.0)	(2.0)	(6.3)	(1.8)	(1.7)	(2.3)	(2.4)	(1.5)	(1.7)	(2.8)	(1.6)	(1.5)	(2.0)
60s (n=13)	MEAN(%)	10.2	10.0	10.8	12.3	11.7	10.6	10.4	11.3	10.2	10.1	10.3	11.9	9.7	10.6	10.6
	SD(%)	(1.3)	(2.1)	(1.4)	(3.2)	(2.4)	(1.8)	(2.2)	(2.7)	(2.4)	(1.8)	(2.2)	(3.9)	(1.6)	(2.6)	(2.8)
70s (n=10)	MEAN(%)	9.1	9.8	9.3	10.6	11.3	10.4	8.6	11.3	11.8	10.6	9.8	11.5	11.1	10.5	11.3
	SD(%)	(1.9)	(1.7)	(1.7)	(1.4)	(2.8)	(2.2)	(2.6)	(2.0)	(2.7)	(3.4)	(2.2)	(3.6)	(3.2)	(1.8)	(1.8)

Table 4-1-1 continued.

%α-ATP

		1	2	3	4	5	6	7	8	9	10	11	12	13	14	15
20s (n=5)	MEAN(%)	14.9	15.9	13.9	14.4	15.1	12.4	14.4	12.8	15.2	13.8	12.2	17.2	14.5	13.0	15.5
	SD(%)	(2.9)	(2.7)	(2.3)	(2.0)	(0.9)	(2.1)	(1.8)	(2.2)	(3.5)	(2.1)	(1.4)	(5.3)	(1.3)	(1.4)	(2.2)
30s (n=20)	MEAN(%)	13.8	14.7	14.2	12.8	13.2	13.4	14.9	13.6	14.0	13.7	14.0	13.4	13.9	13.9	14.2
	SD(%)	(2.7)	(2.3)	(1.7)	(2.4)	(2.5)	(2.1)	(2.1)	(2.4)	(2.6)	(2.7)	(2.1)	(3.0)	(2.4)	(2.1)	(2.5)
40s (n=3)	MEAN(%)	13.4	13.2	17.4	13.2	14.6	13.3	15.7	14.2	15.5	15.6	13.9	13.3	14.5	13.6	14.9
	SD(%)	(1.6)	(1.1)	(4.5)	(2.3)	(2.0)	(2.2)	(2.4)	(4.0)	(2.4)	(1.3)	(2.5)	(1.7)	(1.5)	(2.2)	(1.1)
50s (n=16)	MEAN(%)	12.9	12.9	13.1	13.4	13.8	12.5	15.2	12.7	14.0	13.1	13.8	13.0	13.4	12.9	14.9
	SD(%)	(3.0)	(2.6)	(1.9)	(2.5)	(3.6)	(2.1)	(3.3)	(2.3)	(2.0)	(1.8)	(2.2)	(3.4)	(2.4)	(2.0)	(3.3)
60s (n=13)	MEAN(%)	13.1	13.8	14.4	14.2	12.8	13.8	14.5	12.9	15.8	14.3	13.0	15.7	15.5	13.0	14.1
	SD(%)	(3.6)	(3.0)	(2.0)	(2.9)	(2.5)	(2.3)	(3.5)	(3.7)	(3.0)	(4.4)	(2.3)	(4.4)	(2.4)	(2.9)	(2.9)
70s (n=10)	MEAN(%)	13.4	15.4	13.6	14.5	12.0	13.9	16.1	12.6	12.1	13.6	15.0	11.4	11.9	13.7	12.0
	SD(%)	(3.6)	(1.8)	(1.6)	(3.6)	(2.1)	(2.5)	(2.9)	(4.0)	(2.6)	(3.8)	(2.7)	(3.4)	(2.2)	(3.9)	(3.7)

%β-ATP

		1	2	3	4	5	6	7	8	9	10	11	12	13	14	15
20s (n=5)	MEAN(%)	10.0	9.9	10.1	9.1	9.0	9.6	8.1	10.1	6.6	11.6	9.1	8.1	8.7	10.6	8.6
	SD(%)	(2.8)	(3.6)	(1.1)	(1.6)	(1.8)	(1.6)	(2.6)	(2.7)	(0.7)	(2.9)	(2.5)	(1.5)	(1.4)	(2.3)	(1.7)
30s (n=20)	MEAN(%)	9.3	9.2	10.3	9.7	10.0	10.3	11.1	9.5	10.7	10.8	10.0	9.4	10.9	10.1	10.9
	SD(%)	(2.3)	(1.6)	(1.8)	(1.5)	(2.2)	(1.4)	(2.1)	(2.4)	(2.1)	(2.9)	(1.9)	(1.6)	(2.2)	(2.3)	(1.6)
40s (n=3)	MEAN(%)	10.6	11.9	9.6	11.2	10.8	11.0	10.3	13.4	11.1	8.1	10.5	14.7	8.8	10.9	10.3
	SD(%)	(0.5)	(2.2)	(0.7)	(0.4)	(2.1)	(1.6)	(2.2)	(2.8)	(1.7)	(0.9)	(2.1)	(1.4)	(0.9)	(1.2)	(2.0)
50s (n=16)	MEAN(%)	10.0	10.1	10.6	11.5	10.3	10.4	11.1	10.3	11.1	10.5	10.8	10.3	10.7	11.3	10.4
	SD(%)	(1.9)	(2.5)	(1.7)	(1.6)	(2.0)	(1.4)	(2.5)	(1.6)	(3.2)	(2.0)	(2.1)	(3.3)	(1.7)	(2.4)	(2.1)
60s (n=13)	MEAN(%)	10.5	9.4	9.4	9.6	11.4	10.4	10.9	8.9	11.2	9.8	10.5	9.1	10.8	9.8	12.0
	SD(%)	(1.5)	(2.3)	(1.5)	(2.7)	(2.5)	(2.2)	(2.2)	(2.8)	(2.0)	(2.2)	(2.4)	(3.0)	(1.5)	(2.4)	(2.3)
70s (n=10)	MEAN(%)	10.2	10.6	9.3	9.3	10.3	8.3	8.9	8.1	8.7	9.4	8.2	9.0	8.0	10.0	9.3
	SD(%)	(2.7)	(3.2)	(2.4)	(2.7)	(2.5)	(2.4)	(2.3)	(2.4)	(2.9)	(2.3)	(2.8)	(4.5)	(2.5)	(2.6)	(2.1)

%total-ATP (%γ-ATP+%α-ATP+%β-ATP)

		1	2	3	4	5	6	7	8	9	10	11	12	13	14	15
20s (n=5)	MEAN(%)	34.7	36.6	33.0	34.2	35.1	32.1	32.7	32.5	32.6	35.6	31.4	35.2	33.0	34.3	36.3
	SD(%)	(2.7)	(3.6)	(2.8)	(2.4)	(1.5)	(1.9)	(1.9)	(4.4)	(3.5)	(4.2)	(1.6)	(2.5)	(3.4)	(2.8)	(2.9)
30s (n=20)	MEAN(%)	33.4	34.7	35.0	33.3	34.7	34.4	35.9	34.0	36.3	34.3	34.1	34.4	34.9	33.9	34.5
	SD(%)	(3.5)	(2.8)	(2.6)	(3.1)	(4.0)	(2.1)	(2.7)	(3.9)	(3.3)	(5.1)	(2.3)	(4.1)	(4.1)	(2.4)	(3.6)
40s (n=3)	MEAN(%)	34.4	35.4	37.2	35.3	37.3	34.9	36.1	36.5	38.2	33.9	34.3	38.9	34.9	34.3	37.4
	SD(%)	(2.5)	(2.9)	(4.2)	(1.7)	(3.7)	(1.4)	(1.5)	(4.0)	(1.3)	(2.4)	(3.7)	(2.4)	(1.5)	(1.0)	(2.4)
50s (n=16)	MEAN(%)	33.5	32.9	33.9	36.5	38.5	33.3	36.6	33.9	36.1	34.0	34.6	34.1	34.2	34.4	37.1
	SD(%)	(2.0)	(2.7)	(1.7)	(3.8)	(4.6)	(3.4)	(3.1)	(2.8)	(2.8)	(2.7)	(2.2)	(3.4)	(3.1)	(2.5)	(2.8)
60s (n=13)	MEAN(%)	33.8	33.3	34.5	36.0	35.9	34.7	35.7	35.1	37.2	34.2	33.8	36.7	36.0	33.5	36.7
	SD(%)	(4.5)	(4.1)	(3.2)	(4.7)	(4.0)	(4.1)	(4.0)	(4.5)	(2.4)	(5.9)	(3.8)	(3.9)	(3.2)	(5.7)	(4.4)
70s (n=10)	MEAN(%)	32.6	35.7	32.2	34.5	33.6	32.6	33.6	31.9	32.6	33.7	33.0	31.6	31.1	34.1	32.6
	SD(%)	(4.7)	(4.3)	(2.5)	(4.6)	(2.9)	(3.1)	(4.9)	(4.1)	(2.8)	(3.7)	(2.8)	(4.9)	(3.6)	(3.4)	(4.2)

Table 4-1-1 continued.

PME/PDE ratio

		1	2	3	4	5	6	7	8	9	10	11	12	13	14	15
20s (n=5)	MEAN	0.29	0.32	0.26	0.24	0.25	0.23	0.27	0.26	0.29	0.28	0.23	0.32	0.27	0.27	0.27
	SD	(0.16)	(0.14)	(0.07)	(0.10)	(0.08)	(0.07)	(0.06)	(0.03)	(0.03)	(0.06)	(0.06)	(0.14)	(0.08)	(0.07)	(0.07)
30s (n=20)	MEAN	0.27	0.25	0.28	0.24	0.26	0.24	0.28	0.27	0.29	0.25	0.29	0.28	0.26	0.23	0.28
	SD	(0.07)	(0.05)	(0.07)	(0.05)	(0.08)	(0.06)	(0.07)	(0.08)	(0.09)	(0.07)	(0.08)	(0.09)	(0.06)	(0.07)	(0.08)
40s (n=3)	MEAN	0.25	0.23	0.25	0.26	0.22	0.19	0.27	0.27	0.30	0.23	0.25	0.26	0.25	0.26	0.25
	SD	(0.07)	(0.07)	(0.04)	(0.03)	(0.03)	(0.05)	(0.04)	(0.03)	(0.02)	(0.02)	(0.02)	(0.06)	(0.09)	(0.01)	(0.04)
50s (n=16)	MEAN	0.22	0.27	0.28	0.34	0.32	0.22	0.28	0.27	0.33	0.22	0.28	0.36	0.26	0.30	0.36
	SD	(0.09)	(0.08)	(0.06)	(0.25)	(0.12)	(0.03)	(0.08)	(0.07)	(0.14)	(0.06)	(0.06)	(0.20)	(0.06)	(0.09)	(0.12)
60s (n=13)	MEAN	0.23	0.22	0.23	0.27	0.36	0.21	0.26	0.26	0.30	0.22	0.26	0.33	0.27	0.33	0.35
	SD	(0.07)	(0.07)	(0.06)	(0.10)	(0.17)	(0.06)	(0.06)	(0.07)	(0.08)	(0.07)	(0.06)	(0.15)	(0.07)	(0.18)	(0.13)
70s (n=10)	MEAN	0.33	0.31	0.31	0.25	0.23	0.23	0.29	0.24	0.26	0.27	0.28	0.36	0.31	0.33	0.28
	SD	(0.13)	(0.12)	(0.11)	(0.13)	(0.07)	(0.04)	(0.10)	(0.07)	(0.07)	(0.09)	(0.09)	(0.42)	(0.18)	(0.23)	(0.11)

PCr/Pi ratio

		1	2	3	4	5	6	7	8	9	10	11	12	13	14	15
20s (n=5)	MEAN	2.29	1.74	1.63	2.13	2.47	2.39	2.46	2.48	2.48	3.42	2.76	3.66	3.17	2.36	2.10
	SD	(1.55)	(0.58)	(0.34)	(1.37)	(1.39)	(1.13)	(0.77)	(0.45)	(1.01)	(1.49)	(1.19)	(2.01)	(1.13)	(0.90)	(1.06)
30s (n=20)	MEAN	1.73	1.79	1.72	2.04	2.03	2.04	2.32	2.62	2.18	2.60	2.58	3.88	2.42	1.86	2.73
	SD	(0.65)	(0.50)	(0.44)	(0.54)	(0.87)	(0.69)	(0.84)	(1.24)	(0.68)	(1.11)	(1.11)	(2.21)	(1.07)	(0.65)	(1.56)
40s (n=3)	MEAN	2.06	1.89	2.09	2.32	2.05	2.71	1.94	2.54	4.26	3.97	2.35	6.44	2.33	2.58	2.11
	SD	(0.45)	(1.08)	(0.28)	(0.67)	(0.69)	(0.37)	(0.47)	(0.56)	(3.04)	(3.03)	(0.47)	(3.78)	(0.62)	(0.80)	(0.13)
50s (n=16)	MEAN	1.78	2.09	1.73	2.36	1.93	2.82	2.42	2.68	2.85	3.18	2.42	3.76	2.93	2.55	2.04
	SD	(0.64)	(0.84)	(0.61)	(1.16)	(0.63)	(1.41)	(0.83)	(0.86)	(1.86)	(1.31)	(0.95)	(2.40)	(1.05)	(1.46)	(0.64)
60s (n=13)	MEAN	2.57	2.45	2.16	2.41	2.13	2.94	2.37	4.41	2.90	3.33	2.70	5.04	2.74	2.91	1.91
	SD	(1.11)	(0.96)	(0.65)	(1.32)	(0.81)	(1.25)	(1.04)	(2.04)	(1.36)	(1.39)	(0.96)	(5.64)	(1.37)	(1.24)	(0.69)
70s (n=10)	MEAN	2.25	2.64	2.71	2.41	2.07	2.69	2.92	3.65	3.89	2.86	2.36	3.38	2.64	2.40	2.21
	SD	(1.16)	(1.41)	(0.69)	(0.83)	(0.62)	(0.89)	(1.33)	(3.25)	(1.69)	(1.25)	(0.89)	(1.44)	(1.01)	(1.01)	(0.97)

pHi

		1	2	3	4	5	6	7	8	9	10	11	12	13	14	15
20s (n=5)	MEAN	7.07	7.01	7.03	6.96	7.00	7.05	7.10	7.03	7.06	7.02	7.09	7.06	7.08	7.02	7.04
	SD	(0.08)	(0.09)	(0.05)	(0.07)	(0.03)	(0.04)	(0.10)	(0.07)	(0.04)	(0.04)	(0.04)	(0.12)	(0.10)	(0.03)	(0.05)
30s (n=20)	MEAN	7.04	7.05	7.04	7.00	7.03	7.04	7.09	7.03	7.05	7.05	7.05	7.01	7.04	7.04	7.03
	SD	(0.04)	(0.03)	(0.04)	(0.03)	(0.03)	(0.03)	(0.11)	(0.05)	(0.08)	(0.05)	(0.04)	(0.06)	(0.05)	(0.02)	(0.04)
40s (n=3)	MEAN	7.05	7.05	7.01	7.03	7.03	7.02	7.12	7.09	7.02	7.04	7.08	7.07	7.01	7.04	7.03
	SD	(0.03)	(0.01)	(0.05)	(0.03)	(0.01)	(0.01)	(0.04)	(0.07)	(0.09)	(0.04)	(0.05)	(0.01)	(0.02)	(0.03)	(0.01)
50s (n=16)	MEAN	7.05	7.03	7.05	7.03	7.04	7.02	7.05	7.05	7.06	7.05	7.05	7.04	7.06	7.04	7.06
	SD	(0.05)	(0.05)	(0.04)	(0.05)	(0.05)	(0.04)	(0.05)	(0.05)	(0.05)	(0.05)	(0.03)	(0.06)	(0.03)	(0.06)	(0.05)
60s (n=13)	MEAN	7.04	7.04	7.02	7.04	7.05	7.02	7.02	7.08	7.06	7.05	7.04	7.07	7.06	7.06	7.09
	SD	(0.04)	(0.03)	(0.03)	(0.05)	(0.07)	(0.03)	(0.06)	(0.05)	(0.07)	(0.07)	(0.05)	(0.05)	(0.04)	(0.07)	(0.08)
70s (n=10)	MEAN	7.03	7.06	7.03	7.02	7.03	7.03	7.06	7.09	7.03	7.01	7.08	7.08	7.05	7.05	7.05
	SD	(0.03)	(0.05)	(0.02)	(0.03)	(0.04)	(0.03)	(0.06)	(0.08)	(0.04)	(0.03)	(0.05)	(0.07)	(0.03)	(0.04)	(0.06)

4.1.6 Examples of the metabolite image and contour map of a healthy individual (54 year-old male).

Figures 4-1-27 to 4-1-60 show metabolite images and contour maps of ^{31}P CSI in a healthy individual shown in 4.1.1 to 4.1.3. Metabolite images were obtained by mapping according to the signal intensity of each metabolite. Contour maps were prepared by indicating contour lines of signal intensity graded at 10% intervals on T_1-weighted images. Comparison between the two images clearly represents changes in the signal intensity and shows that the distribution of signal intensity is nearly symmetric in healthy individuals.

R 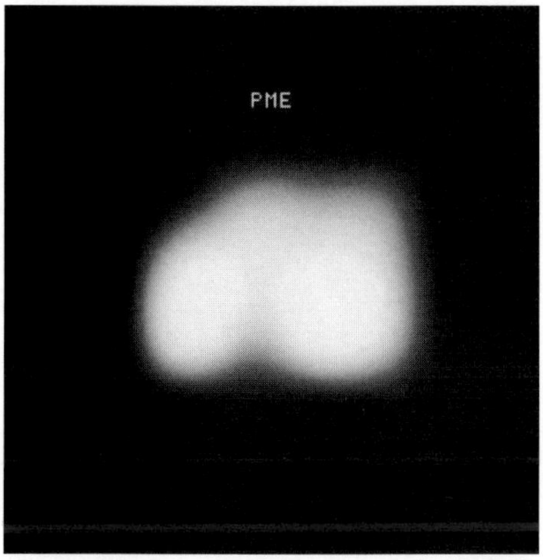 L

Fig. 4-1-27 Coronal PME metabolite image.

R 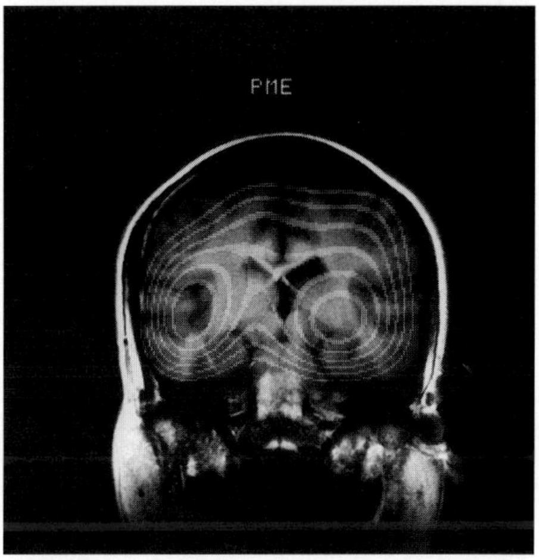 L

Fig. 4-1-28 Coronal PME contour map superimposed on T_1-weighted image (500/15).

R 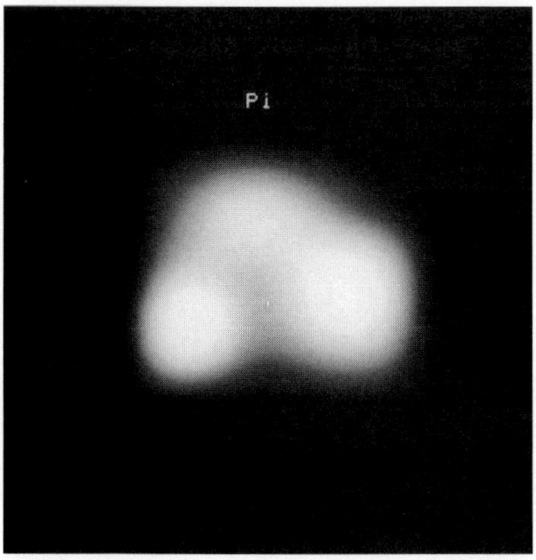 L

Fig. 4-1-29 Coronal Pi metabolite image.

R 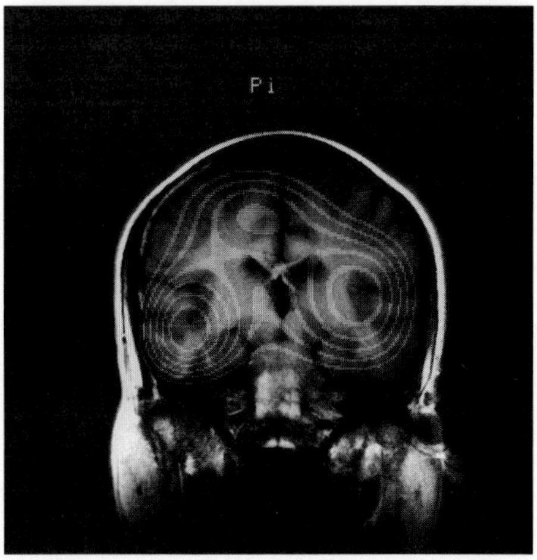 L

Fig. 4-1-30 Coronal Pi contour map superimposed on T_1-weighted image (500/15).

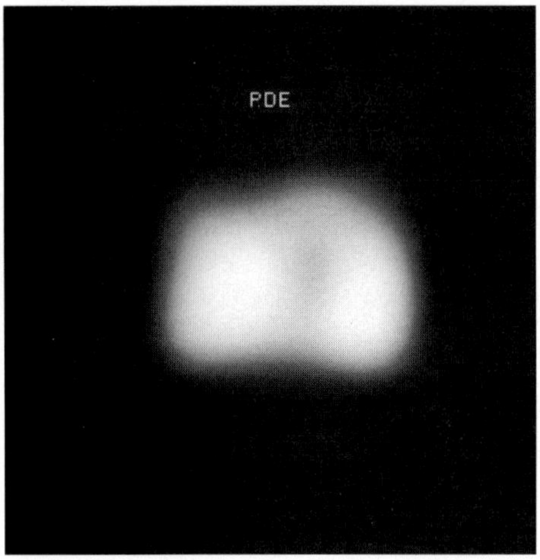

Fig. 4-1-31 Coronal PDE metabolite image.

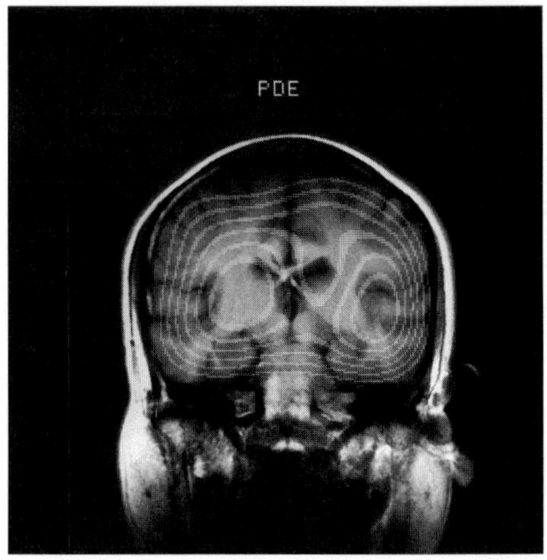

Fig. 4-1-32 Coronal PDE contour map superimposed on T_1-weighted image (500/15).

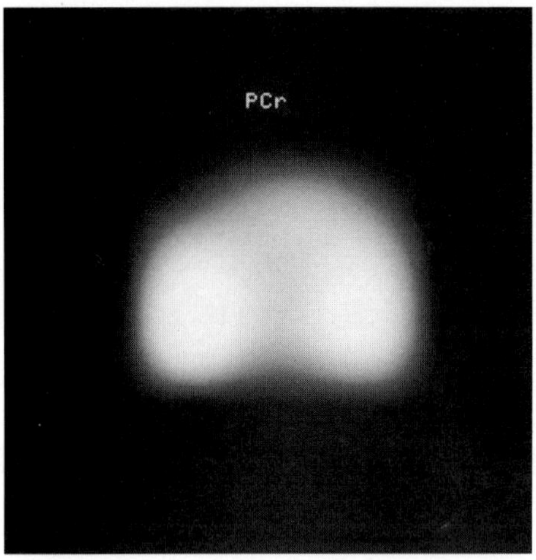

Fig. 4-1-33 Coronal PCr metabolite image.

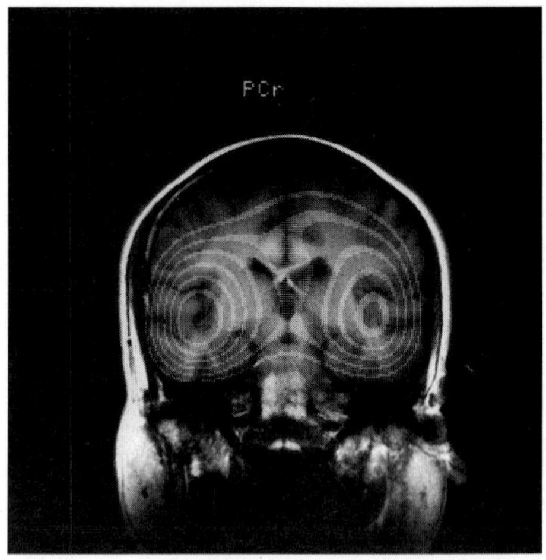

Fig. 4-1-34 Coronal PCr contour map superimposed on T_1-weighted image (500/15).

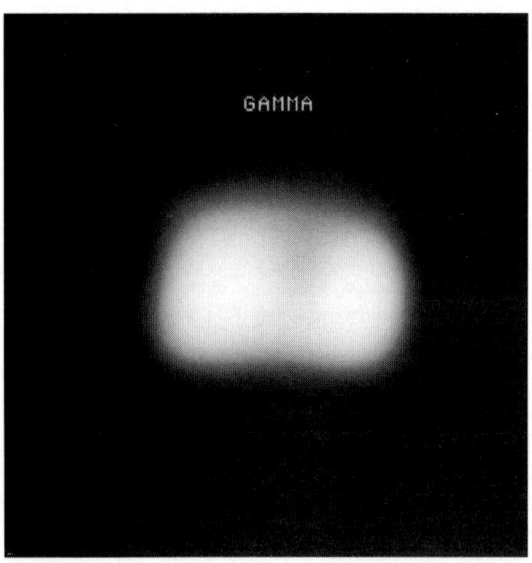

Fig. 4-1-35 Coronal γ-ATP metabolite image.

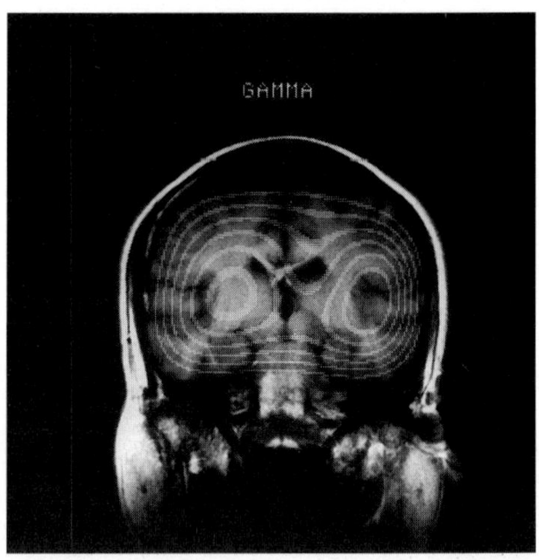

Fig. 4-1-36 Coronal γ-ATP contour map superimposed on T_1-weighted image (500/15).

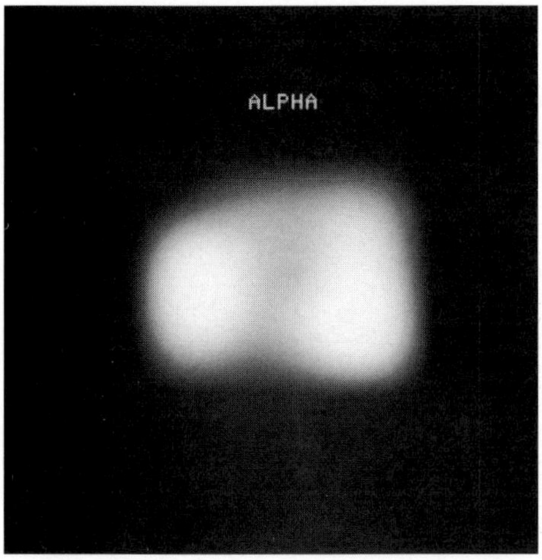

Fig. 4-1-37 Coronal α-ATP metabolite image.

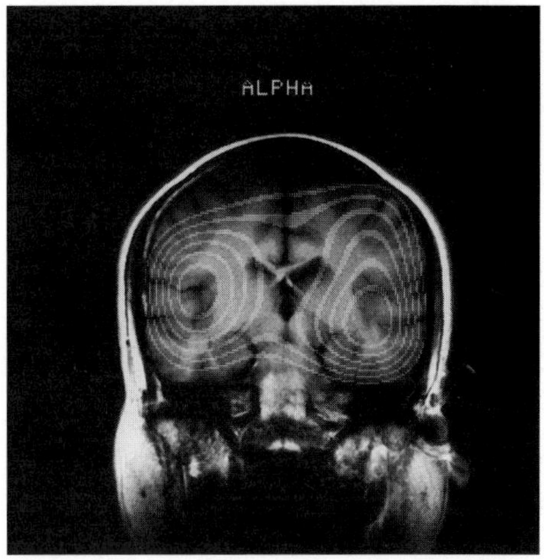

Fig. 4-1-38 Coronal α-ATP contour map superimposed on T_1-weighted image (500/15).

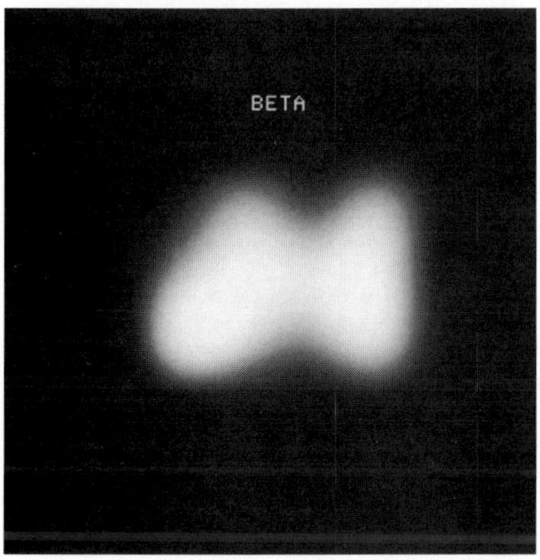

Fig. 4-1-39 Coronal β-ATP metabolite image.

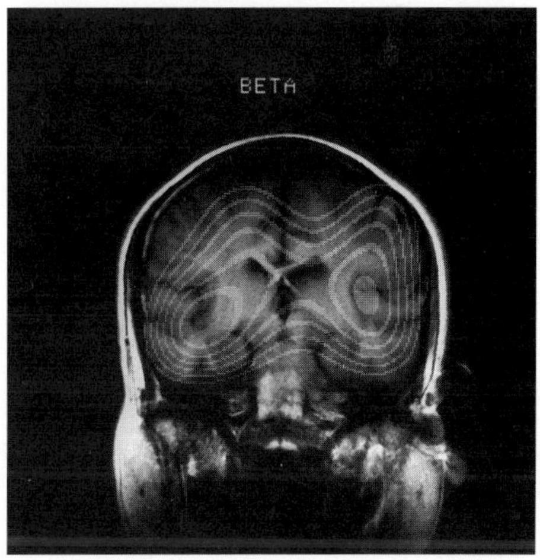

Fig. 4-1-40 Coronal β-ATP contour map superimposed on T_1-weighted image (500/15).

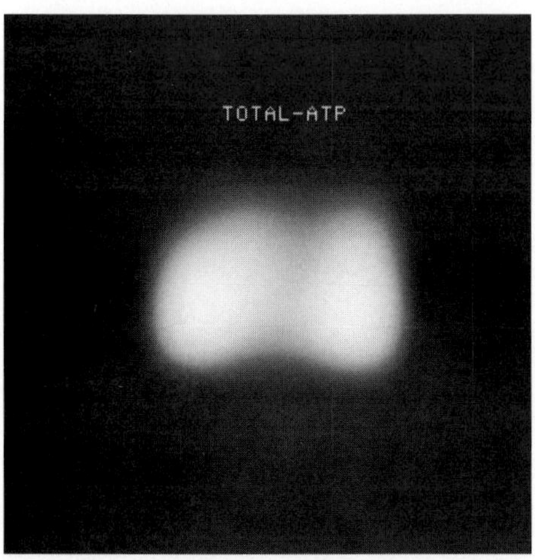

Fig. 4-1-41 Coronal total ATP metabolite image.

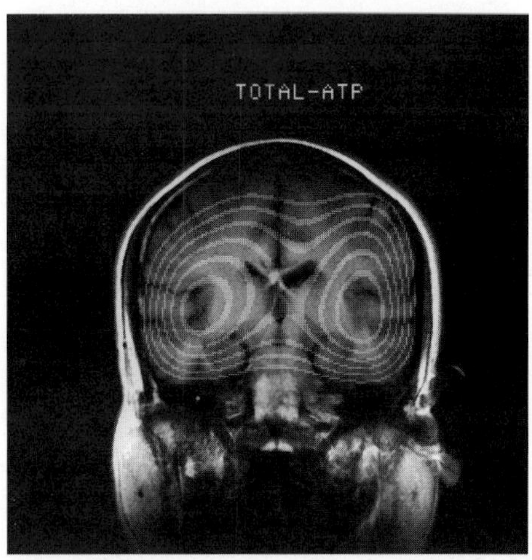

Fig. 4-1-42 Coronal total ATP contour map superimposed on T_1-weighted image (500/15).

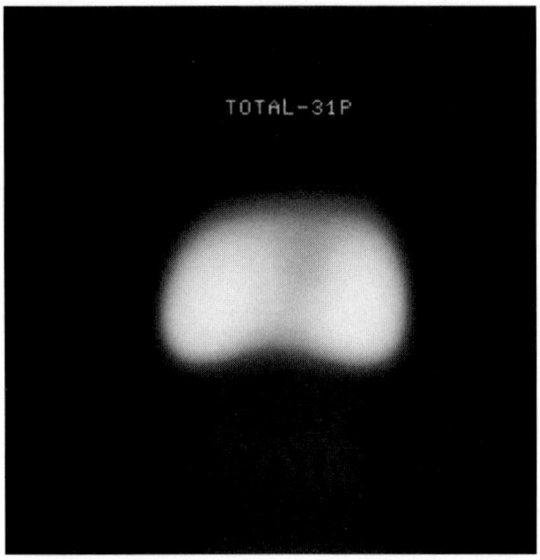

Fig. 4-1-43 Coronal ^{31}P metabolite image.

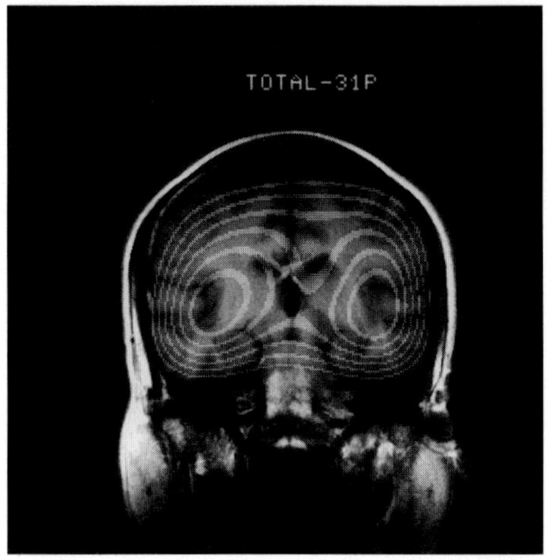

Fig. 4-1-44 Coronal ^{31}P contour map superimposed on T_1-weighted image (500/15).

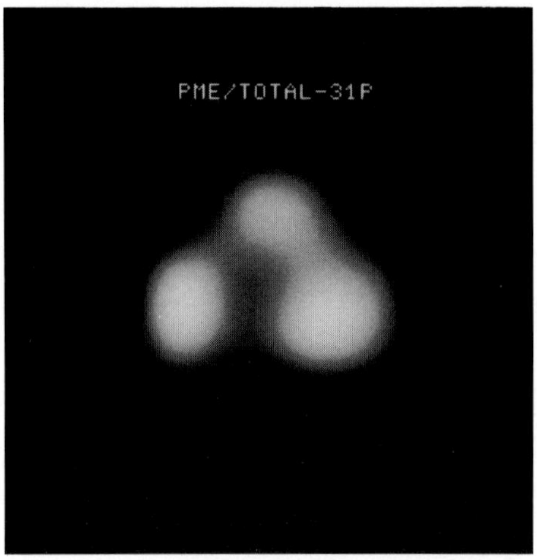

Fig. 4-1-45 Coronal PME/^{31}P metabolite image.

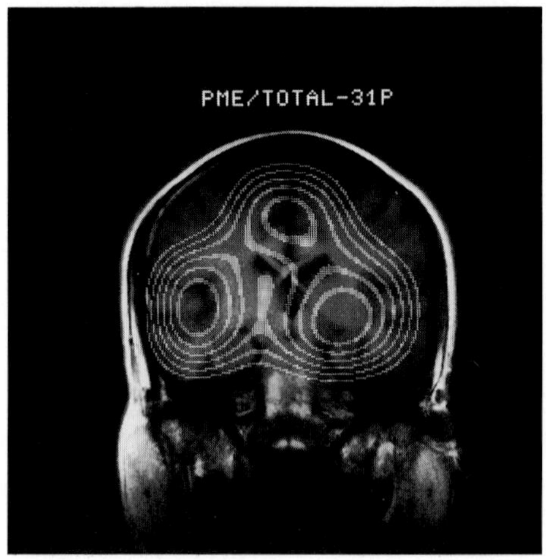

Fig. 4-1-46 Coronal PME/^{31}P contour map superimposed on T_1-weighted image (500/15).

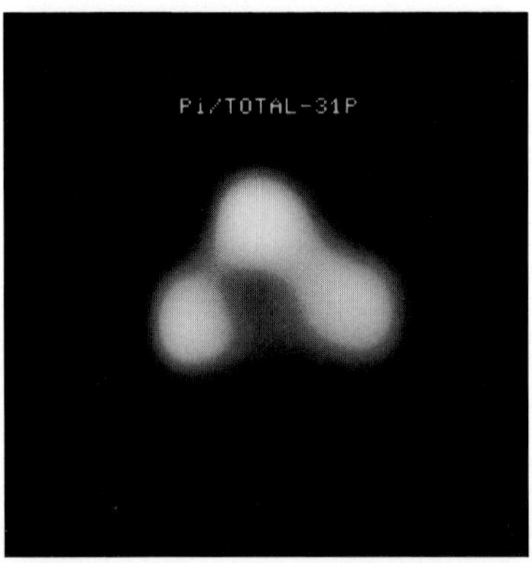

Fig. 4-1-47 Coronal Pi/^{31}P metabolite image.

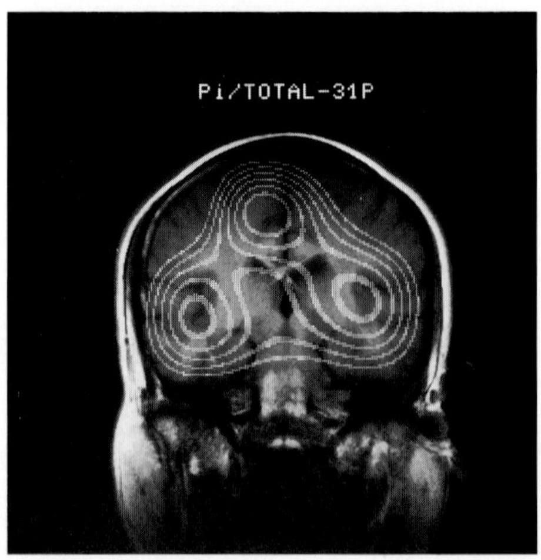

Fig. 4-1-48 Coronal Pi/^{31}P contour map superimposed on T_1-weighted image (500/15).

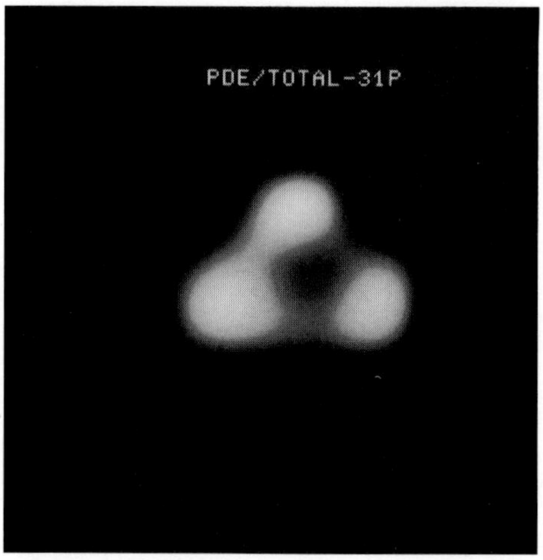

Fig. 4-1-49 Coronal PDE/^{31}P metabolite image.

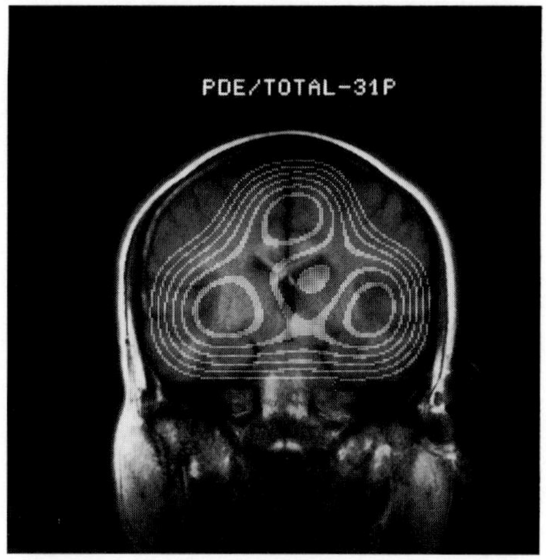

Fig. 4-1-50 Coronal PDE/^{31}P contour map superimposed on T_1-weighted image (500/15).

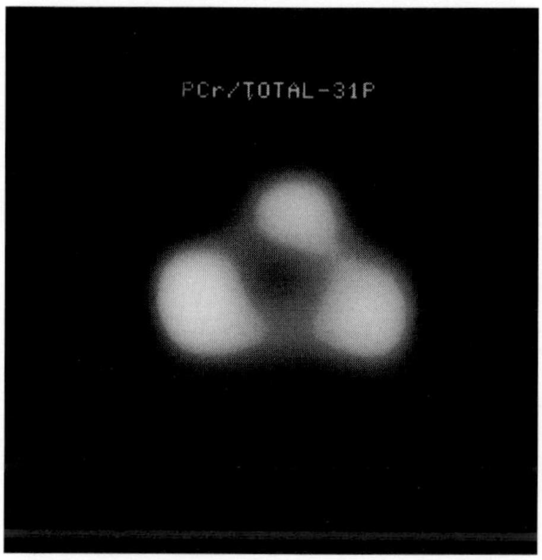

Fig. 4-1-51 Coronal PCr/^{31}P metabolite image.

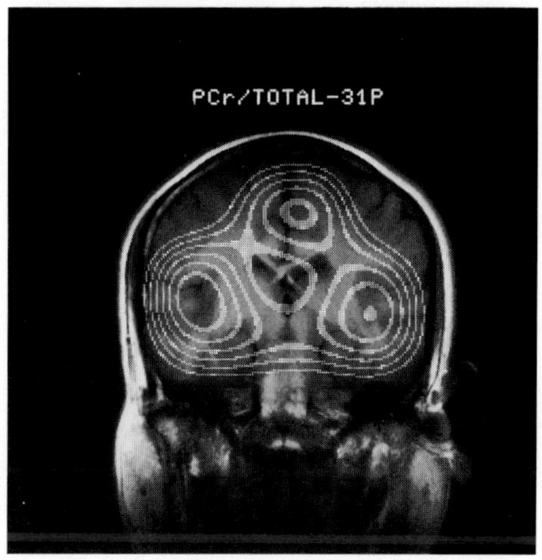

Fig. 4-1-52 Coronal PCr/^{31}P contour map superimposed on T_1-weighted image (500/15).

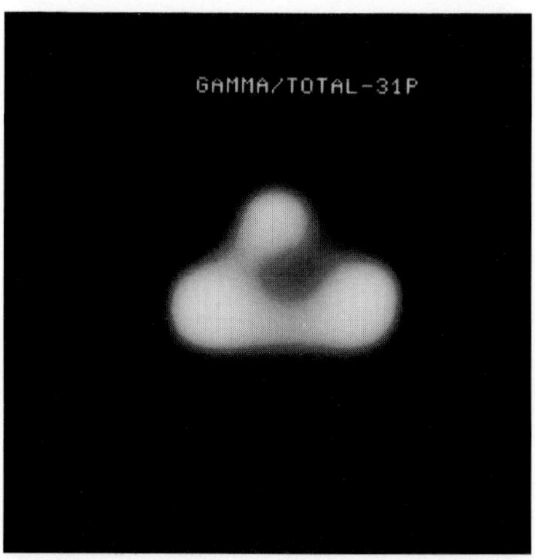

Fig. 4-1-53 Coronal γ-ATP/^{31}P metabolite image.

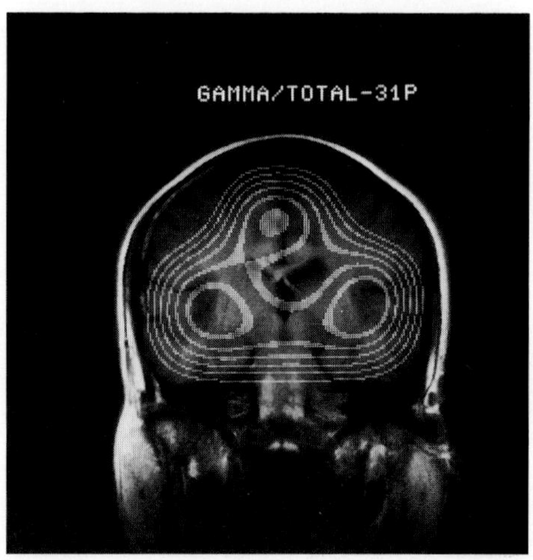

Fig. 4-1-54 Coronal γ-ATP/^{31}P contour map superimposed on T_1-weighted image (500/15).

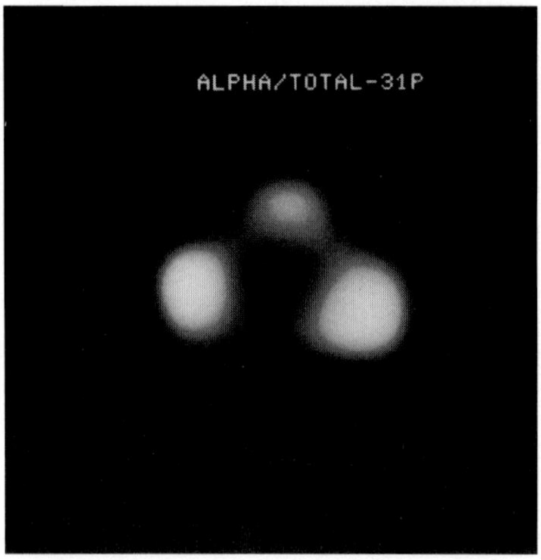

Fig. 4-1-55 Coronal α-ATP/^{31}P metabolite image.

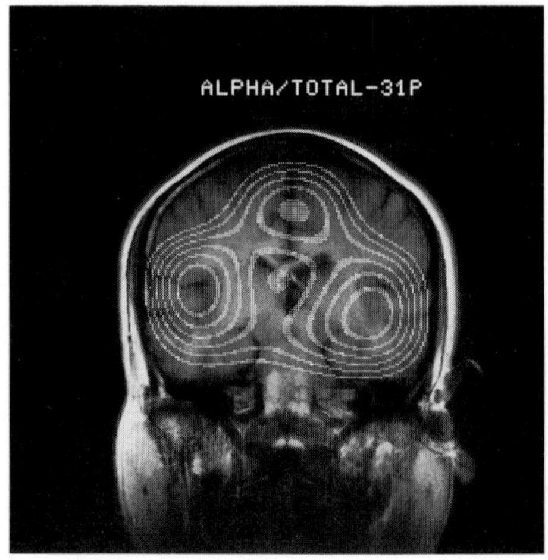

Fig. 4-1-56 Coronal α-ATP/^{31}P contour map superimposed on T_1-weighted image (500/15).

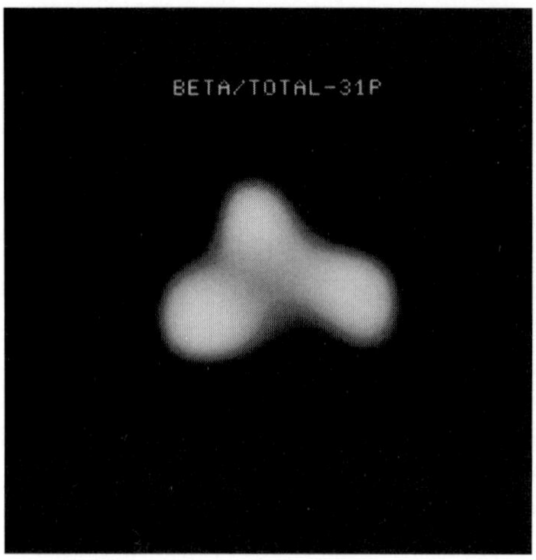

Fig. 4-1-57 Coronal β-ATP/^{31}P metabolite image.

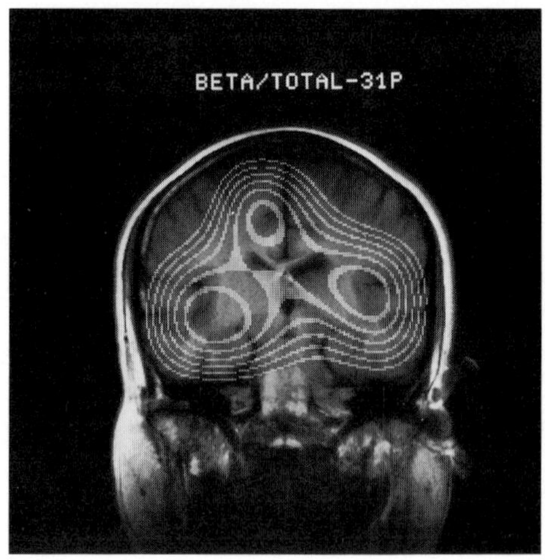

Fig. 4-1-58 Coronal β-ATP/^{31}P contour map superimposed on T_1-weighted image (500/15).

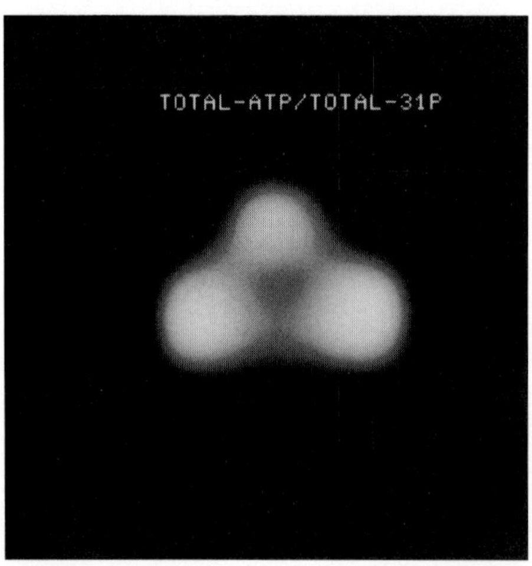

Fig. 4-1-59 Coronal total-ATP/^{31}P metabolite image.

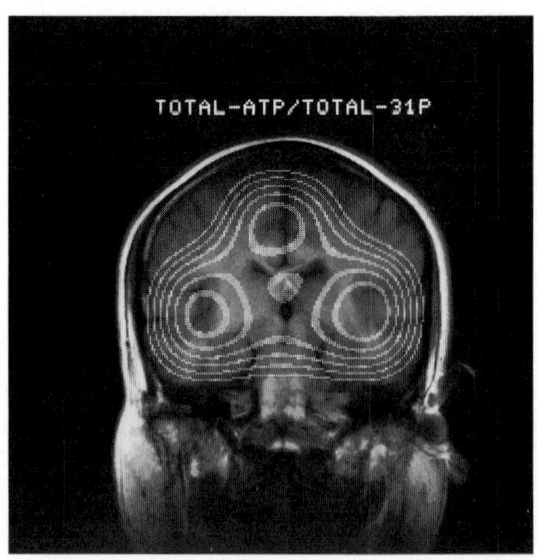

Fig. 4-1-60 Coronal total-ATP/^{31}P contour map superimposed on T_1-weighted image (500/15).

4.2 ^{1}H MRS by the single voxel method

In this volume, ^{1}H spectra are obtained by using two pulse sequences of PRESS (point resolved spectroscopy) and STEAM (stimulated echo acquisition mode). Pulse sequences of PRESS are TR = 1500 ms and TE = 135 ms or 270 ms, and those of STEAM are TR = 2000 ms and TE = 60 ms. The resonances of *N*-acetylaspartate (NAA), creatine plus phosphocreatine (Cr), and choline containing .compounds (Cho) were obtained with high reliability of both methods. In this volume, peak ratios of these metabolites were evaluated.

4.2.1 Examples of the ^{1}H spectrum of the basal ganglia in a healthy individual

Figures 4-2-1 and 2 show voxels ($3\times3\times3$ cm^3 by PRESS; $2.5\times2.5\times2.5$ cm^3 by STEAM) placed in the basal ganglia, which are superimposed on T_1-weighted images. Figures 4-2-3 and 4 show ^{1}H spectra obtained by PRESS, and Figures 4-2-5 and 6 show those obtained by STEAM.

L 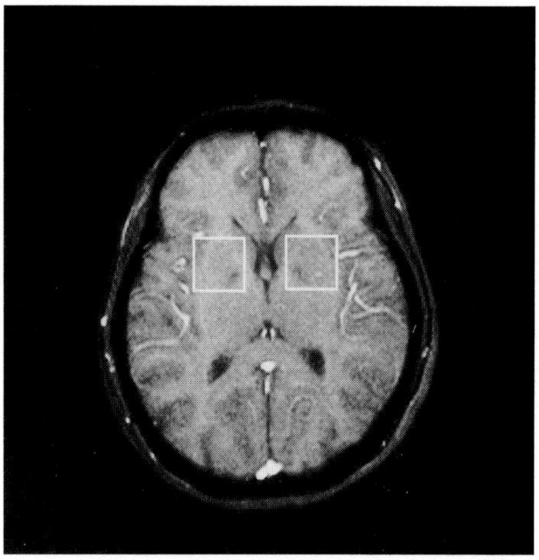 R

Fig. 4-2-1 Voxel superimposed on axial T_1-weighted image (500/15). The voxel with size of $3\times3\times3$ cm^3 is placed in the basal ganglia regions.

R 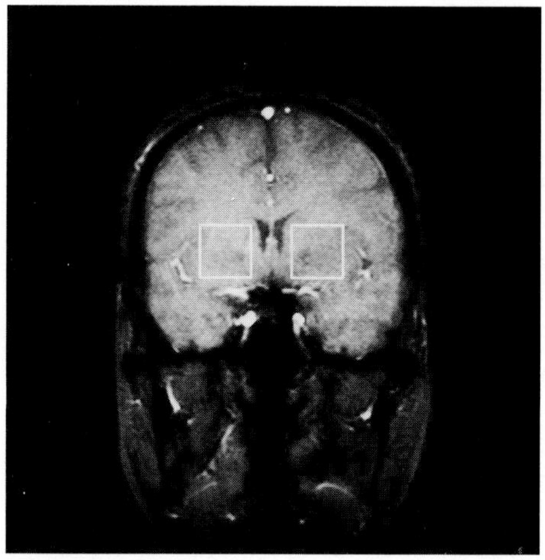 L

Fig. 4-2-2 Voxel superimposed on coronal T_1-weighted image (500/15). The voxel with size of $3\times3\times3$ cm^3 is placed in the basal ganglia regions.

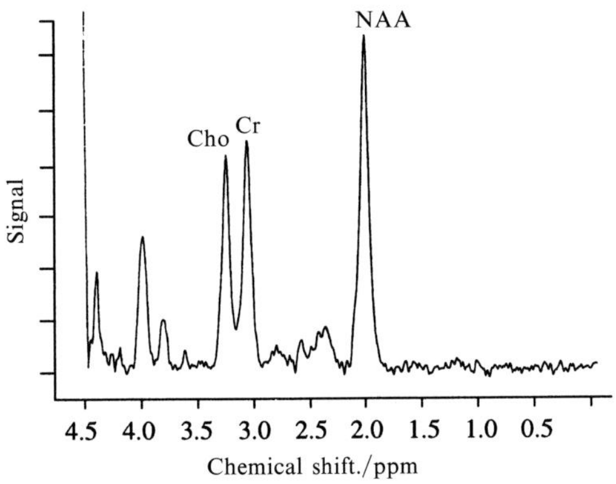

Fig. 4-2-3 ^{1}H spectrum of right basal ganglia region. PRESS (1,500/135)

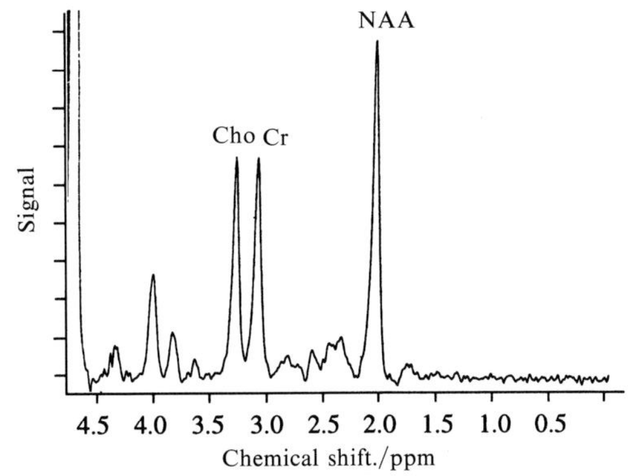

Fig. 4-2-4 ^{1}H spectrum of left basal ganglia region. PRESS (1,500/135)

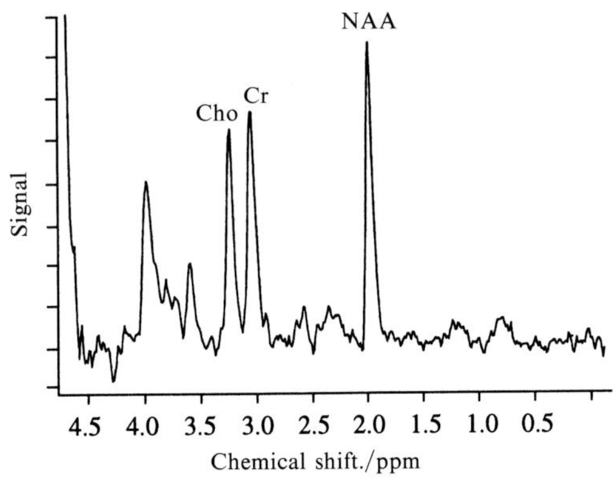

Fig. 4-2-5 ^{1}H spectrum of right basal ganglia region. STEAM (2,000/60)

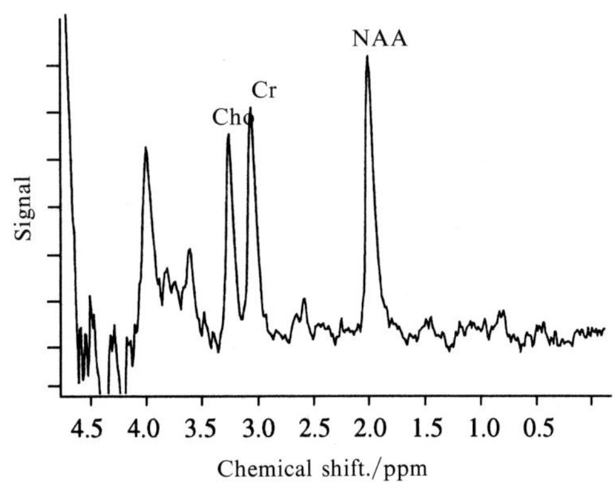

Fig. 4-2-6 ^{1}H spectrum of left basal ganglia region. STEAM (2,000/60)

4.2.2 Mean peak ratios in the ^1H spectrum of the basal ganglia regions in healthy individuals

Table 4-2-1 shows the peak ratios in the ^1H spectra of the basal ganglia regions obtained by PRESS in 11 healthy controls (mean age 41 ± 11 years). Figure 4-2-7 shows them as a bar graph.

Table 4-2-2 shows the peak ratios in the ^1H spectra of the basal ganglia regions obtained by STEAM in 12 healthy controls (mean age 38 ± 7 years). Figure 4-2-8 shows them as a bar graph.

Table 4-2-1 Peak ratios of NAA/Cho, NAA/Cr, NAA/(Cho+Cr) and Cho/Cr in the basal ganglia regions. PRESS (1,500/135)

		NAA/Cho	NAA/Cr	NAA/(Cho+Cr)	Cho/Cr
Left	Mean	1.85	1.68	0.88	0.92
	SD	0.37	0.21	0.14	0.08
Right	Mean	1.60	1.46	0.76	0.92
	SD	0.30	0.24	0.13	0.08

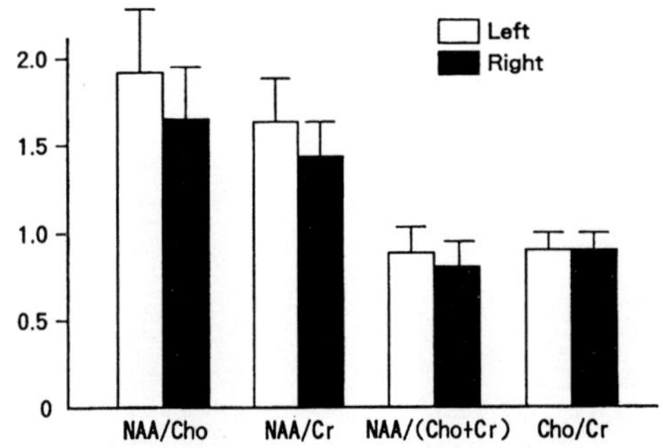

Fig. 4-2-7 Peak ratios of NAA/Cho, NAA/Cr, NAA/(Cho+Cr) and Cho/Cr in the basal ganglia regions. PRESS (1,500/135)

Table 4-2-2 Peak ratios of NAA/Cho, NAA/Cr, NAA/(Cho+Cr) and Cho/Cr in the basal ganglia regions. STEAM (2,000/60)

		NAA/Cho	NAA/Cr	NAA/(Cho+Cr)	Cho/Cr
Left	Mean	2.04	1.52	0.87	0.74
	SD	0.29	0.29	0.14	0.06
Right	Mean	1.91	1.32	0.78	0.70
	SD	0.38	0.20	0.13	0.08

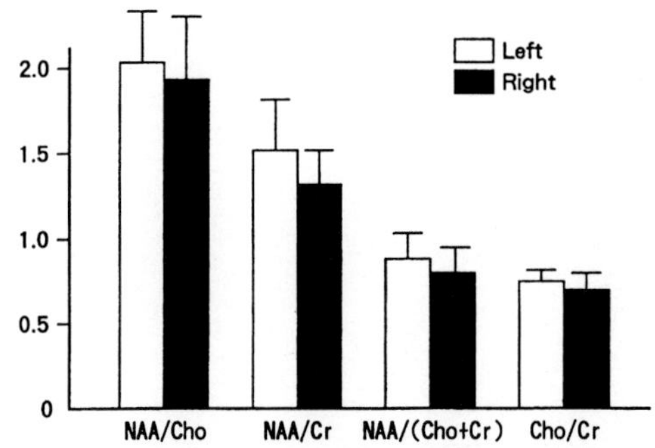

Fig. 4-2-8 Peak ratios of NAA/Cho, NAA/Cr, NAA/(Cho+Cr) and Cho/Cr in the basal ganglia regions. STEAM (2,000/60)

4.2.3 Examples of ^{1}H spectra in mesial temporal lobes in a healthy individual

Figures 4-2-9 and 10 show voxels ($3 \times 3 \times 3$ cm^3 by PRESS; $2.5 \times 2.5 \times 2.5$ cm^3 by STEAM) determined in mesial temporal lobes on T_1-weighted images. Figures 4-2-11 and 12 show ^1H spectra obtained by PRESS, and Figures 4-2-13 and 14 show ^1H spectra obtained by STEAM.

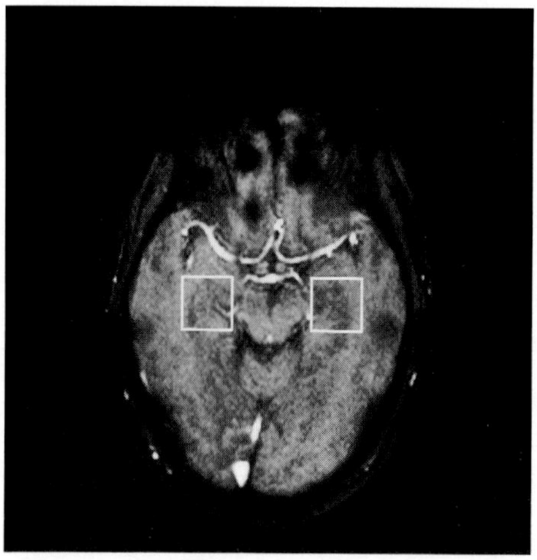

Fig. 4-2-9 Voxel superimposed on axial T_1-weighted image (500/15). The voxel with size of $3 \times 3 \times 3$ cm^3 is placed in the mesial temporal regions.

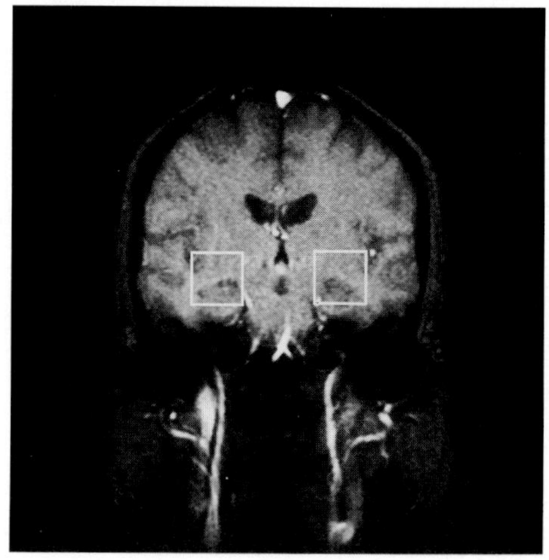

Fig. 4-2-10 Voxel superimposed on coronal T_1-weighted image (500/15). The voxel with size of $3 \times 3 \times 3$ cm^3 is placed in the mesial temporal regions.

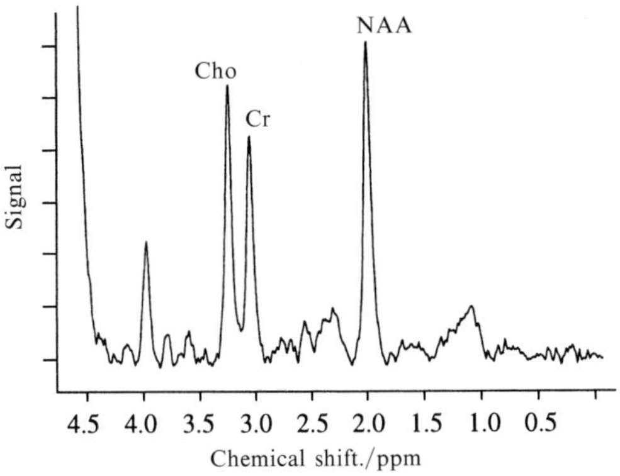

Fig. 4-2-11 ¹H spectrum of right mesial temporal lobe. PRESS (1,500/135)

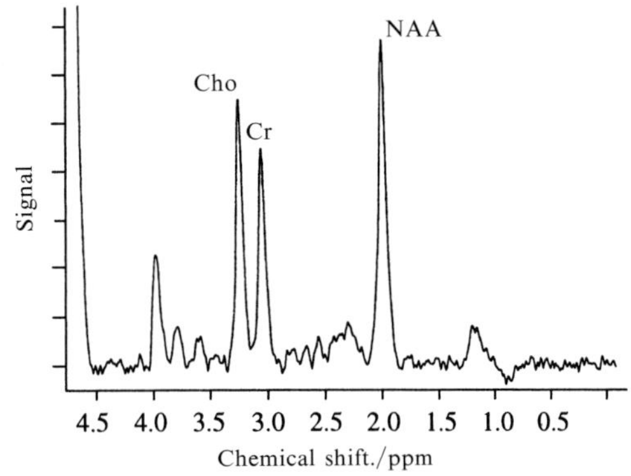

Fig. 4-2-12 ¹H spectrum of left mesial temporal lobe. PRESS (1,500/135)

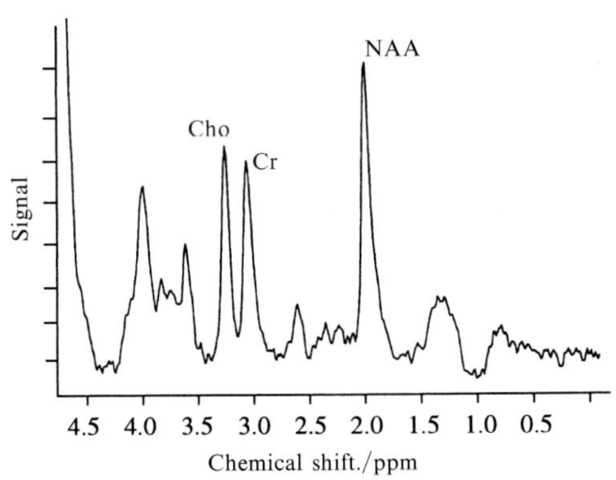

Fig. 4-2-13 ¹H spectrum of right mesial temporal lobe. STEAM (2,000/60)

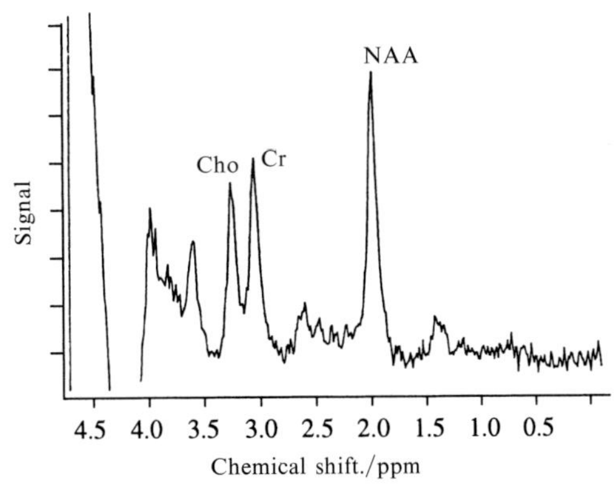

Fig. 4-2-14 ¹H spectrum of left mesial temporal lobe. STEAM (2,000/60)

4.2.4 Mean peak ratios in ^{1}H spectra in mesial temporal lobes in healthy individuals

Table 4-2-3 shows peak ratios in ^{1}H spectra obtained by PRESS in mesial temporal lobes in 10 healthy controls (mean age 42 ± 8 years), and Figure 4-2-15 shows them as a bar graph. Table 4-2-4 shows peak ratios in ^{1}H spectra obtained by STEAM in mesial temporal lobes in 12 healthy controls (mean age 32 ± 12 years), and Figure 4-2-16 shows them as a bar graph.

Table 4-2-3 Peak ratios of NAA/Cho, NAA/Cr, NAA/(Cho+Cr) and Cho/Cr in the mesial temporal regions. PRESS (1,500/135)

		NAA/Cho	NAA/Cr	NAA/(Cho+Cr)	Cho/Cr
Left	Mean	1.45	1.50	0.73	1.04
	SD	0.19	0.23	0.09	0.15
Right	Mean	1.56	1.60	0.79	1.04
	SD	0.32	0.25	0.13	0.11

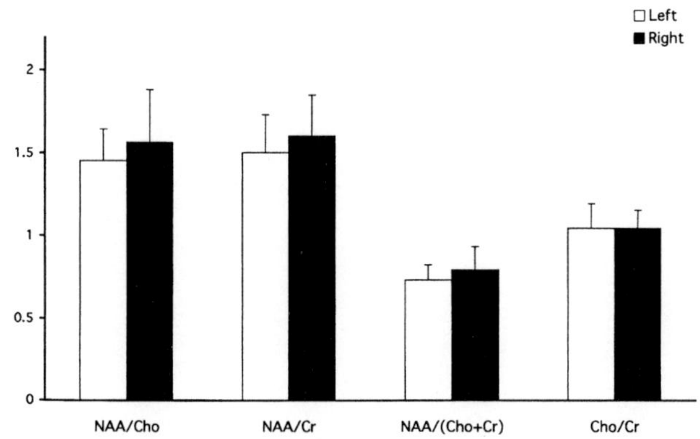

Fig. 4-2-15 Peak ratios of NAA/Cho, NAA/Cr, NAA/(Cho+Cr) and Cho/Cr in the mesial temporal regions. PRESS (1,500/135)

Table 4-2-4 Peak ratios of NAA/Cho, NAA/Cr, NAA/(Cho+Cr) and Cho/Cr in the mesial temporal regions. STEAM (2,000/60)

		NAA/Cho	NAA/Cr	NAA/(Cho+Cr)	Cho/Cr
Left	Mean	1.78	1.30	0.75	0.74
	SD	0.29	0.16	0.10	0.08
Right	Mean	1.90	1.49	0.83	0.82
	SD	0.32	0.22	0.16	0.15

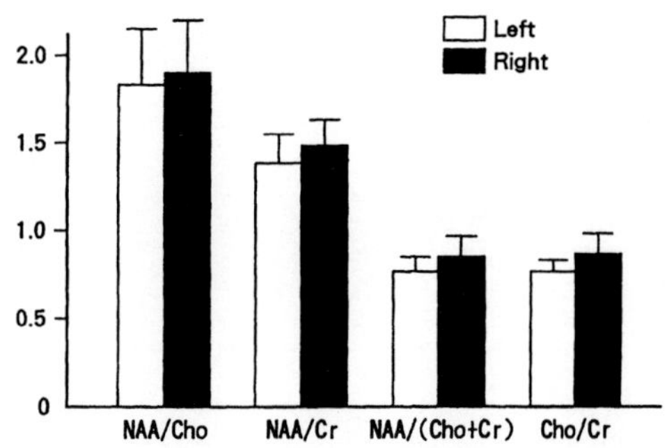

Fig. 4-2-16 Peak ratios of NAA/Cho, NAA/Cr, NAA/(Cho+Cr) and Cho/Cr in the mesial temporal regions. STEAM (2,000/60)

PART II

CLINICAL

APPLICATIONS

Chapter 5 Brain Tumors

Masahiro Sasahira

5.1 CHARACTERISTICS OF THE SPECTRUM

5.1.1 ^{31}P MRS of brain tumors

(1) ***Quantity of phosphorus compounds:*** An increase in PME and a decrease in PCr are generally reported in tumors by ^{31}P MRS. However, various patterns can be observed depending on the stage of the growth and type of tumor.[1] PME is a precursor of cell membrane phospholipids, and a high PME level indicates enhanced synthesis of cell membrane phospholipids, and a decrease in PCr indicates anaerobic metabolism in the tumor.[2,3] Table 1-1 summarizes our findings by 2D- CSI, and Table 1-2 summarizes findings by ^{31}P MRS in reported cases of brain tumor.[4] Among phosphorus compounds, decreases in PCr and PDE and increases in PME are frequently reported. Regarding the contents of phosphorus compounds in various tumors, Arnold et al.[5] observed that PCr and PDE were reduced more markedly in meningioma than in glioma and that PME was increased more markedly in pituitary adenoma. In our cases, (1) ^{31}P was lower in tumors except in meningioma, (2) PCr was reduced in all tumors, (3) ATP was significantly high in meningioma but was lower in glioblastoma, malignant lymphoma, epidermoid, and chondrosarcoma, (4) Pi was high in glioblastoma, metastatic tumor, malignant lymphoma, epidermoid, and chondrosarcoma but was low in other tumors, (5) PME was high in ependymoma, glioblastoma, and malignant lymphoma but low in astrocytoma and chondrosarcoma, and (6) PDE was reduced in all tumors; the contents of phosphorus compounds differed among tumors. On the other hand, Hubesch et al.[6] measured the absolute quantity of phosphorus compounds, and reported that PCr, PDE, and PME were reduced in brain tumors by 20-70% compared with normal tissue but that Pi showed little reduction. This report is interesting in that a high PME level, which has often been documented, was not observed, but the authors suggested that the T_1 value in a normal subject was used as that of the tumor, that T_1 signals of the tumor are weakened by the saturation effect, and that glioma was observed frequently in this series of patients as its possible causes.

(2) ***Intratumoral pH:*** The intracellular pH of

Table. 1-1 Tumor/normal brain ratios of brain tumors

Histology	No.	total ^{31}P	PCr	ATP	Pi	PDE	PME	pHi
Astrocytoma	5	0.80±0.17	0.87±0.25	1.17±0.61	0.88±0.27	0.73±0.21	0.80±0.23	7.067±0.036 :
Ependymoma	1	0.79	0.62	0.96	0.55	0.58	1.27	7.067 *
Glioblastoma	9	0.88±0.22	0.80±0.29	0.86±0.32	1.38±0.67	0.79±0.34 :	1.31±0.90	7.141±0.063⁺ *
Meta.	3	0.89±0.27 *	0.83±0.23	1.04±0.31 *	1.58±1.00	0.77±0.14	0.96±0.55	7.132±0.015 •
Malig. lymp.	1	0.77	0.36	0.68	1.43	0.41	2.49	7.124
Meningioma	9	1.02±0.12	0.17±0.18 •	1.25±0.33 :	1.07±0.42	0.94±0.22	1.04±0.34	7.134±0.104 •
Epidermoid	2	0.88±0.08	0.88±0.19	0.82±0.17	2.24±0.33	0.78±0.16	0.99±0.21	7.092±0.042 :
Chondrosar.	1	0.68	0.53	0.63	2.68	0.92	0.34	7.168

meta. : metastatic tumor, malig.lymp. : malignant lymphoma, chondrosar. : chondrosaroma

⁺ ; $p<0.001$, • ; $p<0.01$, : ; $p<0.05$ vs normal brain, * ; $p<0.05$

Table. 1-2 Reports of ^{31}P MRS with brain tumors

Author	Year	Method	No.	Remarks
Zimmerman	1985	Surface coil	1	PCr/ATP ↓
Segebarth	1987	ISIS	3	PME ↑, PCr ↓, PCr/ATP ↓, Pi ↓ ; monitor
Arnold	1987	ISIS	1	monitor
Thomsen	1988	Surface coil	8	no characteristic pattern of spectra
Heindel	1988	ISIS	43	PCr ↓, PDE ↓, PME ↑ ; monitor
Arnold	1989	ISIS	7	monitor
Ross	1989	CSI	1	monitor
Sutton	1990	DRESS	14	PCr/Pi is good indicator as malignancy
Sasahira	1990	CSI	12	^{31}P ↓, PCr ↓, PME ↑
Hubesch	1990	ISIS	13	quantitation of metabolites. PME ↓, PDE ↓, PCr ↓, ATP ↓, PCr/Pi ↓, PCr/ATP ↓, pHi ↑
Arnold	1991	ISIS	13	LGA (resembled normal spectra), GLI (PDE ↓, PCr ↓, PME ↑, pHi ↑), MEN (PDE ↓, PCr ↓, Pi ↓, pHi ↑) PIT (PME ↑, PDE ↓, PCr ↓, Pi ↓, pHi ↑)
Sasahira	1992	CSI	30	^{31}P ↓, PCr ↓, PME ↑, pHi ↑ ; monitor
Kamata	1992	ISIS	12	PCr/ATP ↓, Pi/ATP ↓

^{31}P : total phosphate, LGA : low grade astrocytoma, GLI : glioblastoma, MEN : meningioma
PIT : pituitary adenoma, monitor : ^{31}P MRS was used for therapeutic monitor
(Asakura. T et al. Med J Kagoshima Univ 46: 29-39, 1994.)

Table. 1-3 ^{31}P MRS as therapeutic monitor

Author	Year	Tumor type	Changes of ^{31}P MRS
Ross	1987	Bone tumors	PME ↓, ATP ↓
Ng	1987	Non-Hodgkin's lymphoma	PDE/ATP ↓, PCr ↑, PDE ↓, pHi ↑
Segebarth	1987	Brain tumors	PCr/ATP ↓, ATP ↓, PCr ↑, PME ↓
Arnold	1987	Brain tumors	PCr ↓, PDE ↓, pHi ↑
Thomsen	1988	Brain tumors	normal spectra pattern
Heindel	1988	Brain tumors	PME ↑, PCr ↑, pHi ↓
Semmler	1988	Superficial tumors	PCr/total^{31}P ↓, NTP /Pi ↓
Brayant	1988	Non-Hodgkin's lymphoma	PME/ATP ↑
Arnold	1989	Brain tumors	pHi change was a good indicator
Ross	1989	Brain tumor	normal pattern
Ng	1989	Superficial tumors	pHi fluctuated
Dewhirst	1990	Sarcomas	PCr/Pi ↓, NTP/Pi ↓, pHi ↓
Karczmar	1991	Superficial tumors	PME/ATP ↓
Smith	1991	Non-Hodgkin's lymphoma	pHi ↑, PDE/ATP ↑
Sasahira	1992	Brain tumors	^{31}P ↓, transient increased Pi, pHi ↓
Redmond	1992	Superficial tumors	Pi ↑, Pi/NTP ↑, Pi/PDE ↑, PME ↓, PME/PCr ↓, PME/NTP ↓, PME/PDE ↓

(Asakura. T et al. *Med J Kagoshima Univ* 46: 29-39, 1994.)

brain tumors is often alkaline.[5–8] In our cases also, astrocytoma, glioblastoma, metastatic tumor, meningioma, and epidermoid were more alkaline than normal brain tissue, and glioblastoma and metastatic tumor were significantly more alkaline than astrocytoma. A possible cause of the enhanced alkalinity of tumor tissues is that the blood-brain barrier is disrupted in brain tumors so that the intratumoral pH approaches the extracellular pH, and that Na^+/H^+ antiporter activity is increased in actively proliferating cells.[6]

(3) ***^{31}P MRS as a means to monitor therapeutic effects on brain tumors***: As a means of monitoring therapeutic effects on brain tumors, ^{31}P MRS allows repeated evaluation of changes in tumor metabolism over a short period of time immediately following treatment and over a prolonged period thereafter. Table 1-3 summarizes reports on changes in tumors including brain tumors as a result of treatments.[4] According to Redmond et al.,[9] who studied superficial tumors, increases in Pi, decreases in PME and ATP, and decreases in pHi were observed following treatment. A decrease in PME indicates reduced synthesis of phosphorylethanolamine and phosphorylcholine, which are important for the formation of the cell membrane, and an increase in Pi indicates changes in energy metabolism in tumor cells. Since there have been few reports of a large series of patients with brain tumors, reported changes in PCr and PME are not consistent and remain controversial.[4] Normalization of the spectrum has been reported along with a reduction in tumor size in some patients.[10] In the author's series,[7,11] malignant lymphomas were reduced in size by treatments, and the spectrum was normalized. In glioma, phosphorus compounds were generally reduced after radiochemotherapy. Furthermore, tumors were observed as high-signal areas by Pi imaging 3 to 17 days after ACNU intra-arterial infusion chemotherapy. These findings are considered to indicate necrosis of the tumor tissue. Arnold et al.[12,13] studied changes in the intratumoral pH associated with BCNU chemotherapy. They considered that alkalization of the intratumoral pH after intra-arterial administration was due to damage to the cell membrane by high concentrations of BCNU, and that acidification after intravenous administration was due to the accumulation of lactic acid and suggested the possibility of the monitoring of adverse reactions to drugs by examination of the intratumoral pH.

5.1.2 ^{1}H MRS of brain tumors

^{1}H MRS on brain tumors clearly exhibits different patterns compared with normal brain tissue.[14] Generally, the patterns are characterized by decreases in NAA and Cr/PCr and by an increase in choline. The increase in choline is striking in

Table. 1-4 ^{1}H MRS of brain tumors

Histology	No.	NAA/Cho	NAA/Cr	Cho/Cr	Cr/Cho
Normal	3	1.86±0.50	1.96±0.41	1.13±0.44	1.11±0.29
Meningioma	5	0.23±0.17*	1.34±0.54	7.32±3.40**	0.19±0.15*
Astrocytoma	2	0.14±0.15**	0.51±0.54**	4.21±0.85**	0.25±0.05**
Glioblastoma	5	0.44±0.27*	0.90±0.36*	2.62±1.64	0.50±0.24**
Ependymoma	1	0.81	4.40	5.45	0.18
Metastatic tumor	2	1.62±1.34	2.19±0.98	1.73±0.87	0.67±0.33
Malig. lymph.	1	0.34	2.38	6.92	0.14
Epidermoid	2	0.60±0.68	0.99±1.13	1.21±0.63	0.96±0.50

malig. lymph. : malignant lymphoma
vs. normal (*<0.01, **<0.05), +<0.05

meningioma, and lactate is increased in malignant tumors such as glioblastoma and metastatic tumor.[15,16] Table 1-4 shows our results. NAA/Cho was reduced in all tumors, and the decrease was significant in meningioma, astrocytoma, and glioblastoma. Among tumors, a significant difference was observed between meningioma and metastatic tumors. NAA/Cr was reduced in all tumors except ependymoma, metastatic tumors, and malignant lymphoma. Cho/Cr was elevated except in epidermoid, and was significantly higher in meningioma and astrocytoma than in normal brain tissue. Among tumors, a significant difference was noted between meningioma and glioblastoma. Cr/Cho was reduced in all tumors, being significantly reduced in meningioma, astrocytoma, and glioblastoma compared with normal brain tissue. Among tumors, significant difference was observed in meningioma compared with glioblastoma, metastatic tumors, and epidermoid. In epidermoid, in particular, the peaks of NAA, Cr/PCr, and choline were very low, and only the peak of lactate was notable, showing a totally different pattern from other tumors.

References

1) Ng, T. C.; Evanochko, W. T.; Hiramoto, R. N. et al. ^{31}P NMR spectroscopy of *in vivo* tumors. *J. Magn. Reson.* 49: 271-286; 1982.

2) Asakura, T.; Sasahira, M. Magnetic resonance spectroscopy and chemical shift imaging of the brain. *Neurosiences* 20: 83 101; 1994.

3) Bottomley, P. A. Human in vivo NMR spectroscopy in diagnostic medicine: Clinical tool or research probe? *Radiology* 170: 1-15; 1989.

4) Asakura, T.; Sasahira, M.; Uchimura, K. et al. ^{31}P magnetic resonance spectroscopy and ^{31}P chemical shift imaging of brain tumors. *Acta Med. Univ. Kagoshima* 46: 29-39; 1994. [Japanese]

5) Arnold, D. L.; Emrich, J. F.; Shoubridge, E. A. et al. Characterization of astrocytomas, meningiomas, and pituitary adenomas by phosphorus magnetic resonance spectroscopy. *J. Neurosurg.* 74: 447-453; 1991.

6) Hubesch, B.; Sappey-Marinier, D.; Roth, K. et al. P-31 MR spectroscopy of normal human brain and brain tumors. *Radiology* 174: 401-409; 1990.

7) Sasahira, M.; Asakura, T.; Uchimura, K. et al. ^{31}P chemical shift imaging of brain tumors and cerebrovascular disease. *Progress in CI* 14: 517-531; 1992. [Japanese]

8) Sutton, L. N.; Lenkinski, R. E.; Cohen, B. H. et al. Localized ^{31}P magnetic resonance spectroscopy of large pediatric brain tumors. *J. Neurosurg.* 72: 65-70; 1990.

9) Redmond, O. M.; Stack, J. P.; O'Connor, N. G. et al. ^{31}P MRS as an early prognostic indicator of patient response to chemotherapy. *Magn. Reson. Med.* 25: 30-44; 1992.

10) Ross, B. D.; Tropp, J.; Derby, K. A. et al. Metabolic response of glioblastoma to adoptive immunotherapy: Detection by phosphorus MR spectroscopy. *J. Comput. Assist. Tomogr.* 13: 189-193; 1989.

11) Sasahira, M.; Uchimura, K.; Terada, K. et al. ^{31}P chemical shift imaging of intracranial tumors. *Neuroradiology* 37 (suppl): 149-150; 1995.

12) Arnold, D. L.; Shoubridge, E. A.; Feindel, W. et al. Metabolic changes in cerebral gliomas within hours of treatment with intra-arterial BCNU demonstrated by phosphorus magnetic resonance spectroscopy. *Can. J. Neurol. Sci.* 14: 570-575; 1987.

13) Arnold, D. L.; Shoubridge, E. A.; Emrich, J. et al. Early metabolic changes following chemotherapy of human gliomas in vivo demonstrated by phosphorus magnetic resonance spectroscopy. *Invest. Radiol.* 24: 958-961; 1989.

14) Demaerel, P.; Johannik, K.; Hecke, P. V. et al. Localized ^{1}H NMR spectroscopy in fifty cases of newly diagnosed intracranial tumors. *J. Comput. Assist. Tomogr.* 15: 67-76; 1991.

15) Frahm, J.; Michaelis, T.; Merboldt, K. D. et al. Improvements in localized proton NMR spectroscopy of human brain. Water suppression, short echo times, and 1 ml resolution. *J. Magn. Resn.* 90: 464-473; 1990.

16) Frahm, J.; Bruhn, H.; Hänicke, W. et al. Localized proton NMR spectroscopy of brain tumors using short-echo time STEAM sequences. *J. Comput. Assist. Tomogr.* 15: 915-922; 1991.

5.2 CASES (1-21)

CASE 1

Case 1: A 51-year-old male

Pituitary adenoma

The patient complained of left retrobulber pain and occipitalgia with a history extending over one year. He was admitted following a 3-month history of thirst and loss of body weight, and was diagnosed as having diabetes mellitus. Computed tomography revealed a pituitary tumor. Neurological examination revealed upper 1/4 hemianopsia. A hormonal examination demonstrated hyperprolactinemia (1400ng/dl). The MRIs in Figures 1-1 and 2 demonstrate a pituitary adenoma occupying the sella turcica. The signal intensity of the tumor is low in the contour maps and metabolite images of ^{31}P, PDE, and PCr are shown in Figures 1-3, 5, and 6. Signal intensity is lower than the surrounding tissues in the metabolite image of PME in Figure 1-4, but is high in the contour map of PME/PDE in Figure 1-7. Figures 1-9 and 1-10 show the spectra of the tumor area and a normal control area. The findings were as mentioned above.

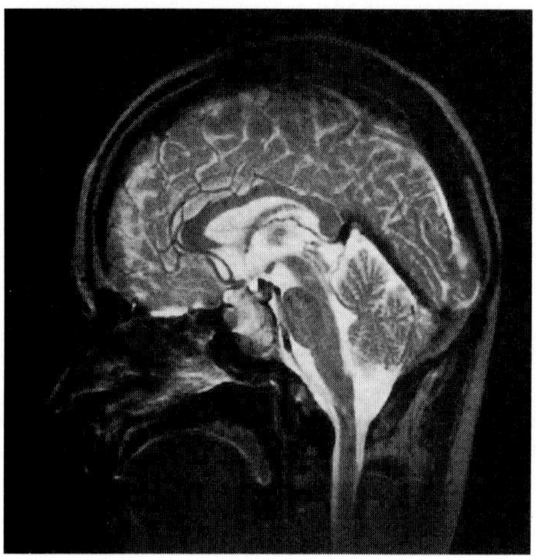

Fig. 1-1 Sagittal T_2-weighted image (2,200/90).

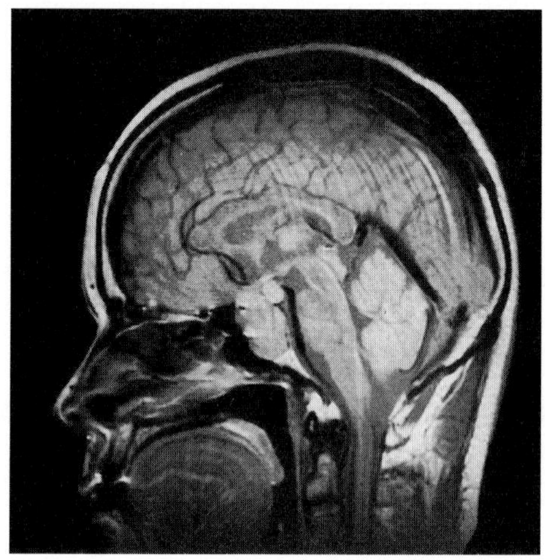

Fig. 1-2 Sagittal proton density-weighted image (2,200/15).

R

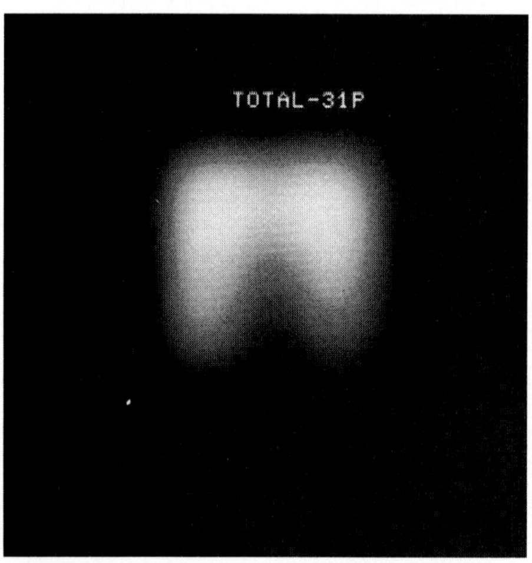

L

Fig. 1-3 Coronal ^{31}P metabolite image.

R

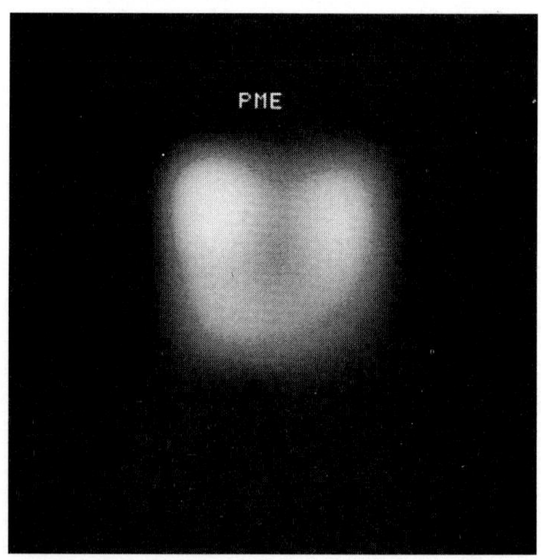

L

Fig. 1-4 Coronal PME metabolite image.

R 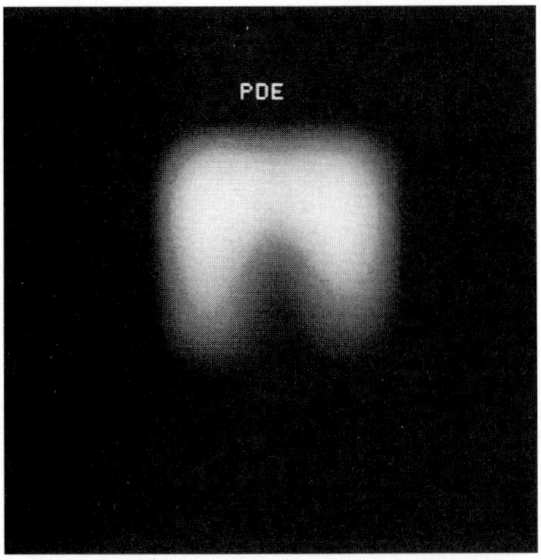 L

Fig. 1-5 Coronal PDE metabolite image.

R 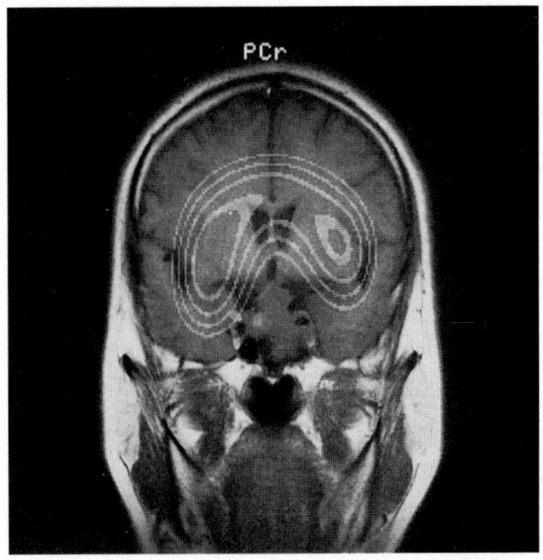 L

Fig. 1-6 Coronal PCr contour map superimposed on T_1 weighted image (500/15).

R 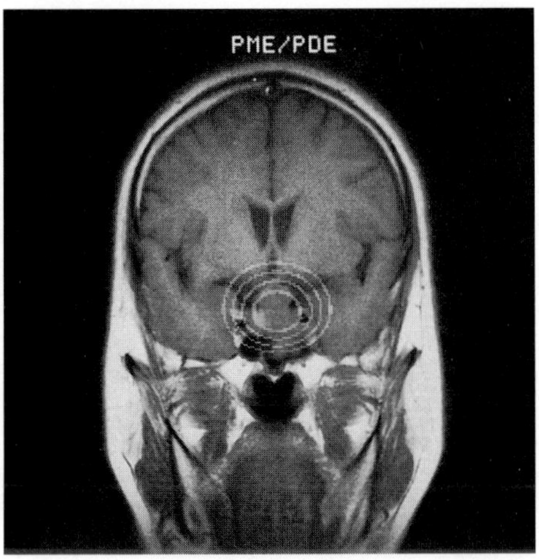 L

Fig. 1-7 Coronal PME/PDE contour map superimposed on T_1-weighted image (500/15).

R 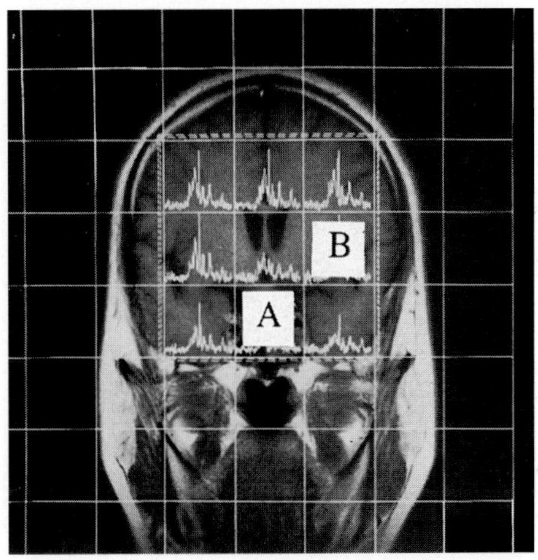 L

Fig. 1-8 T_1-weighted image showing the position of $3 \times 3 \times 4$ cm^3 voxels A and B.

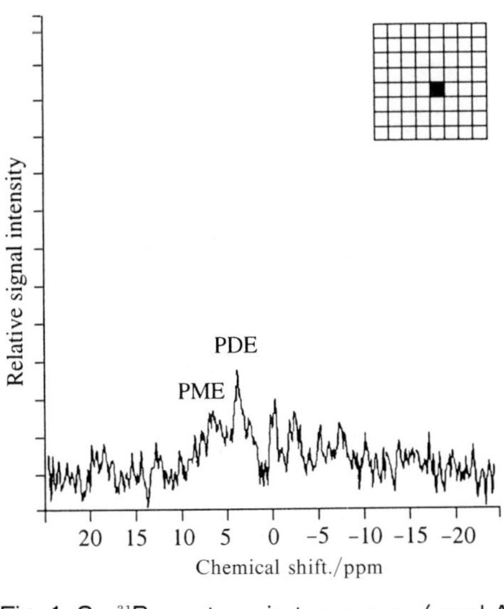

Fig. 1-9 ^{31}P spectrum in tumor area (voxel A).

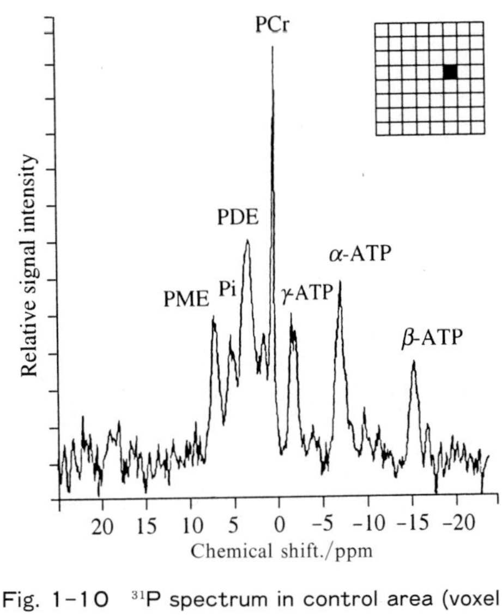

Fig. 1-10 ^{31}P spectrum in control area (voxel B).

CASE 2

Case 2: A 26-year-old male

Pituitary adenoma

On admisson the patient complained of having headaches for 11 months and was diagnosed as having a brain tumor and hydrocephalus. The neurological examination was normal. In the MRIs in Figures 2-1 and 2, a pituitary tumor occupying the sella turcica and extending to the suprasellar region is observed. The tumor is represented as a low-signal intensity area in the contour maps of ^{31}P, total ATP, and Pi in Figures 2-3, 4, and 6. Its signal intensity is lower than in the surrounding tissues in the contour map of PME in Figure 2-5, but is high in the contour map of PME/PDE in Figure 2-7. Figures 2-9 and 2-10 show the spectra of a normal control area and the tumor area. The peak of PME shows an increase in the tumor part.

L 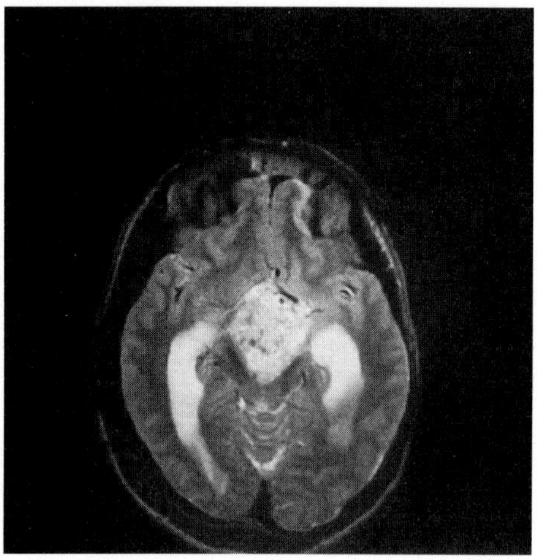 R

Fig. 2-1 Axial T_2-weighted image (2,200/90).

L 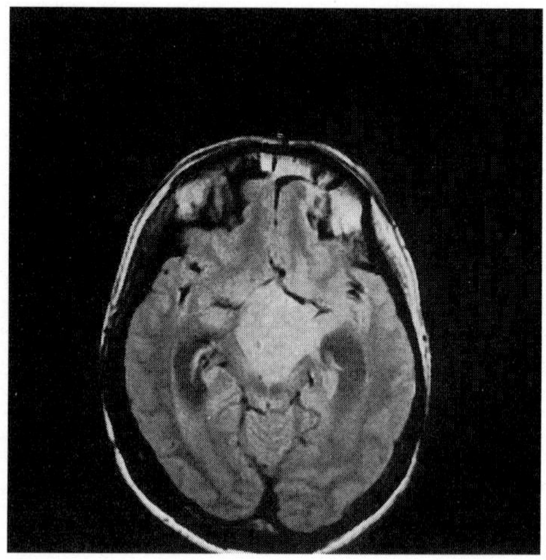 R

Fig. 2-2 Axial proton density-weighted image (2,200/15).

R 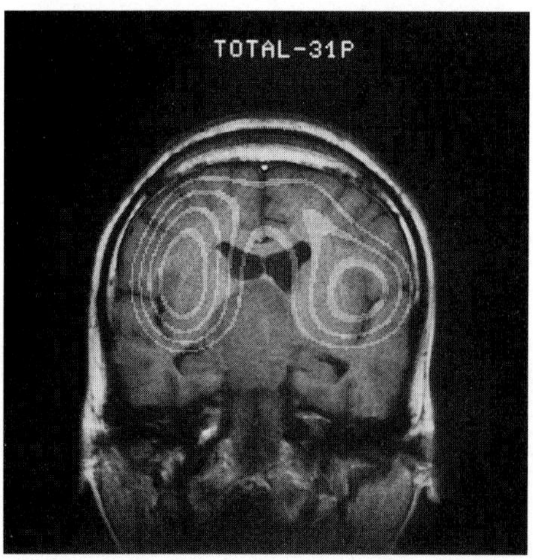 L

Fig. 2-3 Coronal ^{31}P contour map superimposed on T_1-weighted image (500/15).

R 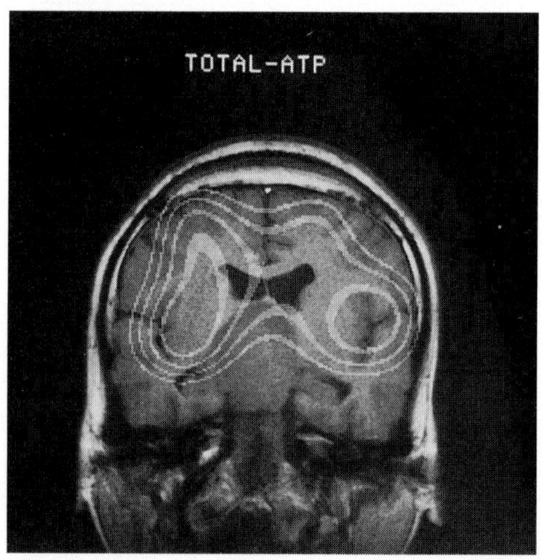 L

Fig. 2-4 Coronal total ATP contour map superimposed on T_1-weighted image (500/15).

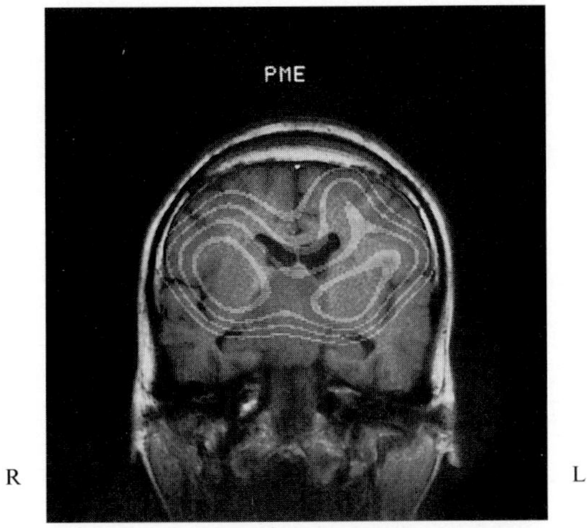

Fig. 2-5 Coronal PME contour map superimposed on T_1-weighted image (500/15).

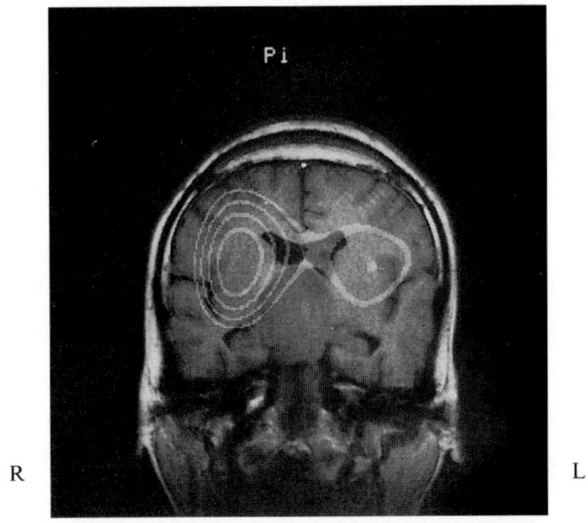

Fig. 2-6 Coronal Pi contour map superimposed on T_1-weighted image (500/15).

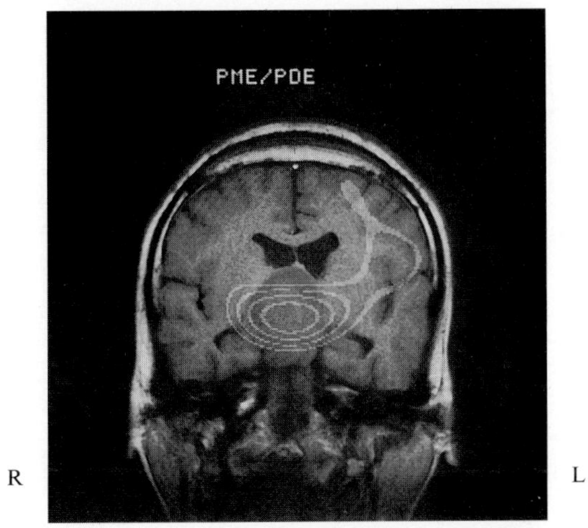

Fig. 2-7 Coronal PME/PDE contour map superimposed on T_1-weighted image (500/15).

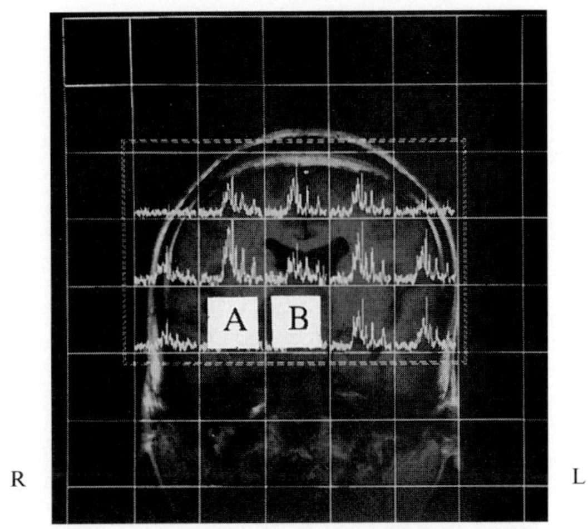

Fig. 2-8 T_1-weighted image showing the position of $3 \times 3 \times 4$ cm^3 voxels A and B.

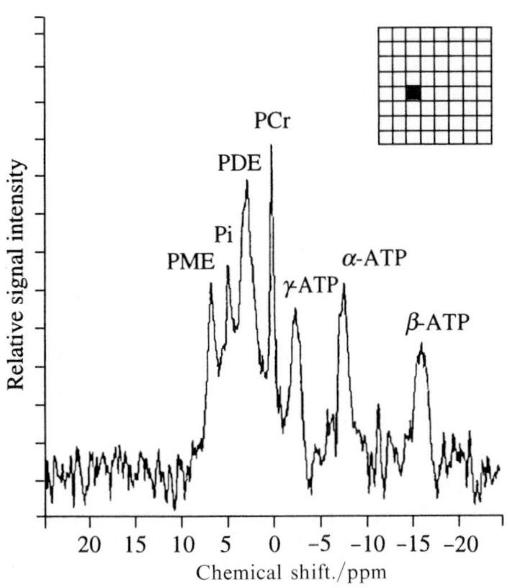

Fig. 2-9 ^{31}P spectrum in control area (voxel A).

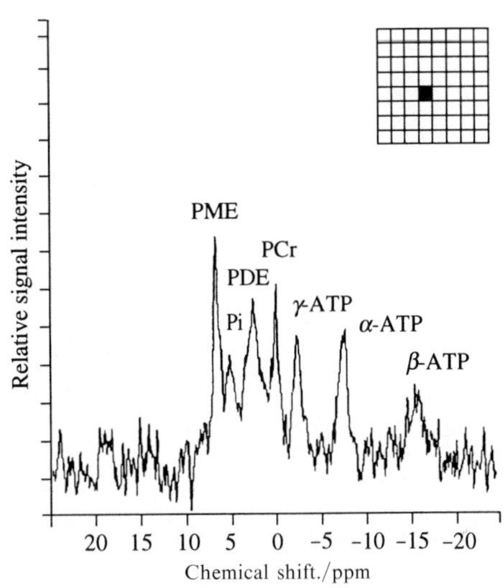

Fig. 2-10 ^{31}P spectrum in tumor area (voxel B).

CASE 3

Case 3: A 33-year-old male

Meningioma

The patient suffered from occipitalgia with a history extending over two months. There were no abnormal neurological findings. Computed tomography demonstrated a left sphenoidal ridge homogenously enhanced mass. A meningioma in the left sphenoidal ridge is observed in the MRIs in Figures 3-1 and 2. The tumor is accompanied by surrounding edema. The ^{31}P contour map in Figure 3-3 represents the tumor as a low-signal intensity area. In the total ATP contour map in Figure 3-4, the signal intensity of the tumor is higher than the surrounding tissues. In the PME and Pi metabolite images in Figures 3-5 and 6, the tumor is a high signal intensity area. Figures 3-9 and 3-10 show the spectra of a normal control area and the tumor area. The findings are as mentioned above.

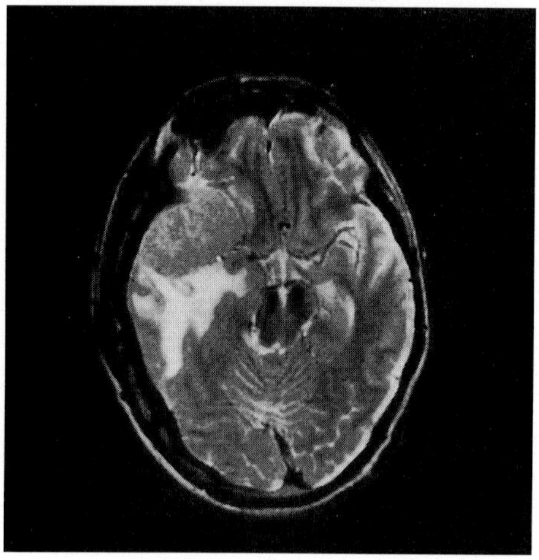

Fig. 3-1 Axial T_2-weighted image (2,200/90).

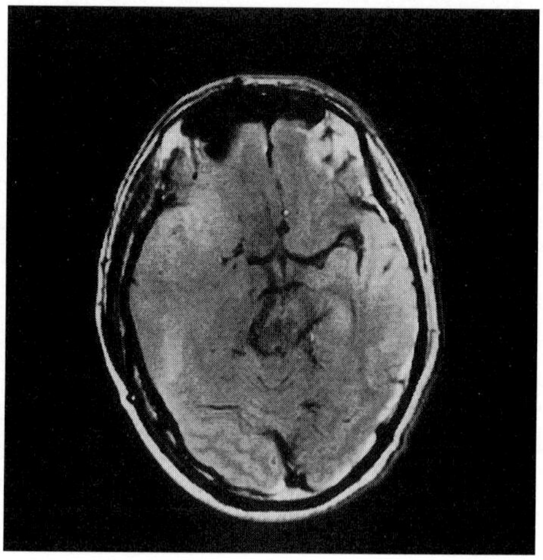

Fig. 3-2 Axial proton density-weighted image (2,200/15).

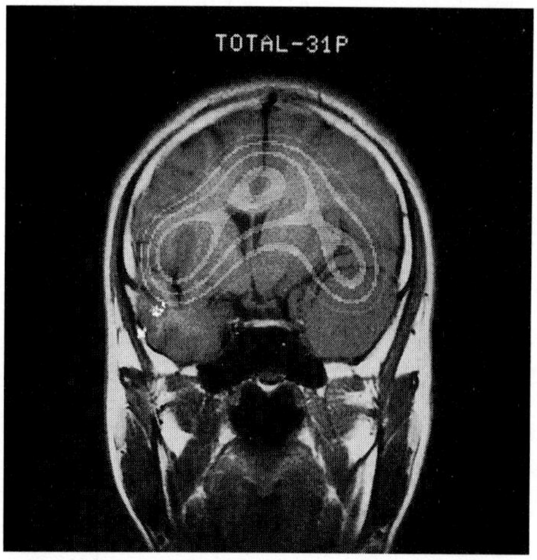

Fig. 3-3 Coronal ^{31}P contour map superimposed on T_1-weighted image (500/15).

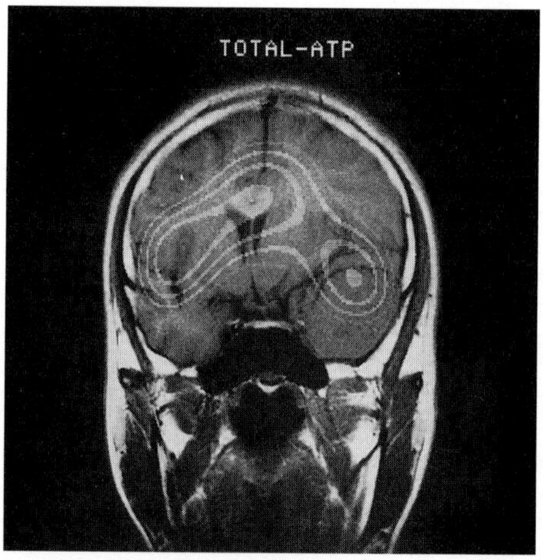

Fig. 3-4 Coronal total ATP contour map superimposed on T_1-weighted image (500/15).

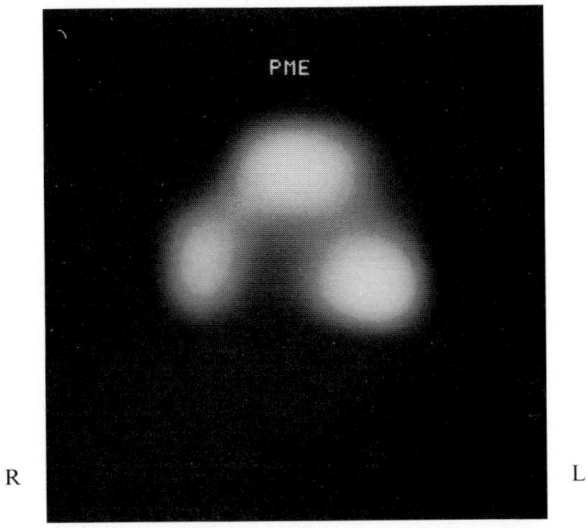

Fig. 3-5 Coronal PME metabolite image.

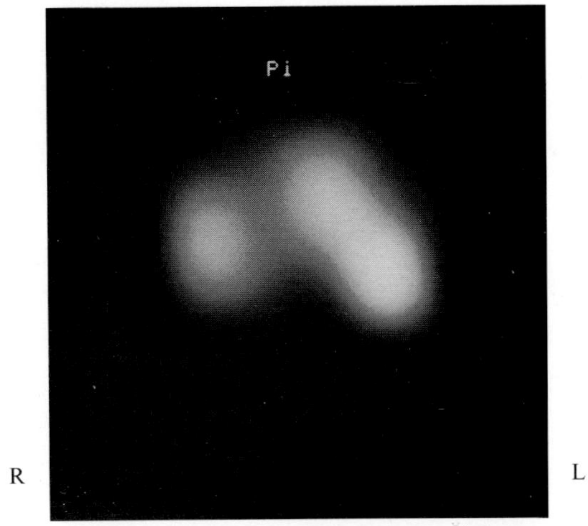

Fig. 3-6 Coronal Pi metabolite image.

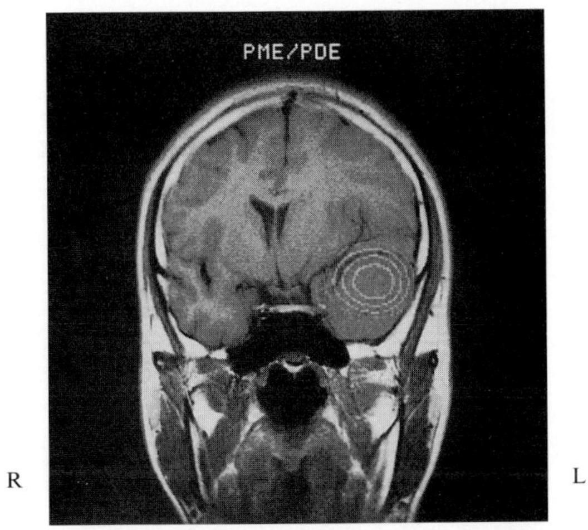

Fig. 3-7 Coronal PME/PDE contour map superimposed on T_1-weighted image (500/15).

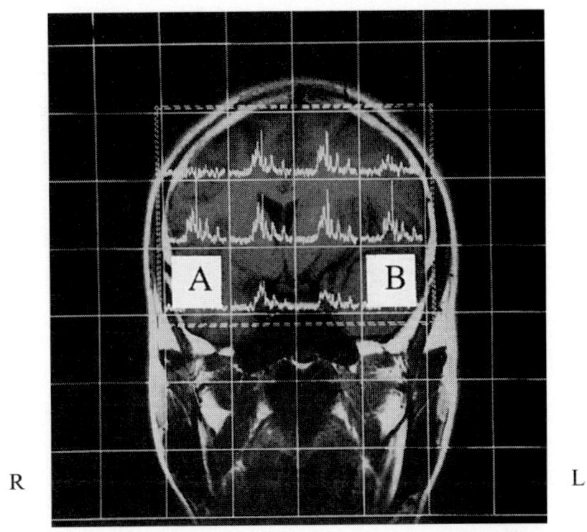

Fig. 3-8 T_1-weighted image showing the position of 3×3×4 cm^3 voxels A and B.

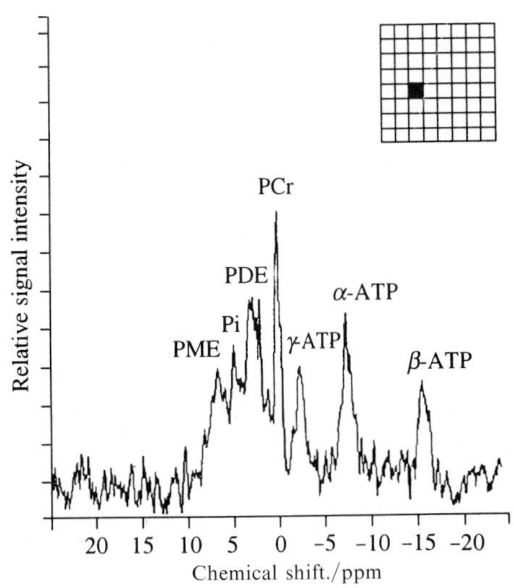

Fig. 3-9 ^{31}P spectrum in control area (voxel A).

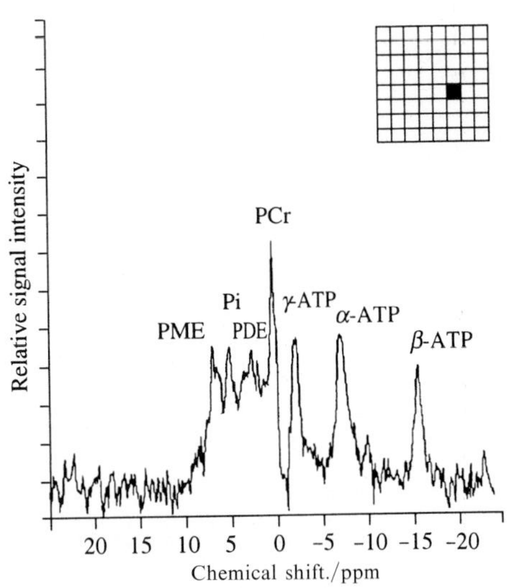

Fig. 3-10 ^{31}P spectrum in tumor area (voxel B).

CASE 4

Case 4: A 69-year-old female

Meningioma

The patient reported disorientaion extending over two months. The neurological examination revealed disorientation, right homonymous hemianopsia, and right hemiparesis. The MRIs in Figures 4-1 and 2 show a giant meningioma in the left occipital region. Edema around the tumor is mild. In the ^{31}P contour map in Figure 4-3, the signal intensity of the tumor is slightly reduced. In the total ATP contour map in Figure 4-4, the signal intensity is increased in the tumor. It is also increased in the PME contour map in Figure 4-5. It is decreased in the PDE and PCr contour maps in Figures 4-6 and 7. Figures 4-9 and 4-10 show the spectra of the tumor area and normal control area. The findings are as mentioned above.

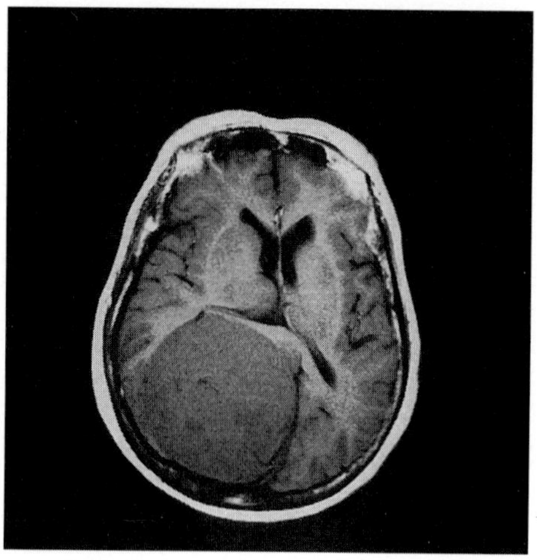

Fig. 4-1 Axial T_1-weighted image (500/15).

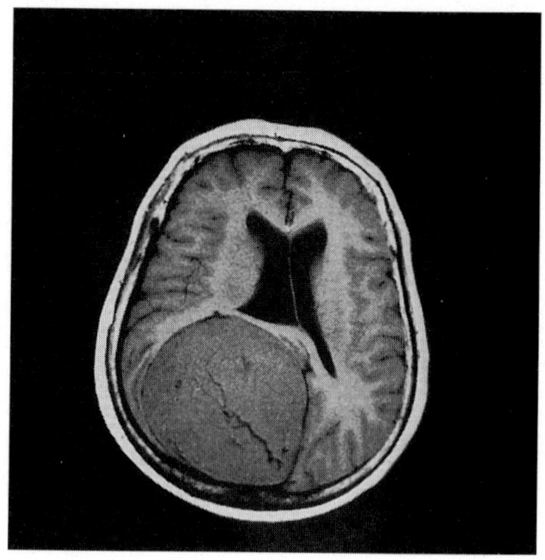

Fig. 4-2 Axial T_1-weighted image (500/15).

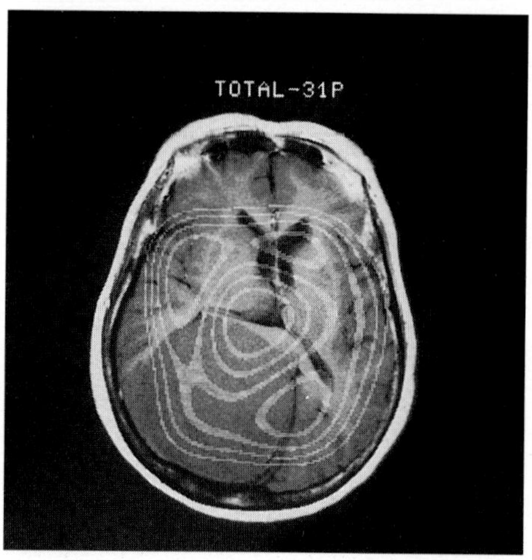

Fig. 4-3 Axial ^{31}P contour map superimposed on T_1-weighted image (500/15).

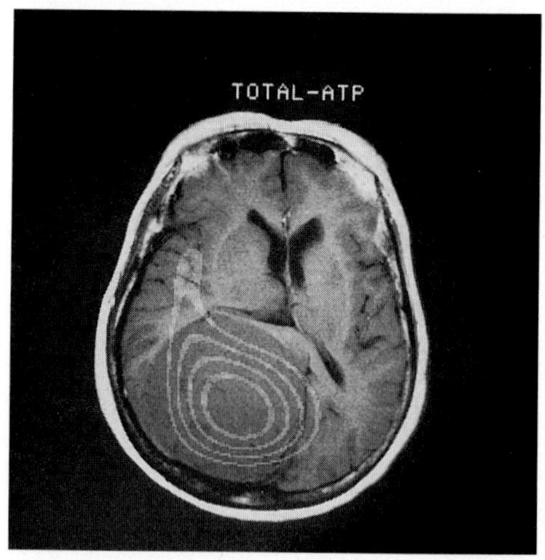

Fig. 4-4 Axial total ATP contour map superimposed on T_1-weighted image (500/15).

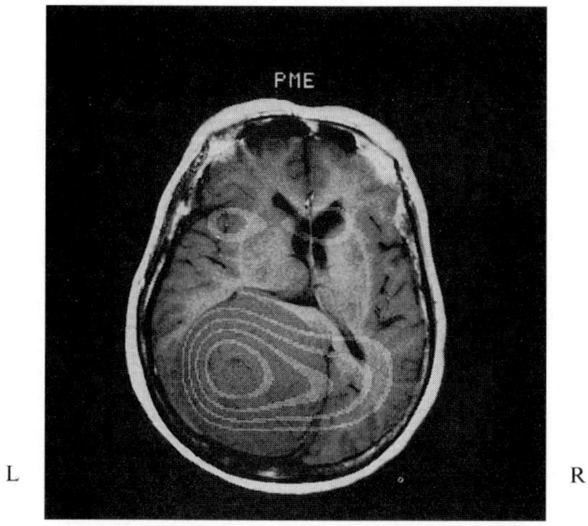

Fig. 4-5 Axial PME contour map superimposed on T_1-weighted image (500/15).

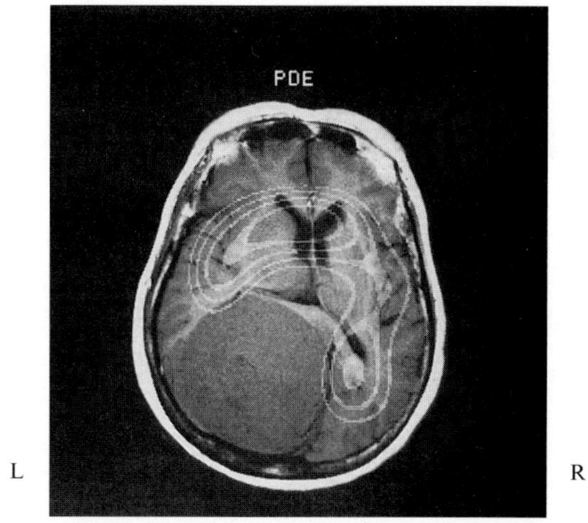

Fig. 4-6 Axial PDE contour map superimposed on T_1-weighted image (500/15).

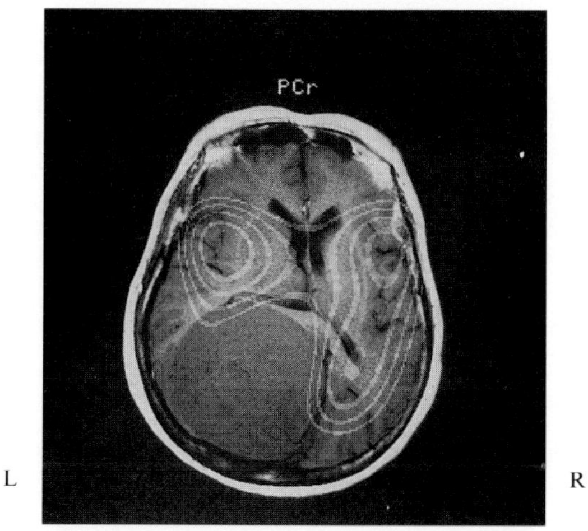

Fig. 4-7 Axial PCr contour map superimposed on T_1-weighted image (500/15).

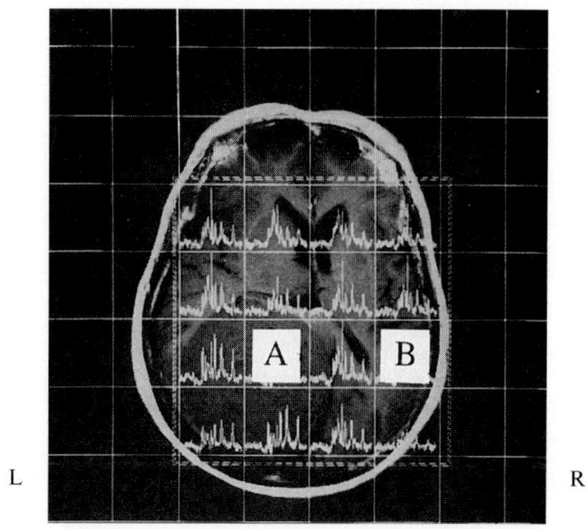

Fig. 4-8 T_1-weighted image showing the position of $3 \times 3 \times 4$ cm^3 voxels A and B.

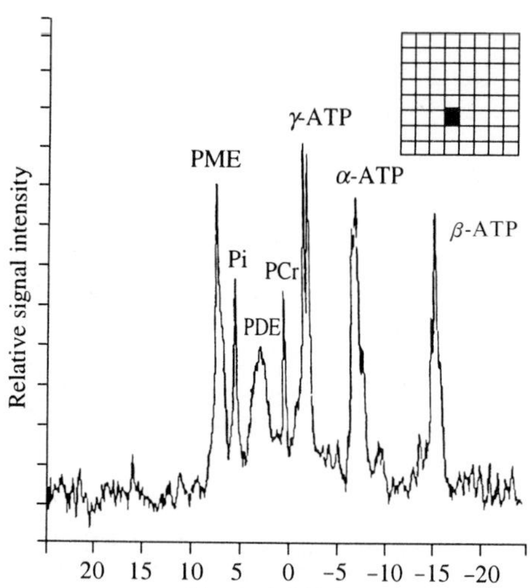

Fig. 4-9 ^{31}P spectrum in tumor area (voxel A).

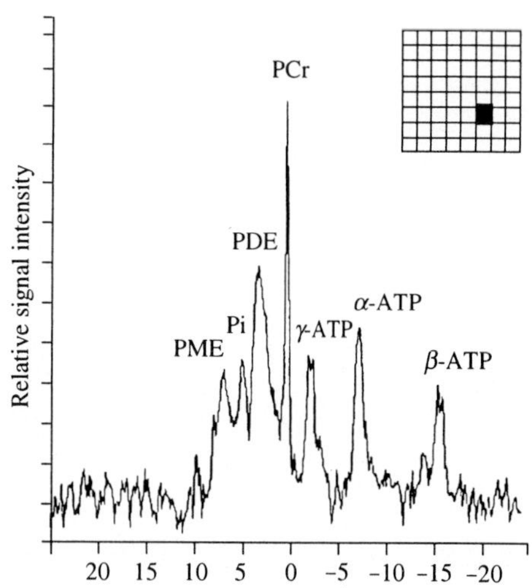

Fig. 4-10 ^{31}P spectrum in control area (voxel B).

CASE 5

Case 5: A 67-year-old female

Meningioma

The patient complained of dizziness and occipital headache. The neurological examination was normal. The MRIs in Figures 5-1 and 2 demonstrate a meningioma in the right posterior fossa. Mild edema is noted around the tumor. The signal intensity of the tumor remains unchanged in the contour maps of ^{31}P, total ATP, PME, and PDE in Figures 5-3, 4, 5, and 7. It is slightly increased in the Pi contour map in Figure 5-6. Figures 5-9 and 5-10 show the spectra of a normal control area and the tumor area. The findings are as mentioned above.

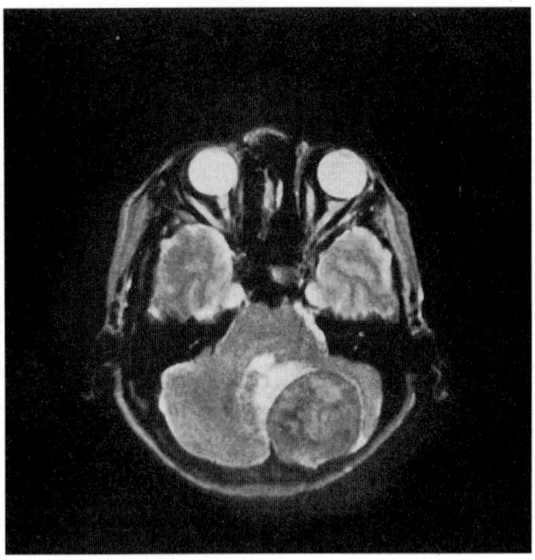

Fig. 5-1 Axial T_2-weighted image (2,200/90).

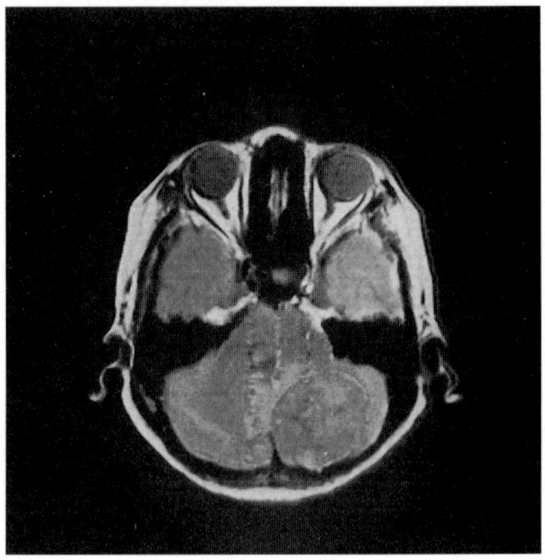

Fig. 5-2 Axial proton density-weighted image (2,200/15).

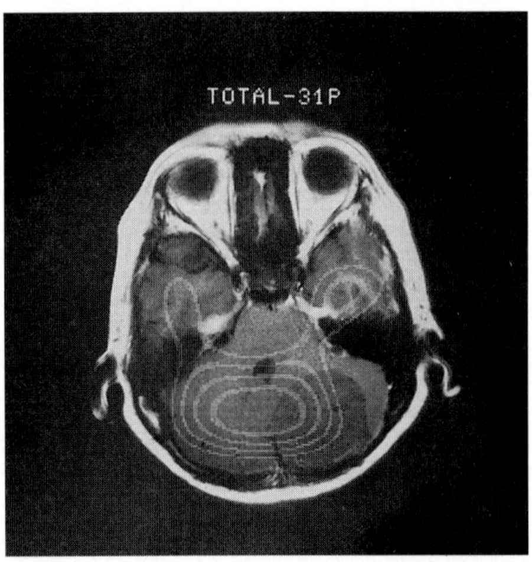

Fig. 5-3 Axial ^{31}P contour map superimposed on T_1- weighted image (500/15).

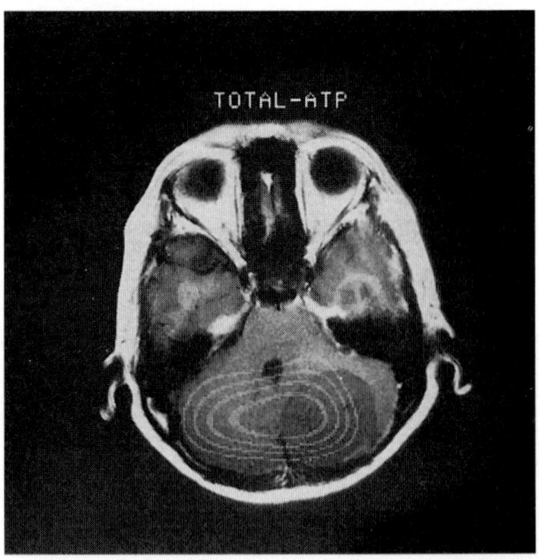

Fig. 5-4 Axial total ATP contour map superimposed on T_1-weighted image (500/15).

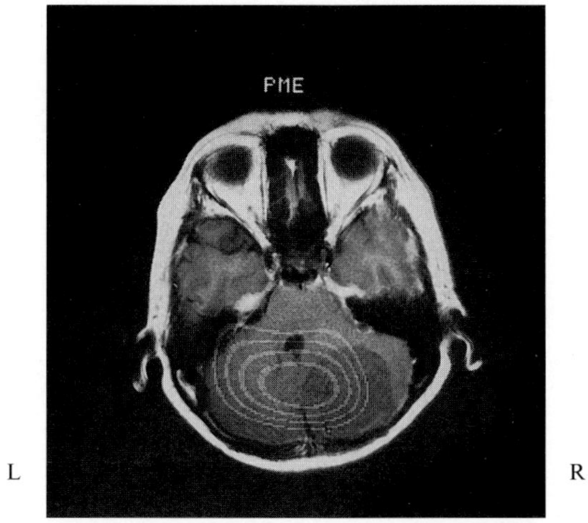

Fig. 5-5 Axial PME contour map superimposed on T_1-weighted image (500/15).

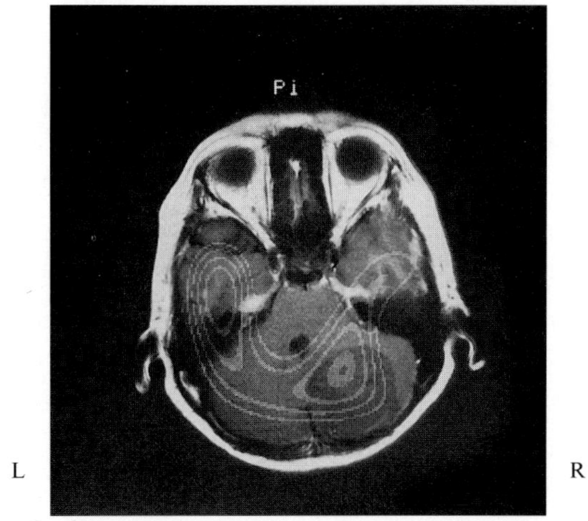

Fig. 5-6 Axial Pi contour map superimposed on T_1-weighted image (500/15).

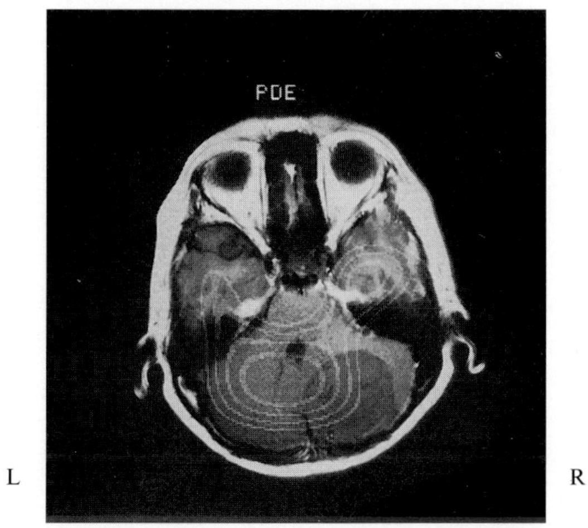

Fig. 5-7 Axial PDE contour map superimposed on T_1-weighted image (500/15).

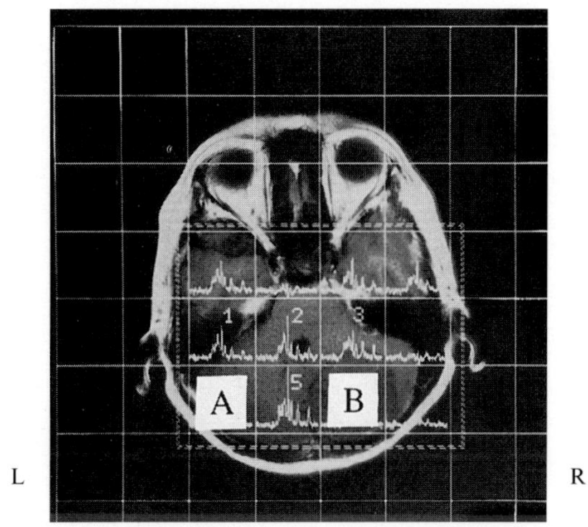

Fig. 5-8 T_1-weighted image showing the position of $3 \times 3 \times 4$ cm^3 voxels A and B.

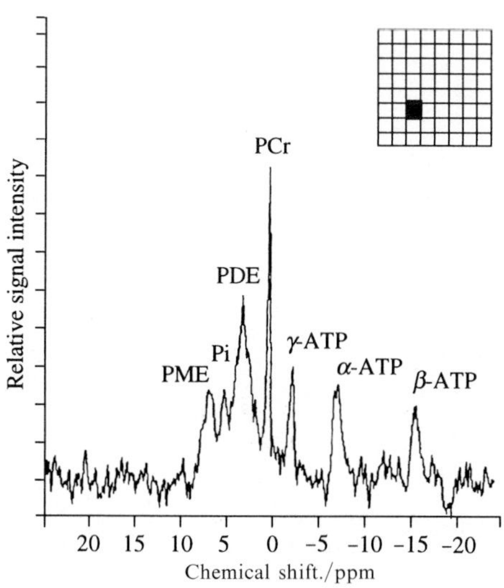

Fig. 5-9 ^{31}P spectrum in control area (voxel A).

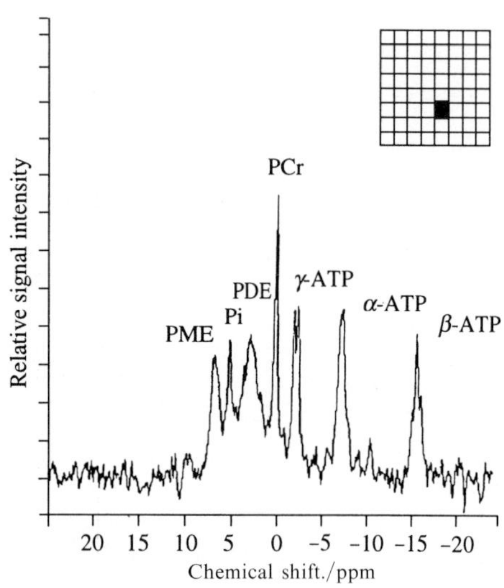

Fig. 5-10 ^{31}P spectrum in tumor area (voxel B).

CASE 6

Case 6: A 46-year-old male

Neurinoma

The patient suffered left visual loss with a history extending over three years. He noticed a loss of left facial sensation and left deafness extending over 6 months. The neurological examination revealed left multiple cranial nerve (I -VIII and IX) palsies. The MRIs in Figures 6-1 and 2 reveal a neurinoma occupying the left middle fossa. Mild brain edema is noted around the tumor. The signal intensity is reduced in the tumor in the ^{31}P, total ATP, PDE contour maps in Figures 6-3, 4, and 7. It is increased in the PME and Pi contour maps in Figures 6-5 and 6. Figures 6-9 and 6-10 show the spectra of a normal control area and the tumor area. The findings are as mentioned above.

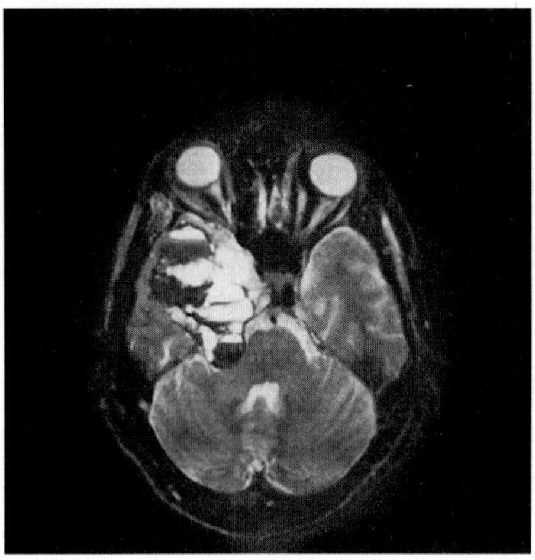

Fig. 6-1 Axial T_2-weighted image (2,200/90).

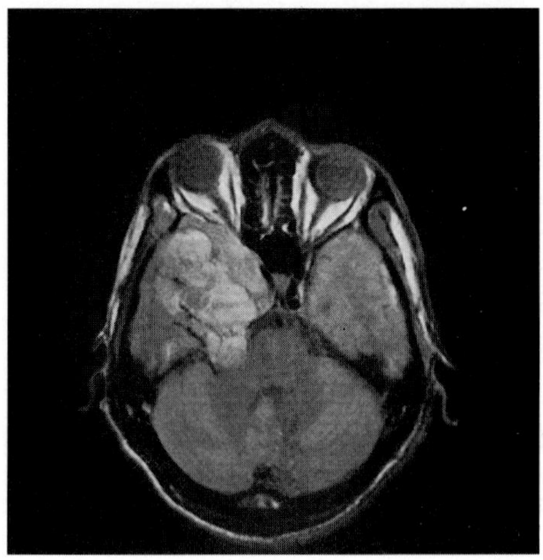

Fig. 6-2 Axial proton density-weighted image (2,200/15).

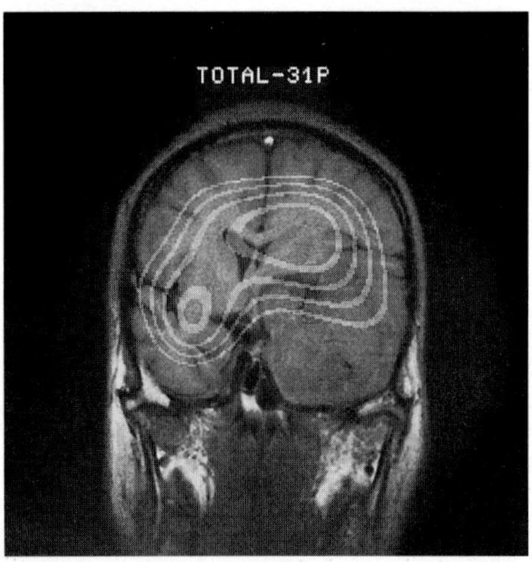

Fig. 6-3 Coronal ^{31}P contour map superimposed on T_1-weighted image (500/15).

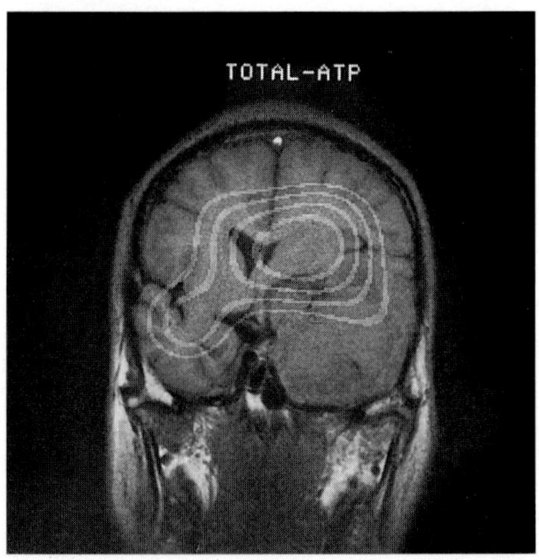

Fig. 6-4 Coronal total ATP contour map superimposed on T_1-weighted image (500/15).

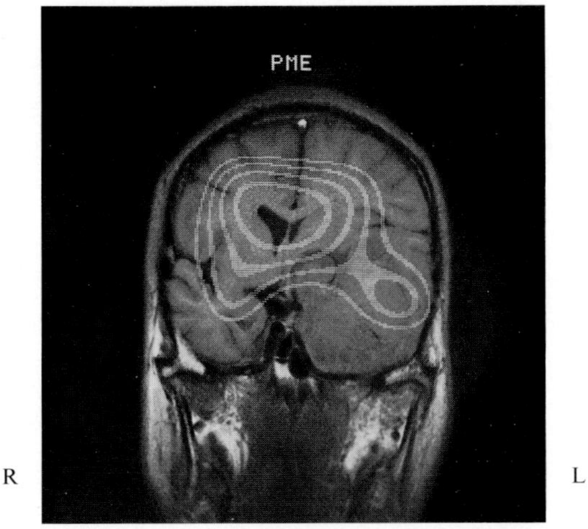

Fig. 6-5 Coronal PME contour map superimposed on T_1-weighted image (500/15).

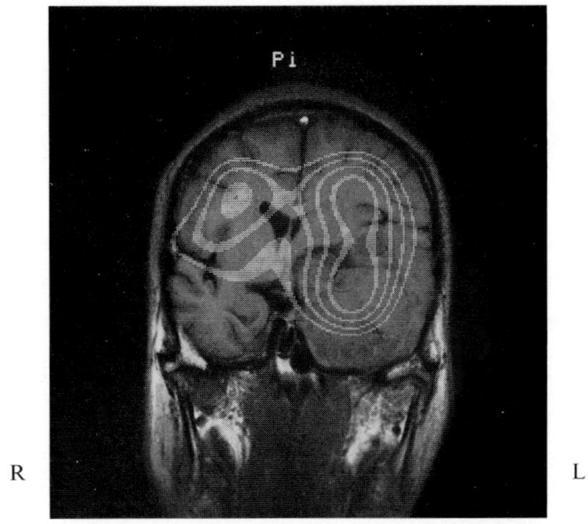

Fig. 6-6 Coronal Pi contour map superimposed on T_1-weighted image (500/15).

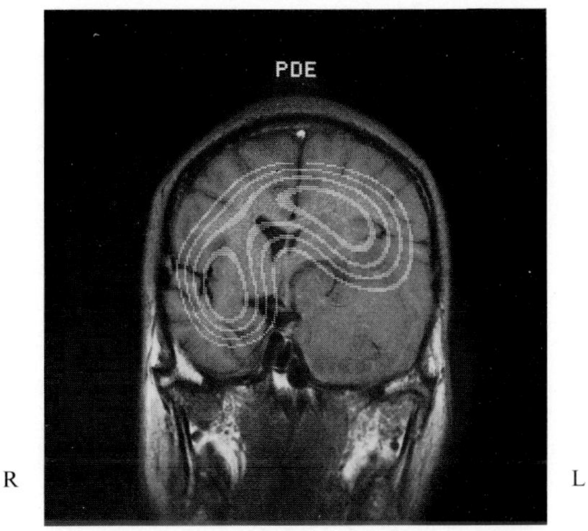

Fig. 6-7 Coronal PDE contour map superimposed on T_1-weighted image (500/15).

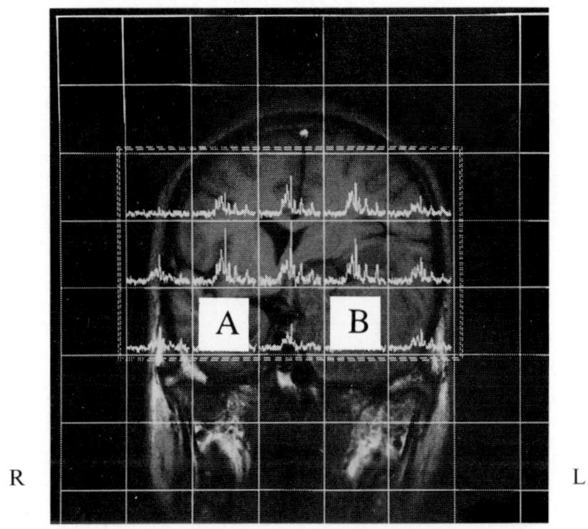

Fig. 6-8 T_1-weighted image showing the position of $3\times3\times4$ cm^3 voxels A and B.

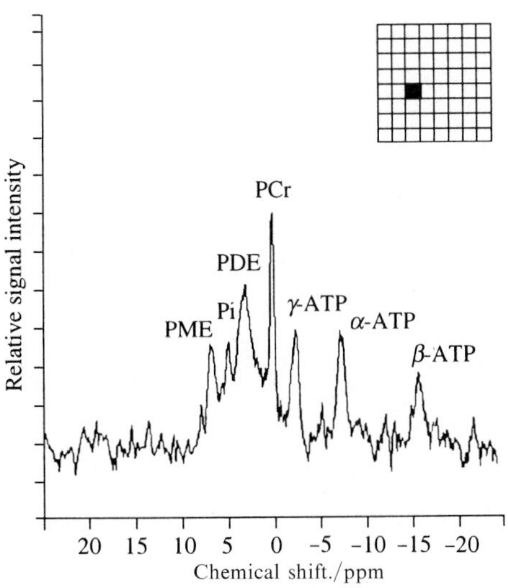

Fig. 6-9 ^{31}P spectrum in control area (voxel A).

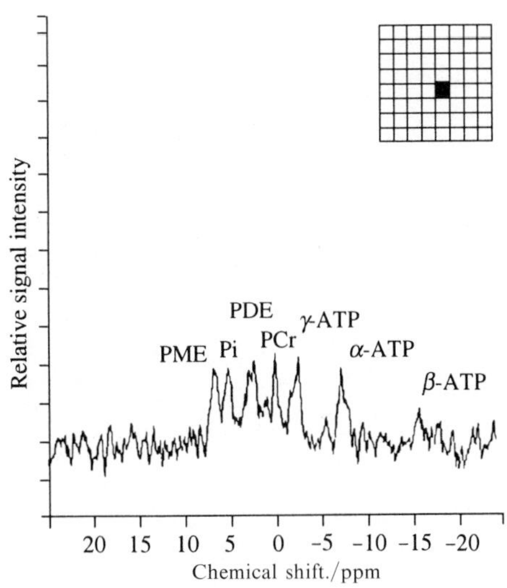

Fig. 6-10 ^{31}P spectrum in tumor area (voxel B).

CASE 7

Case 7: A 67-year-old male

Epidermoid

The patient complained of dizziness with a history extending over seven months. The neurological examination revealed truncal ataxia. The MRIs in Figures 7-1 and 2 demonstrate an epidermoid in the posterior fossa and the median part of the cerebellum. Mild edema is noted around the tumor. The signal intensity of the tumor is slightly reduced in the ^{31}P, total ATP, and PDE contour maps in Figures 7-3, 4, and 7. It is increased in the tumor area in the PME and Pi contour maps in Figures 7-5 and 6. Figures 7-9 and 7-10 show the spectra of the tumor area and normal control area, respectively. The findings are as mentioned above.

L 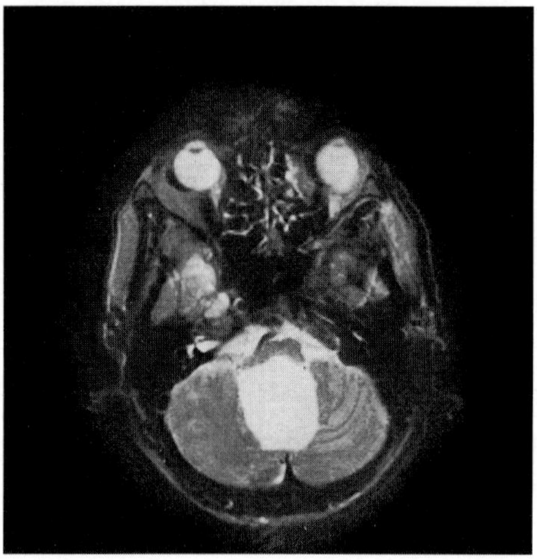 R

Fig. 7-1 Axial T_2-weighted image (2,200/90).

L 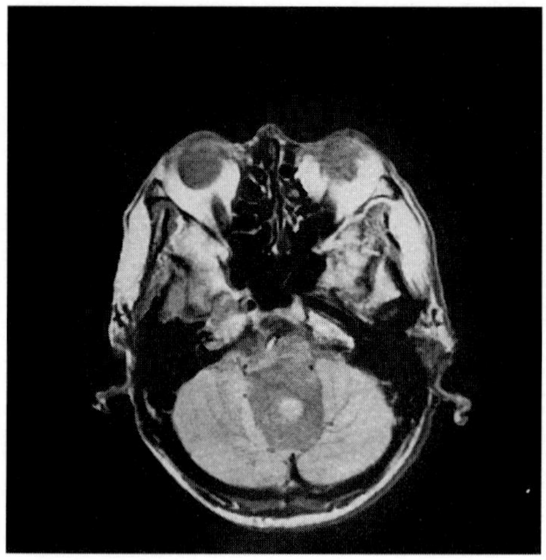 R

Fig. 7-2 Axial proton density-weighted image (2,200/15).

L 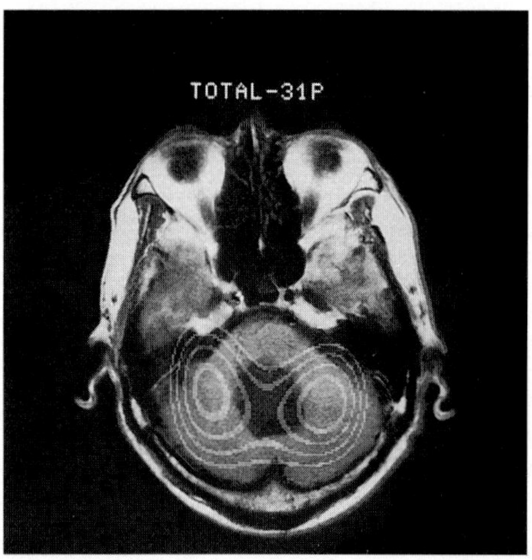 R

Fig. 7-3 Axial ^{31}P contour map superimposed on T_1-weighted image (500/15).

L 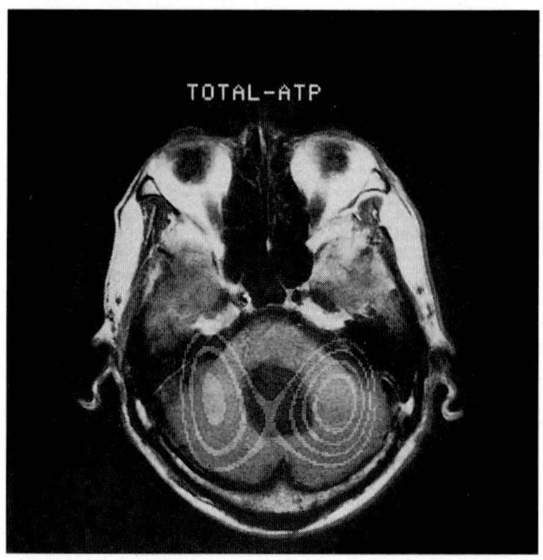 R

Fig. 7-4 Axial total ATP contour map superimposed on T_1-weighted image (500/15).

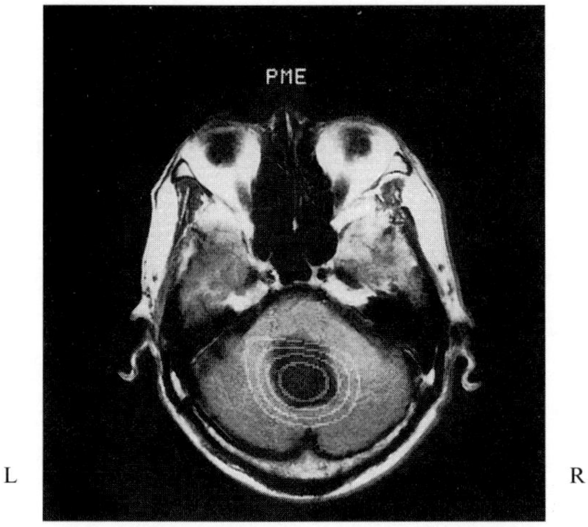

Fig. 7-5 Axial PME contour map superimposed on T_1-weighted image (500/15).

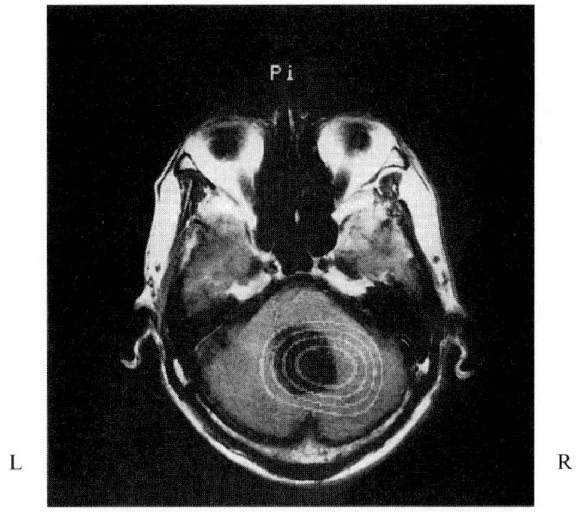

Fig. 7-6 Axial Pi contour map superimposed on T_1-weighted image (500/15).

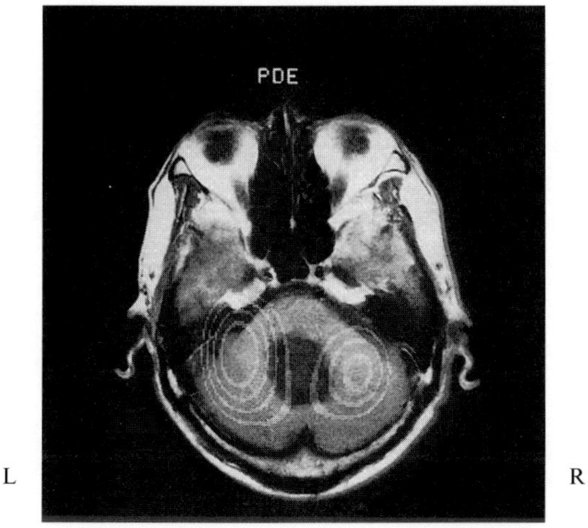

Fig. 7-7 Axial PDE contour map superimposed on T_1-weighted image (500/15).

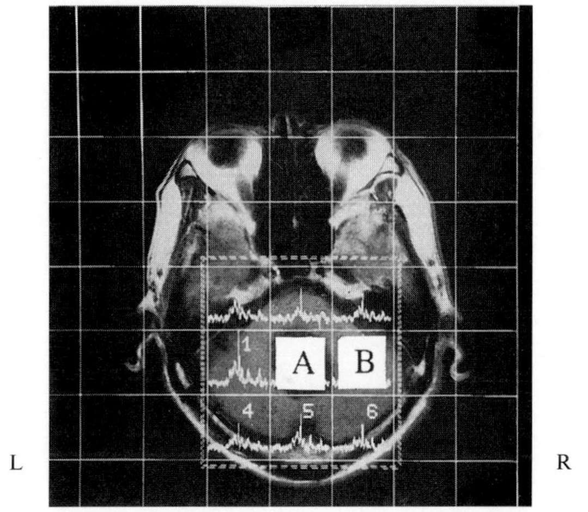

Fig. 7-8 T_1-weighted image showing the position of $3 \times 3 \times 4$ cm^3 voxels A and B.

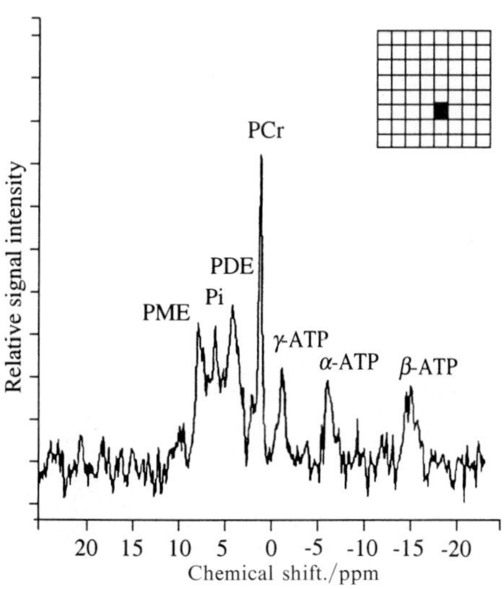

Fig. 7-9 ^{31}P spectrum in tumor area (voxel A).

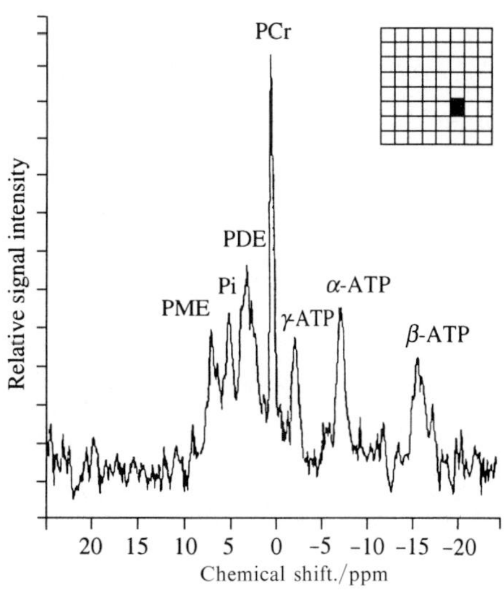

Fig. 7-10 ^{31}P spectrum in control area (voxel B).

CASE 8

Case 8: A 53-year-old male

Astrocytoma (grade I)

The patient suffered a syncopal attack with a history extending over two years and nine months. He visited a hospital because of these attacks. The neurological examination was normal. The MRIs in Figures 8-1 and 2 show a tumor in the left temporal area. Mild brain edema is noted around the tumor. The signal intensity of the tumor area is slightly reduced in the ^{31}P, total ATP, and PDE contour maps in Figures 8-3, 4, and 7. It is slightly reduced in the tumor area in the PME contour map in Figure 8-5. The signal intensity is slightly higher in the tumor area than in the surrounding tissues in the Pi contour map in Figure 8-6. Figures 8-9 and 8-10 show the spectra of the normal control area and the tumor area. The findings are as described above.

L 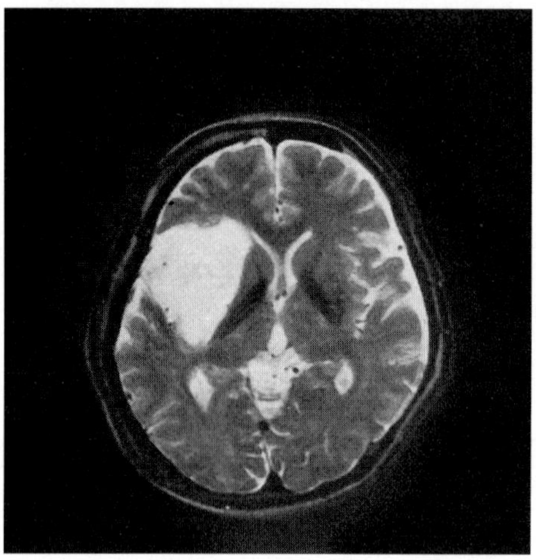 R

Fig. 8-1 Axial T_2-weighted image (2,200/90).

L 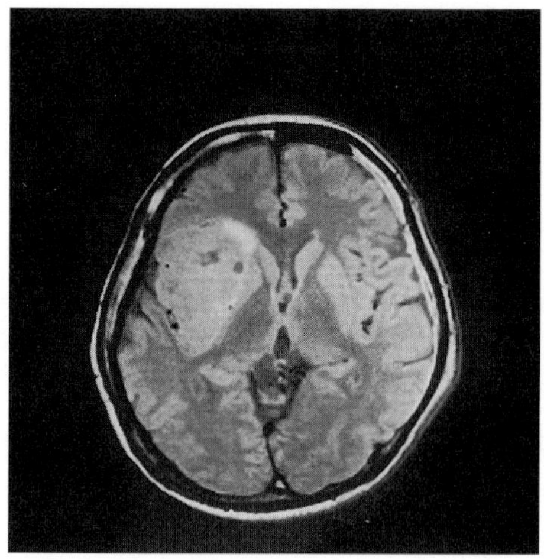 R

Fig. 8-2 Axial proton density-weighted image (2,200/15).

R 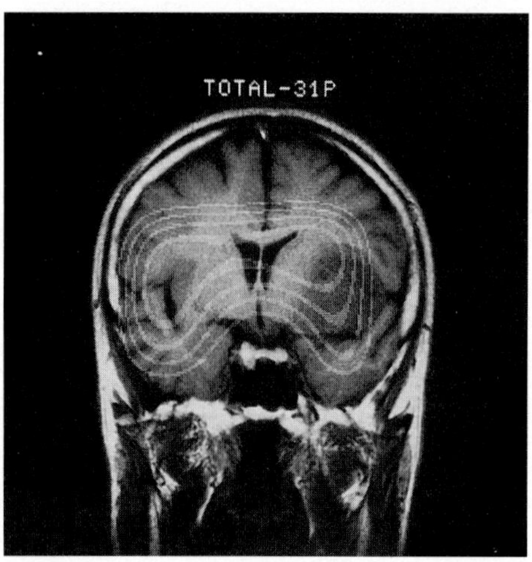 L

Fig. 8-3 Coronal ^{31}P contour map superimposed on T_1-weighted image (500/15).

R 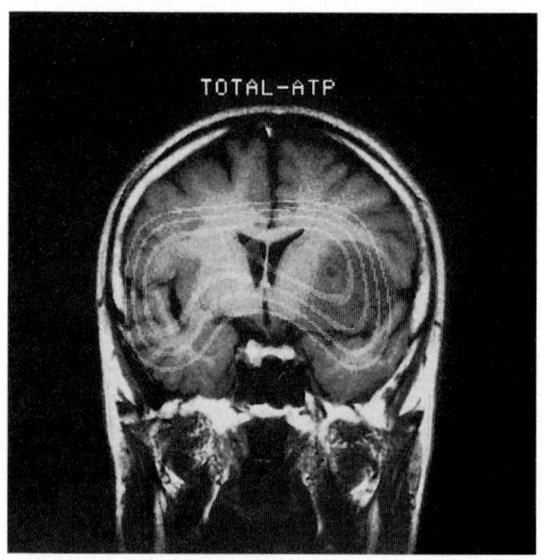 L

Fig. 8-4 Coronal total ATP contour map superimposed on T_1-weighted image (500/15).

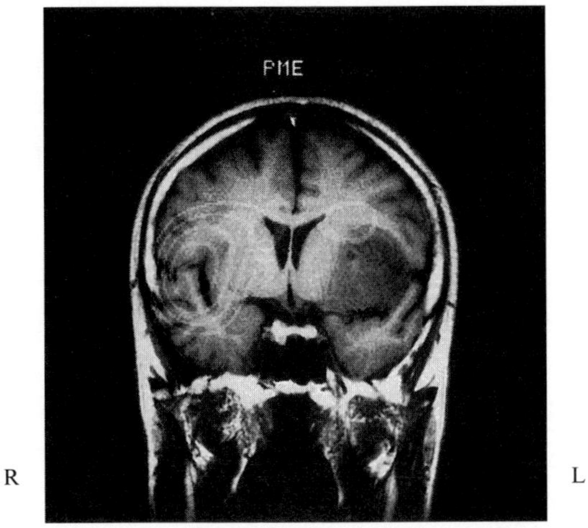

Fig. 8-5 Coronal PME contour map superimposed on T_1-weighted image (500/15).

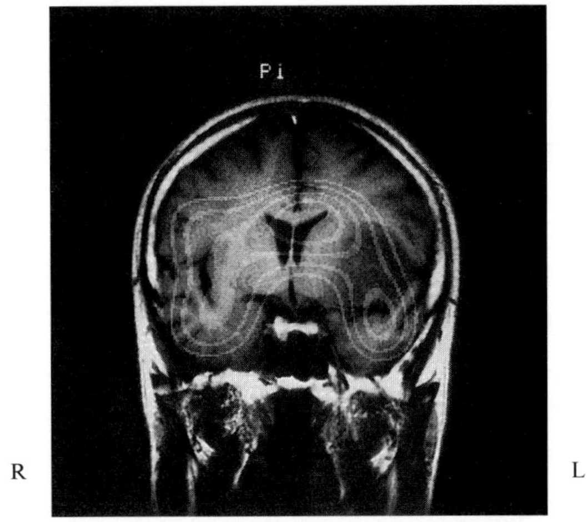

Fig. 8-6 Coronal Pi contour map superimposed on T_1-weighted image (500/15).

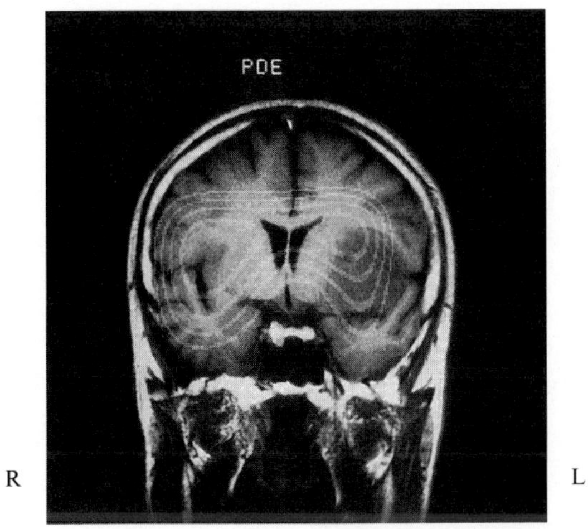

Fig. 8-7 Coronal PDE contour map superimposed on T_1-weighted image (500/15).

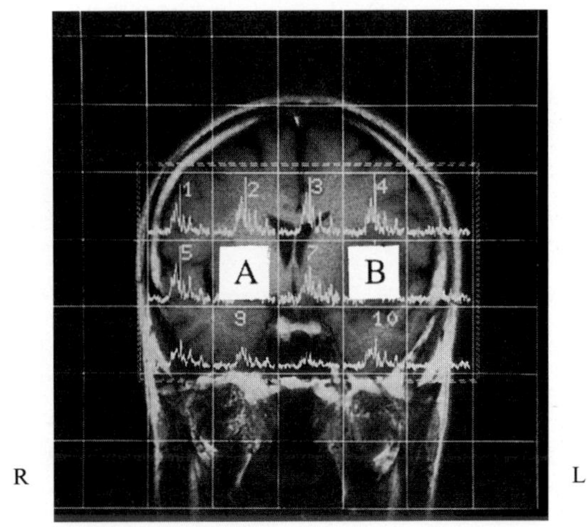

Fig. 8-8 T_1-weighted image showing the position of $3 \times 3 \times 4\ cm^3$ voxels A and B.

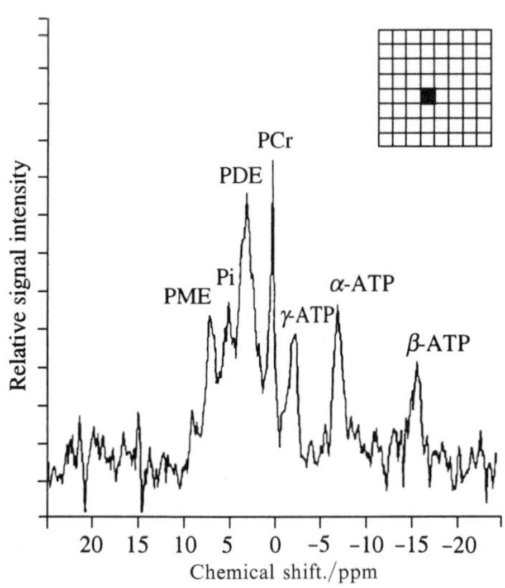

Fig. 8-9 ^{31}P spectrum in control area (voxel A).

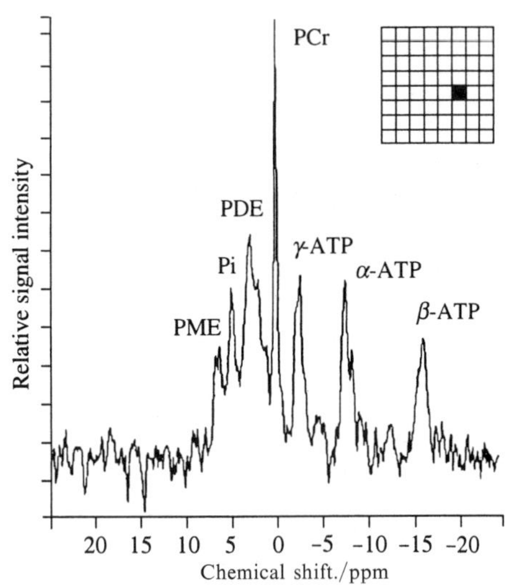

Fig. 8-10 ^{31}P spectrum in tumor area (voxel B).

CASE 9

Case 9: A 35-year-old female

Astrocytoma (grade II)

Evaluations before and after ACNU chemotherapy

The patient suffered from convulsions with a history extending over 15 years. She was diagnosed as having a brain tumor, but she refused therapy 7 years ago. She complained of right hemiparesis and frequent attacks of seizures and visited a hospital. Radiation therapy was performed 4 years ago. She complained of right hemiparesis again one year ago and again received radiation therapy. She noticed worsening right hemiparesis and was readmitted. Intra-arterial infusion of ACNU was performed for recurrent brain tumor. Figure 9-1 shows the spectra of 16× 16 voxels of a patient with astrocytoma grade II of the bilateral thalamus. Figure 9-2 shows changes in MRI from before to after intra-arterial infusion of ACNU. No enlargement of the tumor is observed, and its size is slightly reduced. Figure 9-3 shows changes in the ^{31}P, PCr, total ATP, Pi, PDE, and PME metabolite images from before to after intra-arterial infusion of ACNU.

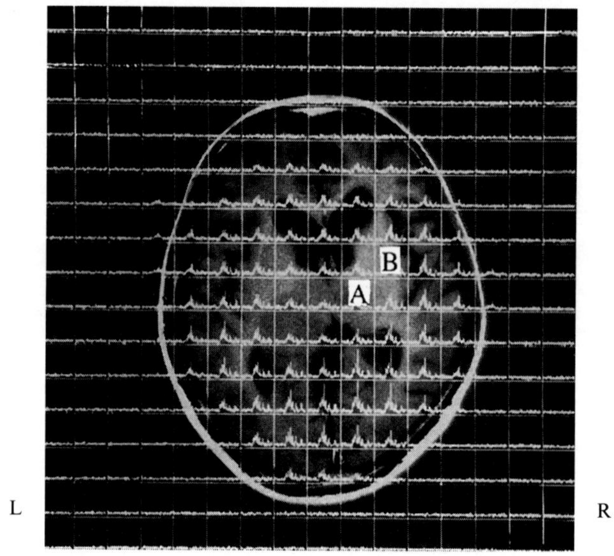

Fig. 9-1 T_1-weighted image showing the position of $1.5 \times 1.5 \times 4$ cm^3 voxels A and B.

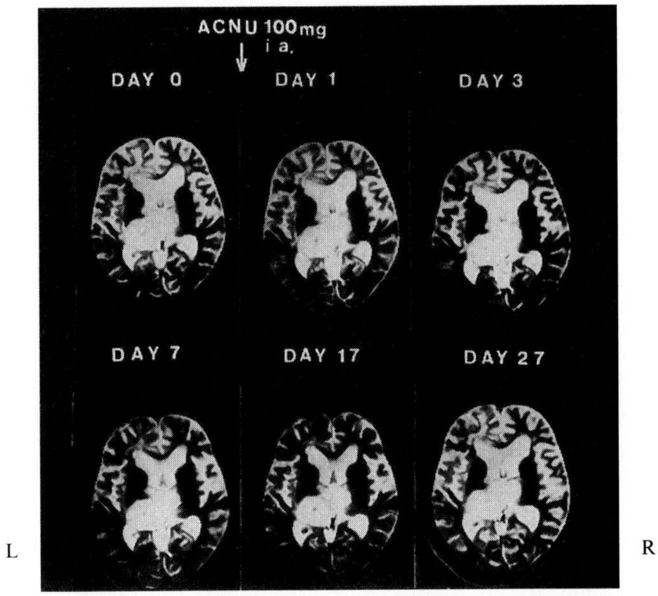

Fig. 9-2 Axial T_2-weighted image (2,200/90) of astrocytoma grade II before and after treatment.

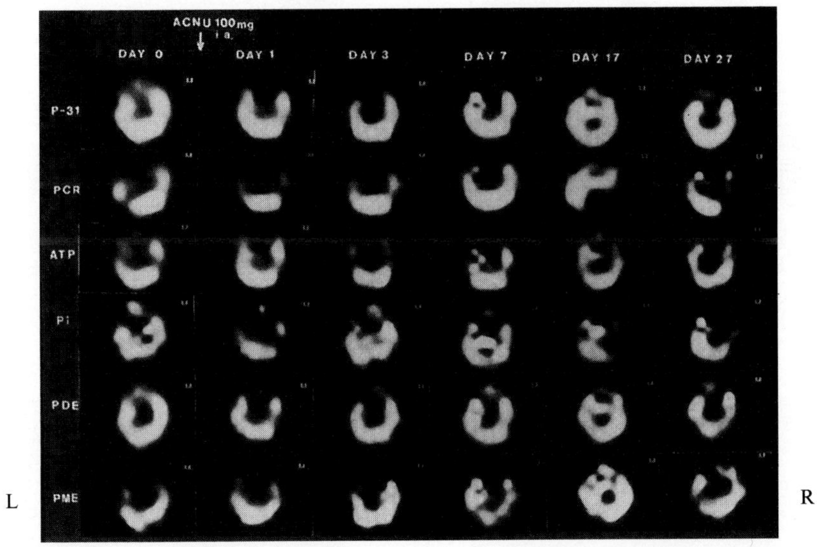

Fig. 9-3 Axial ^{31}P metabolite images of astrocytoma grade II before and after treatment.

Astrocytoma (grade II)

Before ACNU therapy

Tumors can be observed in the bilateral thalami in the MRIs in Figures 9-4 and 5. Mild brain edema is noted around the tumor. The signal intensity of the tumor area is reduced in the ^{31}P, total ATP, PME, PDE, and PCr metabolite images in Figures 9-6, 7, 8, 10, and 11. It is slightly increased in the Pi metabolite image in Figure 9-9. Figures 9-13 and 9-12 show the spectra of the tumor area and normal control area. The findings are as described above.

L 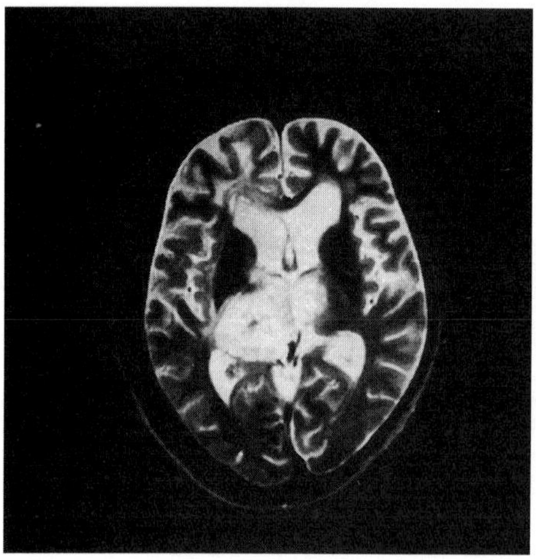 R

Fig. 9-4 Axial T_2-weighted image (2,200/90).

L 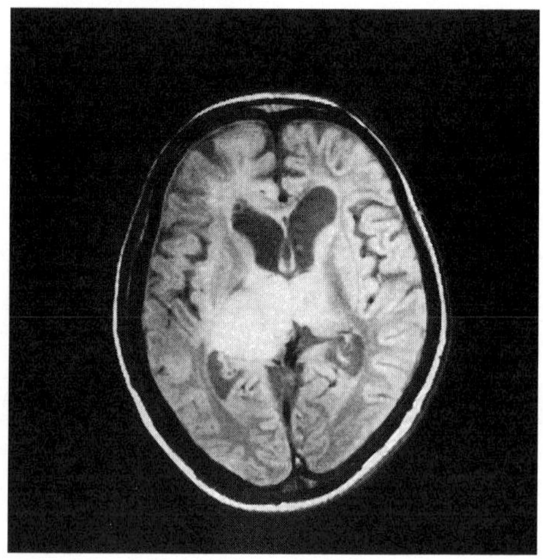 R

Fig. 9-5 Axial proton density-weighted image (2,200/15).

L 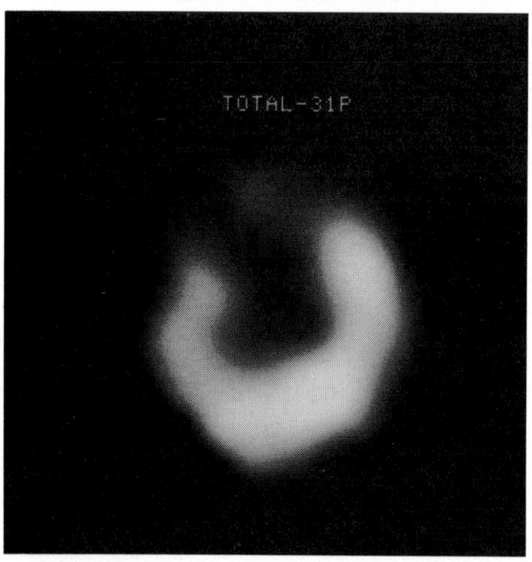 R

Fig. 9-6 Axial ^{31}P metabolite image.

L 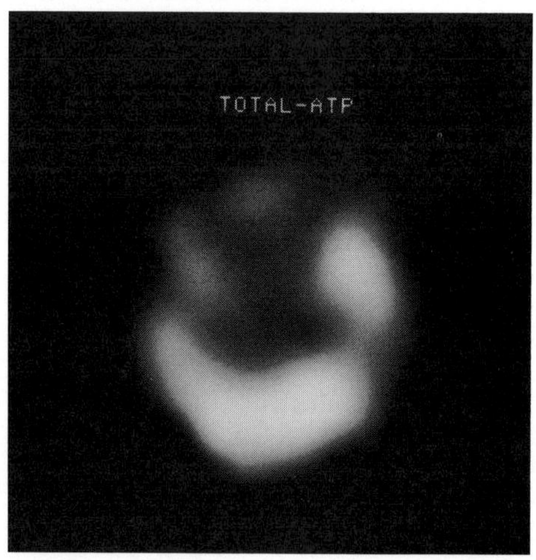 R

Fig. 9-7 Axial total ATP metabolite image.

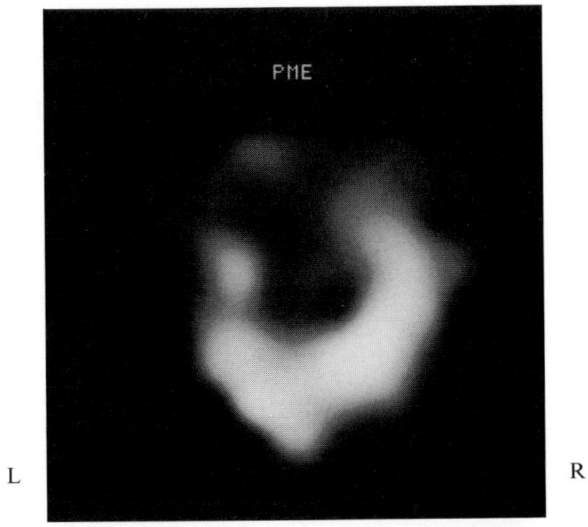

Fig. 9-8 Axial PME metabolite image.

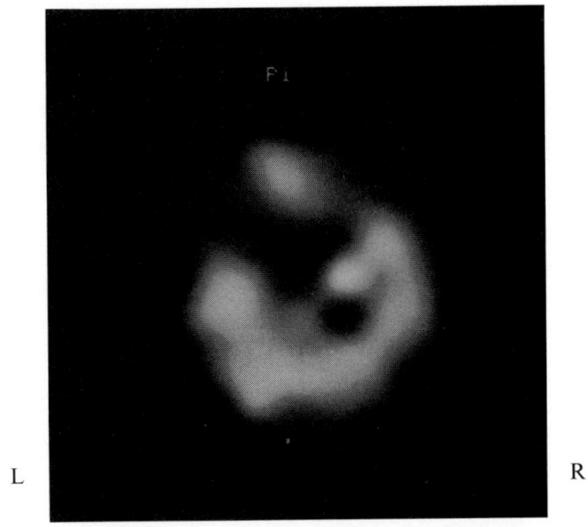

Fig. 9-9 Axial Pi metabolite image.

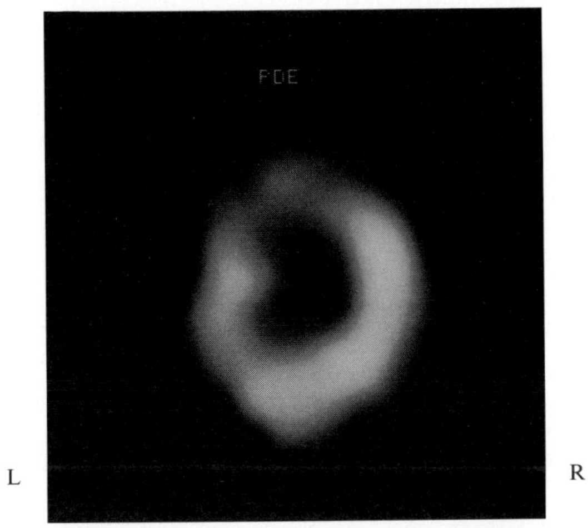

Fig. 9-10 Axial PDE metabolite image.

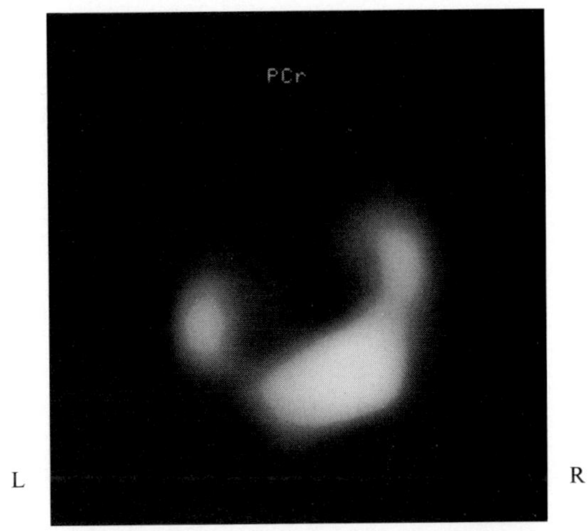

Fig. 9-11 Axial PCr metabolite image.

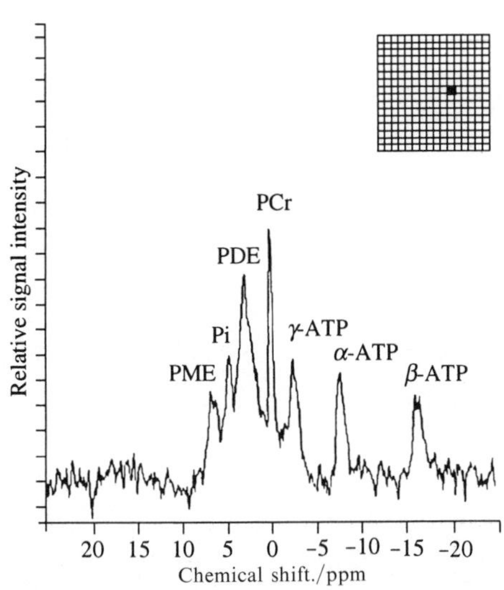

Fig. 9-12 ³¹P spectrum in control area (voxel B).

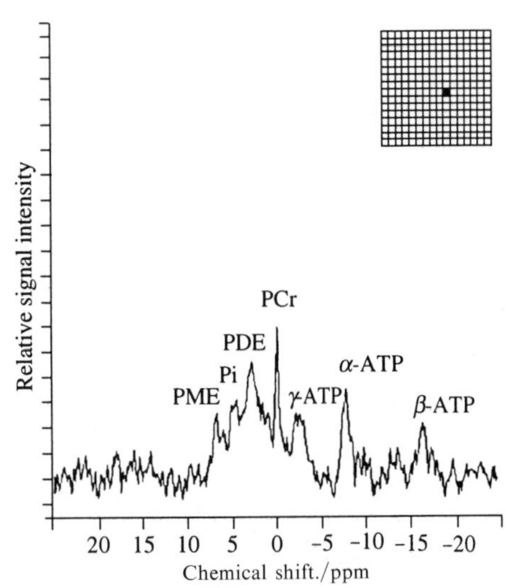

Fig. 9-13 ³¹P spectrum in tumor area (voxel A).

Astrocytoma (**grade** II)

1 day after ACNU therapy

Tumors can be observed in the bilateral thalami in the MRIs in Figures 9-14 and 15. Mild brain edema is noted around the tumor. The signal intensity of the tumor area is reduced in the ^{31}P, total ATP, PDE, and PCr metabolite images in Figures 9-16, 17, 20, and 21. It is slightly increased in the tumor area in the PME and Pi metabolite images in Figures 9-18 and 19. Figures 9-23 and 9-22 show the spectra of the tumor area and normal control area. The findings are as described above.

L 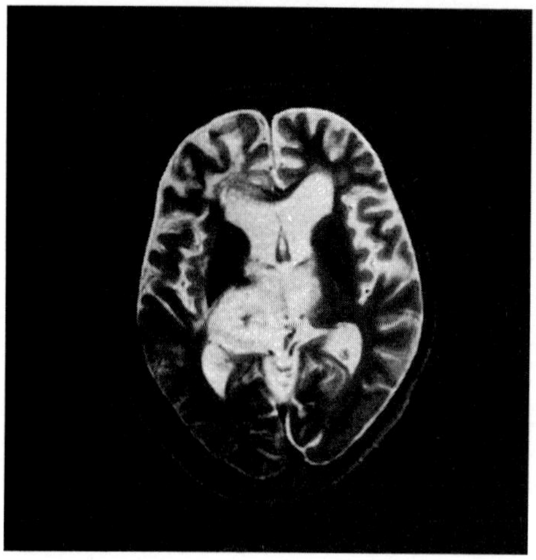 R

Fig. 9-14 Axial T_2-weighted image (2,200/90).

L 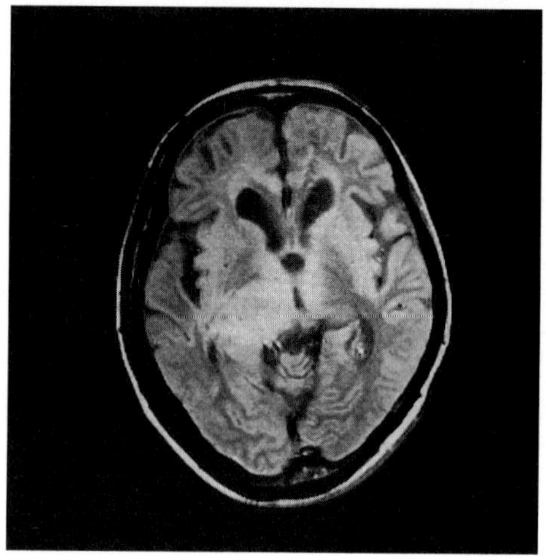 R

Fig. 9-15 Axial proton density-weighted image (2,200/15).

L 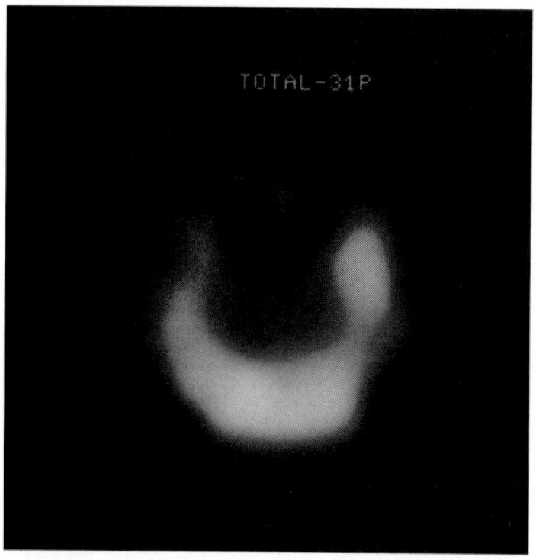 R

Fig. 9-16 Axial ^{31}P metabolite image.

L 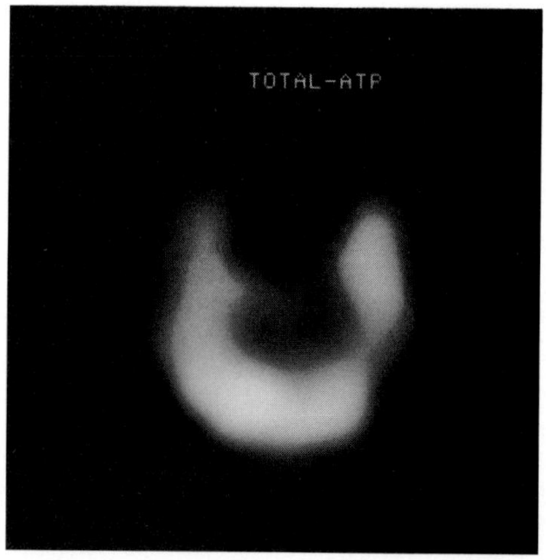 R

Fig. 9-17 Axial total ATP metabolite image.

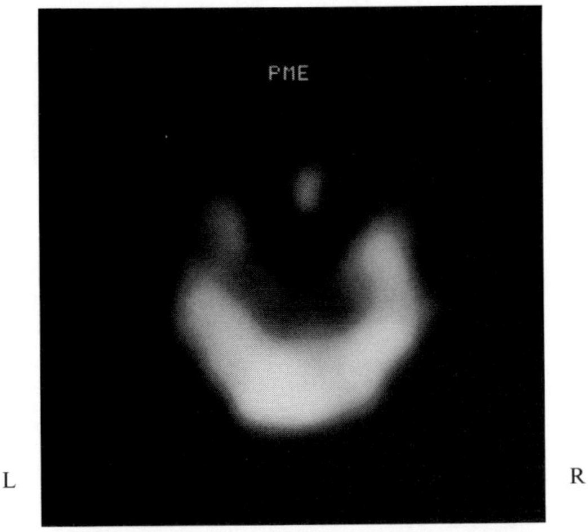

Fig. 9-18 Axial PME metabolite image.

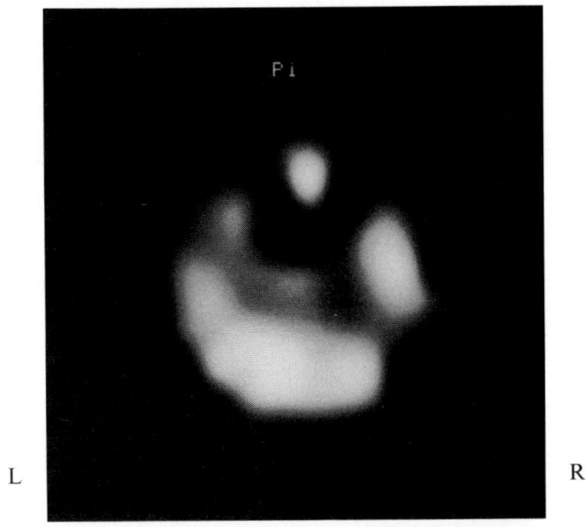

Fig. 9-19 Axial Pi metabolite image.

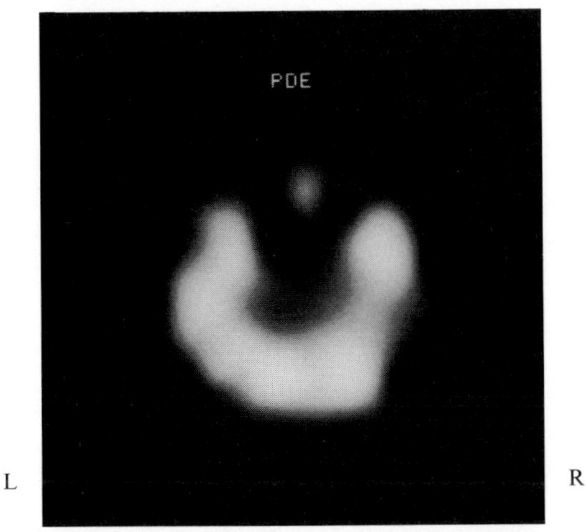

Fig. 9-20 Axial PDE metabolite image.

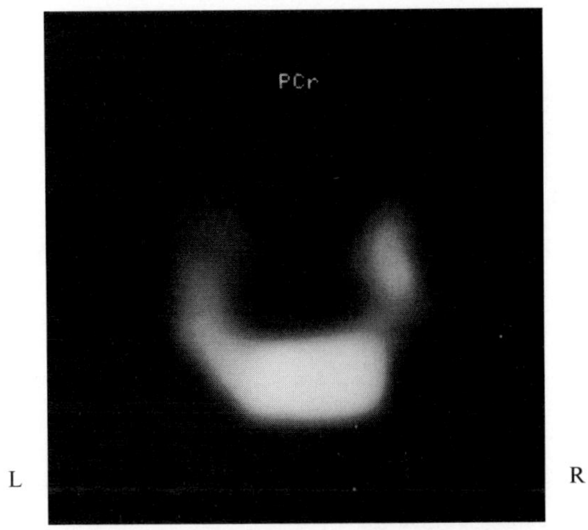

Fig. 9-21 Axial PCr metabolite image.

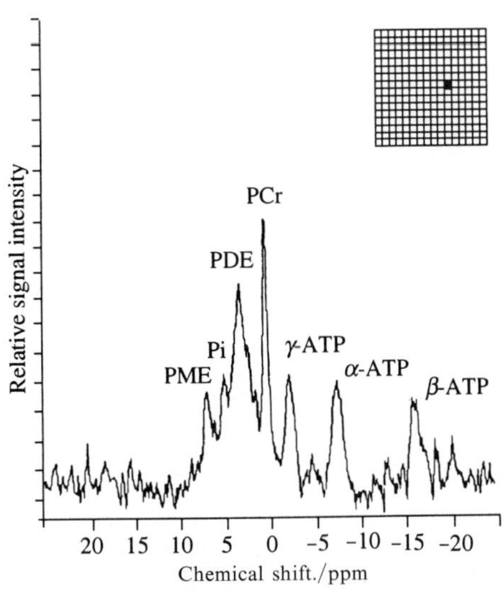

Fig. 9-22 ^{31}P spectrum in control area (voxel B).

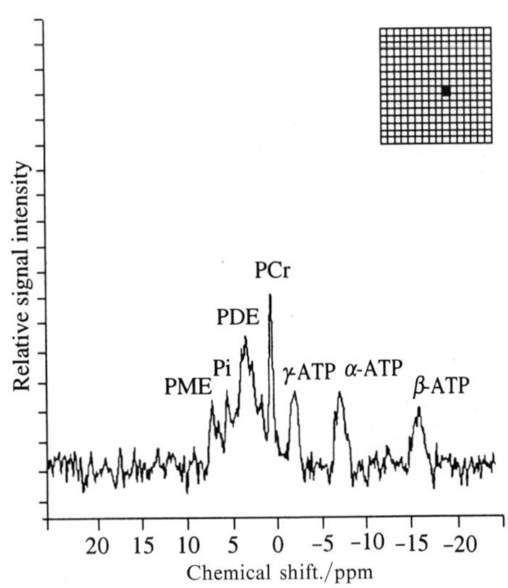

Fig. 9-23 ^{31}P spectrum in tumor area (voxel A).

Astrocytoma (grade II)

3 days after ACNU therapy

Tumors can be observed in the bilateral thalami in the MRIs in Figures 9-24 and 25. Mild brain edema is noted around the tumor. The signal intensity of the tumor area is reduced in the ^{31}P, total ATP, PDE, and PCr metabolite images in Figures 9-26, 27, 30, and 31. It is slightly decreased in the tumor area in the PME metabolite image in Figures 9-28 but is slightly increased in the Pi metabolite image in Figure 9-29. Figures 9-33 and 9-32 show the spectra of the tumor area and normal control area. The findings are as described above.

L 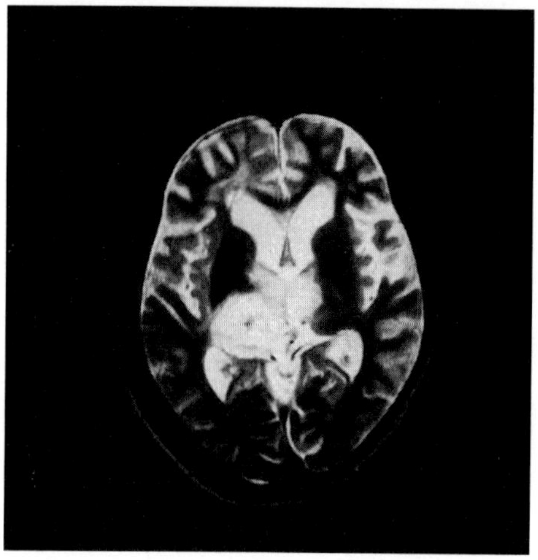 R

Fig. 9-24 Axial T_2-weighted image (2,200/90).

L 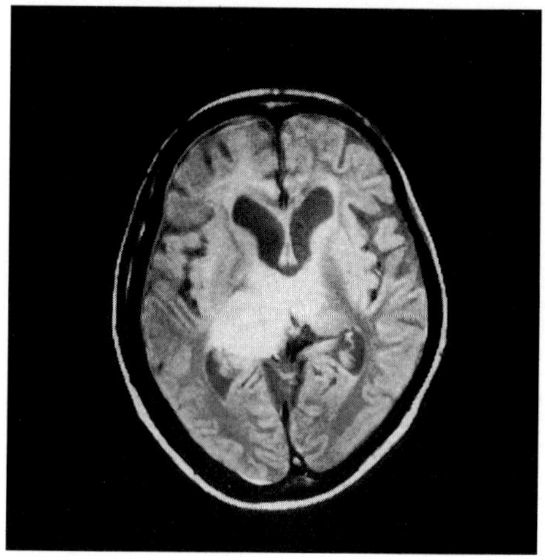 R

Fig. 9-25 Axial proton density-weighted image (2,200/15).

L 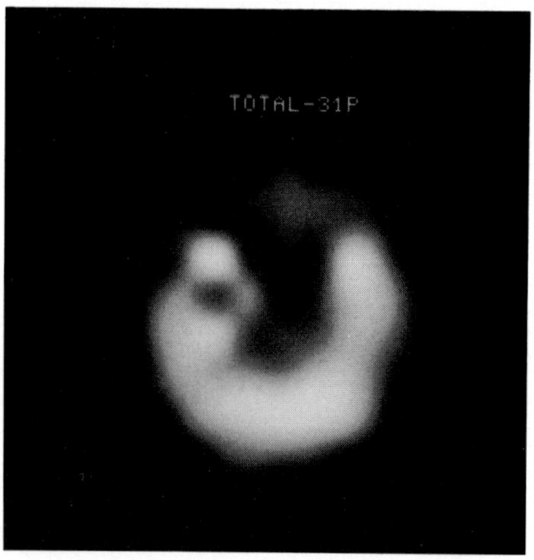 R

Fig. 9-26 Axial ^{31}P metabolite image.

L 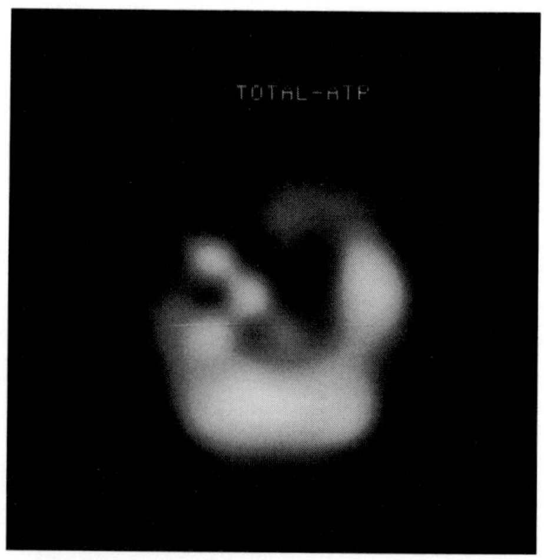 R

Fig. 9-27 Axial total ATP metabolite image.

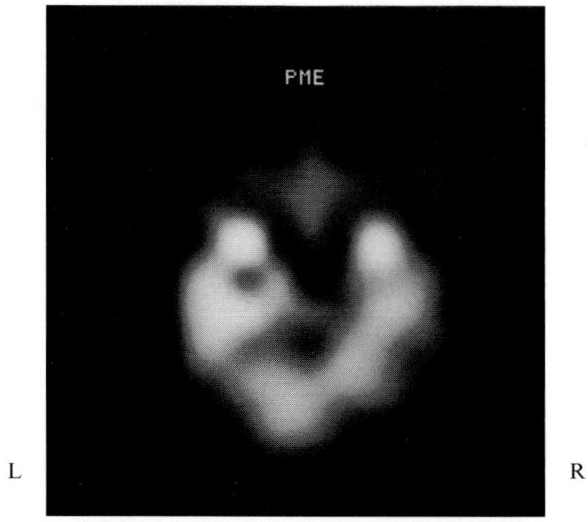

Fig. 9-28 Axial PME metabolite image.

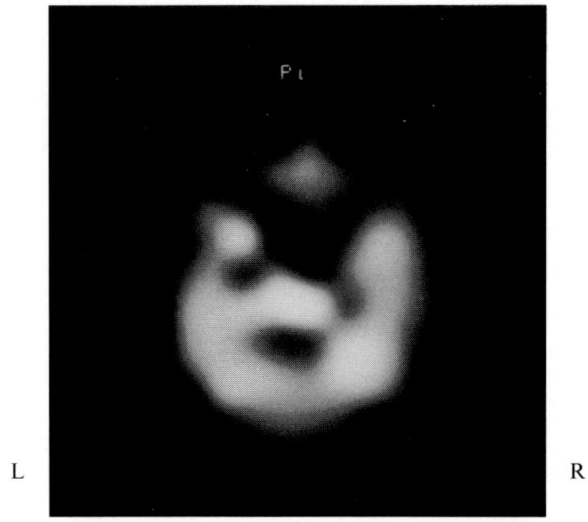

Fig. 9-29 Axial Pi metabolite image.

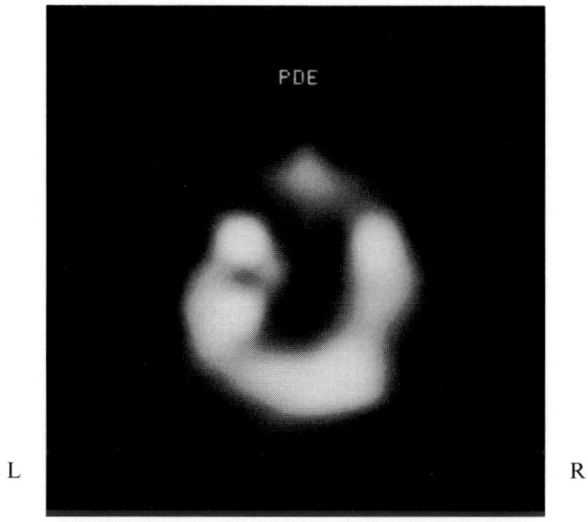

Fig. 9-30 Axial PDE metabolite image.

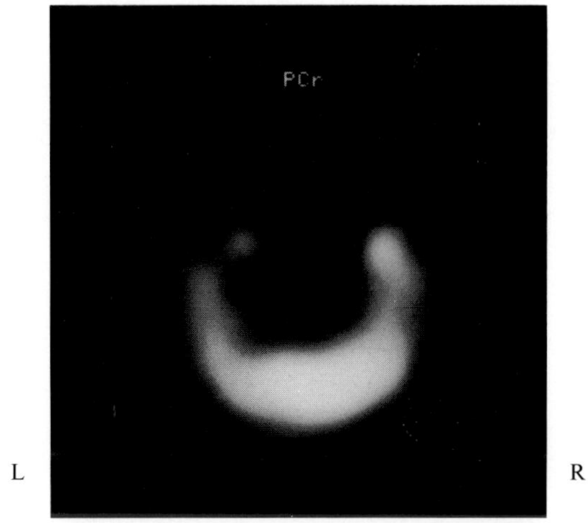

Fig. 9-31 Axial PCr metabolite image.

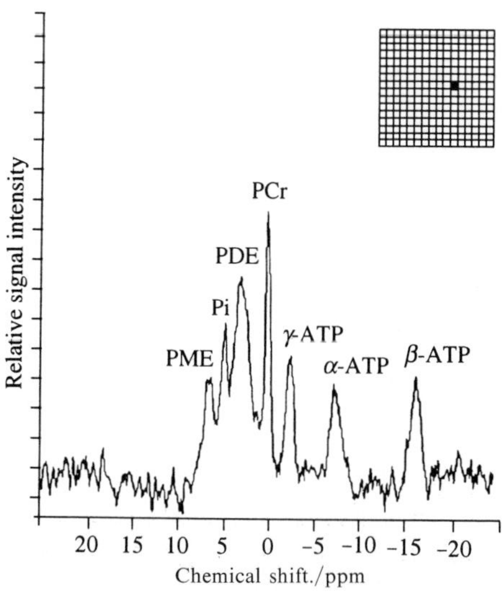

Fig. 9-32 ^{31}P spectrum in control area (voxel B).

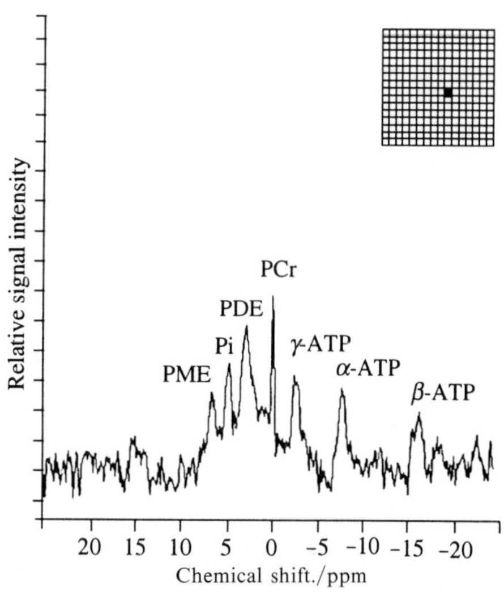

Fig. 9-33 ^{31}P spectrum in tumor area (voxel A).

Astrocytoma (grade II)

7 days after ACNU therapy

Tumors can be observed in the bilateral thalami in the MRIs in Figures 9-34 and 35. Mild brain edema is noted around the tumor. The tumors have begun to decrease slightly in size. The signal intensity of the tumor area is reduced in the ^{31}P, total ATP, PME, PDE, and PCr metabolite images in Figures 9-36, 37, 38, 40, and 41. It is increased in the Pi metabolite image in Figure 9-39. Figures 9-43 and 9-42 show the spectra of the tumor area and normal control area. The findings are as described above.

L 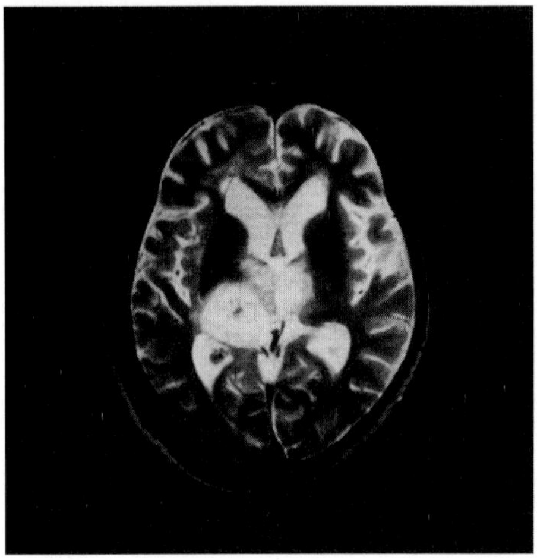 R

Fig. 9-34 Axial T_2-weighted image (2,200/90).

L 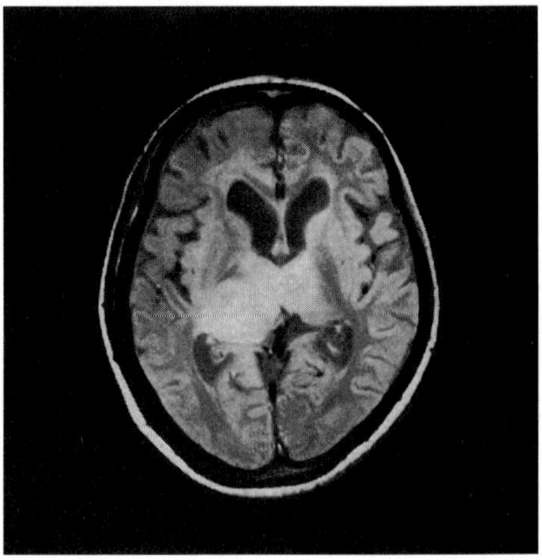 R

Fig. 9-35 Axial proton density-weighted image (2,200/15).

L 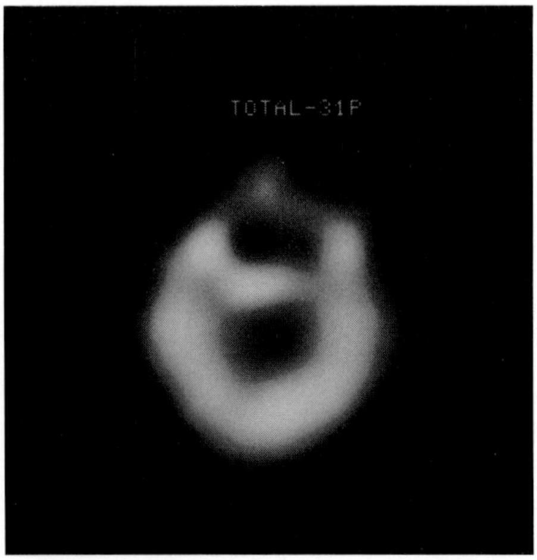 R

Fig. 9-36 Axial ^{31}P metabolite image.

L 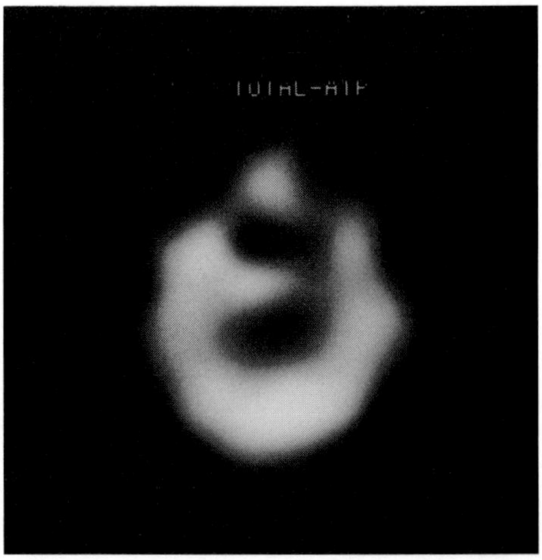 R

Fig. 9-37 Axial total ATP metabolite image.

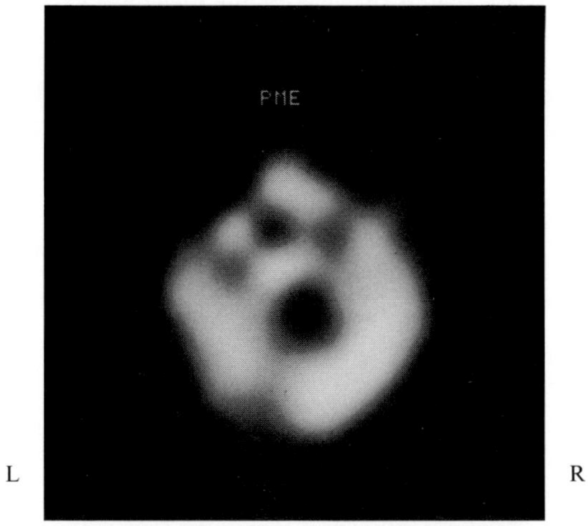

Fig. 9-38 Axial PME metabolite image.

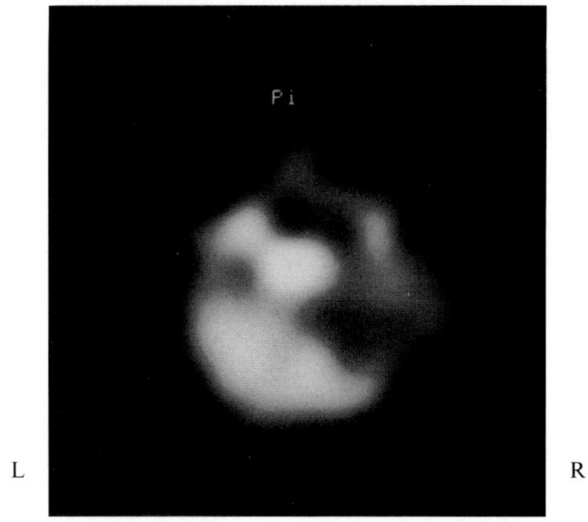

Fig. 9-39 Axial Pi metabolite image.

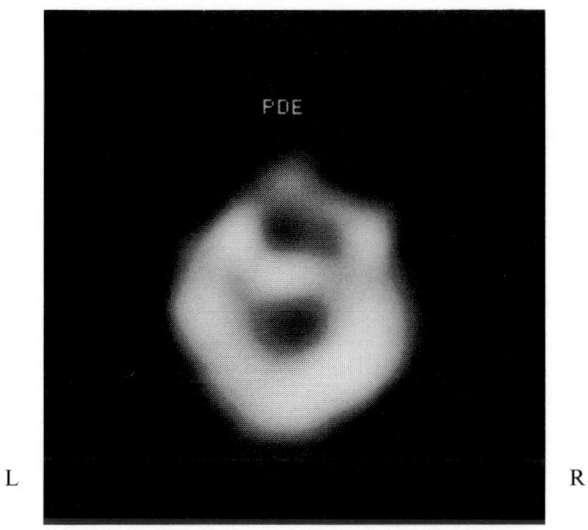

Fig. 9-40 Axial PDE metabolite image.

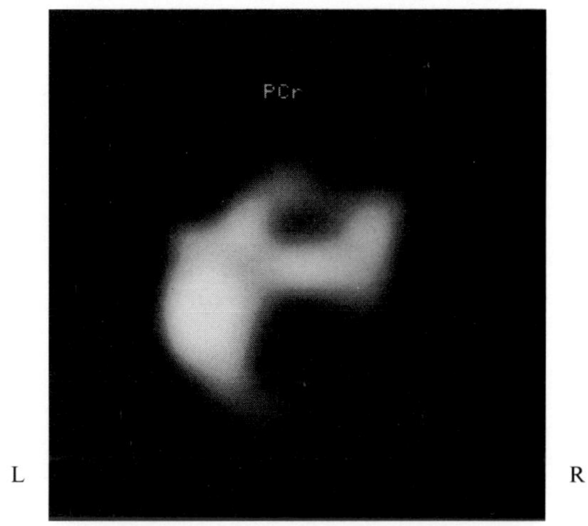

Fig. 9-41 Axial PCr metabolite image.

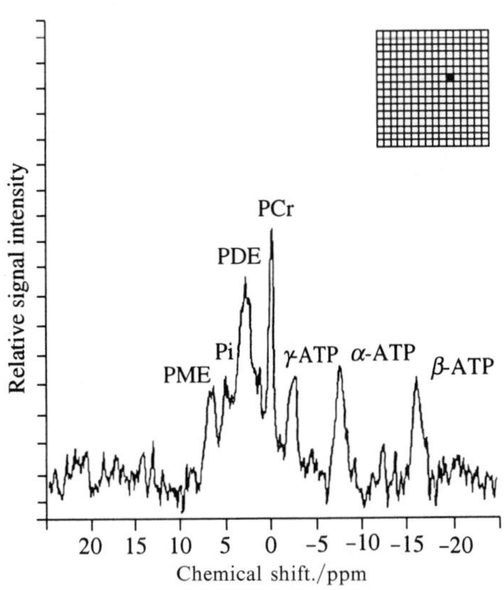

Fig. 9-42 ^{31}P spectrum in control area (voxel B).

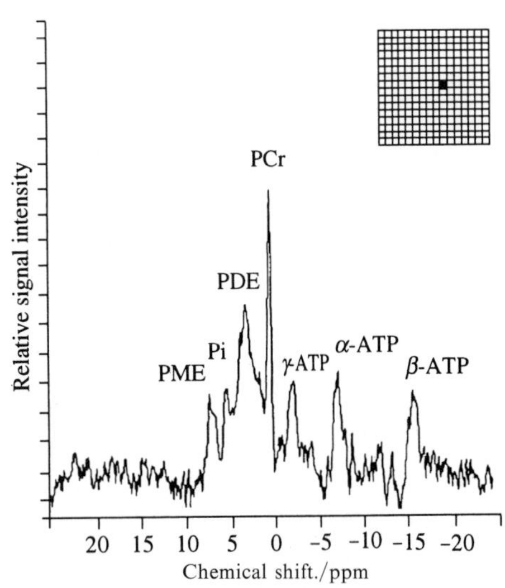

Fig. 9-43 ^{31}P spectrum in tumor area (voxel A).

Astrocytoma (**grade** II)

17 days after ACNU therapy

Tumors can be observed in the bilateral thalami in the MRIs in Figures 9-44 and 45. The tumor area has decreased. Mild brain edema is noted around the tumor. The signal intensity of the tumor area is reduced in the ^{31}P, total ATP, PME, PDE, and PCr metabolite images in Figures 9-46, 47, 48, 50, and 51. It is slightly increased in the Pi metabolite image in Figure 9-49. Figures 9-53 and 9-52 show the spectra of the tumor area and normal control area. The findings are as described above.

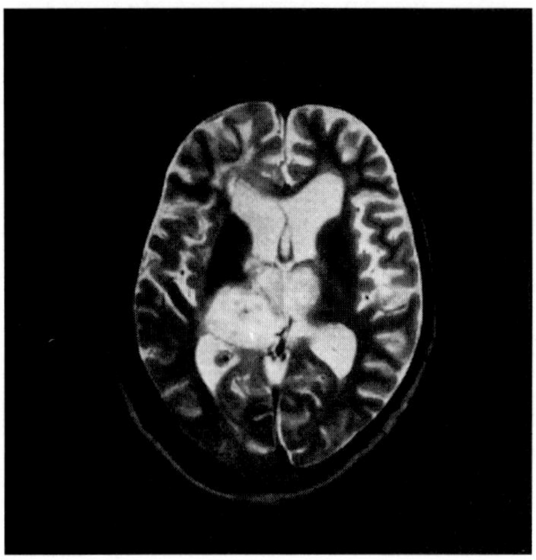

Fig. 9-44 Axial T_2-weighted image (2,200/90).

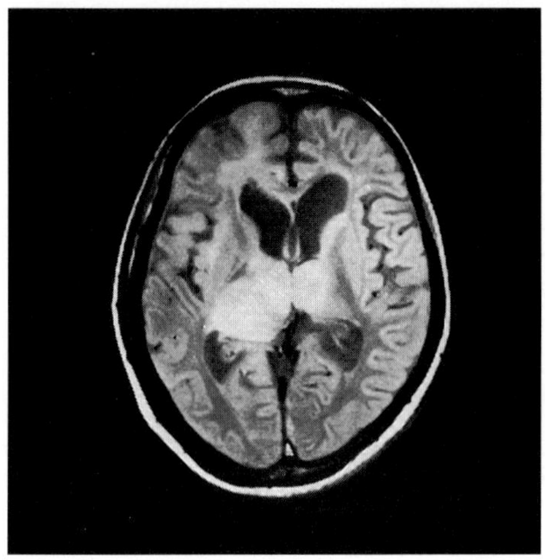

Fig. 9-45 Axial proton density-weighted image (2,200/15).

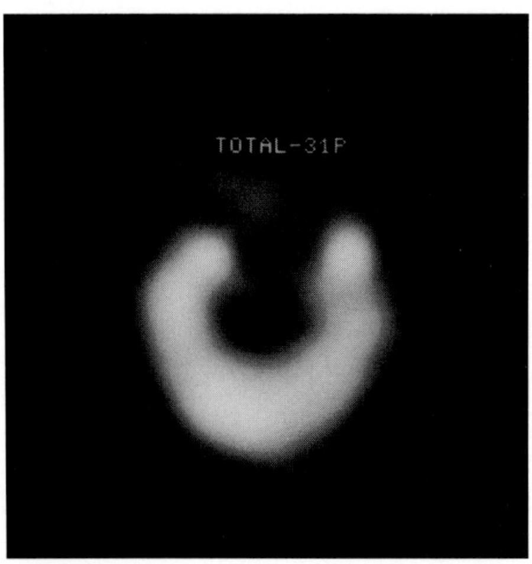

Fig. 9-46 Axial ^{31}P metabolite image.

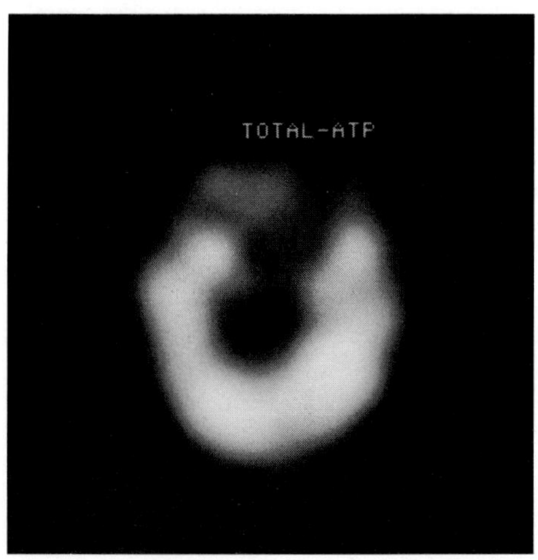

Fig. 9-47 Axial total ATP metabolite image.

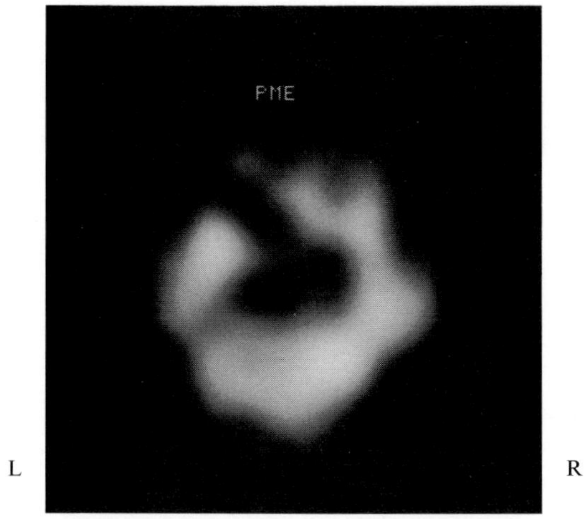

Fig. 9-48 Axial PME metabolite image.

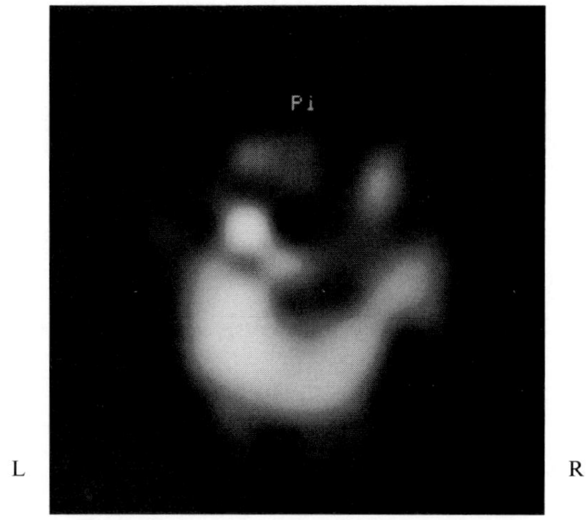

Fig. 9-49 Axial Pi metabolite image.

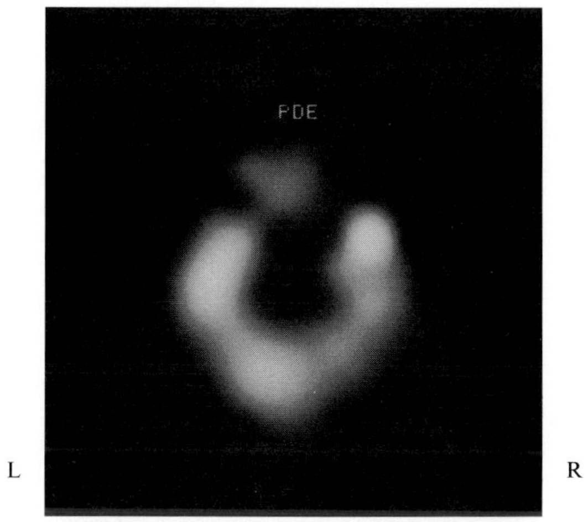

Fig. 9-50 Axial PDE metabolite image.

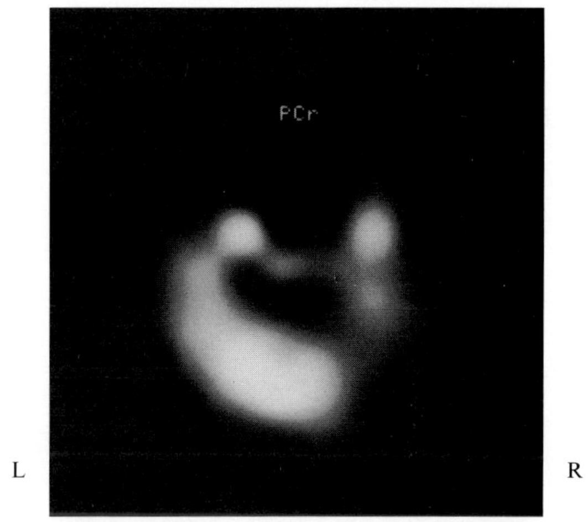

Fig. 9-51 Axial PCr metabolite image.

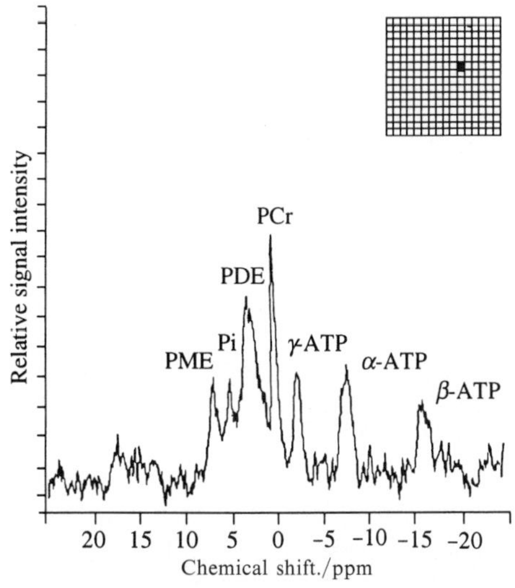

Fig. 9-52 ^{31}P spectrum in control area (voxel B).

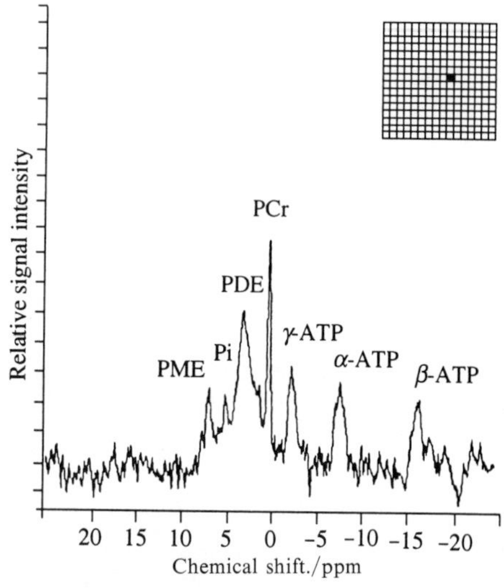

Fig. 9-53 ^{31}P spectrum in tumor area (voxel A).

Astrocytoma (grade II)

16 months after ACNU therapy

A tumor can be observed in the left thalamus in the MRIs in Figures 9-54 and 55. An extension of the tumor is noted in the left frontal lobe. Brain edema is observed around the tumor. The signal intensity of the tumor area is lower than in the surrounding tissues in the ^{31}P, total ATP, PME, PDE, and PCr metabolite images in Figures 9-56, 57, 58, 60, and 61. It is slightly increased in the tumor area in the Pi metabolite image in Figure 9-59. Figures 9-63 and 62 show the spectra of the tumor area and a normal control area. The findings are as described above.

L 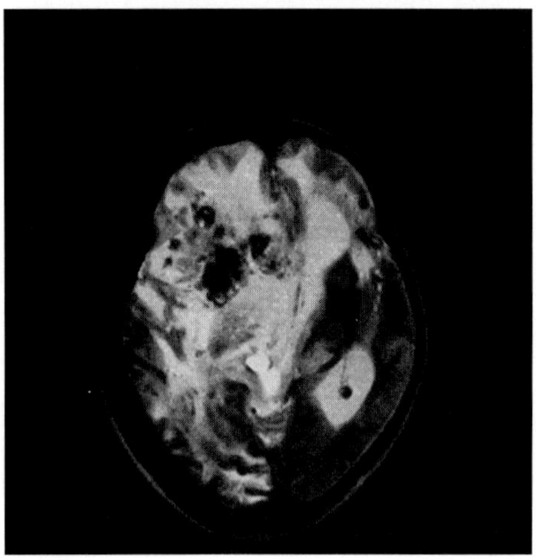 R

Fig. 9-54 Axial T_2-weighted image (2,200/90).

L 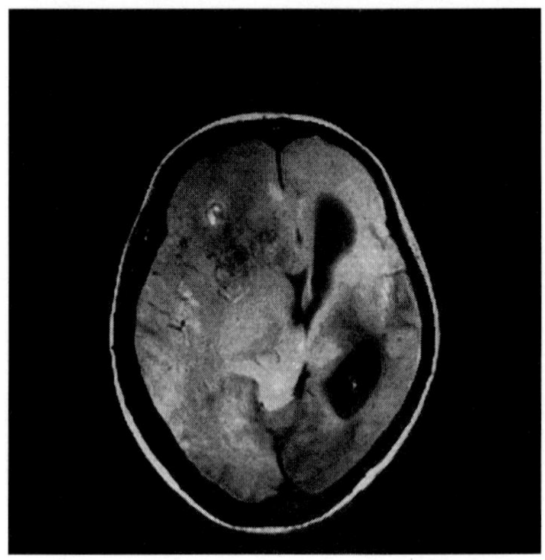 R

Fig. 9-55 Axial proton density-weighted image (2,200/15).

L 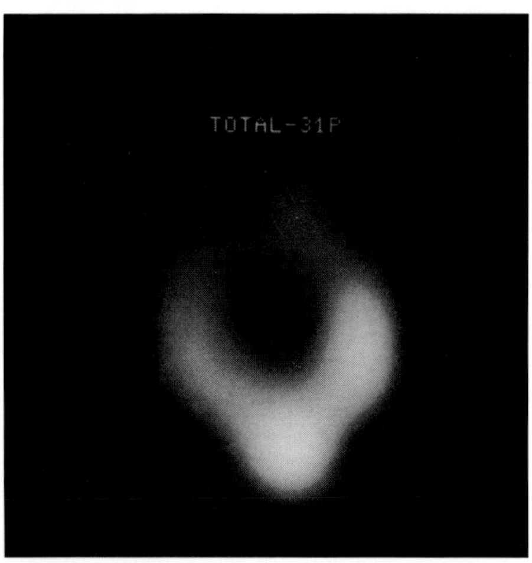 R

Fig. 9-56 Axial ^{31}P metabolite image.

L 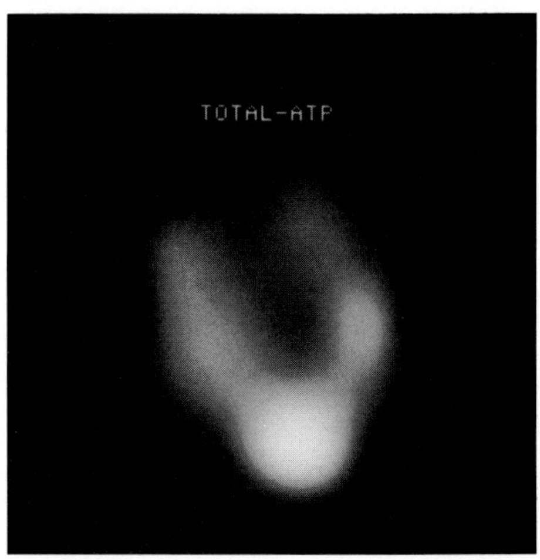 R

Fig. 9-57 Axial total ATP metabolite image.

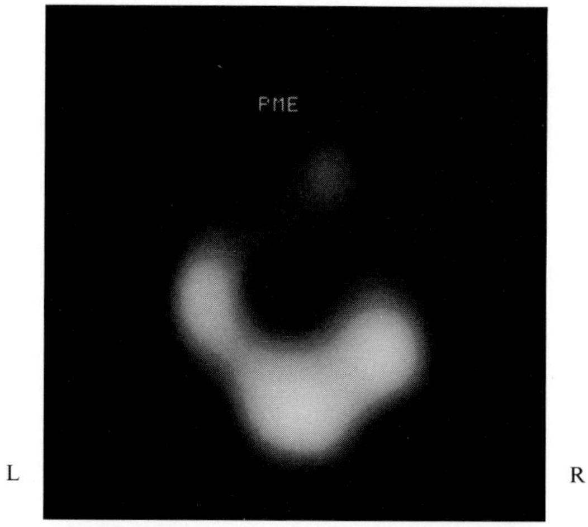

Fig. 9-58 Axial PME metabolite image.

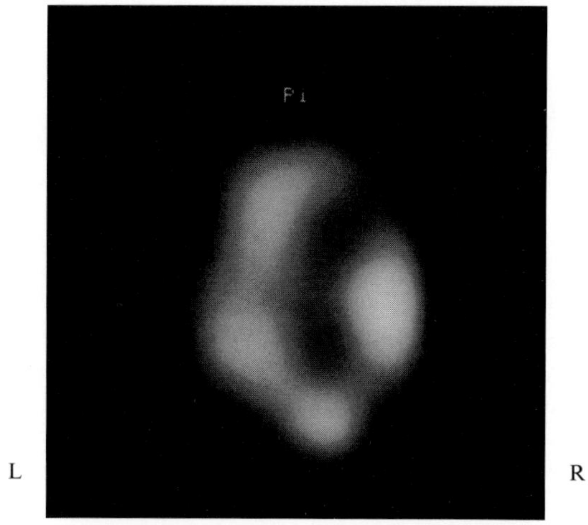

Fig. 9-59 Axial Pi metabolite image.

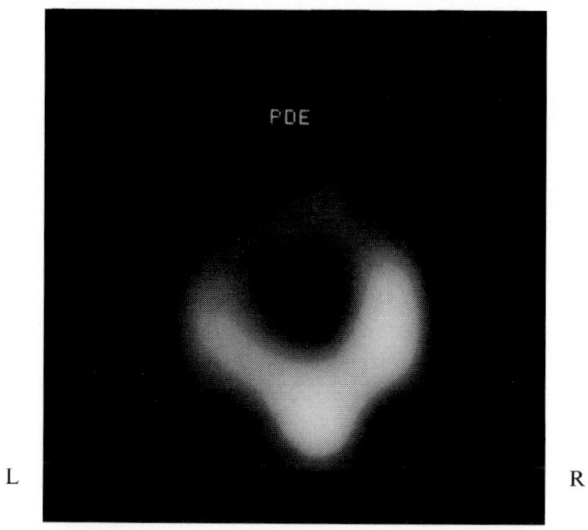

Fig. 9-60 Axial PDE metabolite image.

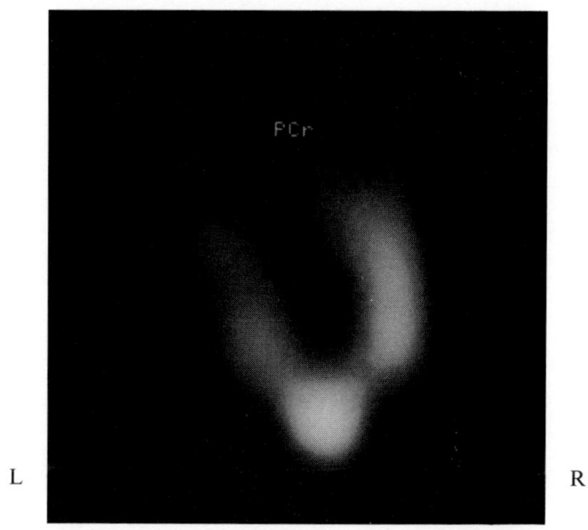

Fig. 9-61 Axial PCr metabolite image.

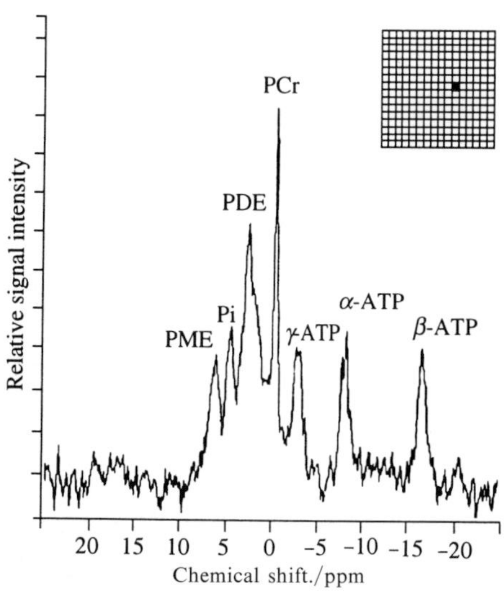

Fig. 9-62 ^{31}P spectrum in control area (Voxel B).

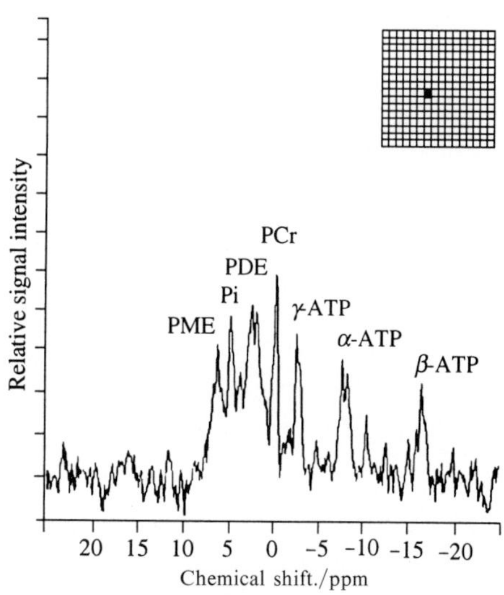

Fig. 9-63 ^{31}P spectrum in tumor area (Voxel A).

CASE 10

Case 10: A 48-year-old male
Astrocytoma (grade Ⅲ)

The patient suffered from right hemiparesis attacks and focal seizures of the right upper extremity and was admitted to the hospital. The neurological examination revealed right hemiparesis, right hemihypesthesia, dementia, and choked disc. Figure 10-1 is a ^{1}H-MRS of the tumor area. A peak of lactic acid is observed, and the peak of NAA is reduced. In the MRIs in Figures 10-2 and 3, a tumor can be observed in the right thalamus, which is seen to extend to the left thalamus. Brain edema is noted around the tumor. In the ^{31}P, total ATP, and PDE contour maps in Figures 10-4, 5, and 8, the signal intensity is reduced in the tumor area compared with the surrounding tissue. It is slightly increased in the tumor area in the PME and Pi contour maps in Figures 10-6 and 7. Figures 10-10 and 10-11 show the spectra of the tumor area and a normal control area. The findings are as described above.

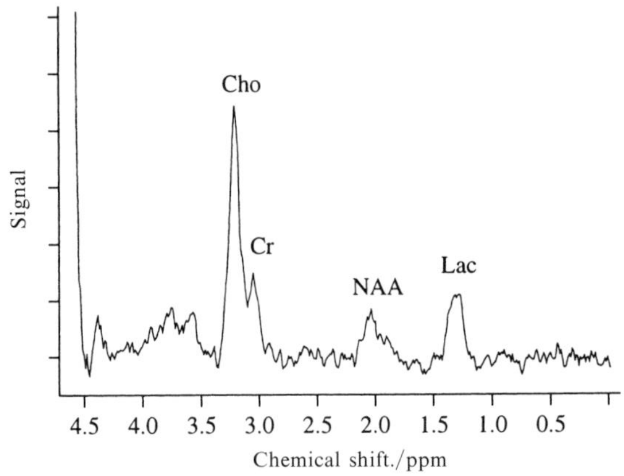

Fig. 10-1 ^{1}H spectrum of brain tumor region. PRESS (1,500/270)

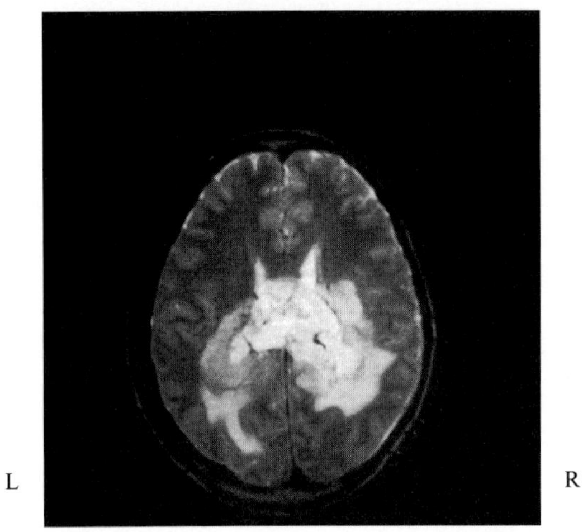

Fig. 10-2 Axial T_2-weighted image (2,200/90).

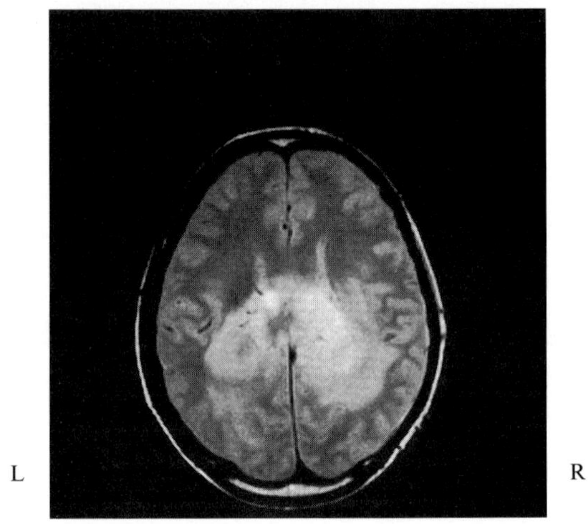

Fig. 10-3 Axial proton density-weighted image (2,200/15).

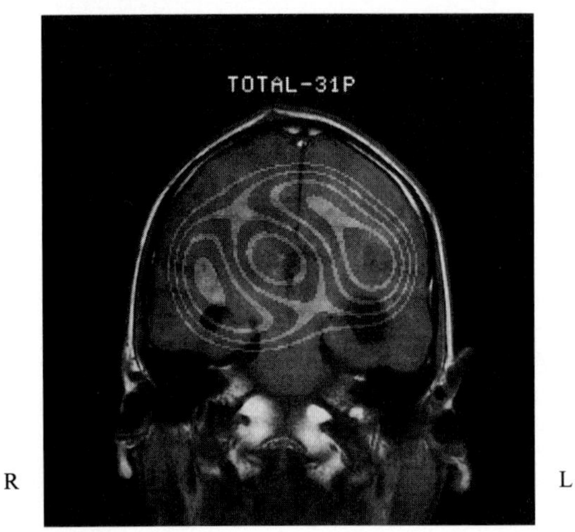

Fig. 10-4 Coronal ^{31}P contour map superimposed on T_1-weighted image (500/15).

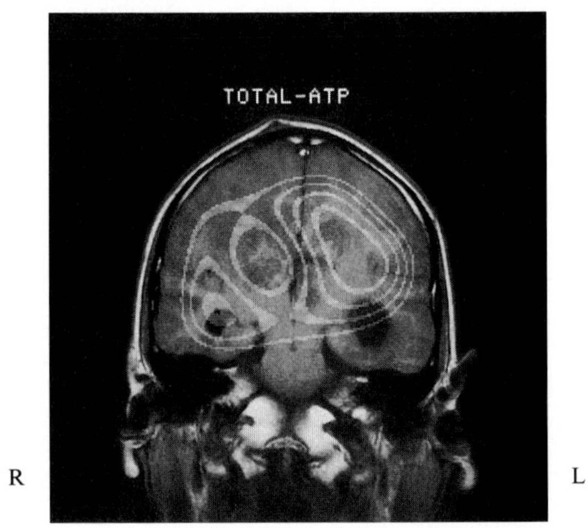

Fig. 10-5 Coronal total ATP contour map superimposed on T_1-weighted image (500/15).

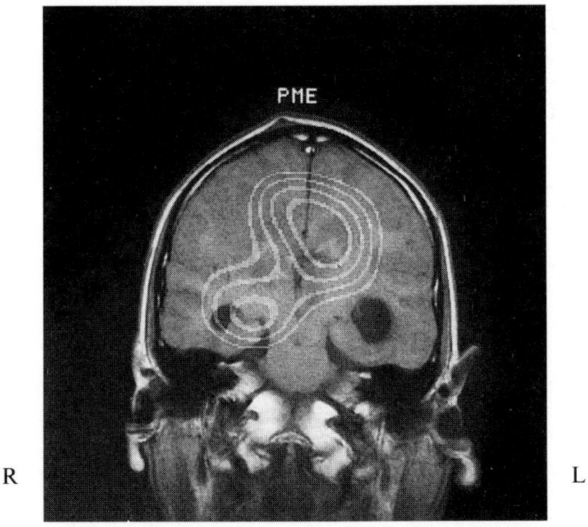

Fig. 10-6 Coronal PME contour map superimposed on T_1-weighted image (500/15).

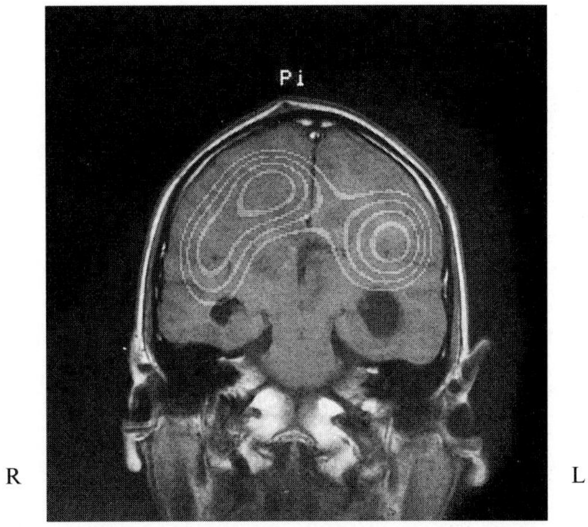

Fig. 10-7 Coronal Pi contour map superimposed on T_1-weighted image (500/15).

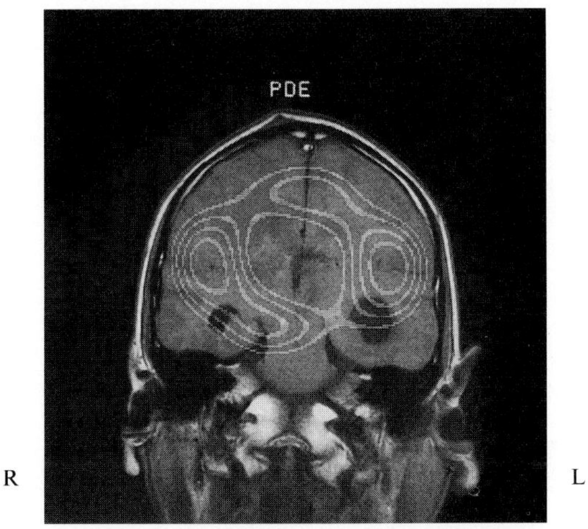

Fig. 10-8 Coronal PDE contour map superimposed on T_1-weighted image (500/15).

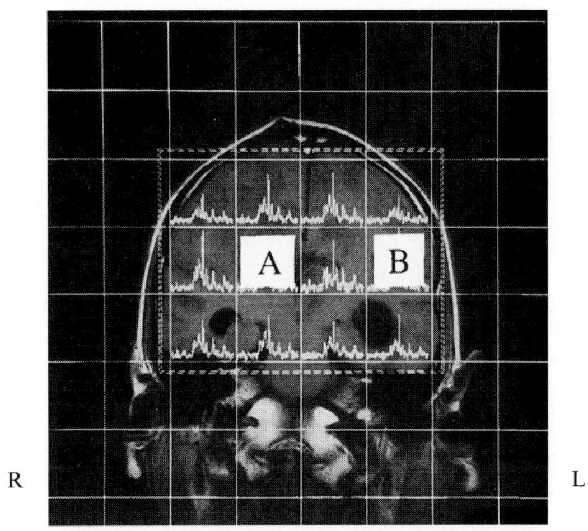

Fig. 10-9 T_1-weighted image showing the position of $3 \times 3 \times 4$ cm^3 voxels A and B.

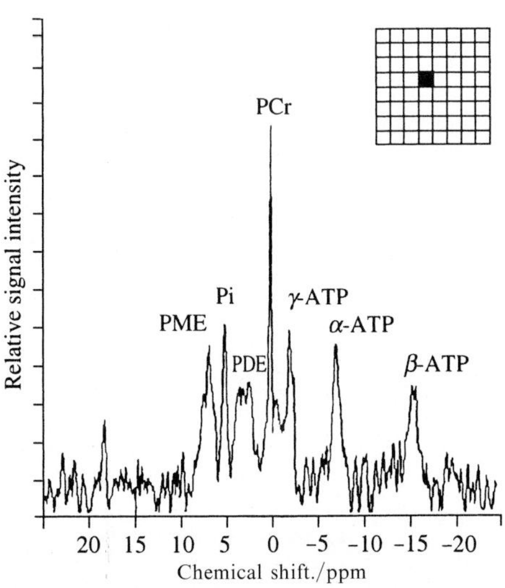

Fig. 10-10 ^{31}P spectrum in tumor area (voxel A).

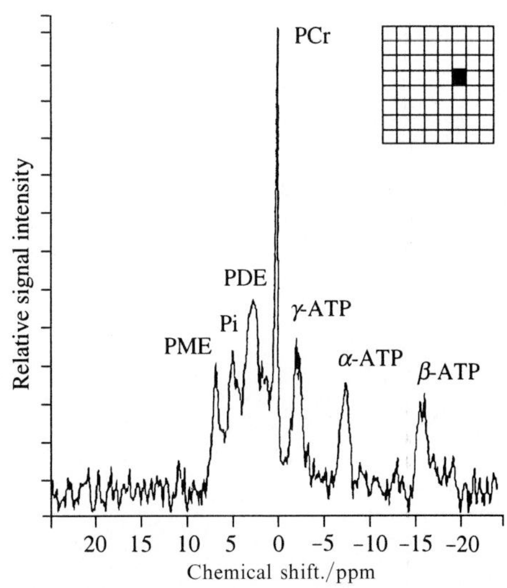

Fig. 10-11 ^{31}P spectrum in control area (voxel B).

CASE 11

Case 11: A 43-year-old male
Astrocytoma (grade III)

The patient suffered from generalized convulsions and took medication for epilepsy with a history extending over 28 years. He had frequent seizure attacks 3 months previously and noticed right hemiparesis. The neurological examination revealed right hemiparesis and right hemihypesthesia. Figure 11-1 shows a ^{1}H-MRS of the tumor area. The peak of choline is high, and that of NAA is low. A peak of lactic acid is noted. This is a typical pattern of malignant tumor in ^{1}H-MRS. In the MRIs in Figures 11-2 and 3, a tumor can be observed in the left parietal lobe. Brain edema is noted around the tumor. The signal intensity is reduced in the tumor area compared with the surrounding tissues in the ^{31}P, total ATP, PCr, and PME metabolite images or the contour map in Figures 11-4, 5, 7, and 8. It is slightly increased in the tumor area in the Pi contour map in Figure 11-6. Figures 11-10 and 11-11 show the spectra of the tumor area and a normal control area. The findings are as described above.

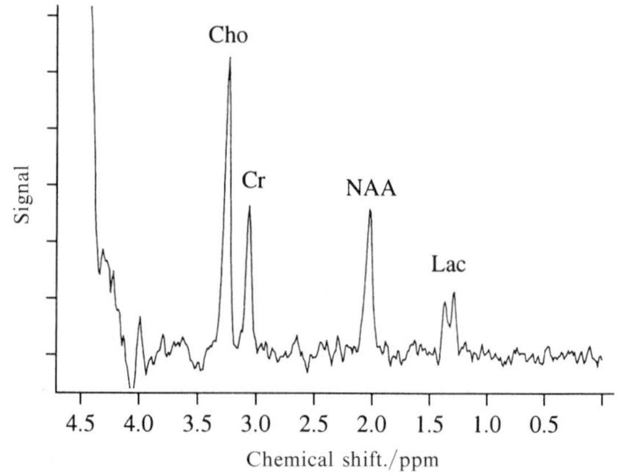

Fig. 11-1 ^{1}H spectrum of brain tumor region. PRESS (1,500/270).

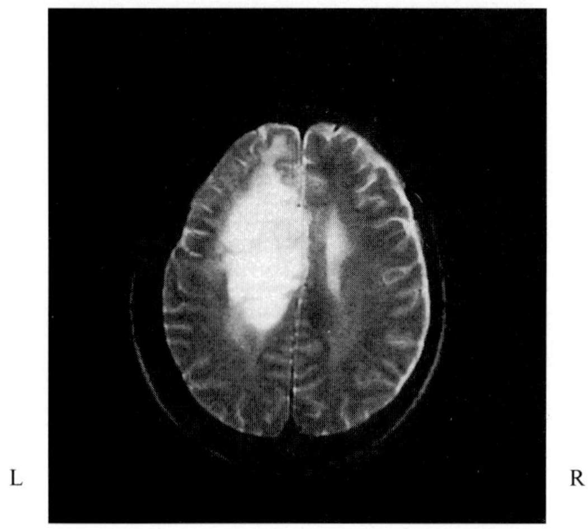

Fig. 11-2 Axial T_2-weighted image (2,200/90).

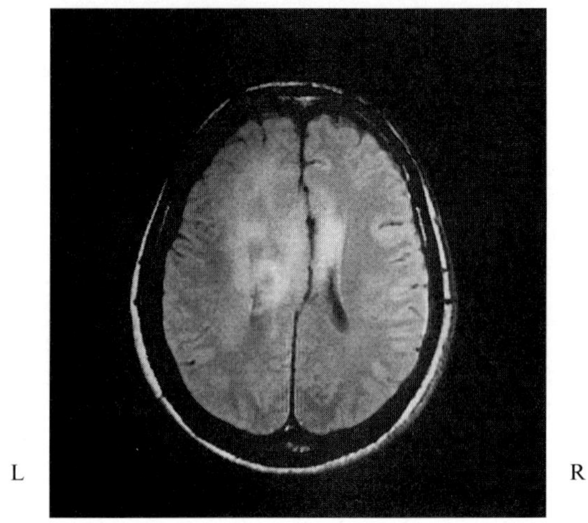

Fig. 11-3 Axial proton density-weighted image (2,200/15).

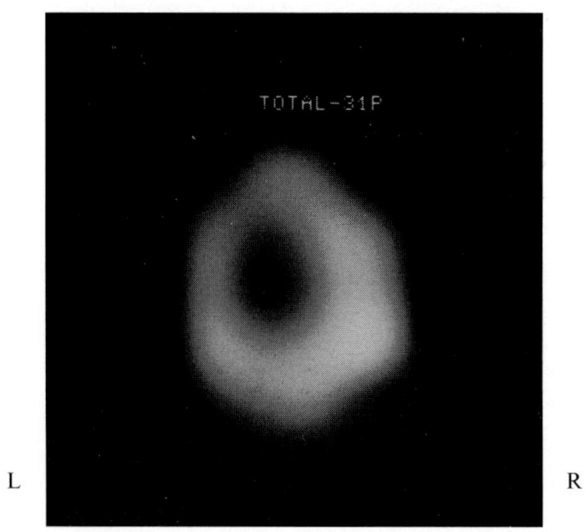

Fig. 11-4 Axial ^{31}P metabolite image.

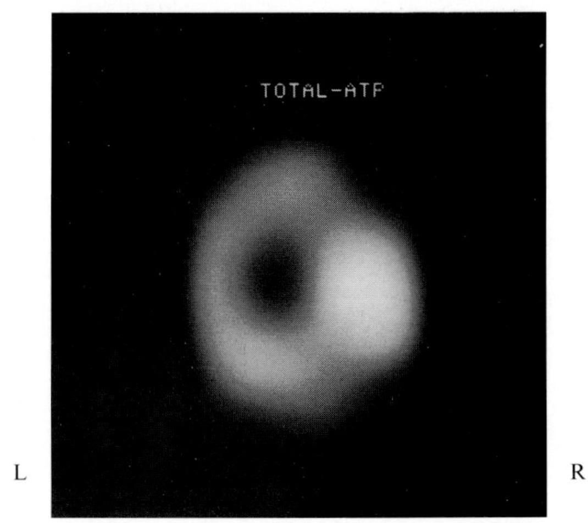

Fig. 11-5 Axial total ATP metabolite image.

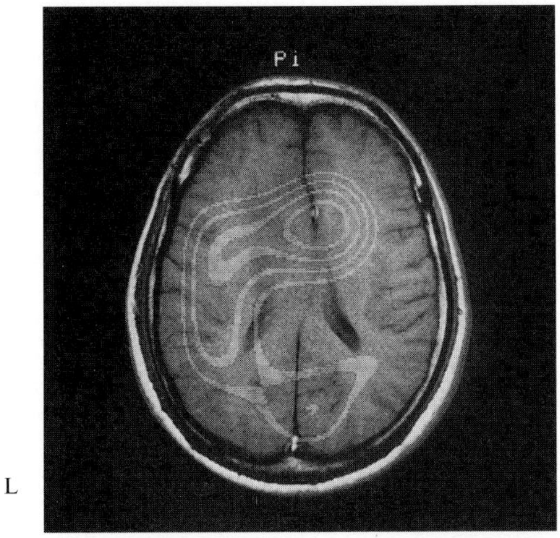

Fig. 11-6 Axial Pi contour map superimposed on T_1-weighted image (500/15).

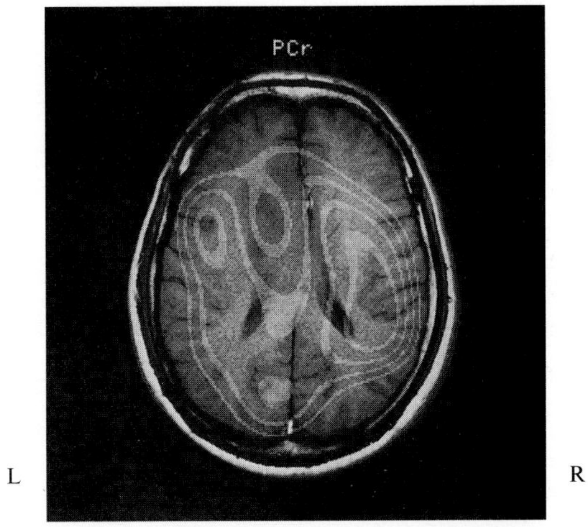

Fig. 11-7 Axial PCr contour map superimposed on T_1-weighted image (500/15).

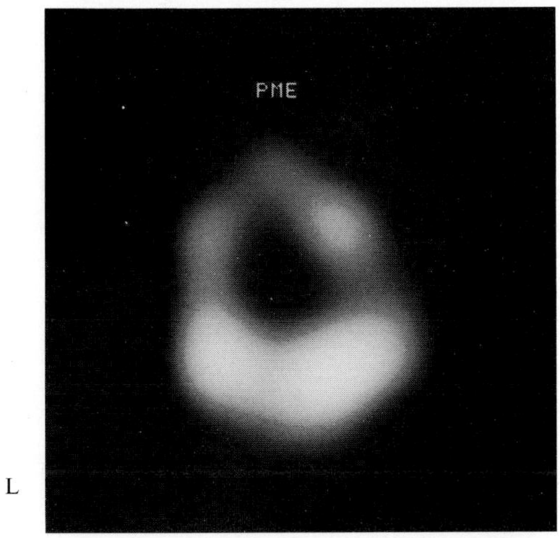

Fig. 11-8 Axial PME metabolite image.

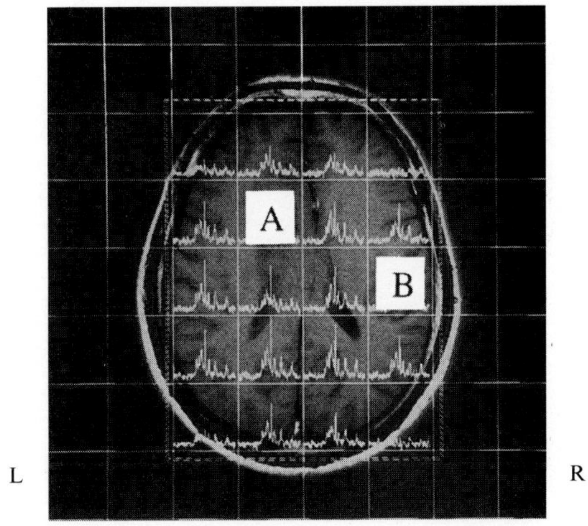

Fig. 11-9 T_1-weighted image showing the position of $3 \times 3 \times 4$ cm^3 voxels A and B.

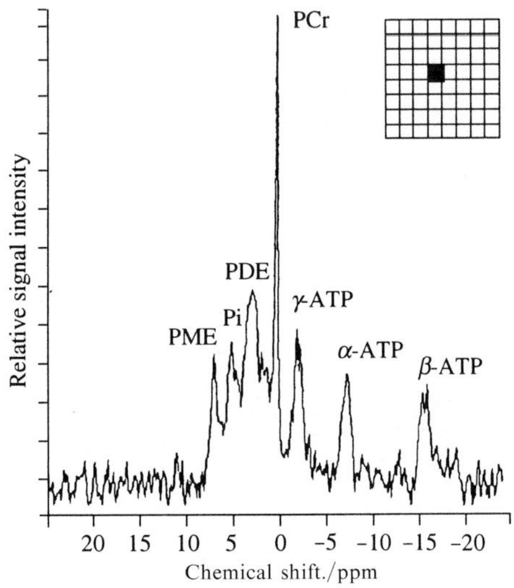

Fig. 11-10 ^{31}P spectrum in tumor area (voxel A).

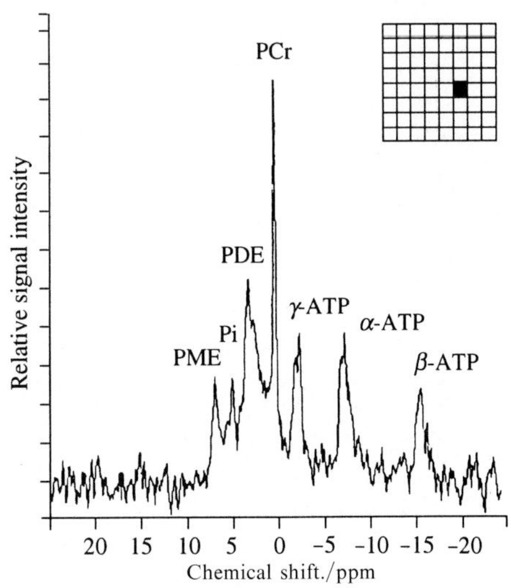

Fig. 11-11 ^{31}P spectrum in control area (voxel B).

20 days after treatment

The MRIs in Figures 11-12 and 13 show a tumor in the left parietal lobe. Brain edema around the tumor has been alleviated. The signal intensity is slightly reduced in the tumor area compared with the surrounding tissues in the ^{31}P, total ATP, PME, and PDE contour maps in Figures 11-14, 15, 16, and 18. It is slightly increased in the tumor area in the Pi contour map shown in Figure 11-17. Figures 11-20 and 11-21 show the spectra of the tumor area and a normal control area. The findings are as described above.

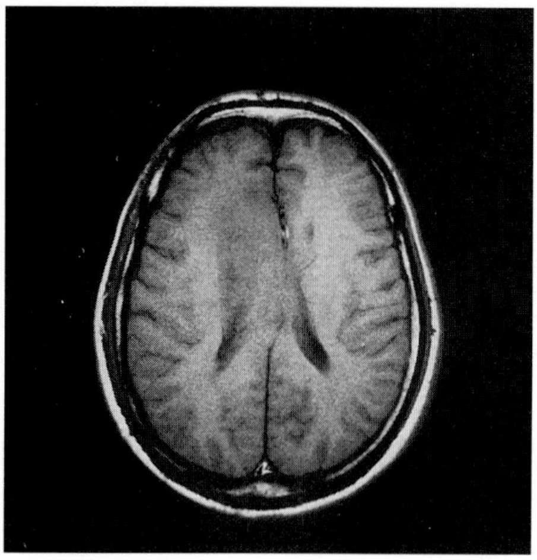

Fig. 11-12 Axial T_1-weighted image (500/15).

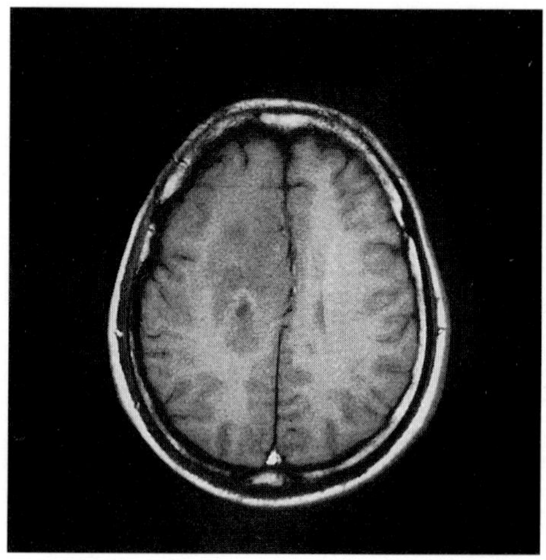

Fig. 11-13 Axial T_1-weighted image (500/15).

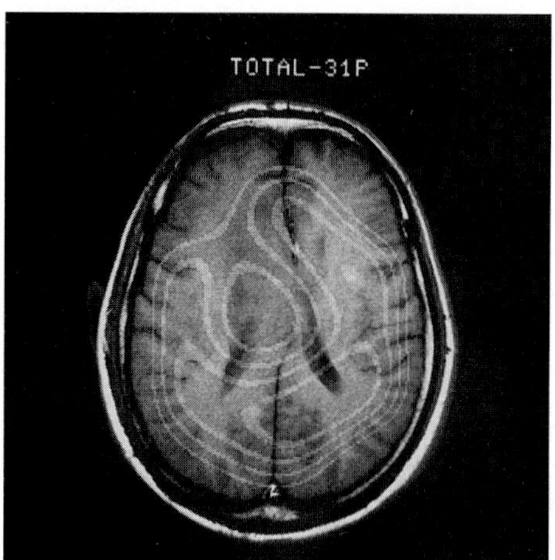

Fig. 11-14 Axial ^{31}P contour map superimposed on T_1-weighted image (500/15).

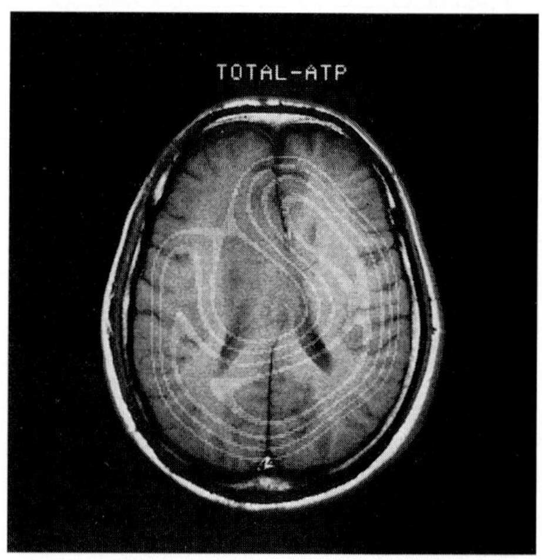

Fig. 11-15 Axial total ATP contour map superimposed on T_1-weighted image (500/15).

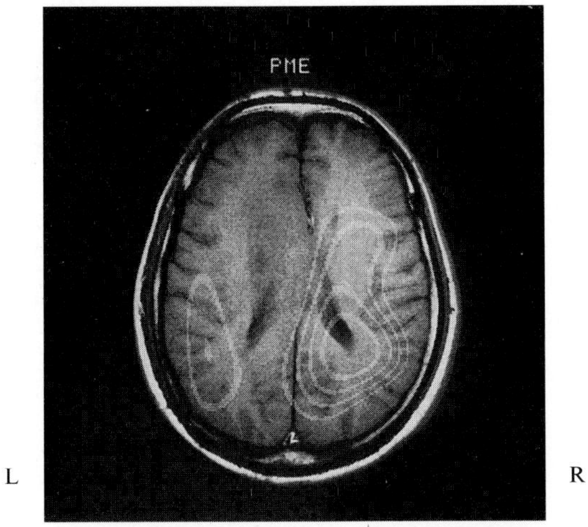

Fig. 11-16 Axial PME contour map superimposed on T_1-weighted image (500/15).

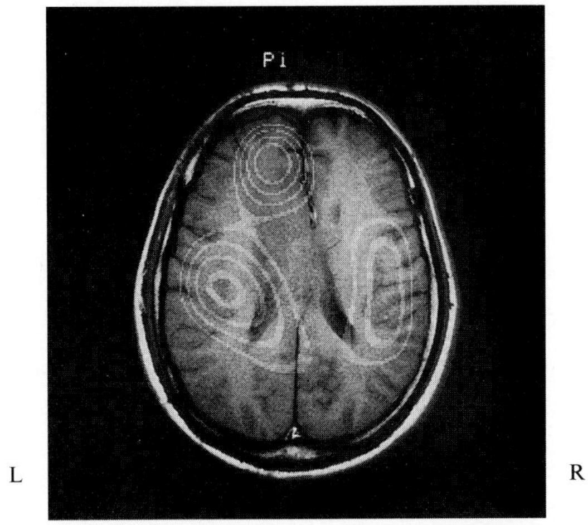

Fig. 11-17 Axial Pi contour map superimposed on T_1-weighted image (500/15).

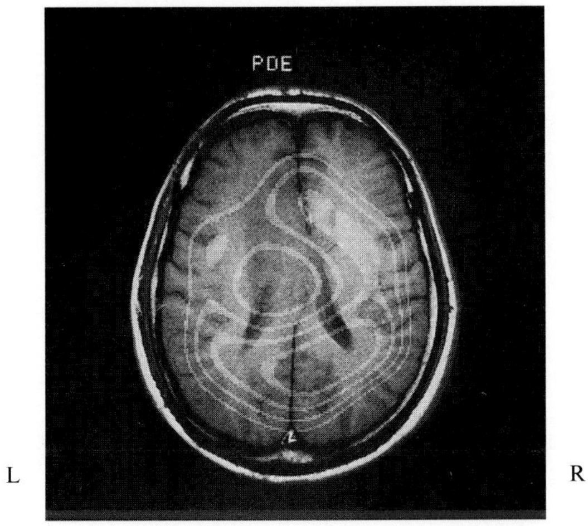

Fig. 11-18 Axial PDE contour map superimposed on T_1-weighted image (500/15).

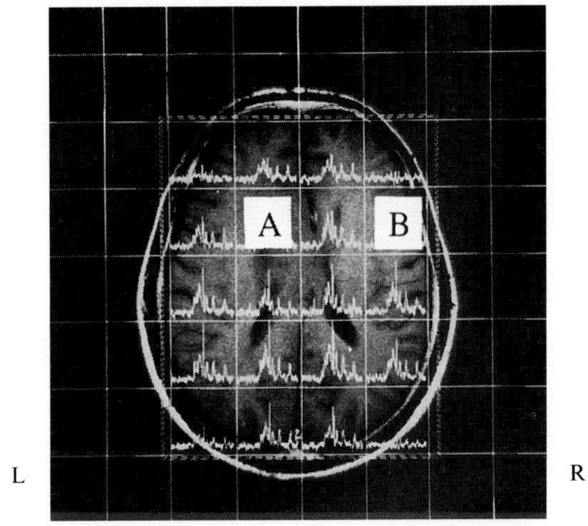

Fig. 11-19 T_1-weighted image showing the position of 3×3×4 cm^3 voxels A and B.

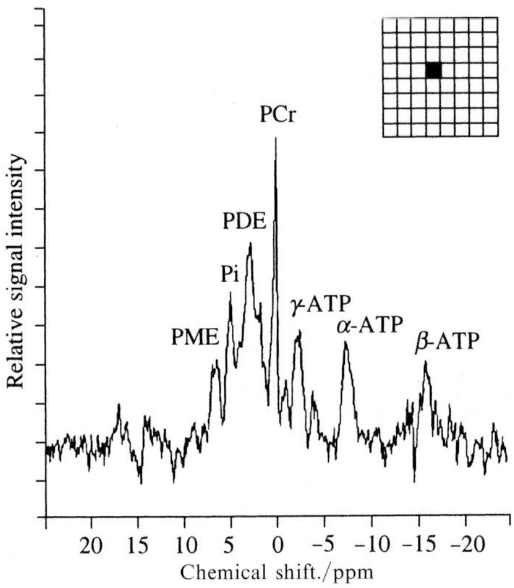

Fig. 11-20 ^{31}P spectrum in tumor area (voxel A).

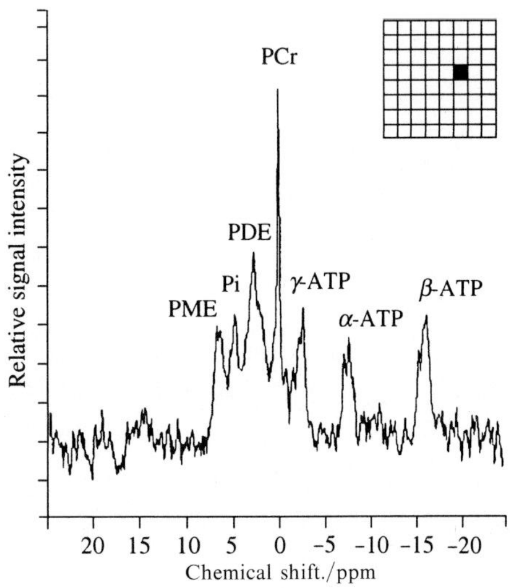

Fig. 11-21 ^{31}P spectrum in control area (voxel B).

CASE 12

Case 12: A 43-year-old female

Astrocytoma (grade III)

The patient suffered generalized convulsions and was admitted to the hospital. The neurological examination revealeda choked disc. The MRIs in Figures 12-1 and 2 show a tumor in the right fronto-temporal area. Brain edema is noted around the tumor. The signal intensity is slightly reduced in the tumor area compared with the surrounding area in the ^{31}P, total ATP, and PDE contour maps in Figures 12-3, 4, and 7. It is high in the tumor area in the PME and Pi contour maps in Figures 12-5 and 6. Figures 12-10 and 12-9 show the spectra of the tumor area and a normal control area. The findings are as described above.

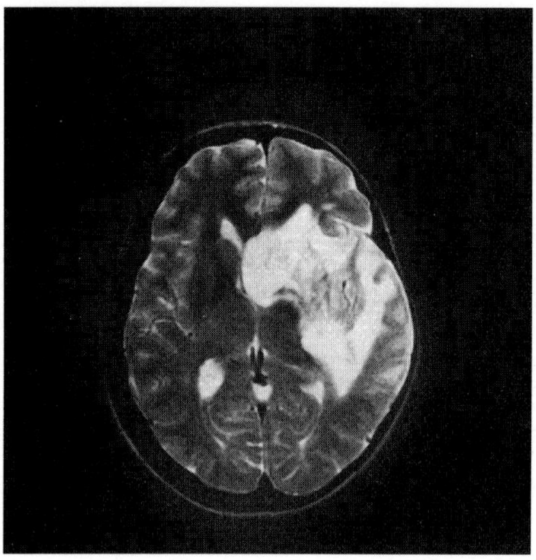

Fig. 12-1 Axial T_2-weighted image (2,200/90).

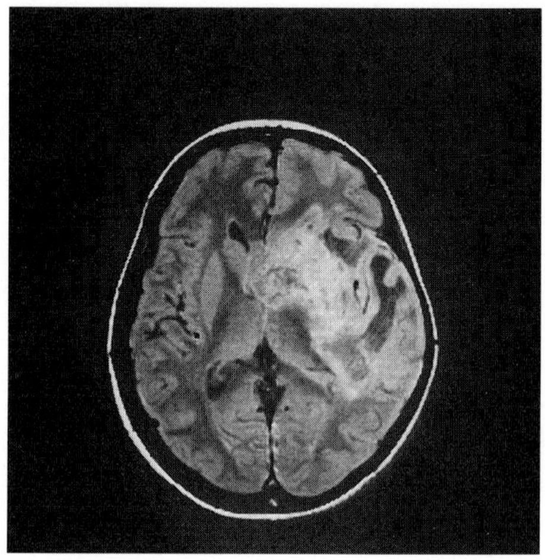

Fig. 12-2 Axial proton density-weighted image (2,200/15).

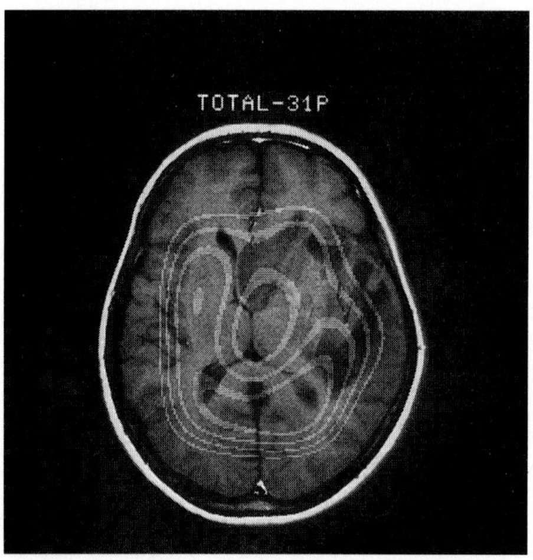

Fig. 12-3 Axial ^{31}P contour map superimposed on T_1-weighted image (500/15).

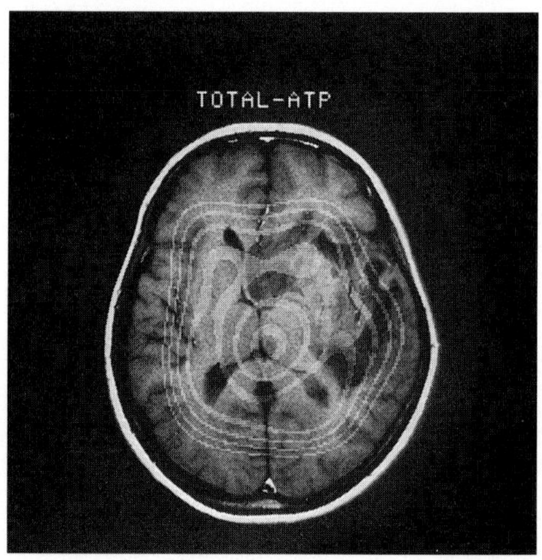

Fig. 12-4 Axial total ATP contour map superimposed on T_1-weighted image (500/15).

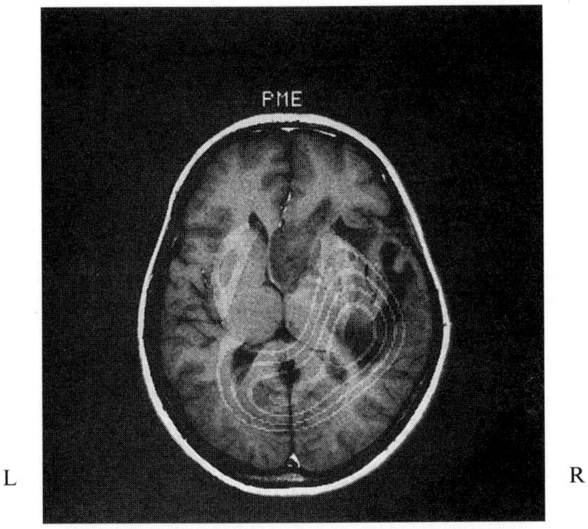

Fig. 12-5 Axial PME contour map superimposed on T_1-weighted image (500/15).

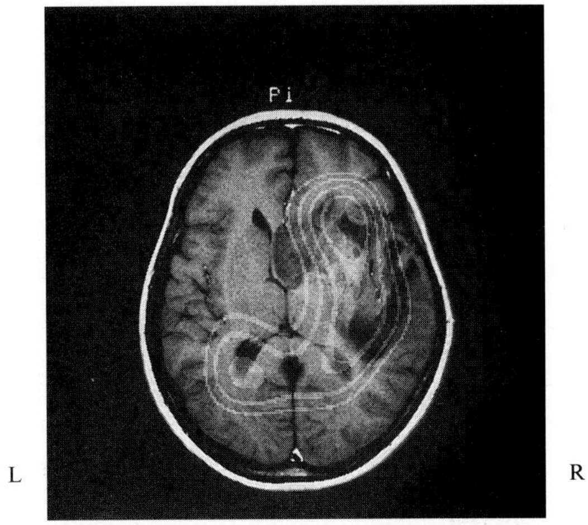

Fig. 12-6 Axial Pi contour map superimposed on T_1-weighted image (500/15).

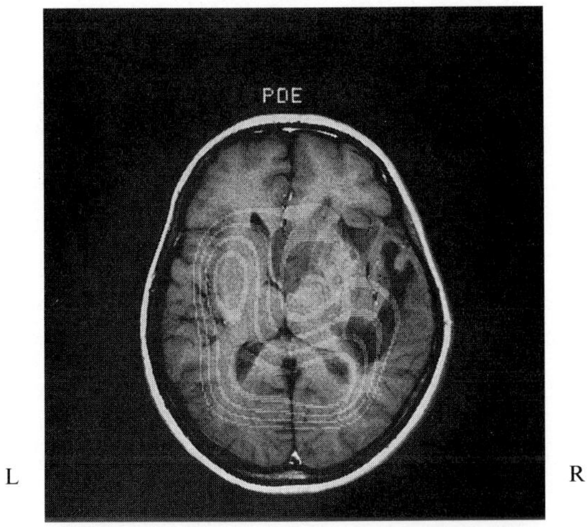

Fig. 12-7 Axial PDE contour map superimposed on T_1-weighted image (500/15).

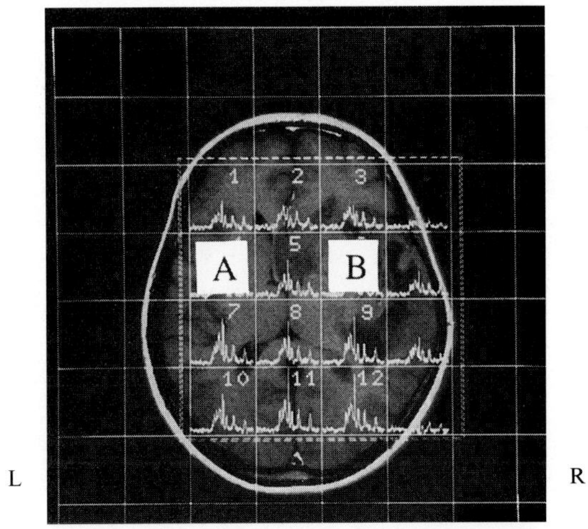

Fig. 12-8 T_1-weighted image showing the position of $3 \times 3 \times 4$ cm^3 voxels A and B.

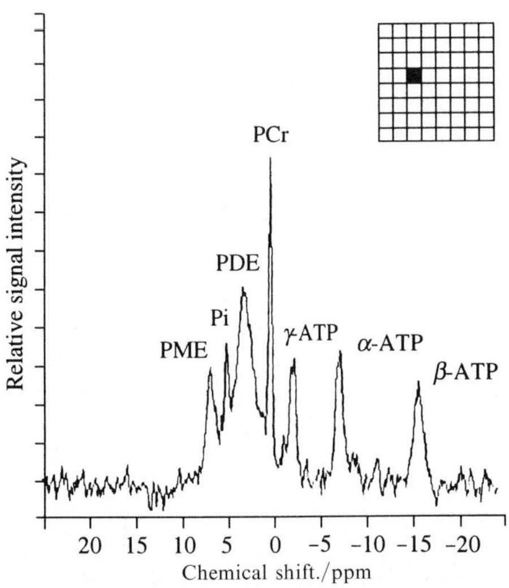

Fig. 12-9 ^{31}P spectrum in control area (voxel A).

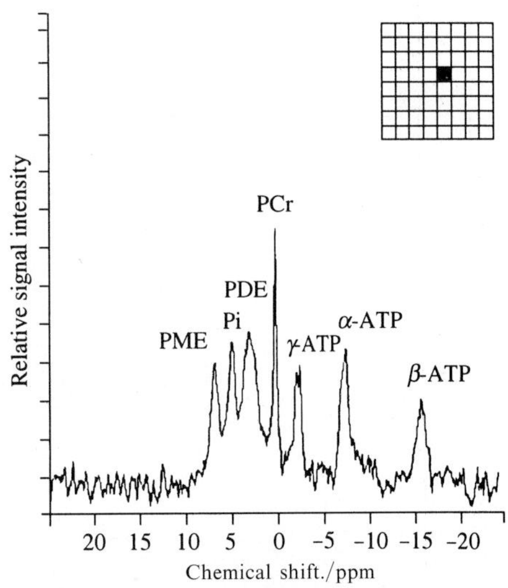

Fig. 12-10 ^{31}P spectrum in tumor area (voxel B).

CASE 13

Case 13: A 73-year-old male
Astrocytoma (grade IV)

The patient exhibited confused speech, and a low density area was found in the left occipital lobe one month previously. He complained of headache and was readmitted to the hospital. The neurological examination revealed disorientation, aphasia, and Gerstman syndrome. The ^{1}H-MRS of the tumor area in Figure 13-1 shows a marked increase in lactic acid and a decrease in NAA. In the MRIs in Figures 13-2 and 3, a tumor can be seen in the left temporal lobe. Tissues around the tumor are markedly edematous. The signal intensity is slightly reduced in the tumor area compared with the surrounding tissues in the ^{31}P and total ATP contour maps in Figures 13-4 and 5. It is increased in the tumor area in the PME and Pi metabolite images in Figures 13-6 and 7 and in the PME/PDE contour map in Figure 13-8. Figures 13-11 and 13-10 show the spectra of the tumor area and a normal control area. The findings are as described above.

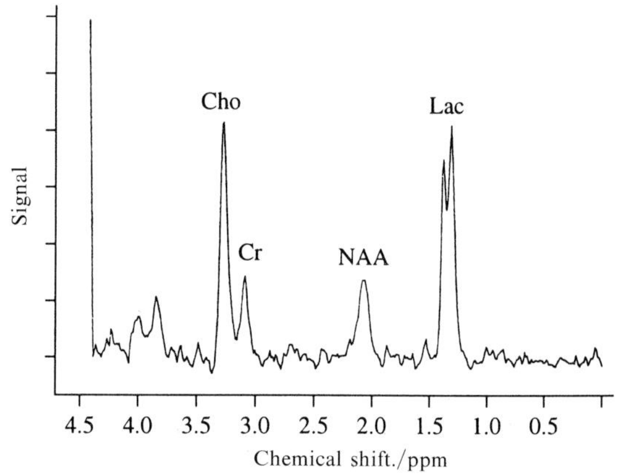

Fig. 13-1 ^{1}H spectrum of brain tumor region. PRESS (1,500/270).

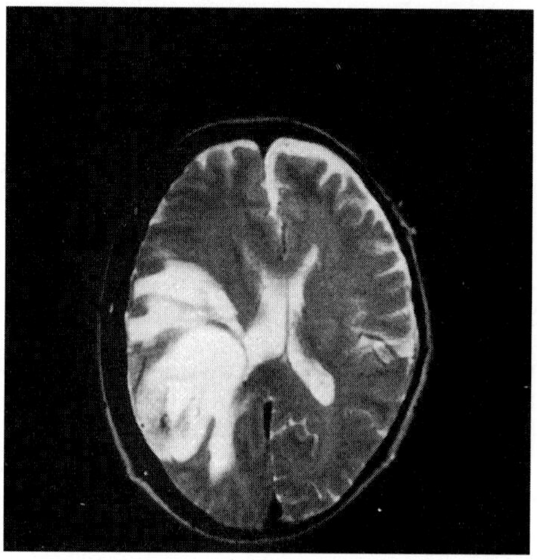

L R

Fig. 13-2 Axial T_2-weighted image (2,200/90).

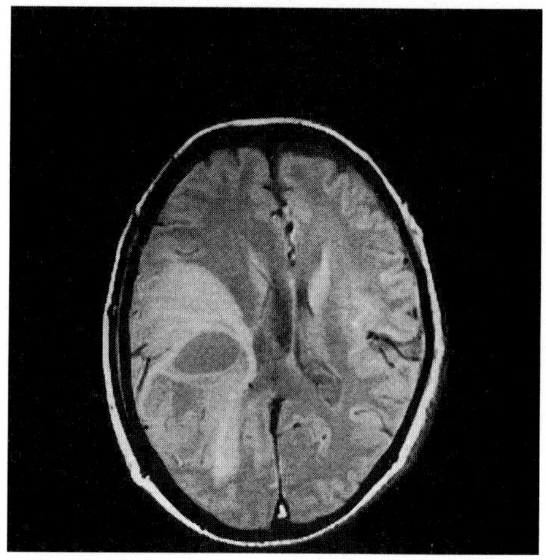

L R

Fig. 13-3 Axial proton density-weighted image (2,200/15).

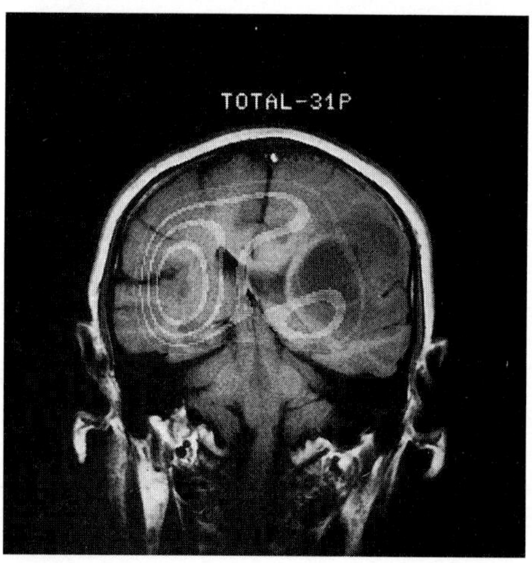

R L

Fig. 13-4 Coronal ^{31}P contour map superimposed on T_1-weighted image (500/15).

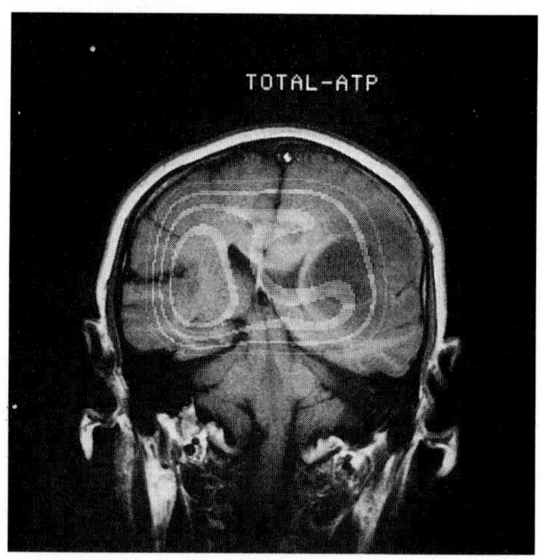

R L

Fig. 13-5 Coronal total ATP contour map superimposed on T_1-weighted image (500/15).

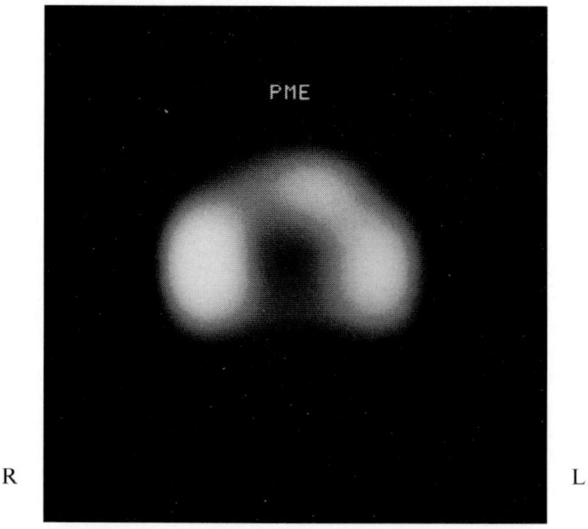

Fig. 13-6 Coronal PME metabolite image.

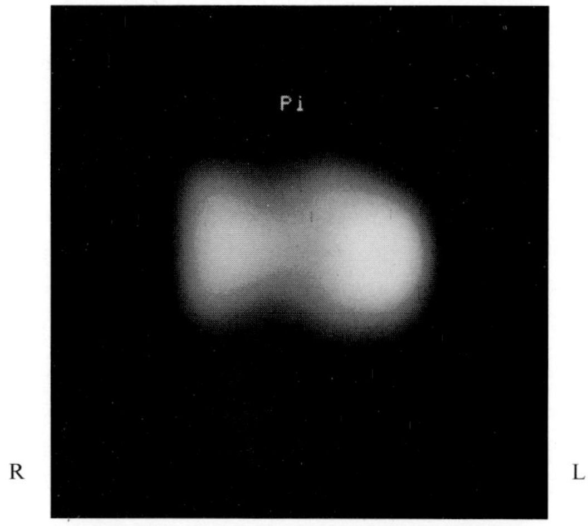

Fig. 13-7 Coronal Pi metabolite image.

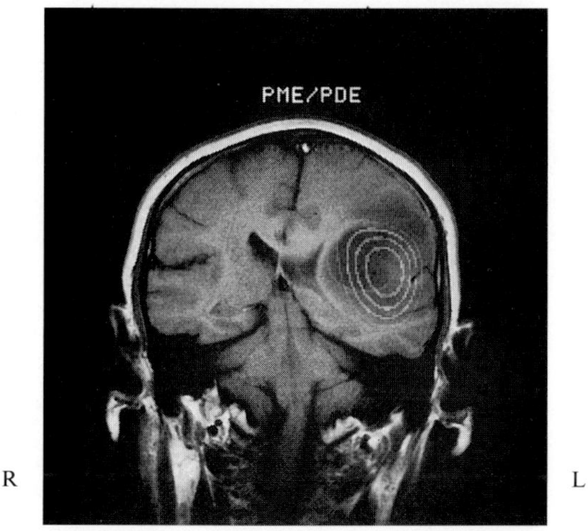

Fig. 13-8 Coronal PME/PDE contour map superimposed on T_1-weighted image (500/15).

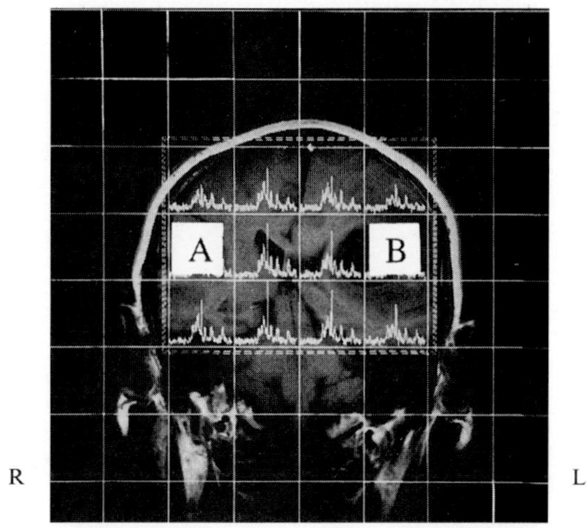

Fig. 13-9 T_1-weighted image showing the position of 3×3×4 cm^3 voxels A and B.

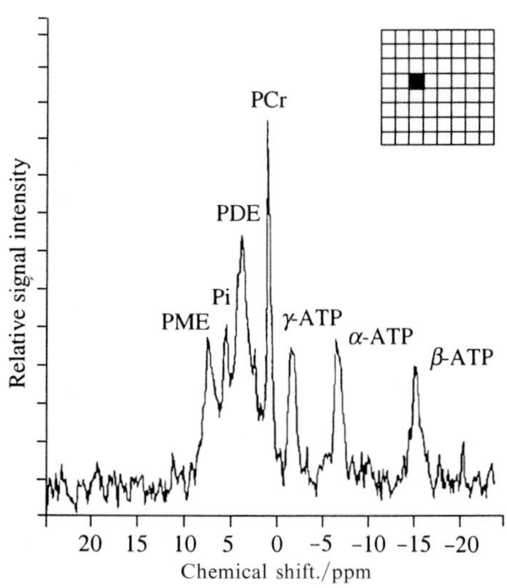

Fig. 13-10 ^{31}P spectrum in control area (voxel A).

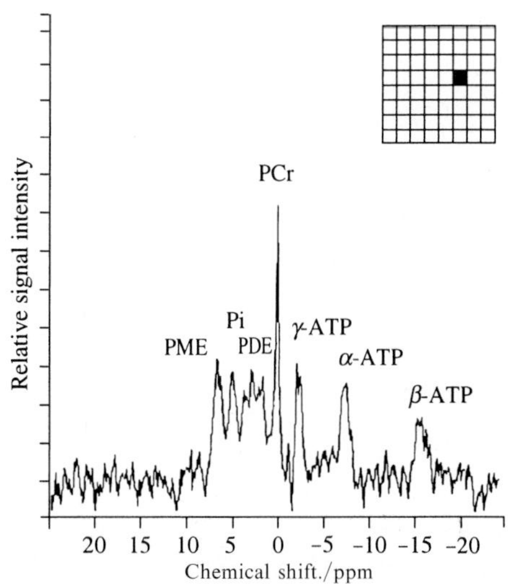

Fig. 13-11 ^{31}P spectrum in tumor area (voxel B).

CASE 14

Case 14: A 41-year-old male

Glioblastoma

The patient suffered an attack of dysthesia and pain in his left forearm with a history extending over one year. He revealed attenuation of attentiveness and was diagnosed with a brain tumor six months previously. Resection of right fronto-parietal tumor (glioblastoma) and chemoradiotherapy were performed. He suffered from a high frequency of generalized convulsions two months previously and underwent resection of the brain tumor and an intra-arterial injection of MCNU. The neurological examination revealed apallic state and left hemiparesis. Enhanced CT in Figure 14-1 shows a tumor with contrast-enhancement in the right frontal region. MRIs in Figures 14-2, 3, and 4 demonstrate a tumor in the right frontal lobe. Marked brain edema is noted around the tumor, and part of the tumor is necrotic. The signal intensity is reduced in the tumor area in the ^{31}P contour map and metabolite image in Figures 14-5 and 6. It is increased in the tumor area in the PME metabolite image in Figure 14-7. In the PME/PDE contour map in Figure 14-8, the signal intensity is high in the tumor area but is low in the center of the tumor due to necrosis. The signal intensity is reduced in the tumor area in PDE metabolite image in Figure 14-9. It is high in the tumor area in the Pi metabolite image in Figure 14-10. Figures 14-14 to 22 are spectra of various parts of the tumor.

L 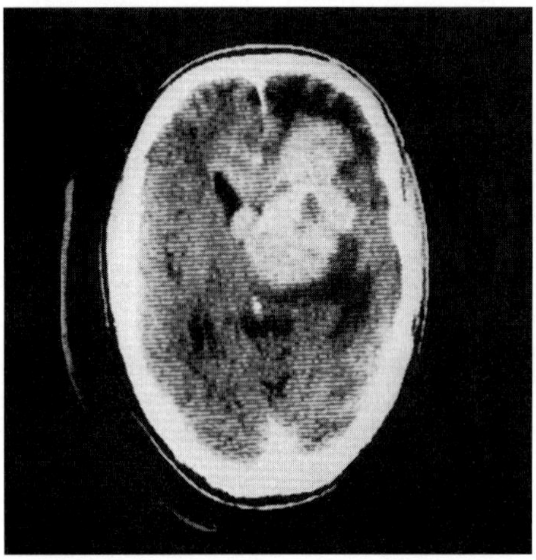 R

Fig. 14-1 Axial enhanced X-CT image.

L 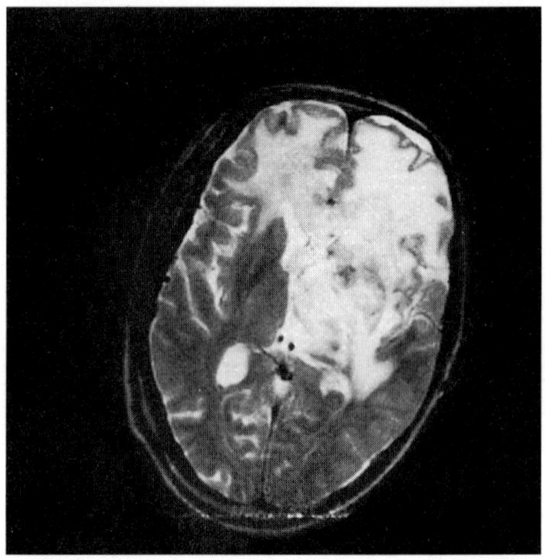 R

Fig. 14-2 Axial T_2-weighted image (2,200/90).

L 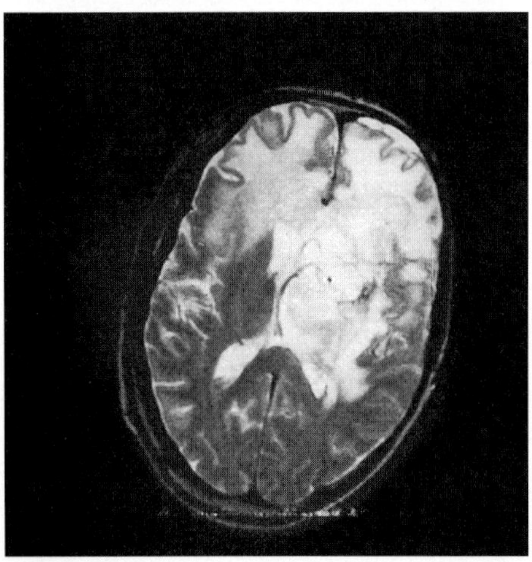 R

Fig. 14-3 Axial T_2-weighted image (2,200/90).

L 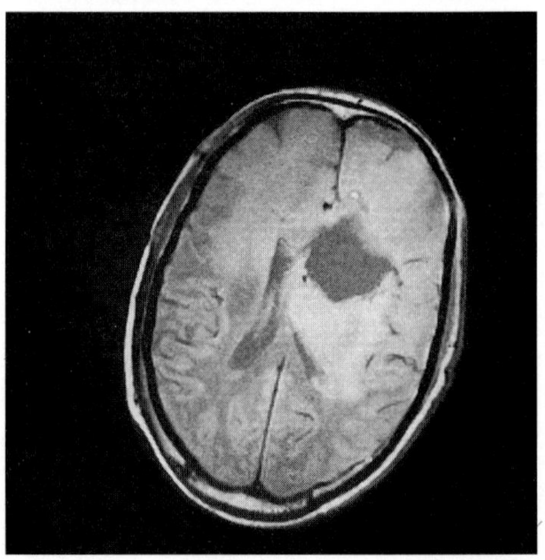 R

Fig. 14-4 Axial proton density-weighted image (2,200/15).

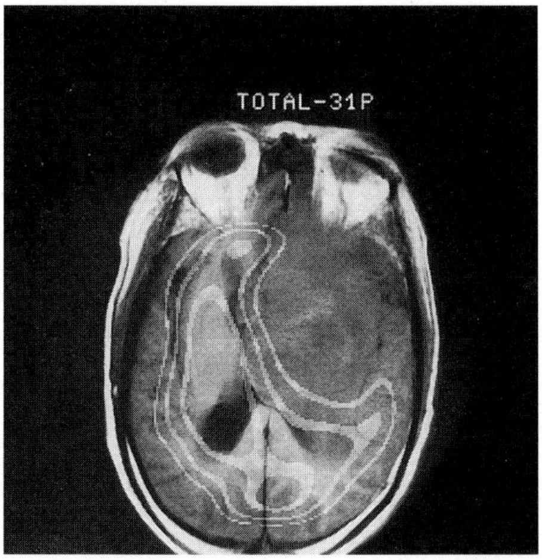

Fig. 14-5 Axial ^{31}P contour map superimposed on T_1-weighted image (500/15).

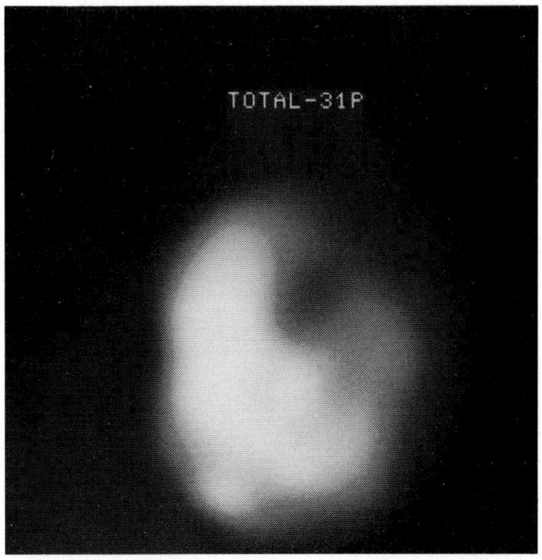

Fig. 14-6 Axial ^{31}P metabolite image.

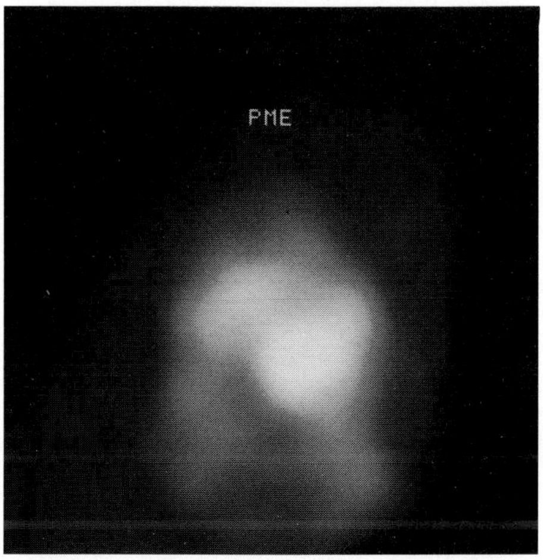

Fig. 14-7 Axial PME metabolite image.

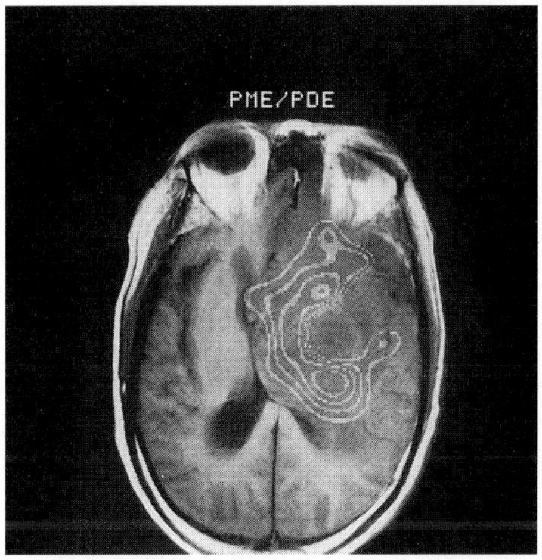

Fig. 14-8 Axial PME/PDE contour map superimposed on T_1-weighted image (500/15).

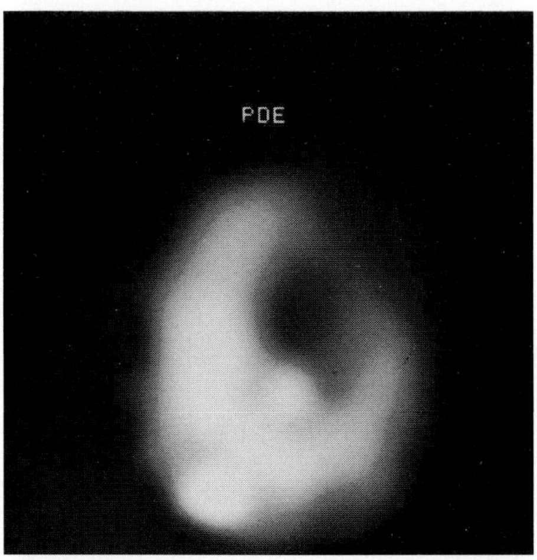

Fig. 14-9 Axial PDE metabolite image.

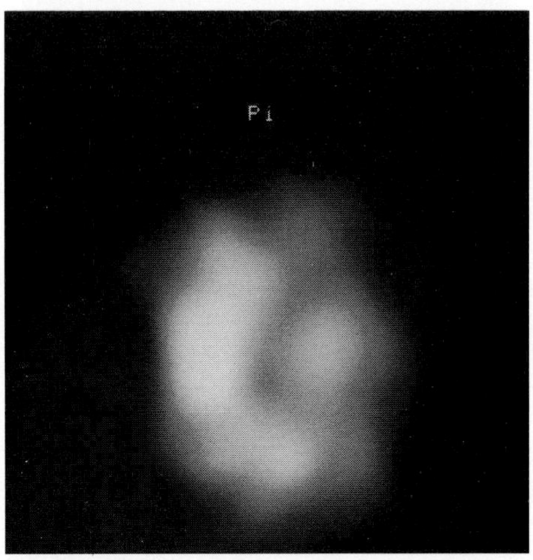

Fig. 14-10 Axial Pi metabolite image.

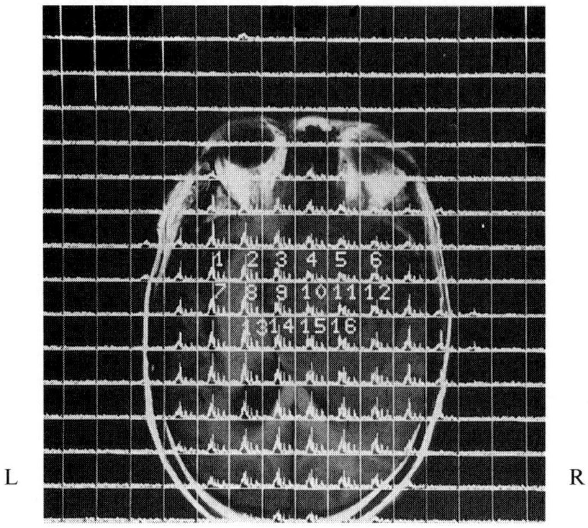

Fig. 14-11 T_1-weighted image showing the position of 1.5×1.5×4 cm^3 voxel.

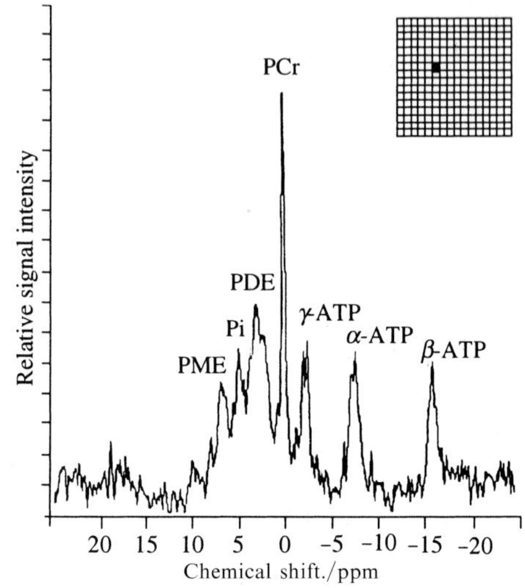

Fig. 14-12 ^{31} spectrum in control area (voxel 1).

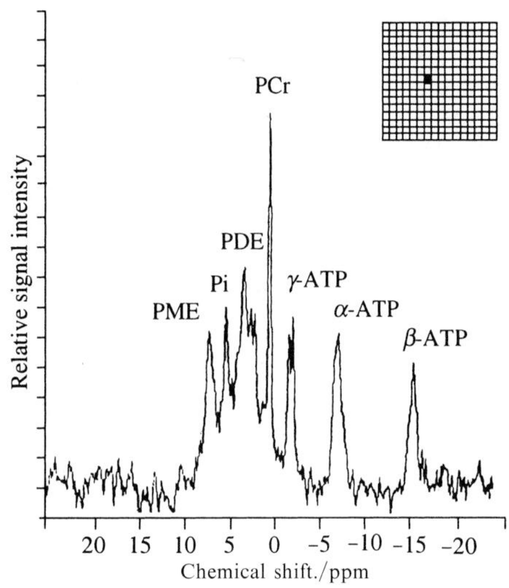

Fig. 14-13 ^{31}P spectrum in control area (voxel 2).

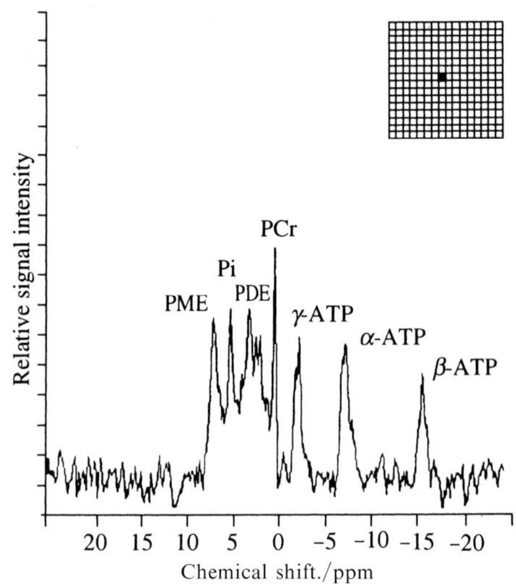

Fig. 14-14 ^{31}P spectrum in tumor area (voxel 3).

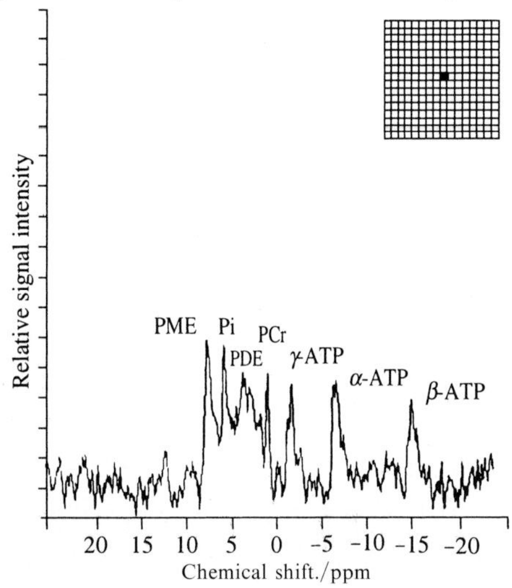

Fig. 14-15 ^{31}P spectrum in tumor area (voxel 4).

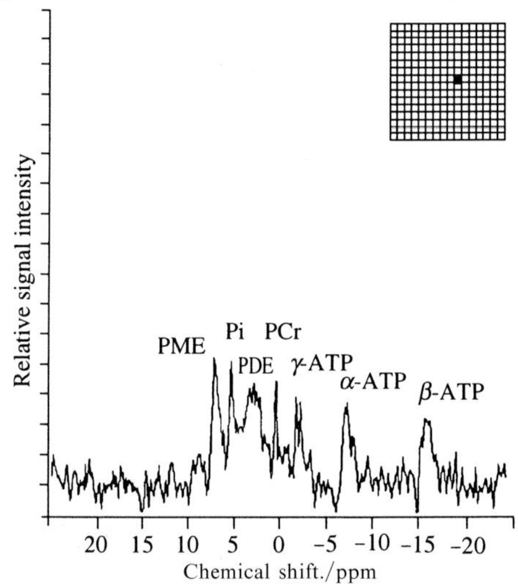

Fig. 14-16 ^{31}P spectrum in tumor area (voxel 5).

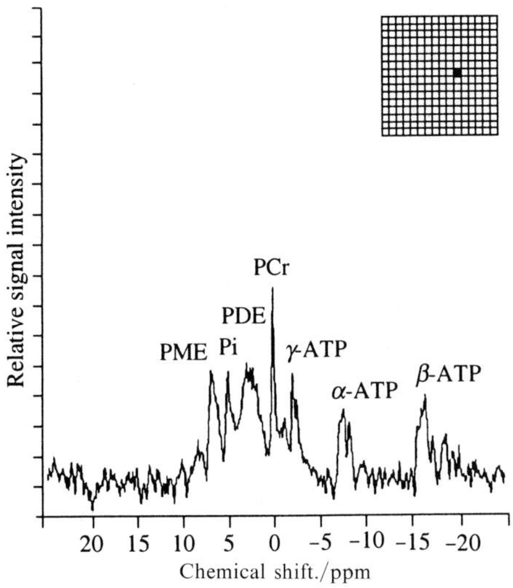

Fig. 14-17 ^{31}P spectrum in tumor area (voxel 6).

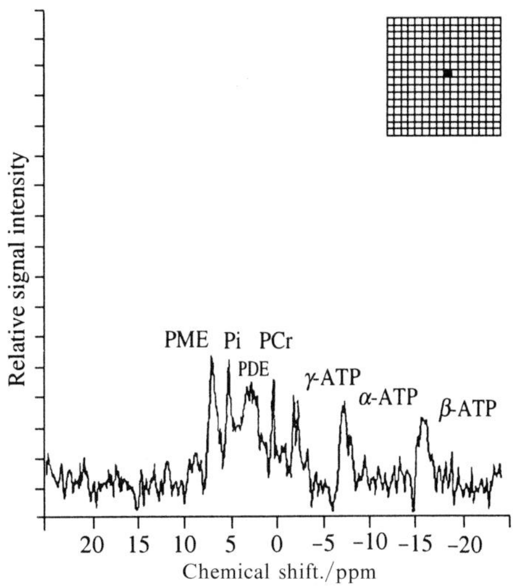

Fig. 14-18 ^{31}P spectrum in tumor area (voxel 10).

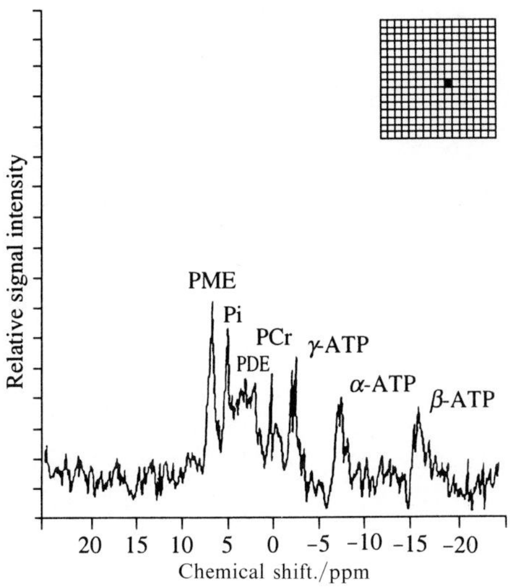

Fig. 14-19 ^{31}P spectrum in tumor area (voxel 11).

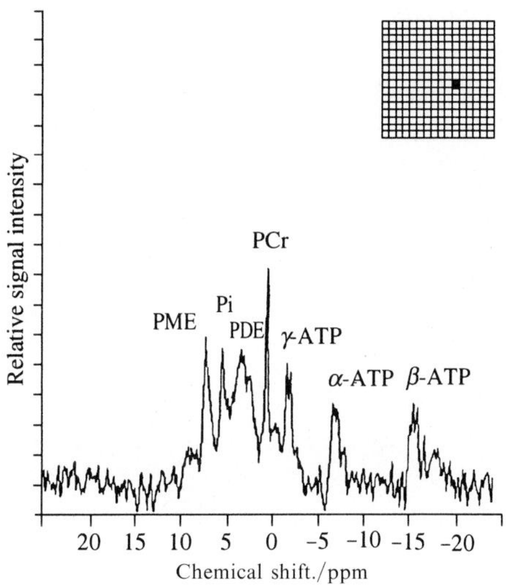

Fig. 14-20 ^{31}P spectrum in tumor area (voxel 12).

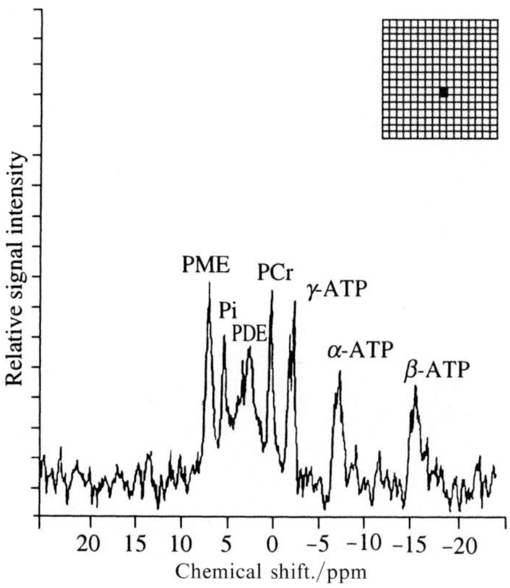

Fig. 14-21 ^{31}P spectrum in tumor area (voxel 15).

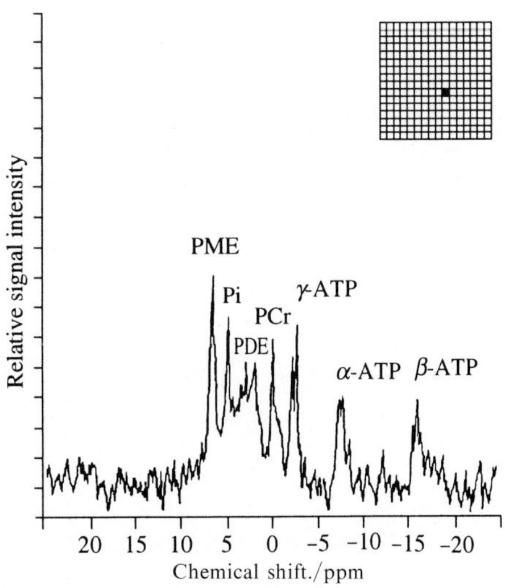

Fig. 14-22 ^{31}P spectrum in tumor area (voxel 16).

CASE 15

Case 15: A 58-year-old male

Glioblastoma

The patient suffered a left visual disturbance one month previously and revealed left hemiparesis 20 days later. The neurological examination revealed left hemiparesis, left homonymous hemianopsia, and dyscalculia. In the MRIs in Figures 15-1 and 2, a tumor is located from the right thalamus to the temporal lobe. Marked edema is noted around the tumor, and part of the tumor is necrotic. The signal intensity is reduced in the tumor area in the ^{31}P, total ATP, PME, and PDE contour maps in Figures 15-3, 4, 5, and 7. It is high in the tumor area in the Pi contour map in Figure 15-6. Figures 15-10 and 15-9 are the spectra of the tumor area and a normal control area.

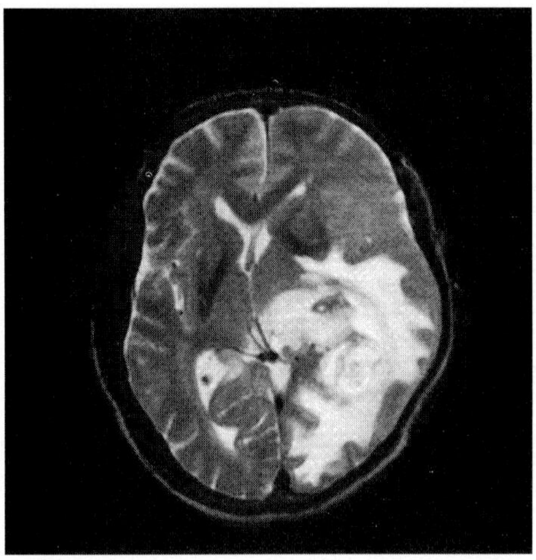

Fig. 15-1 Axial T_2-weighted image (2,200/90).

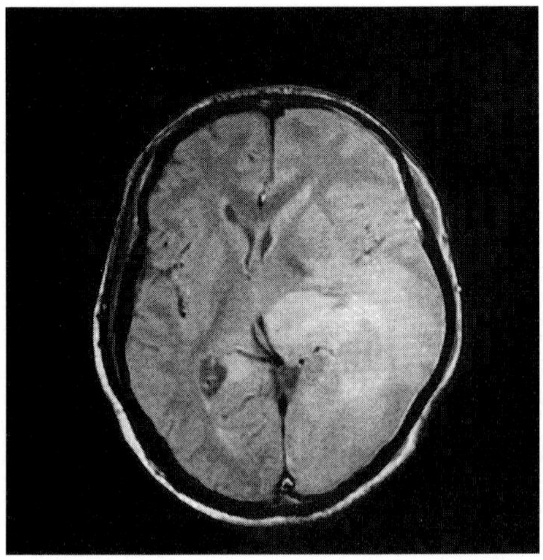

Fig. 15-2 Axial proton density-weighted image (2,200/15).

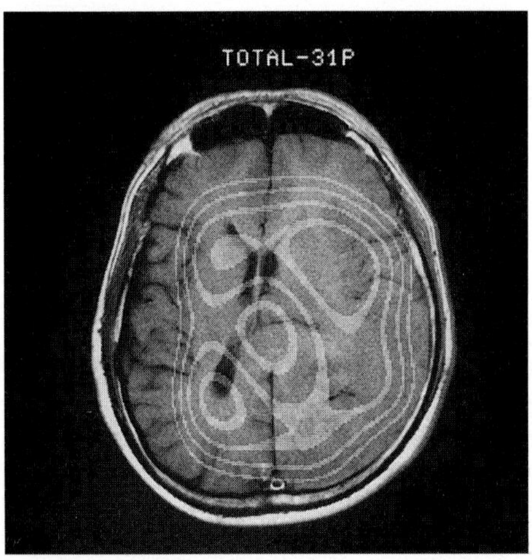

Fig. 15-3 Axial ^{31}P contour map superimposed on T_1-weighted image (500/15).

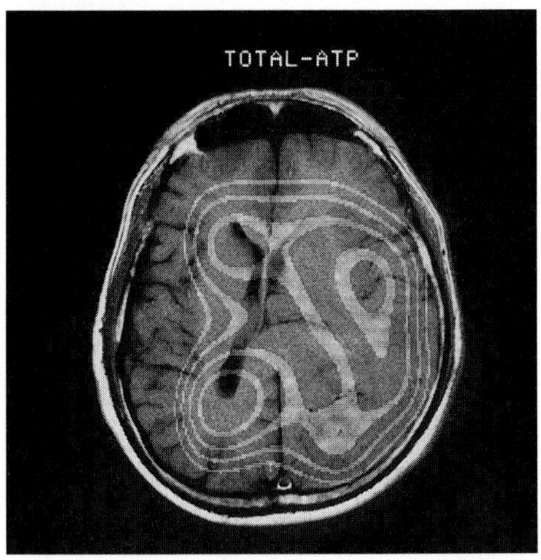

Fig. 15-4 Axial total ATP contour map superimposed on T_1-weighted image (500/15).

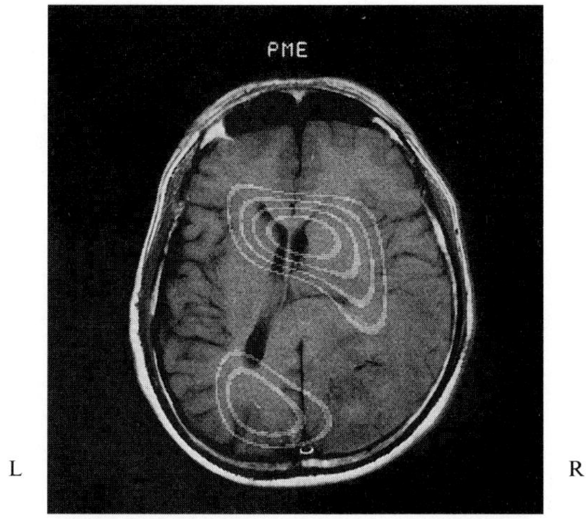

Fig. 15-5 Axial PME contour map superimposed on T_1-weighted image (500/15).

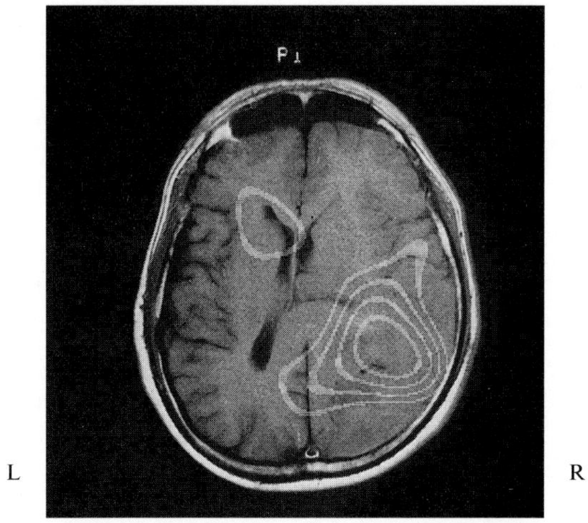

Fig. 15-6 Axial Pi contour map superimposed on T_1-weighted image (500/15).

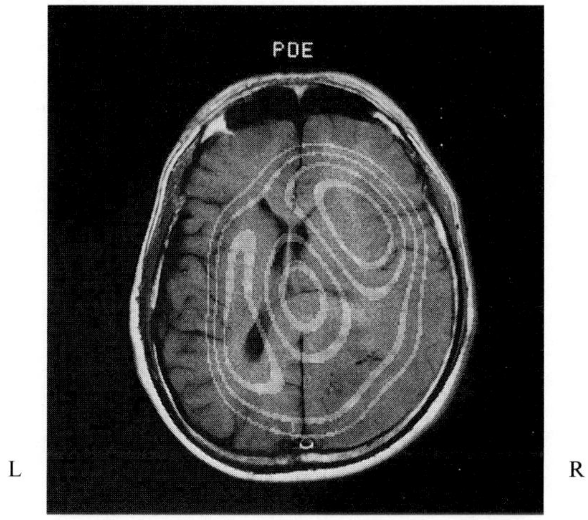

Fig. 15-7 Axial PDE contour map superimposed on T_1-weighted image (500/15).

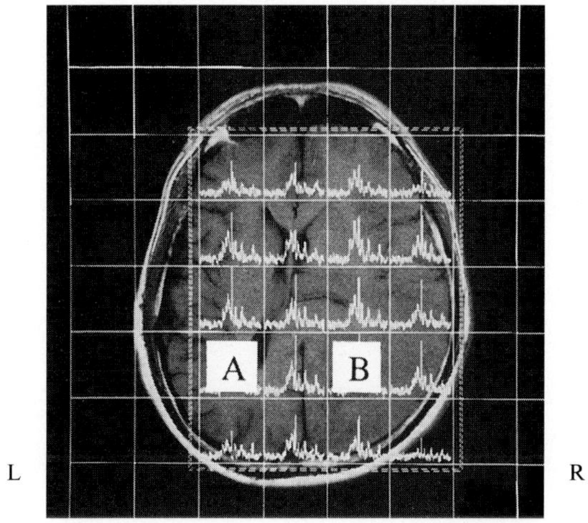

Fig. 15-8 T_1-weighted image showing the position of $3 \times 3 \times 4$ cm^3 voxels A and B.

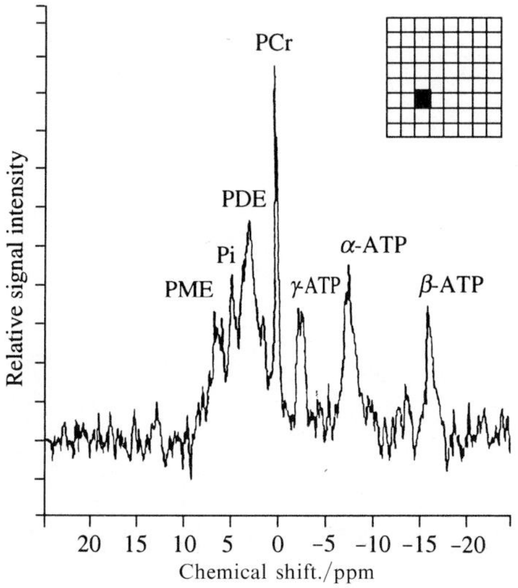

Fig. 15-9 ^{31}P spectrum in control area (voxel A).

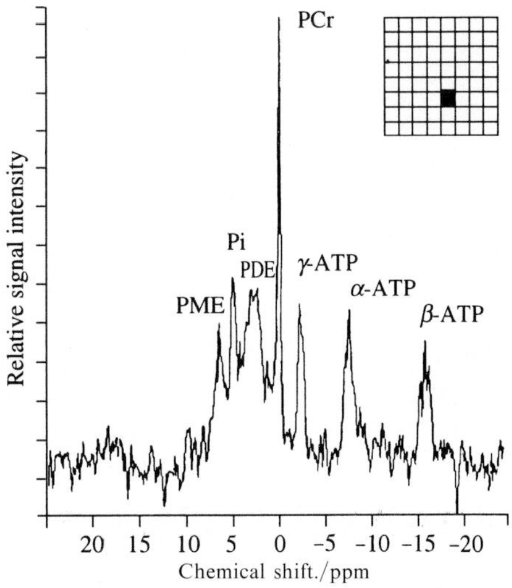

Fig. 15-10 ^{31}P spectrum in tumor area (voxel B).

CASE 16

Case 16: A 11-year-old male

Oligodendroglioma

The patient revealed right hemiparesis six months previously. The neurological examination revealed right hemiparesis. The MRIs in Figures 16-1 and 2 show a tumor extending from the left caudate nucleus to the right corona radiata. No brain edema is noted around the tumor. The signal intensity is slightly reduced in the tumor area in the ^{31}P, total ATP, PME, Pi, and PDE contour maps and metabolite image in Figures 16-3, 4, 5, 6, and 7. Figures 16-9 and 16-10 show the spectra of the tumor area and a normal control area.

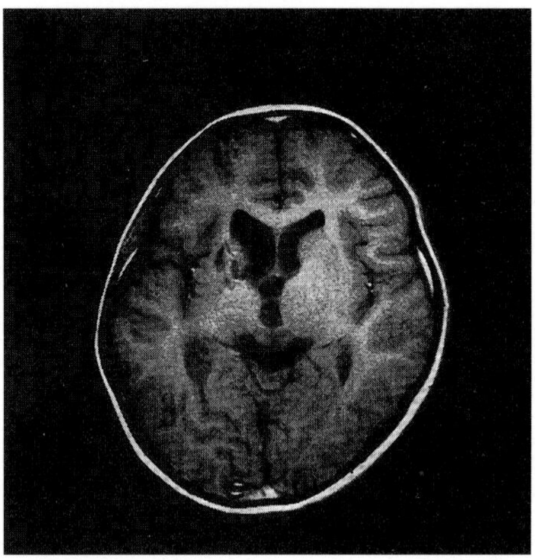

Fig. 16-1 Axial T_1-weighted image (500/15).

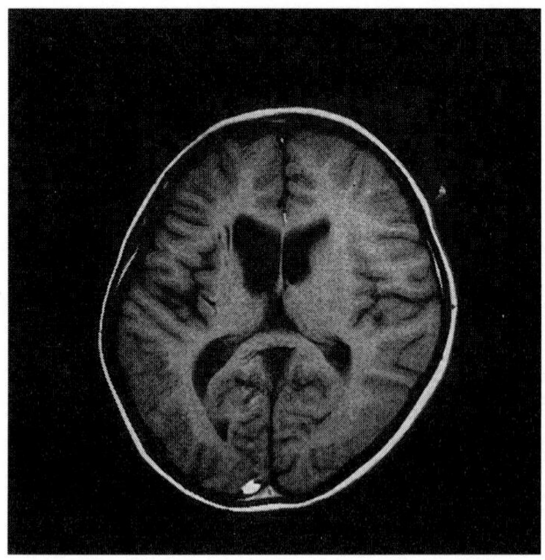

Fig. 16-2 Axial T_1-weighted image (500/15).

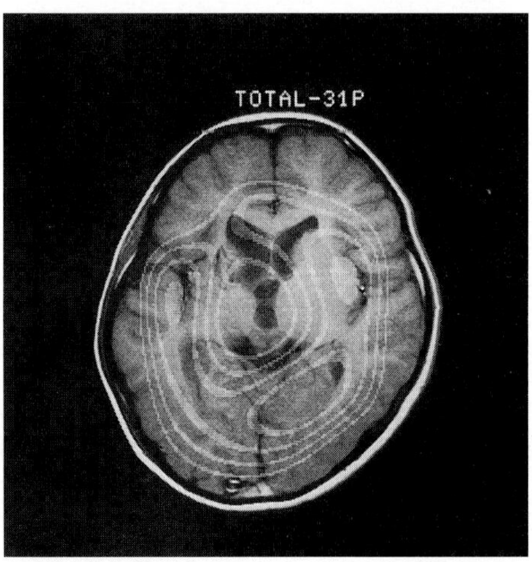

Fig. 16-3 Axial ^{31}P contour map superimposed on T_1-weighted image (500/15).

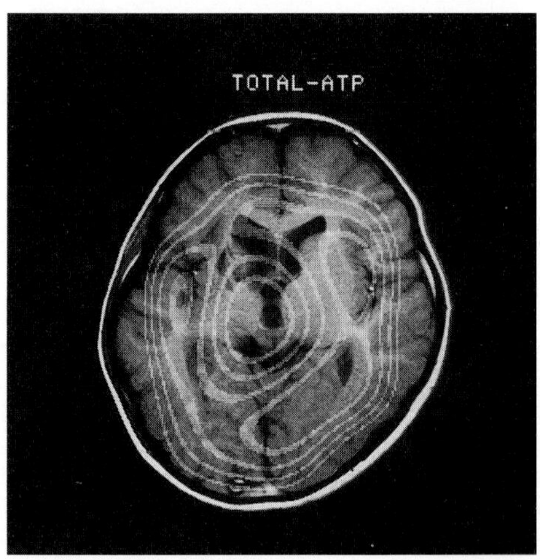

Fig. 16-4 Axial total ATP contour map superimposed on T_1-weighted image (500/15).

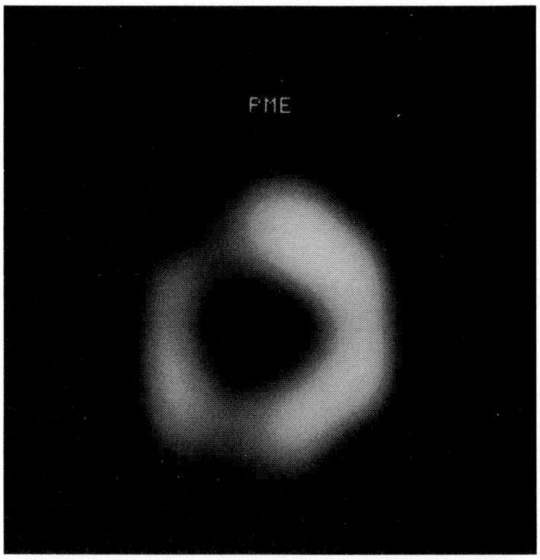

Fig. 16-5 Axial PME metabolite image.

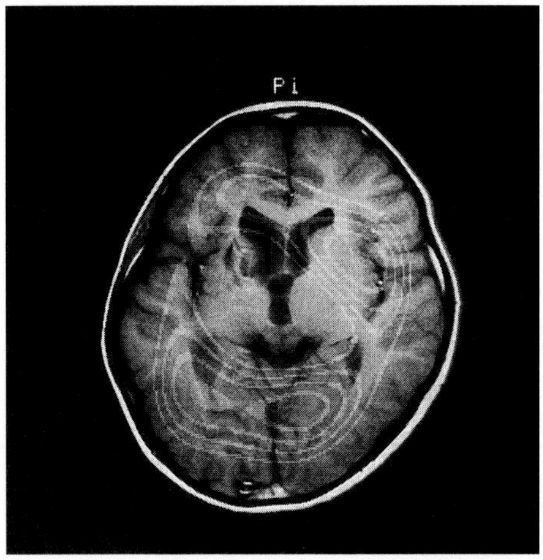

Fig. 16-6 Axial Pi contour map superimposed on T_1-weighted image (500/15).

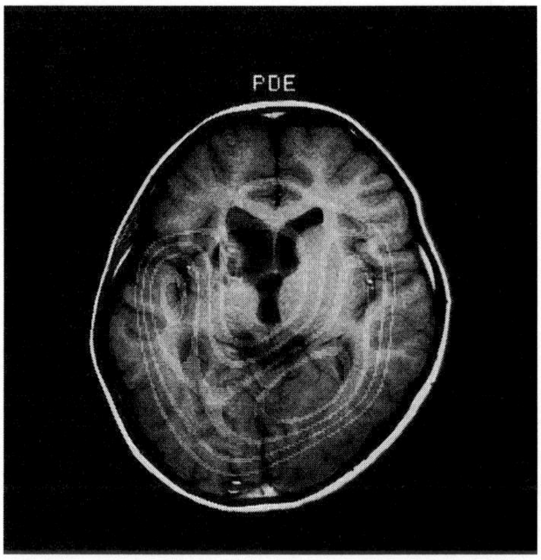

Fig. 16-7 Axial PDE contour map superimposed on T_1-weighted image (500/15).

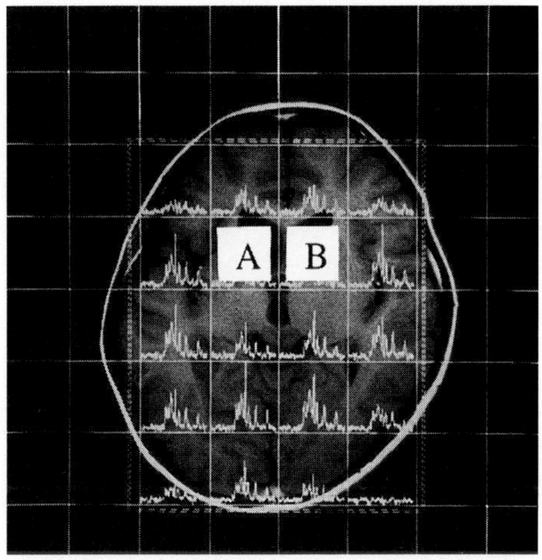

Fig. 16-8 T_1-weighted image showing the position of $3 \times 3 \times 4$ cm^3 voxels A and B.

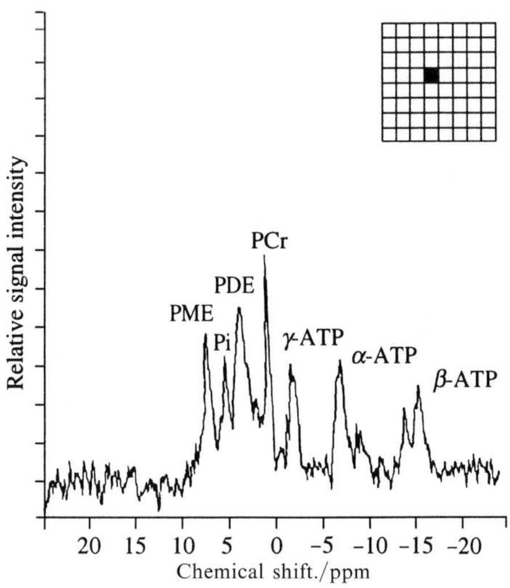

Fig. 16-9 ^{31}P spectrum in tumor area (voxel A).

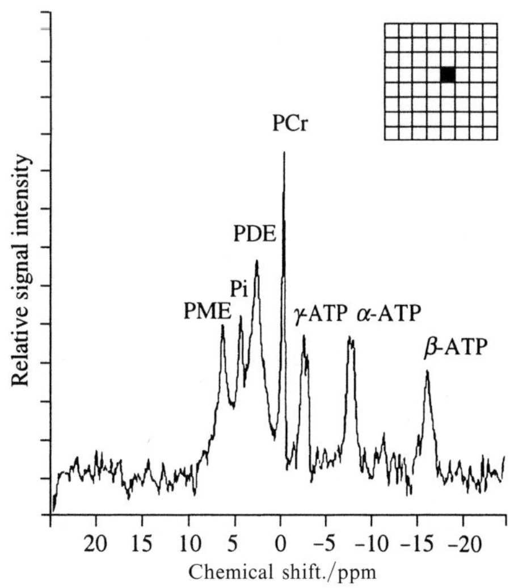

Fig. 16-10 ^{31}P spectrum in control area (voxel B).

CASE 17

Case 17: A 62-year-old male

Metastatic brain tumor (from the rectum)

The patient underwent resection of colon cancer (adenocarcinoma) three years previously. He suffered lower abdominal pain and back pain and was diagnosed as having a metastatic liver tumor one month previously. He revealed left hemiparesis and was diagnosed with a metastatic brain tumor. The neurological examination revealed left hemiparesis. The MRIs in Figures 17-1 and 2 show a tumor in the right occipital lobe. Marked brain edema is noted around the tumor. The signal intensity is slightly reduced in the tumor area in the ^{31}P, total ATP, and PDE contour maps in Figures 17-3, 4, and 7. It is high in the tumor area in the PME and Pi contour maps in Figures 17-5 and 6. Figures 17-10 and 17-9 show the spectra of the tumor area and a normal control area. The findings are as described above.

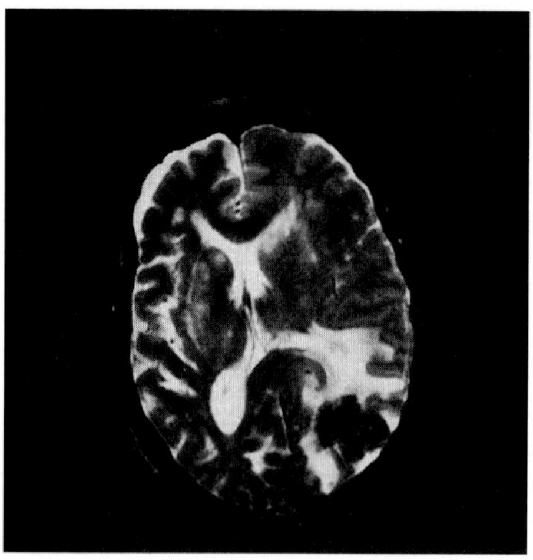

Fig. 17-1 Axial T_2-weighted image (2,200/90).

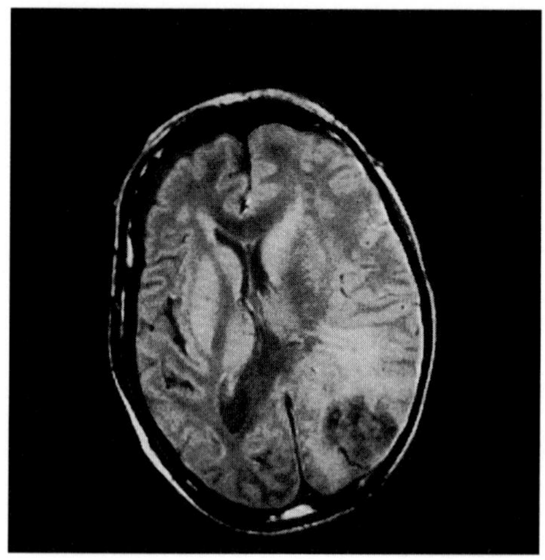

Fig. 17-2 Axial proton density-weighted image (2,200/15).

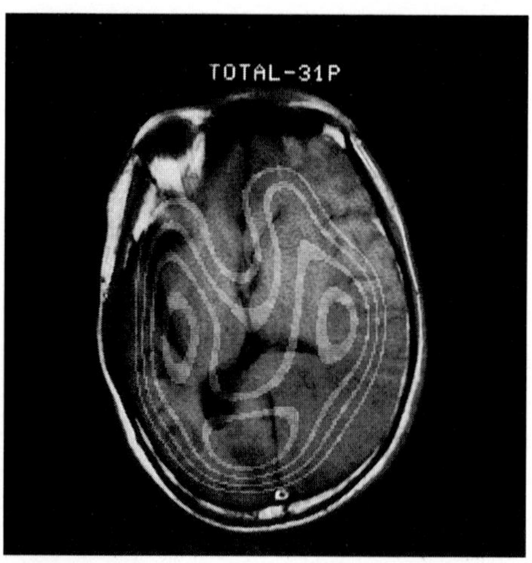

Fig. 17-3 Axial ^{31}P contour map superimposed on T_1-weighted image (500/15).

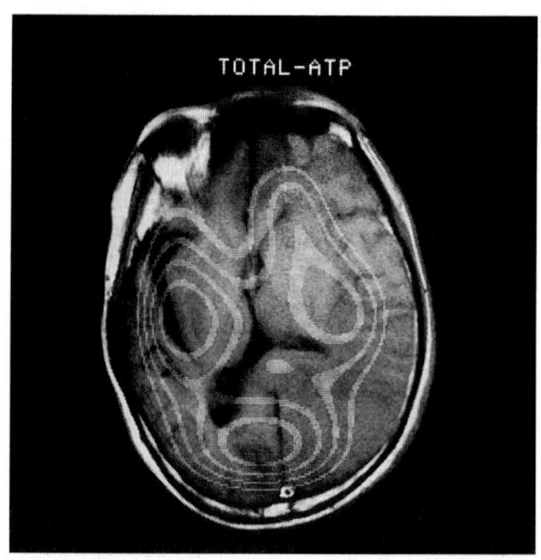

Fig. 17-4 Axial total ATP contour map superimposed on T_1-weighted image (500/15).

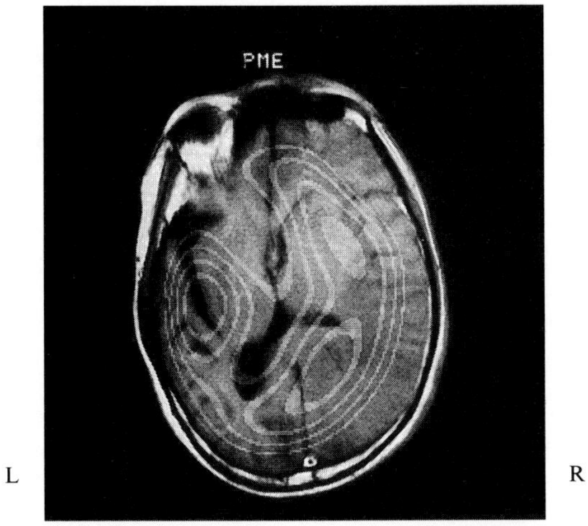

Fig. 17-5 Axial PME contour map superimposed on T_1-weighted image (500/15).

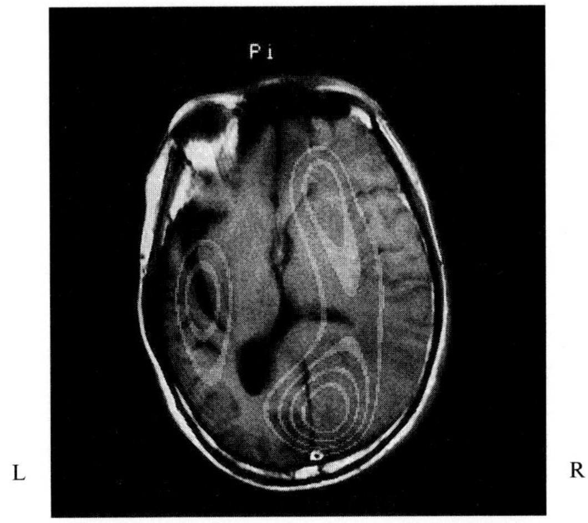

Fig. 17-6 Axial Pi contour map superimposed on T_1-weighted image (500/15).

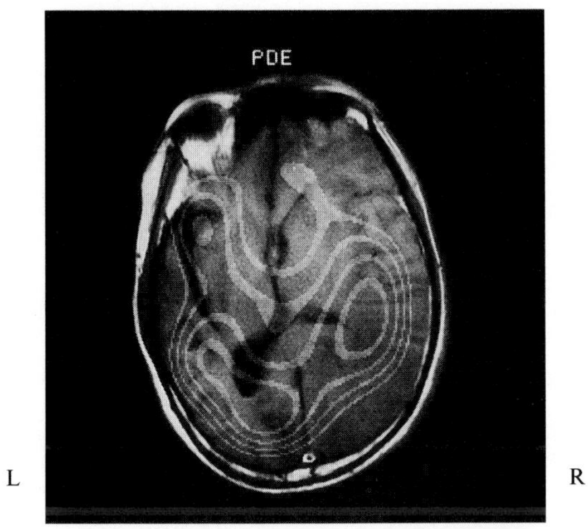

Fig. 17-7 Axial PDE contour map superimposed on T_1-weighted image (500/15).

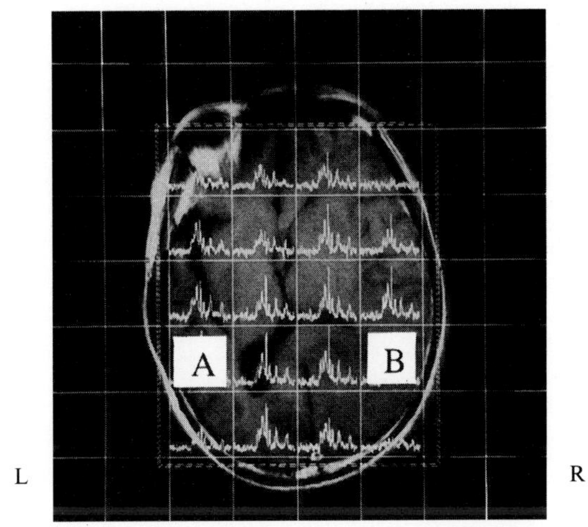

Fig. 17-8 T_1-weighted image showing the position of $3 \times 3 \times 4$ cm^3 voxels A and B.

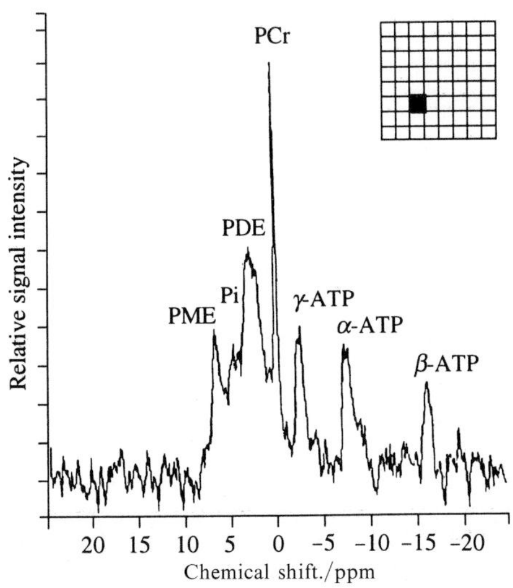

Fig. 17-9 ^{31}P spectrum in control area (voxel A).

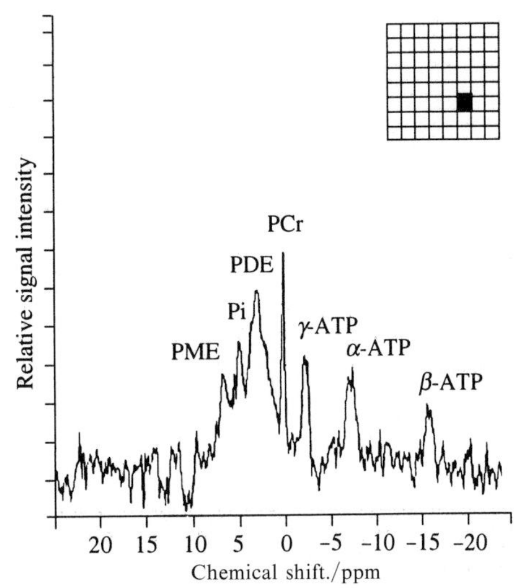

Fig. 17-10 ^{31}P spectrum in tumor area (voxel B).

CASE 18

Case 18: A 62-year-old male

Metastatic brain tumor (from the lung)

The patient suffered motor weakness of the left lower extremity three months previously and noticed motor weakness of the left upper extremity two and a half months later. The neurological examination revealed left hemiperesis. Computed tomography demonstrated multiple tumor (left cerebellar hemisphere, left occipital, and right frontal). Chest X-ray revealed a lung tumor. The MRIs in Figures 18-1 and 2 show a tumor in the right fronto-parietal region. Marked edema is noted around the tumor. The signal intensity is slightly reduced in the tumor area compared with the surrounding tissues in the ^{31}P, PDE, and β-ATP metabolite images in Figures 18-3, 6, and 7. It is slightly increased in the PME metabolite image in Figure 18-4. It is high in the tumor area in the Pi metabolite image in Figure 18-5. Figures 18-10 and 18-9 show the spectra of the tumor area and a normal control area. The findings are as described above.

L 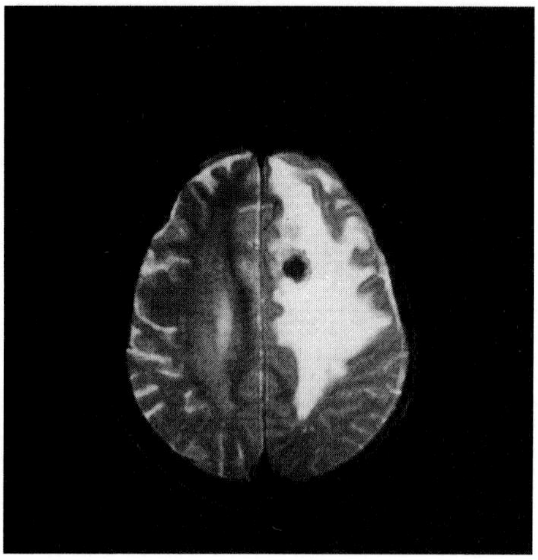 R

Fig. 18-1 Axial T_2-weighted image (2,200/90).

L 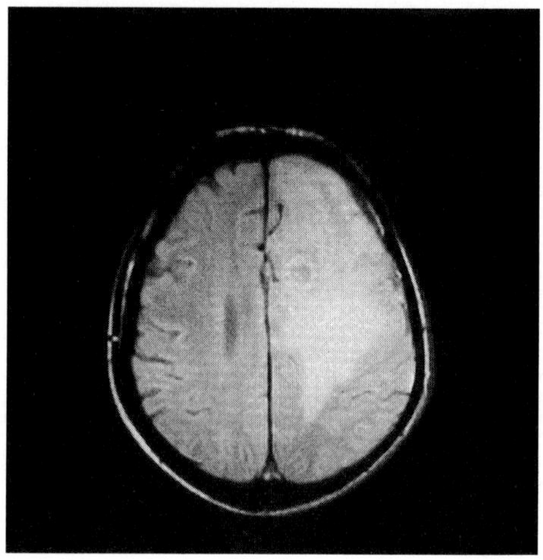 R

Fig. 18-2 Axial proton density-weighted image (2,200/15).

L 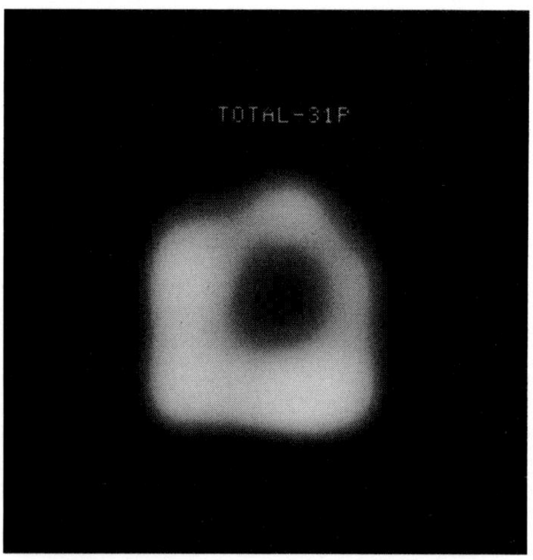 R

Fig. 18-3 Axial ^{31}P metabolite image.

L 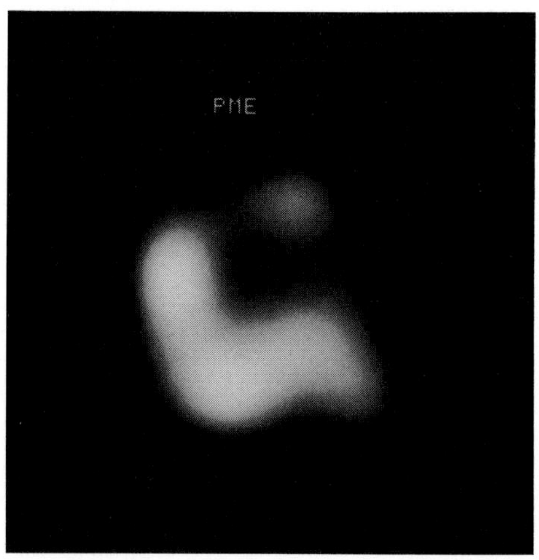 R

Fig. 18-4 Axial PME metabolite image.

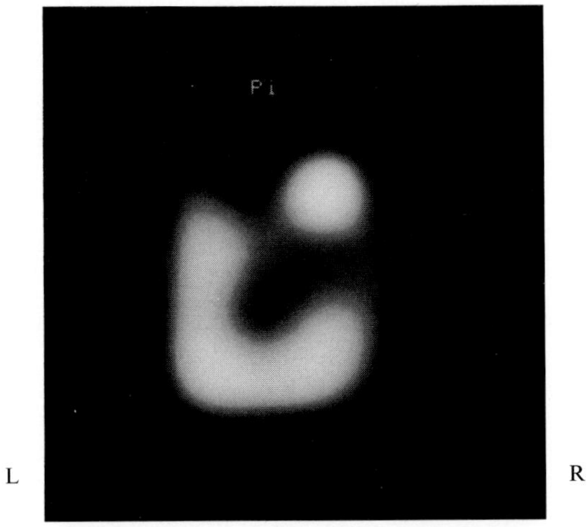

Fig. 18-5 Axial Pi metabolite image.

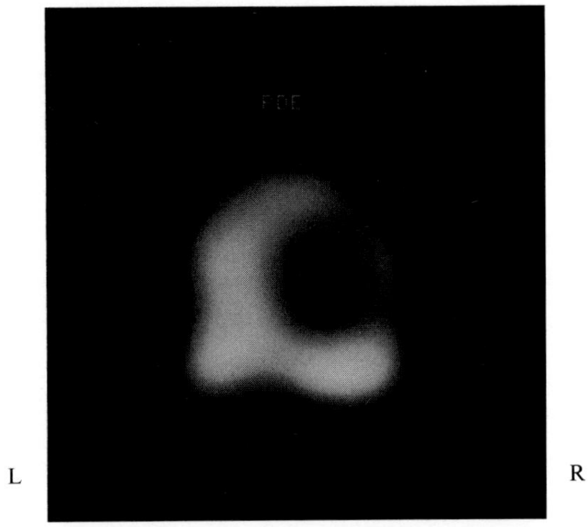

Fig. 18-6 Axial PDE metabolite image.

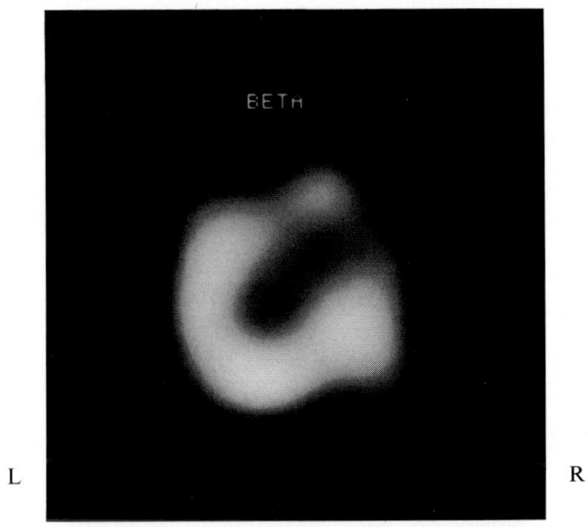

Fig. 18-7 Axial β-ATP metabolite image.

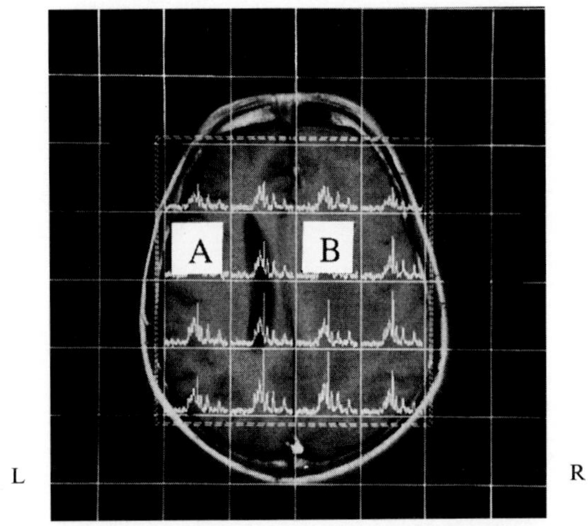

Fig. 18-8 T_1-weighted image showing the position of $3 \times 3 \times 4$ cm^3 voxels A and B.

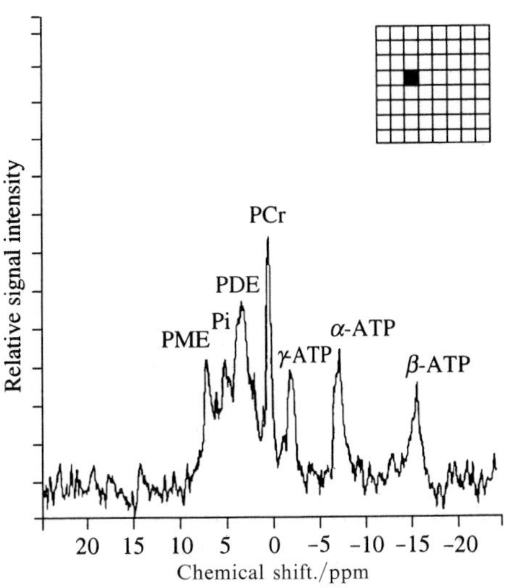

Fig. 18-9 ^{31}P spectrum in control area (voxel A).

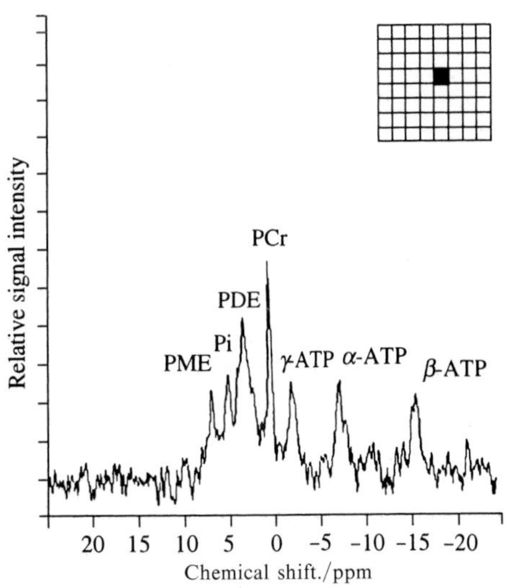

Fig. 18-10 ^{31}P spectrum in tumor area (voxel B).

CASE 19

Case 19: An 80-year-old male

Metastatic brain tumor (from the lung)

The patient suffered occipitalgia. The neurological examination revealed disorientation, motor aphasia, and right hemiparesis. Chest X-ray demonstrated a lung tumor. The MRIs in Figures 19-1 and 2 show a tumor in the left temporal lobe. Marked brain edema is noted around the tumor. The signal intensity is slightly reduced in the tumor area compared with the surrounding tissues in the ^{31}P, PDE, and PCr metabolite images shown in Figures 19-3, 6, and 7. It is slightly high in the PME metabolite image in Figure 19-4. It is high in the tumor area in the Pi metabolite image in Figure 19-5. Figures 19-9 and 19-10 show the spectra of the tumor area and a normal control area. The findings are as described above.

L 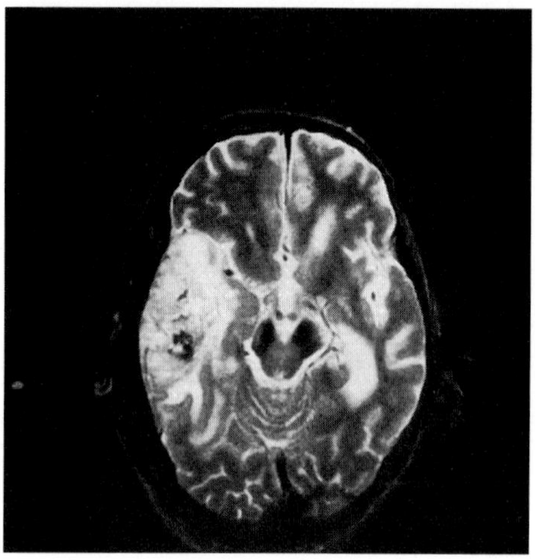 R

Fig. 19-1 Axial T_2-weighted image (2,200/90).

L 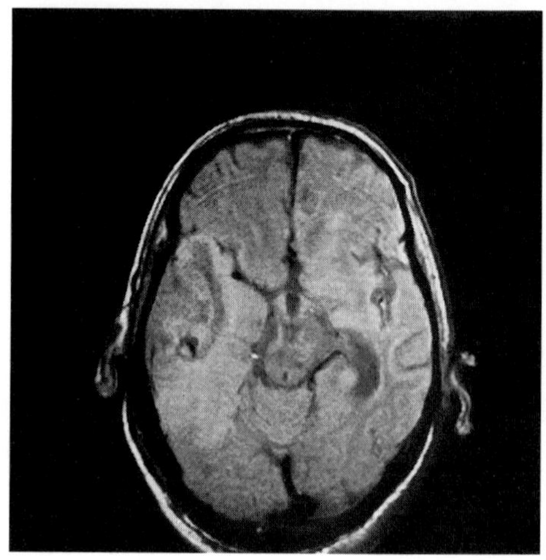 R

Fig. 19-2 Axial proton density-weighted image (2,200/15).

L 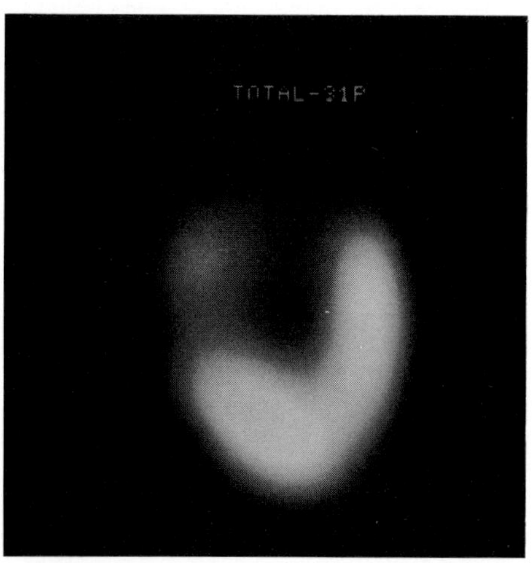 R

Fig. 19-3 Axial ^{31}P metabolite image.

L 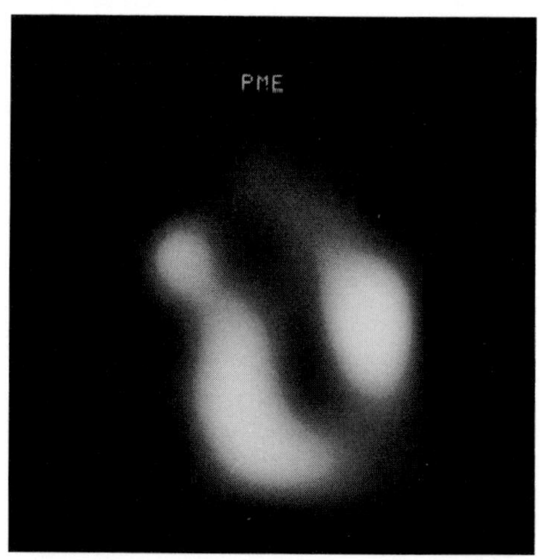 R

Fig. 19-4 Axial PME metabolite image.

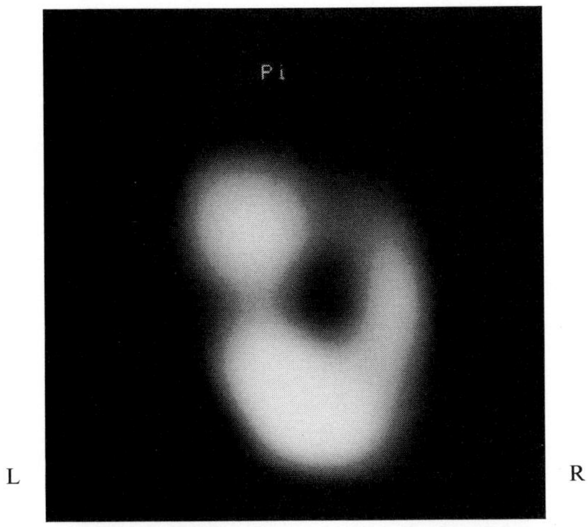

Fig. 19-5 Axial Pi metabolite image.

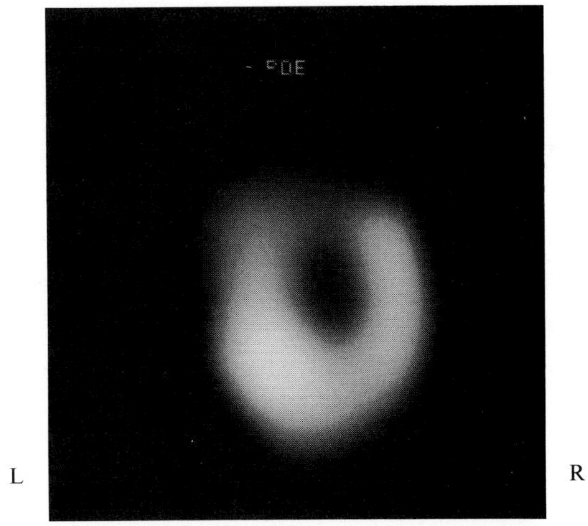

Fig. 19-6 Axial PDE metabolite image.

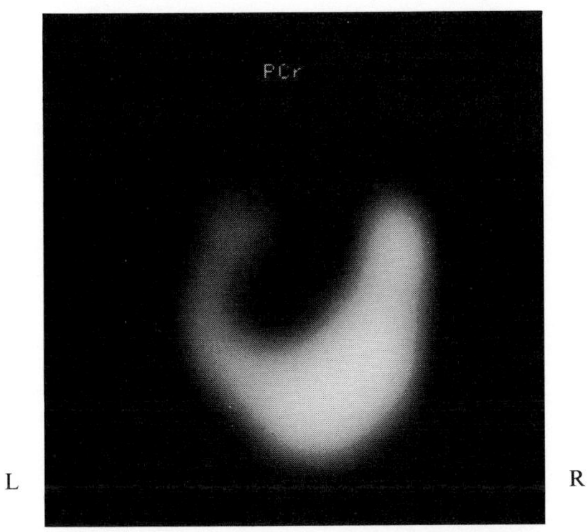

Fig. 19-7 Axial PCr metabolite image.

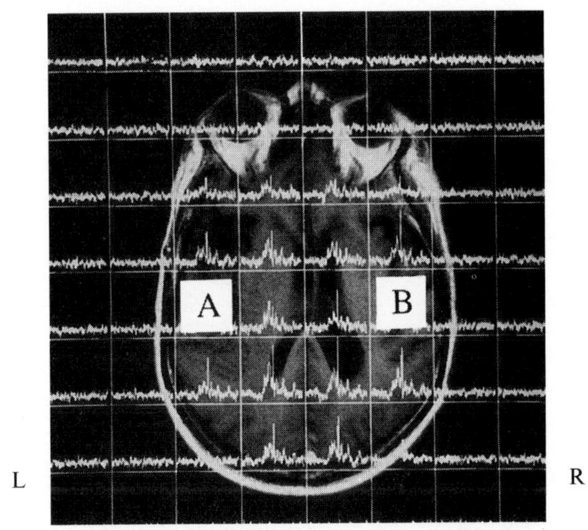

Fig. 19-8 T_1-weighted image showing the position of $3 \times 3 \times 4$ cm^3 voxels A and B.

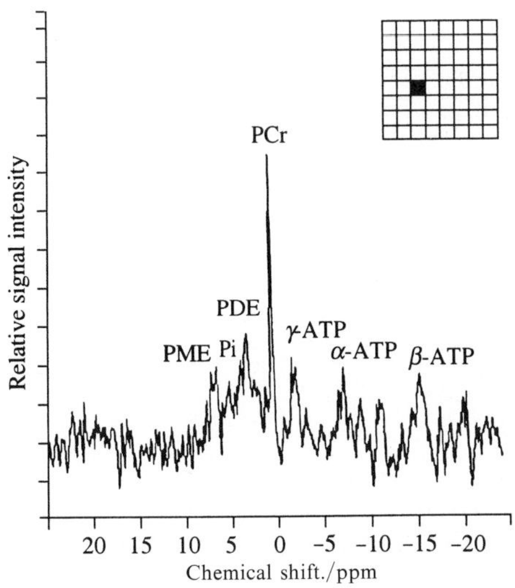

Fig. 19-9 ^{31}P spectrum in tumor area (voxel A).

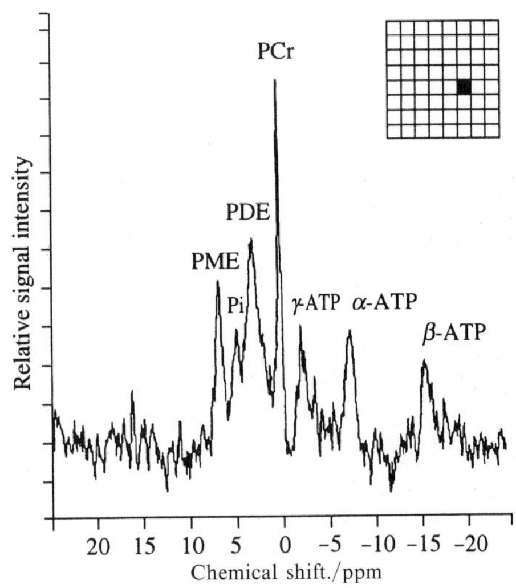

Fig. 19-10 ^{31}P spectrum in control area (voxel B).

CASE 20

Case 20: A 37-year-old-female

Chondrosarcoma

The patient suffered transient diplopia 11 months previously. She complained of right temporal headache and right hypesthesia of the face. The neurological examination revealed right hypesthesia of the face. The MRIs in Figures 20-1 and 2 show a tumor in the right temporal lobe. Brain edema around the tumor is mild. The signal intensity is reduced in the tumor area compared with the surrounding tissues in the ^{31}P, total ATP, PME, Pi, and PDE contour maps in Figures 20-3, 4, 5, 6, and 7. Figures 20-9 and 20-10 show the spectra of the tumor area and a normal control area. The findings are as described above.

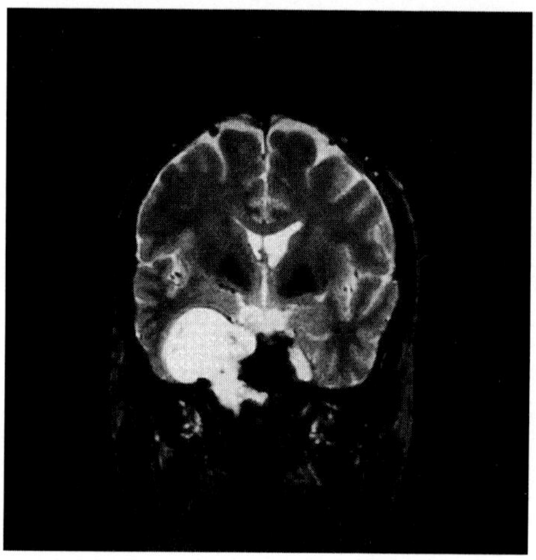

Fig. 20-1 Coronal T_2-weighted image (2,200/90).

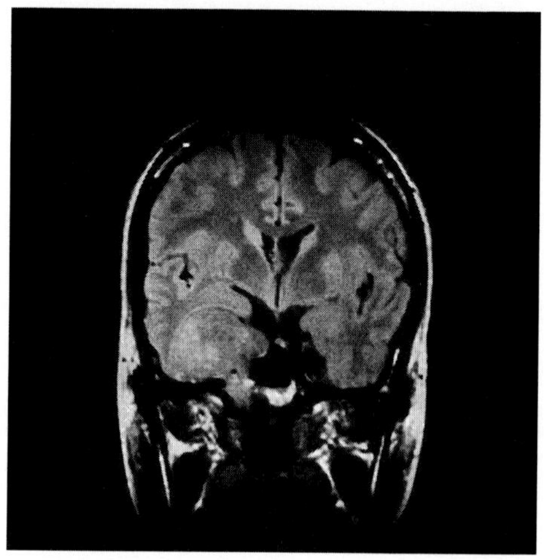

Fig. 20-2 Coronal proton density-weighted image (2,200/15).

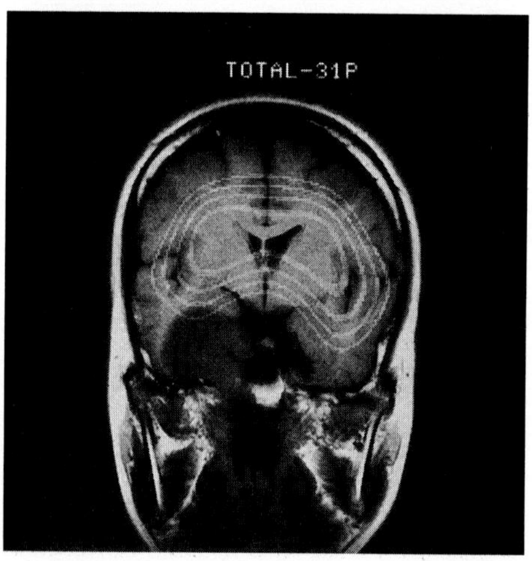

Fig. 20-3 Coronal ^{31}P contour map superimposed on T_1-weighted image (500/15).

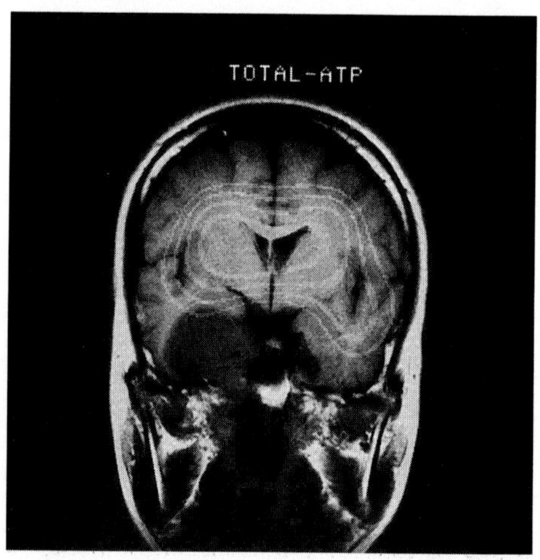

Fig. 20-4 Coronal total ATP contour map superimposed on T_1-weighted image (500/15).

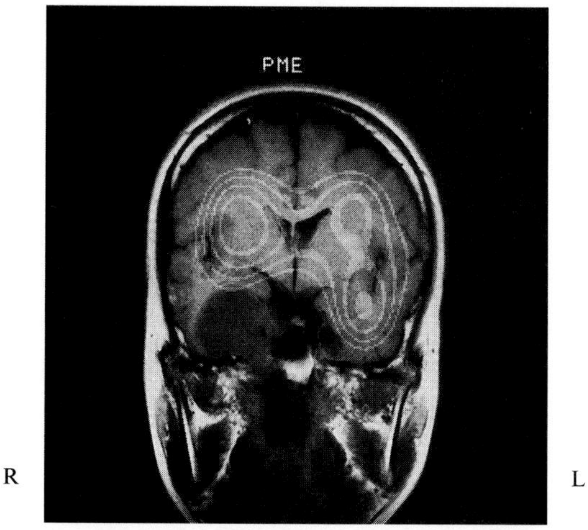

Fig. 20-5 Coronal PME contour map superimposed on T_1-weighted image (500/15).

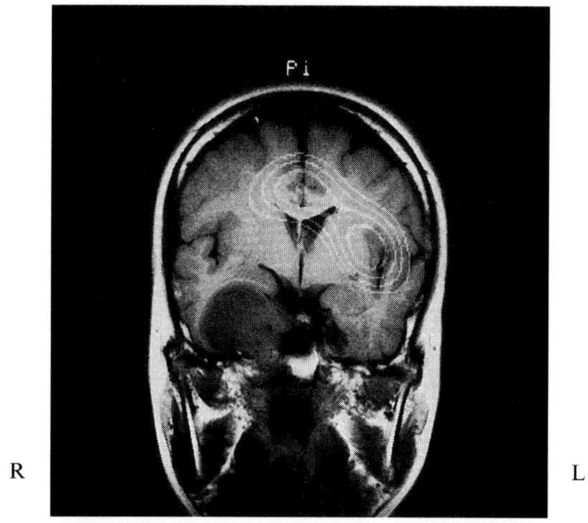

Fig. 20-6 Coronal Pi contour map superimposed on T_1-weighted image (500/15).

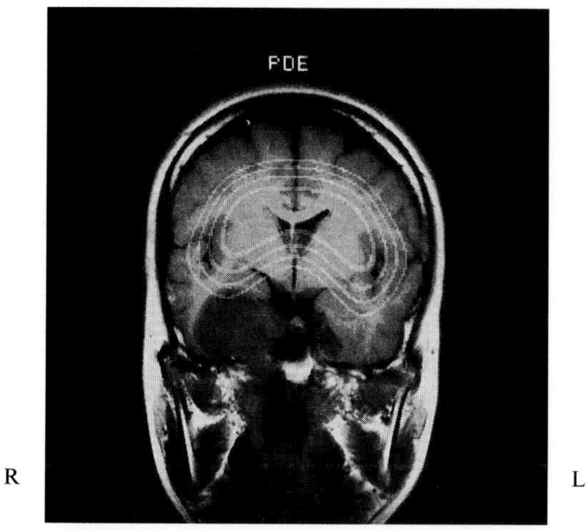

Fig. 20-7 Coronal PDE contour map superimposed on T_1-weighted image (500/15).

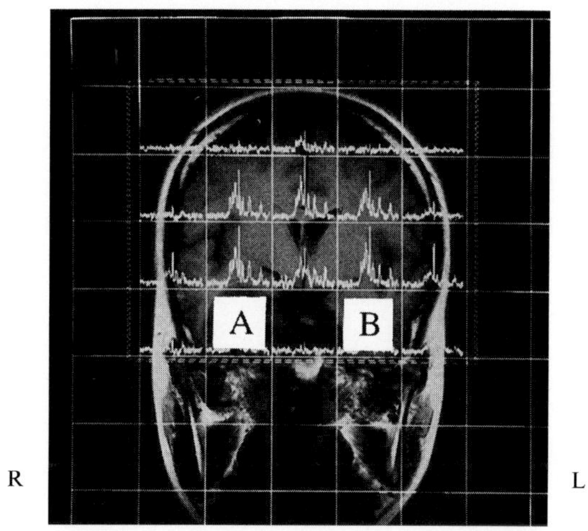

Fig. 20-8 T_1-weighted image showing the position of 3×3×4 cm^3 voxels A and B.

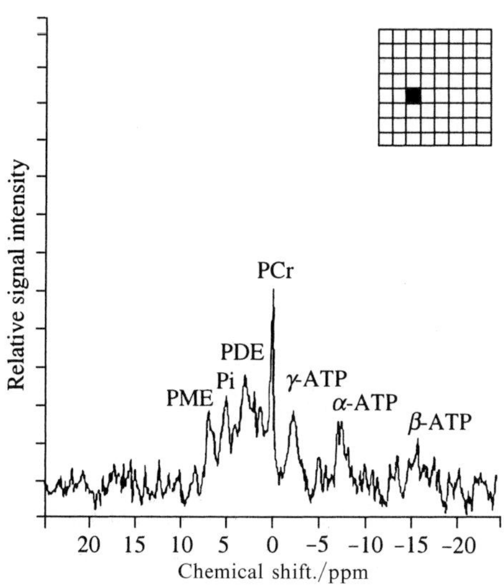

Fig. 20-9 ^{31}P spectrum in tumor area (voxel A).

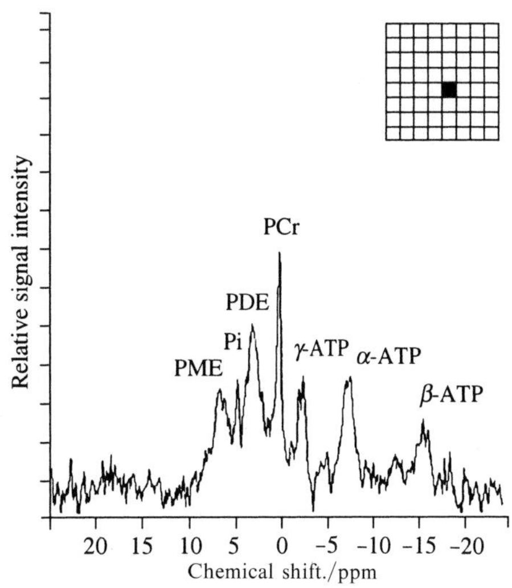

Fig. 20-10 ^{31}P spectrum in control area (voxel B).

CASE 21

Case 21: A 71-year-old male

Mucocele

The patient suffered syncopal attacks and was admitted to the hospital. The neurolgical examination was normal. He had a long history of pansinusitis but did not undergo any treatment. The MRIs in Figures 21-1 and 2 show a tumor in the right base of the skull. Mild brain edema is noted around the tumor. The signal intensity is reduced in the tumor area in the ^{31}P, total ATP, PME, Pi, and PDE contour maps and metabolite images in Figures 21-3, 4, 5, 6, and 7. Figures 21-10 and 9 show the spectra of the lesion and a normal control area. The findings are as described above.

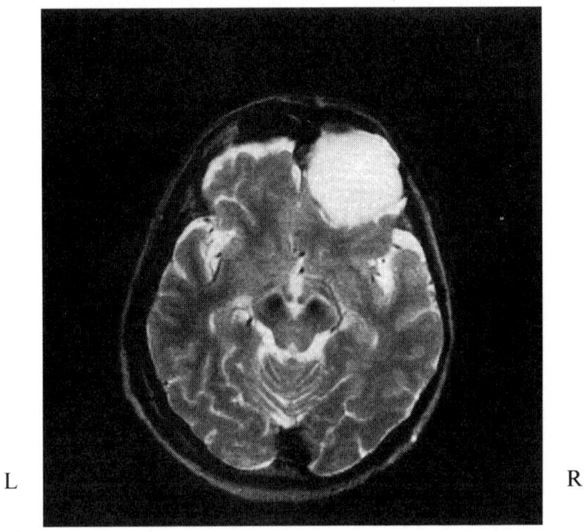

Fig. 21-1 Axial T_2-weighted image (2,200/90).

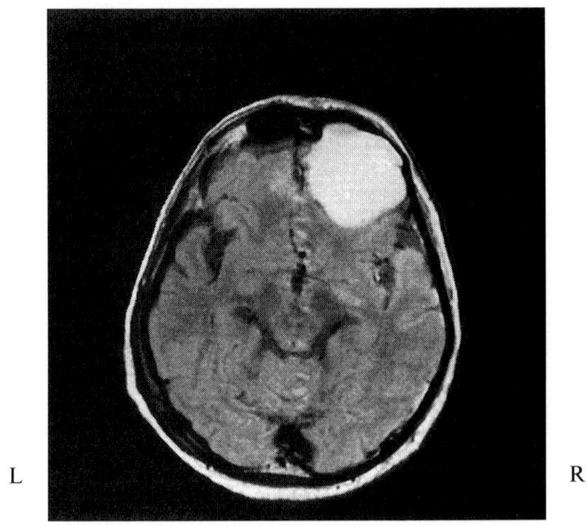

Fig. 21-2 Axial proton density-weighted image (2,200/15).

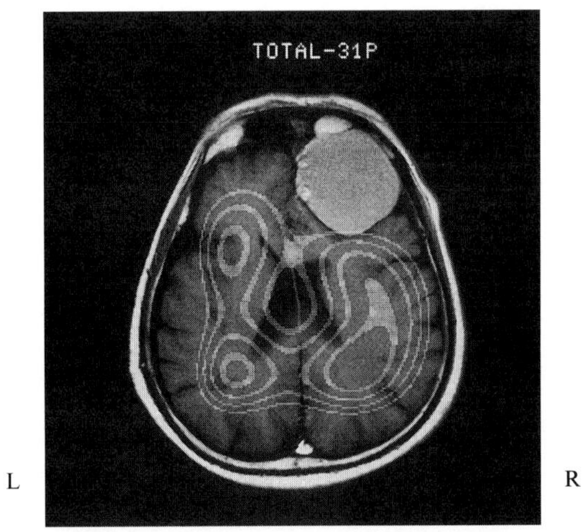

Fig. 21-3 Axial ^{31}P contour map superimposed on T_1-weighted image (500/15).

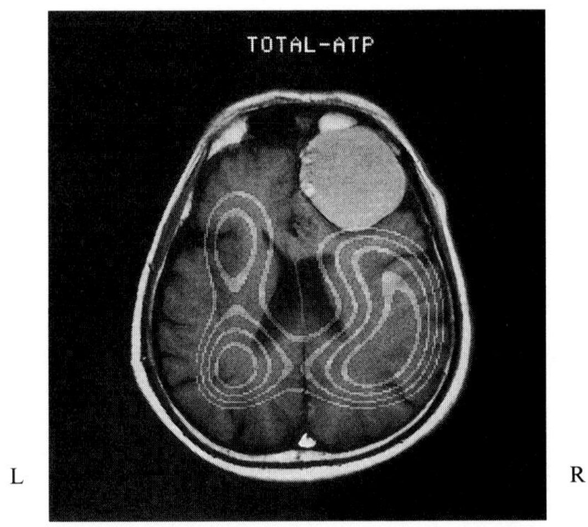

Fig. 21-4 Axial total ATP contour map superimposed on T_1- weighted image (500/15).

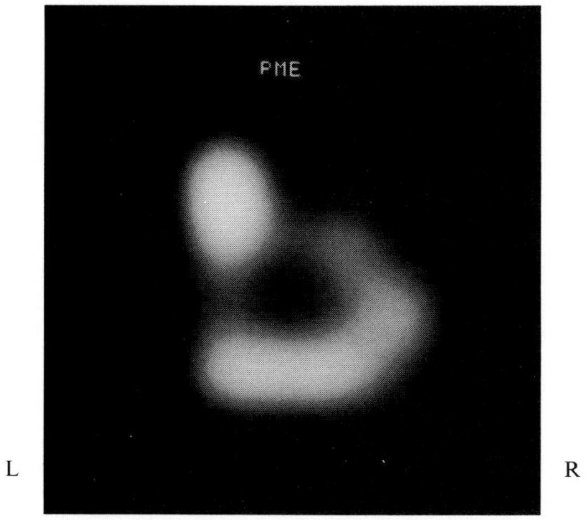

Fig. 21-5 Axial PME metabolite image.

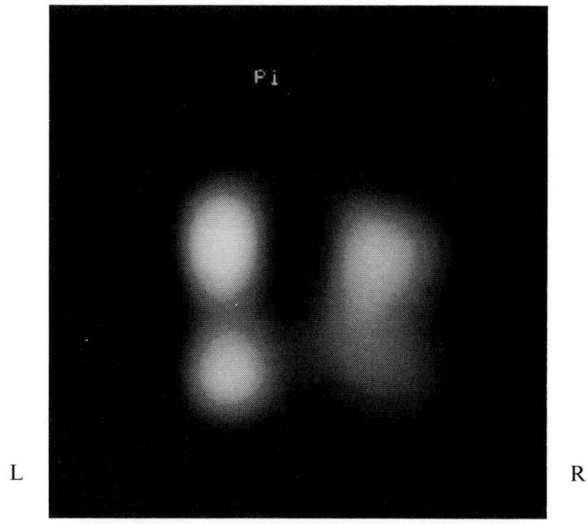

Fig. 21-6 Axial Pi metabolite image.

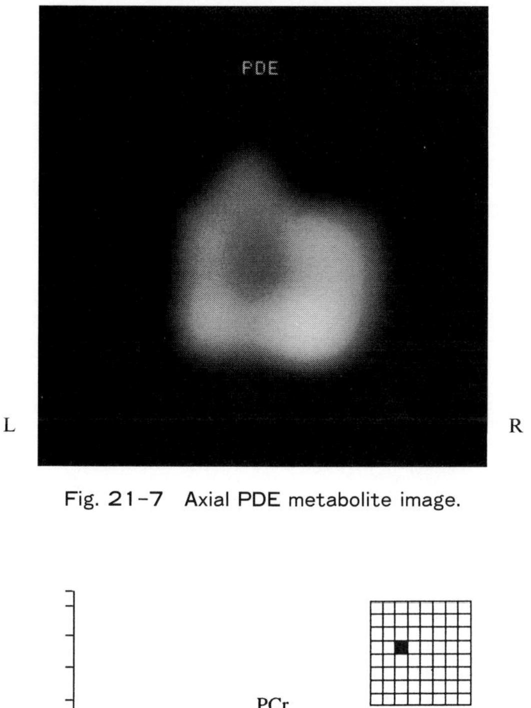

Fig. 21-7 Axial PDE metabolite image.

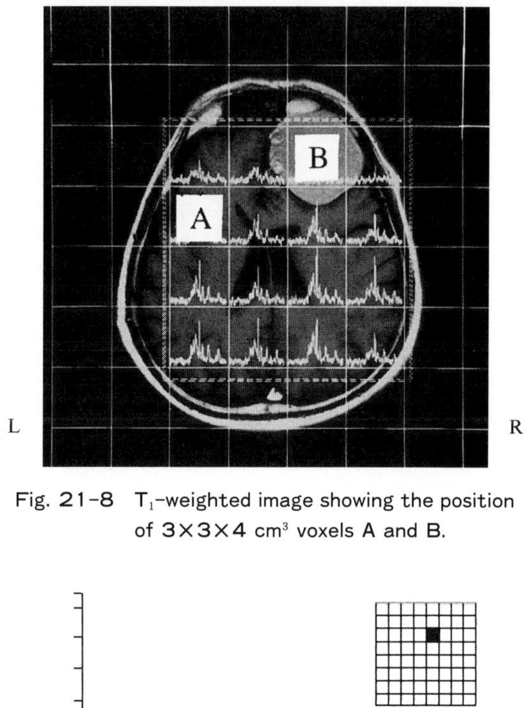

Fig. 21-8 T_1-weighted image showing the position of $3 \times 3 \times 4$ cm^3 voxels A and B.

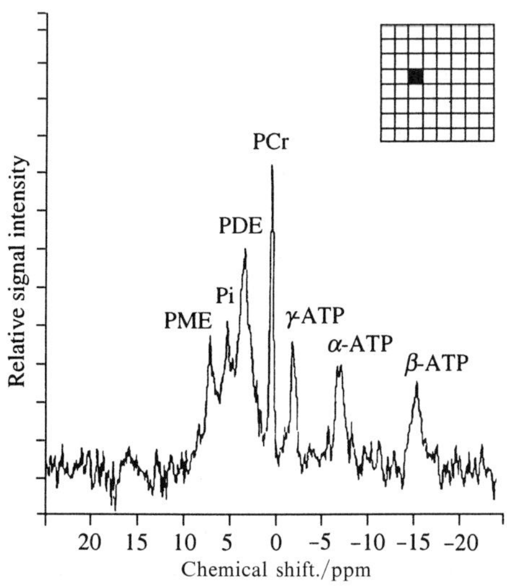

Fig. 21-9 ^{31}P spectrum of control area (voxel A).

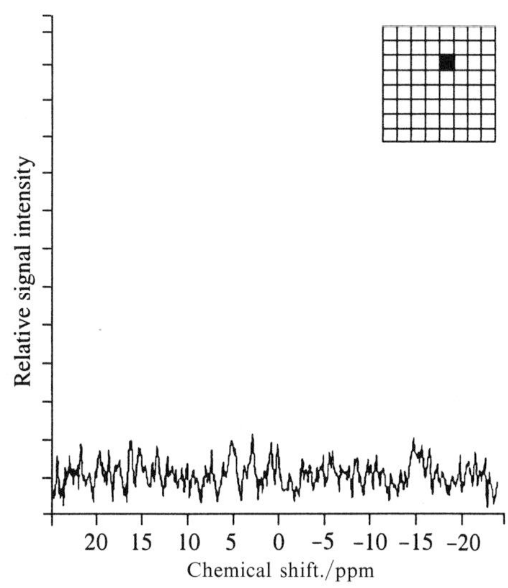

Fig. 21-10 ^{31}P spectrum of tumor area (voxel B).

5.3 EVALUATION OF THE EFFECTS OF RADIOTHERAPY AND CHEMOTHERAPY ON BRAIN TUMORS

CASE 22

4 cases: 1 case of glioblastoma and 3 cases of astrocytoma (grade III)

Figures 22-1, 2, 3, and 4 are examples from patient 1. The findings in the tumor area and normal control areas before and after treatment and at follow-up are compared. All patients were treated by radiotherapy (56-60 Gy) and ACNU chemotherapy. Figures 22-5 to 10 show changes in the tumor/normal ratio of various phosphorus compounds and pHi. The responsiveness of the tumor is observed graphically.

L 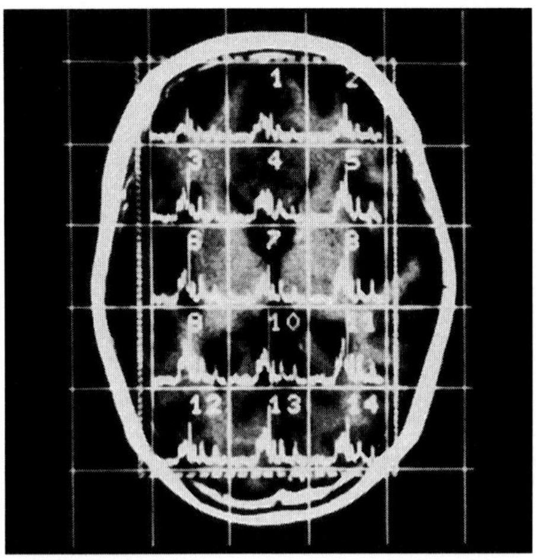 R

Fig. 22-1 T_1-weighted image showing the position of 3×3×4 cm^3 voxel.

L 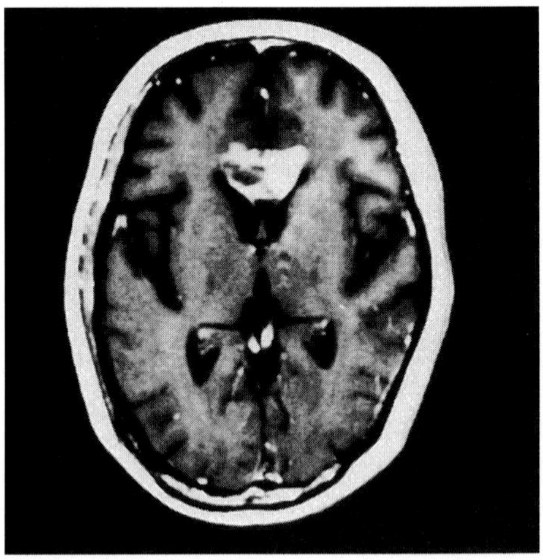 R

Fig. 22-2 Axial enhanced T_1 weighted image (500/15).

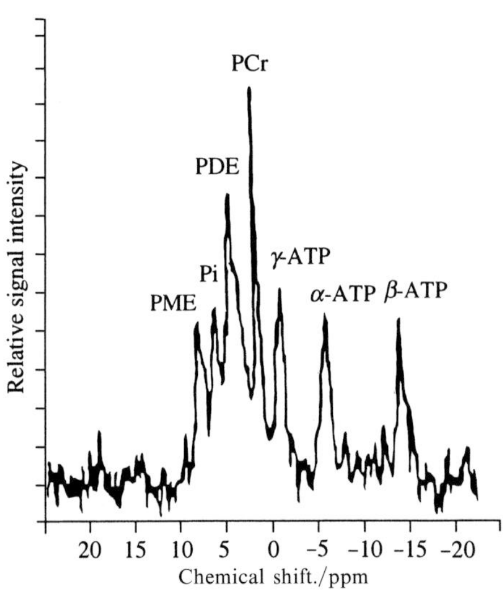

Fig. 22-3 ^{31}P spectrum of control area.

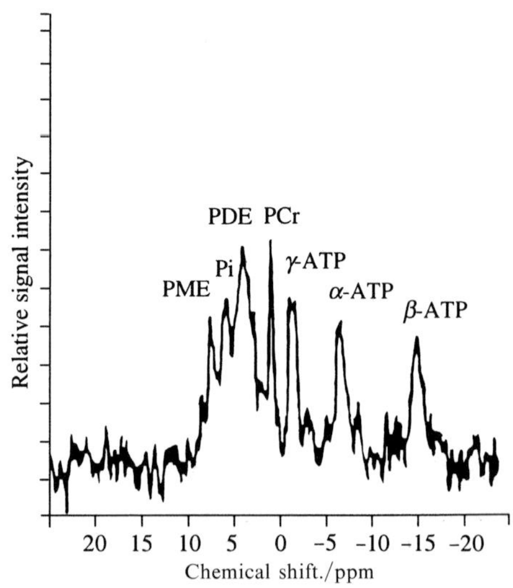

Fig. 22-4 ^{31}P spectrum of tumor area.

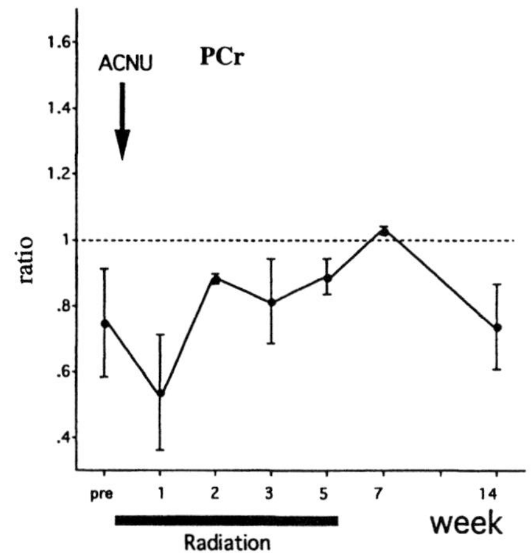

Fig. 22-5 PCr changes due to therapy.

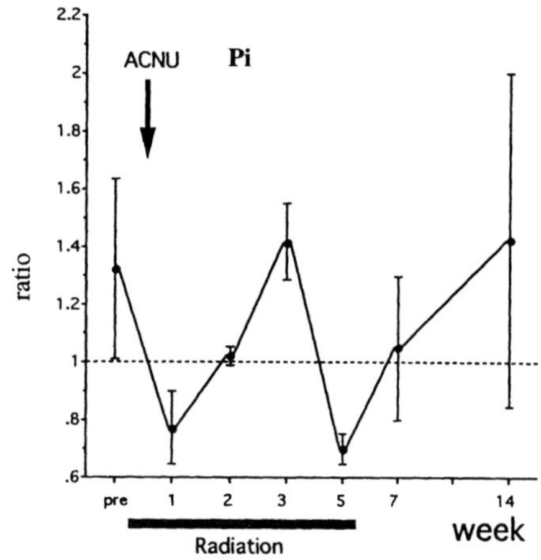

Fig. 22-6 Pi changes due to therapy.

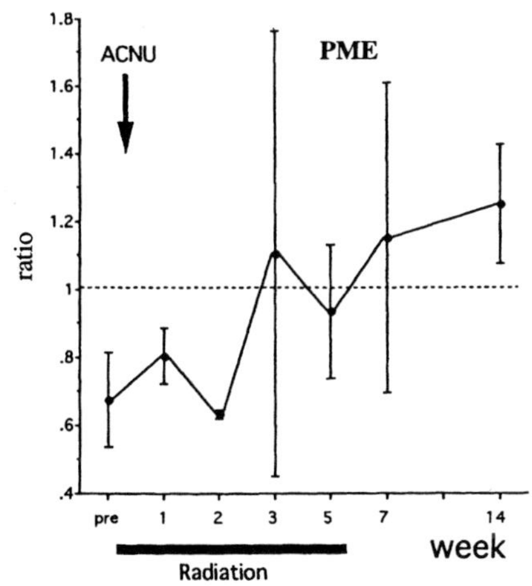

Fig. 22-7 PME changes due to therapy.

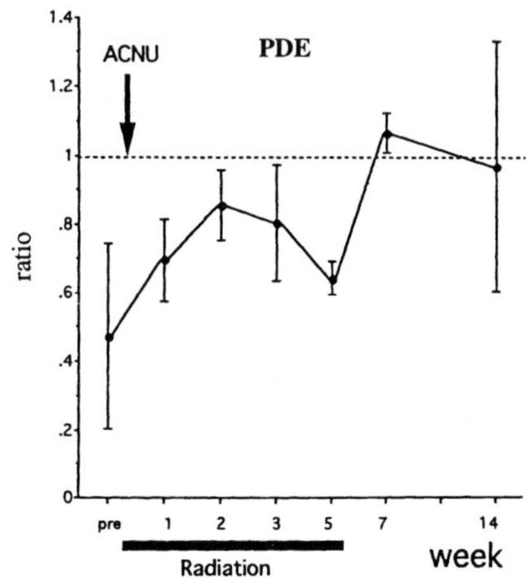

Fig. 22-8 PDE changes due to therapy.

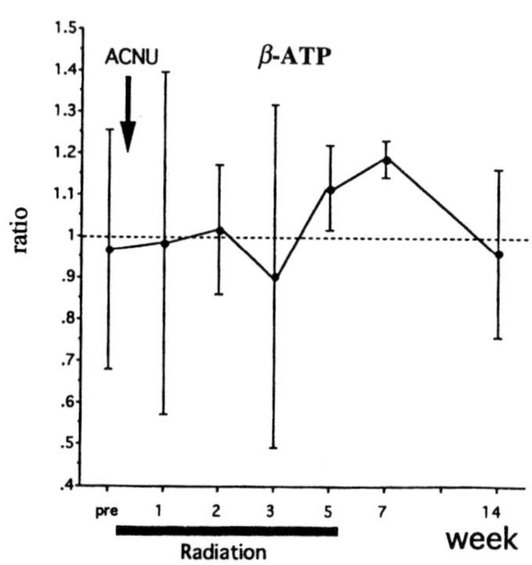

Fig. 22-9 β-ATP changes due to therapy.

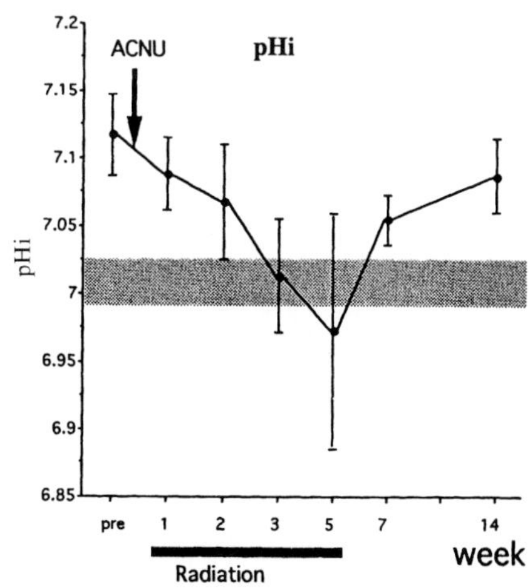

Fig. 22-10 pHi changes due to therapy.

5.4 EVALUATION OF THE EFFECTS OF RADIOTHERAPY FOR BRAIN TUMORS ON NORMAL BRAIN TISSUE

CASE 23

6 cases: 5 cases of glioma and 1 case of metastatic brain tumor

Figures 23-1, 2, 3, and 4 are examples from patient 1. Findings in the normal area before, 7 weeks after, and 16 weeks after radiotherapy were compared. The results were expressed as percentages and compared with those in healthy individuals. Figures 23-5 to 10 show changes in the treated/normal ratios of various phosphorus compounds and pHi. Pi increased transiently, PDE increased, and intracellular pH decreased transiently and increased thereafter. A pattern of metabolic disturbance similar to that in ischemia was observed from the very early stage of radiotherapy. This examination is useful for assessment of the damage to normal brain tissues.

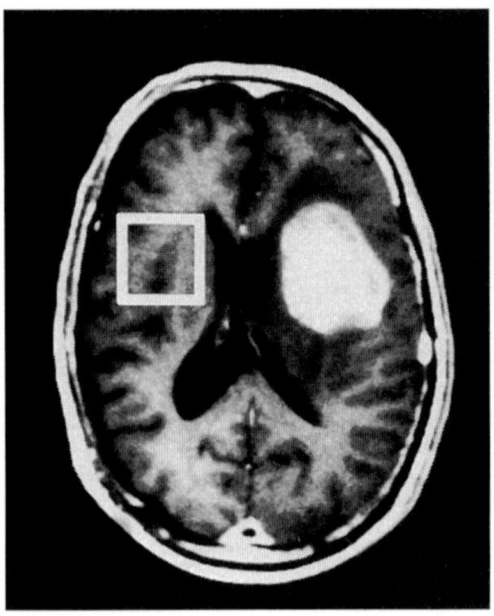

Fig. 23-1 ^{31}P spectra obtained in voxel in the normal area to the tumor. Voxel size : 3×3×4 cm³.

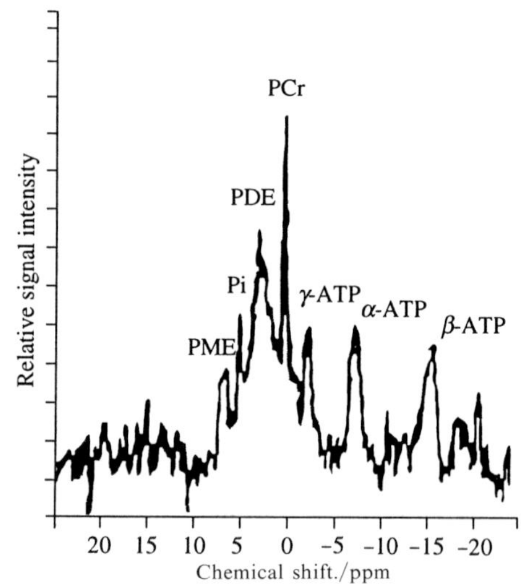

Fig. 23-2 ^{31}P spectrum before radiation.

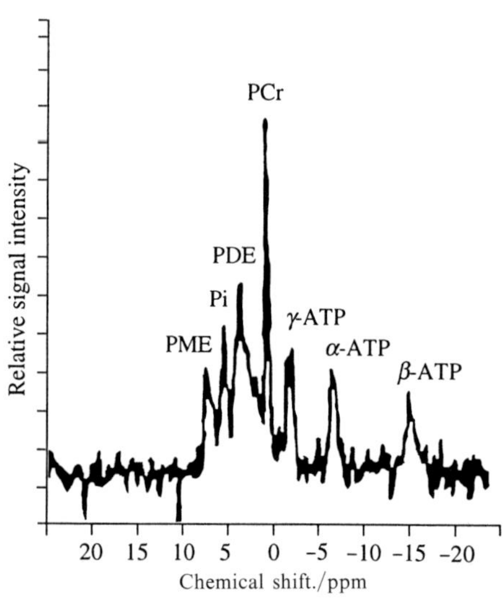

Fig. 23-3 ^{31}P spectrum after 7 weeks of radiation.

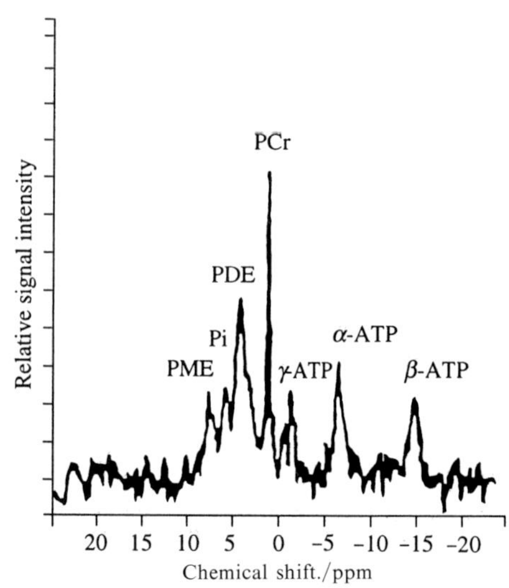

Fig. 23-4 ^{31}P spectrum after 16 weeks of radiation.

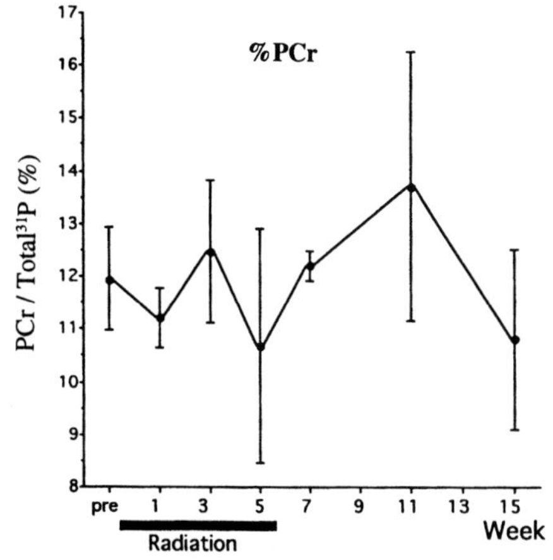

Fig. 23-5 Changes of %PCr due to therapy.

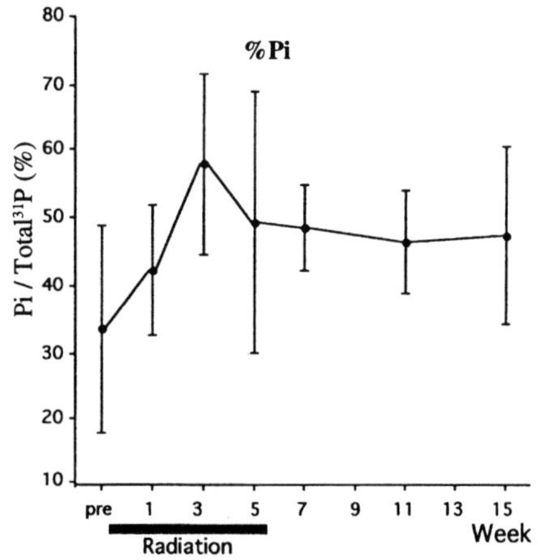

Fig. 23-6 Changes of %Pi due to therapy.

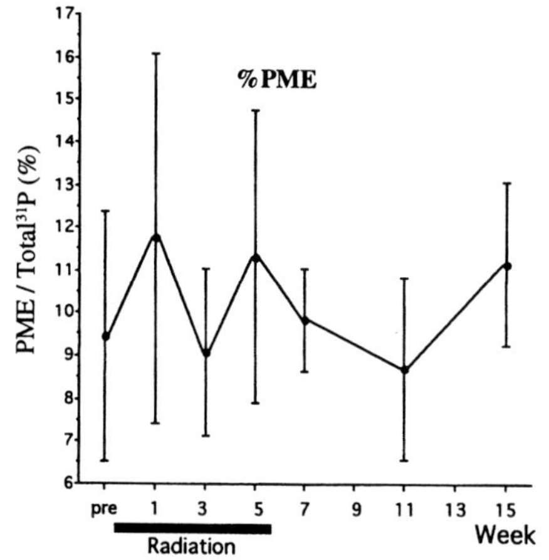

Fig. 23-7 Changes of %PME due to therapy.

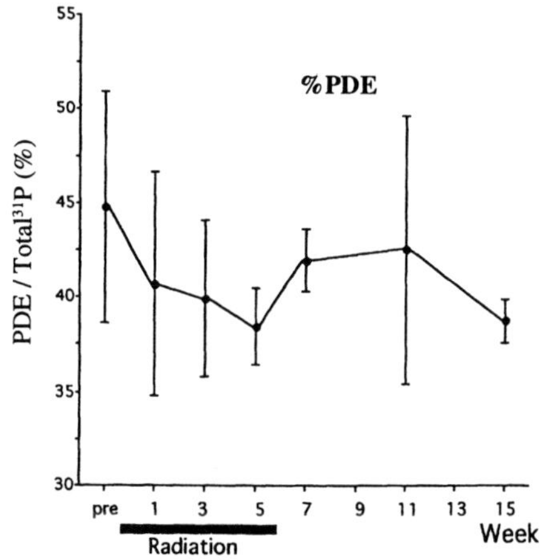

Fig. 23-8 Changes of %PDE due to therapy.

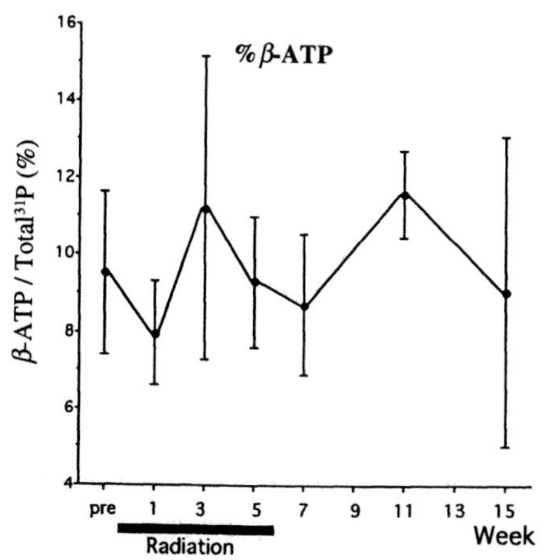

Fig. 23-9 Changes of %β-ATP due to therapy.

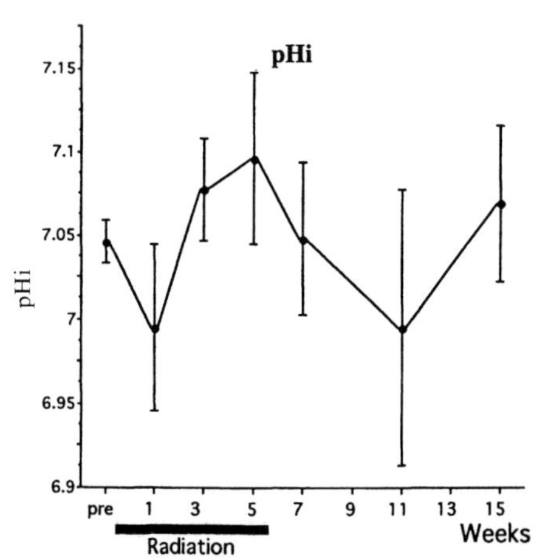

Fig. 23-10 Changes of pHi due to therapy.

Chapter 6 Cerebral Infarction

Kousaku Terada

6.1 CHARACTERISTICS OF THE SPECTRUM

Cerebral infarction is a pathologic condition in which aerobic metabolism in brain cells is suddenly replaced by anaerobic metabolism due to disruption to the cerebral circulation which causes damage to brain tissues. These changes can be observed by ^{31}P-MRS as changes in ATP and PCr, which are high energy phosphates, and Pi produced by their degradation.

A marked increase in Pi, decreases in PCr and ATP, and a decrease in the intracellular pH can be observed by ^{31}P-MRS from the early stage of cerebral infarction. Such changes can be observed immediately after the stroke, when cerebral infarction cannot be detected clearly by CT or MRI.[1] This marked increase in Pi is due to the shift from impaired aerobic glycolysis to anaerobic glycolysis, and to the accumulation of Pi produced by hydrolysis of ATP without reutilization. In addition, PCr and ATP are reduced due to the decrease in high energy phosphates. Pi decreases gradually thereafter, and signal intensities of ^{31}P-NMR are generally reduced in the chronic stage. This is considered to be due to a decrease in the number of cells or the activity of cells in the foci of cerebral infarction.[2–4]

Intracellular pH becomes acidosis in the ischemic brain early in the stroke and a transition toward and into alkalosis occurs within a few days. Chronic cerebral infarction demonstrates essentially normal intracellular pH or minimally alkalotic values.[5] This acidosis in the acute stage is considered to be caused primarily by accumulation of lactic acid, which is a product of anaerobic glycolysis. However, according to studies using ^{1}H-MRS, lactic acid persists even in subacute and chronic cerebral infarction, when acidosis has shifted to alkalosis, and changes in the amount of lactic acid are not necessarily associated with those in the intracellular pH.[6] Although the cause of this alkaline shift of the intracellular pH remains unclear, involvement of the increase in extracellular fluid, proliferation of glial cells or infiltration of phagocytes (which have higher intracellular pH than neurons), and changes in the buffering mechanism via the Na^+/H^+ antiporter system in and out of the cells have been suggested.[7–8] It has also been speculated that lactate is observed over a long period despite the alkalotic intracellular pH, because the production of lactate from pyruvate mediated by phosphofructokinase is promoted in alkalosis.[6]

^{31}P-MRS is a very useful method of examination, because it allows non-invasive and serial observation of changes in energy metabolism in brain tissues in cerebral infarction. These changes can be observed by ^{31}P-MRS even when no morphological changes are detected by CT or MRI. Therefore, this method is extremely useful for the analysis of the pathogenesis and may be applicable to evaluation of the indication of vascular reconstructive surgery or the assessment of therapeutic effects.

REFERENCES

1) Sasahira, M.; Uchimura, K.; Yatsushiro, K. et al. Early detection of cerebral infarction by ^{31}P spectroscopic imaging. *Neuroradiology* 32: 43–46; 1990.
2) Bottomley, P. A.; Drayer, B. P.; Smith, L. S. Chronic

adult cerebral infarction studied by phosphorus NMR spectroscopy. *Radiology* 160: 763–766; 1986.

3) Houkin, K.; Nakada, T.; Suzuki, N. et al. ^{31}P magnetic resonance spectroscopy of chronic cerebral infarction in rats. *NMR Biomed*. 2: 83–86; 1989.

4) Uchimura, K. A clinical study on the energy metabolism and intracellular pH in human brain with cerebral infarction ; Detection by ^{31}P-magnetic resonance spectroscopy. *Med. J. Kagoshima Univ*. 42: 223–244 ; 1990.

5) Chopp, M.; Chen, H.; Linde, A. M. Q. V. et al. Time course of postischemic intracellular alkalosis reflects the duration of ischemia. *J. Cereb. Blood Flow Metab.* 10: 860–865; 1990.

6) Hugg, J. W.; Duijn, J. H.; Matson, G. B. et al. Elevated lactate and alkalosis in chronic human brain infarction observed by ^{1}H and ^{31}P MR spectroscopic imaging. *J. Cereb. Blood Flow Metab*. 12: 734–744; 1992.

7) Levine, S. R.; Helpern, J. A.; Welch, K. M. A. et al. Human focal cerebral ischemia: Evaluation of brain pH and energy metabolism with P-31 NMR spectroscopy. *Radiology* 185: 537–544; 1992.

8) Sappey-Marinier, D.; Hubesch, B.; Matson, G. B. et al. Decreased phosphorus metabolite concentrations and alkalosis in chronic cerebral infarction. *Radiology* 182: 29–34; 1992.

9) Asakura, T.; Sasahira, M. Magnetic resonance spectroscopy and chemical shift imaging of the brain. *Neurosciences* 20: 83–101; 1994.

10) Terada, K.; Moriya, N.; Fujimoto, T. et al. ^{31}P chemical shift imaging in cerebral ischemic disorders. *Abstracts of 51st Annual Meeting of the Japan Neurosurgical Society. Book 2. Kagoshima* p. 198; 1992.

6.2 CASES (24-35)

CASE 24

CASE 24: A 69-year-old male

Cerebral infarction of the left and right occipital lobes (5 hours and 1 year after the stroke)

The patient presented with sudden onset of right hemiparesis and consciousness disturbance. He had an episode of hypertension, atrial fibrillation, and right temporooccipital infarction 12 months previous.

The MRIs in Figures 24-1 and 2 show an old cerebral infarction in the right occipital lobe, but no infarcted area is observed in the left occipital lobe. Figures 24-3 to 10 show ^{31}P-MRS's taken during this period. In the contour maps in Figures 24-3, 4, 5, 6, and 7, the signal intensities of ^{31}P, ATP, Pi, PDE, and PCr are all low in the right occipital lobe, where the old cerebral infarction is located. However, in the left occipital lobe, where infarction immediately after the stroke is located, the signal intensities of Pi are markedly increased whereas the signal intensities of ATP, PCr, and PDE are decreased, so the signal intensities of ^{31}P are not changed. Figure 24-9 shows the ^{31}P spectrum of the area of acute infarction in the left occipital lobe. Figure 24-10 shows the ^{31}P spectrum of the area of chronic infarction in the right occipital lobe. Note the strikingly high signal intensities of Pi and low signal intensities of other components immediately after the stroke of cerebral infarction.

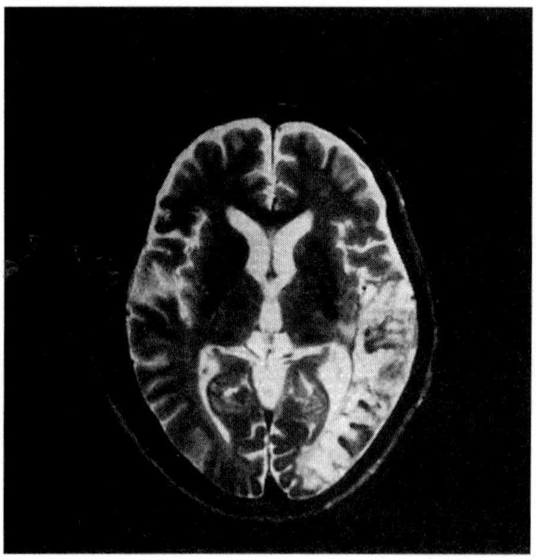

Fig. 24-1 Axial T_2-weighted image (2,200/90).

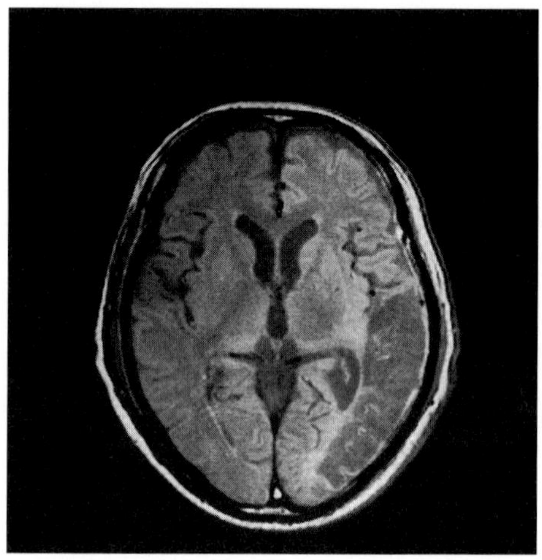

Fig. 24-2 Axial proton density-weighted image (2,200/15).

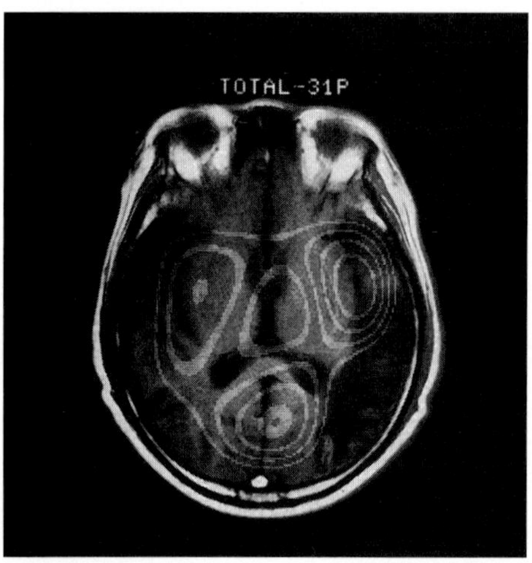

Fig. 24-3 Axial ^{31}P contour map superimposed on T_1-weighted image (500/15).

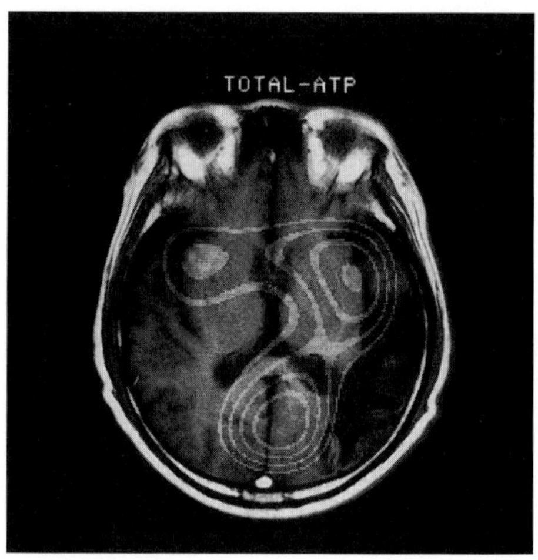

Fig. 24-4 Axial total ATP contour map superimposed on T_1-weighted image (500/15).

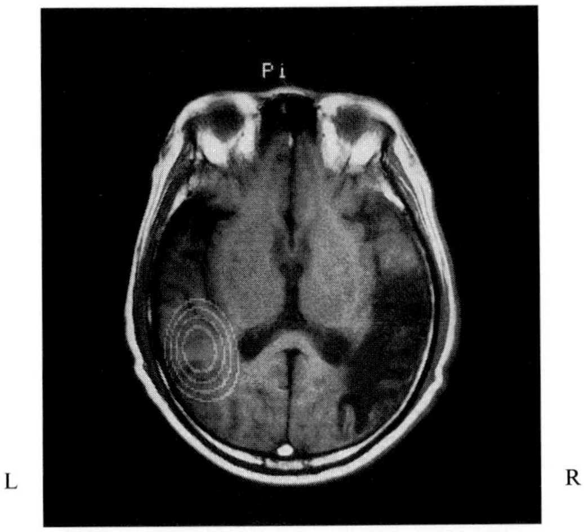

Fig. 24-5 Axial Pi contour map superimposed on T_1-weighted image (500/15).

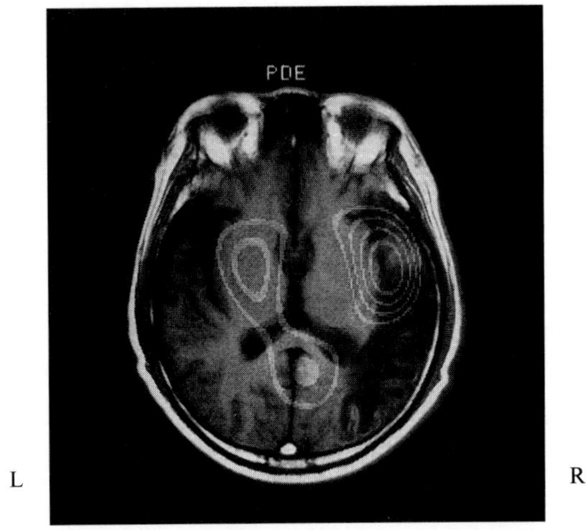

Fig. 24-6 Axial PDE contour map superimposed on T_1-weighted image (500/15).

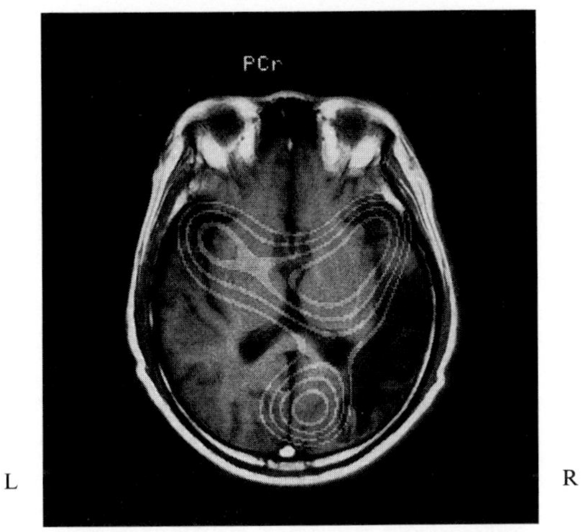

Fig. 24-7 Axial PCr contour map superimposed on T_1-weighted image (500/15).

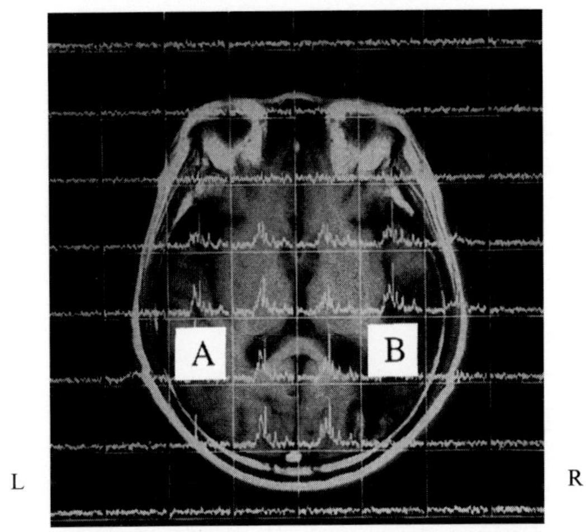

Fig. 24-8 T_1-weighted image showing the position of 3×3×4 cm^3 voxels A and B.

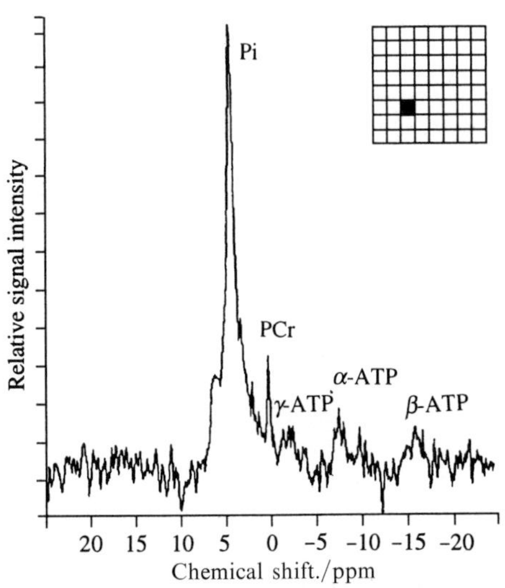

Fig. 24-9 ^{31}P spectrum of left occipital infarcted area (voxel A). (Acute stage.)

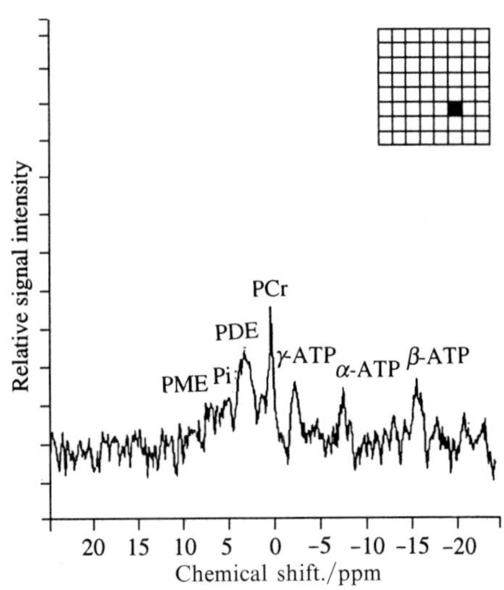

Fig. 24-10 ^{31}P spectrum of right occipital infarcted area (voxel B). (Chronic stage.)

CASE 25

CASE 25: A 78-year-old female

Cerebral infarction of the right temporal and occipital lobes (2 days after the stroke)

The patient presented with sudden onset of left hemiparesis and consciousness disturbance. She had a past history of hypertension, atrial fibrillation, and right occipital infarction that occurred several years previous.

The MRIs in Figures 25-1 and 2 show a wide area of cerebral infarction from the right temporal to the occipital lobe. In the ^{31}P, ATP, PME, and PDE metabolite images in Figures 25-3, 4, 5, and 7, the signal intensity is reduced in the infarcted area. In the Pi contour map shown in Figure 25-6, the infarcted area is observed as a high-signal intensity area. Figure 25-9 shows ^{31}P spectrum obtained in an area opposite the infarcted area, and Figure 25-10 shows the ^{31}P spectrum of the infarcted area. Note the high Pi peak and low peaks of other components in the spectrum of the infarcted area.

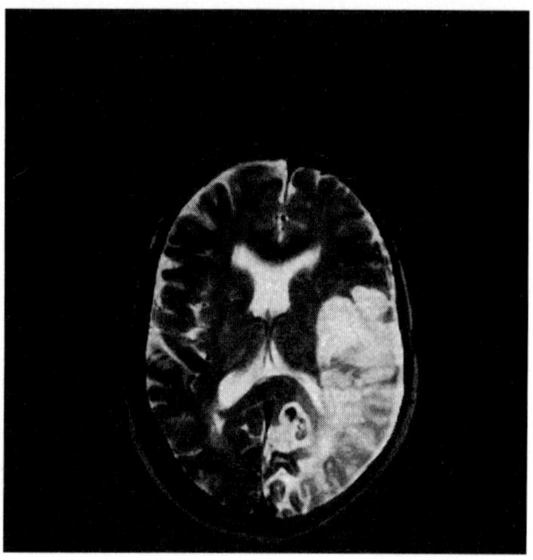

Fig. 25-1 Axial T_2-weighted image (2,200/90).

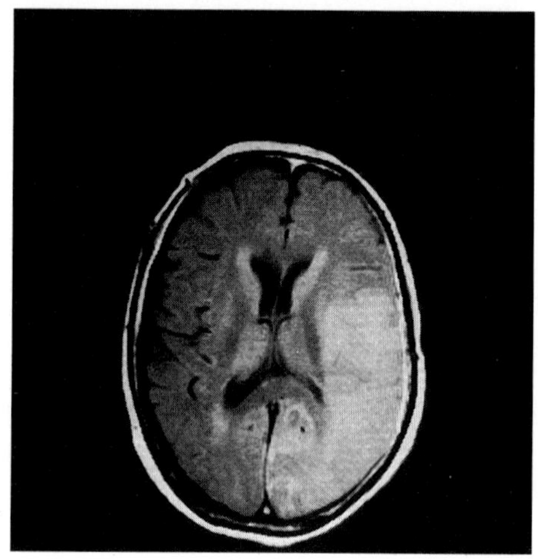

Fig. 25-2 Axial proton density-weibghted image (2,200/15).

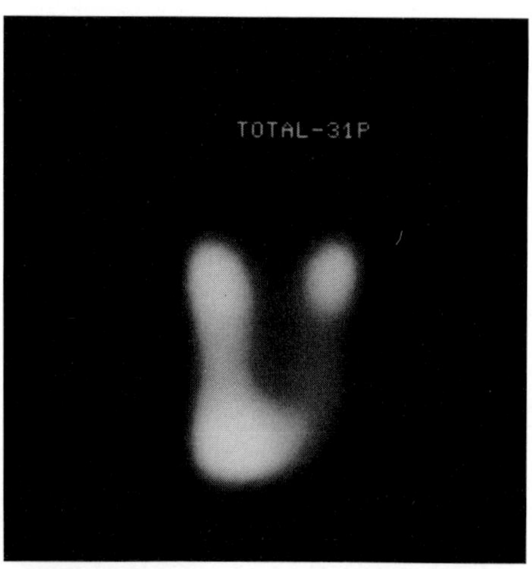

Fig. 25-3 Axial ^{31}P metabolite image.

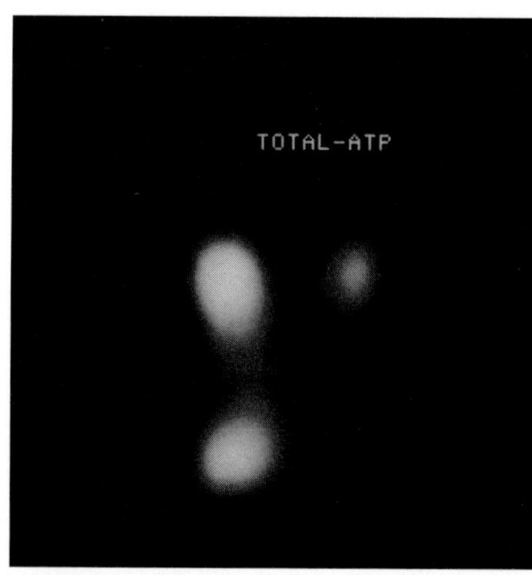

Fig. 25-4 Axial total ATP metabolite image.

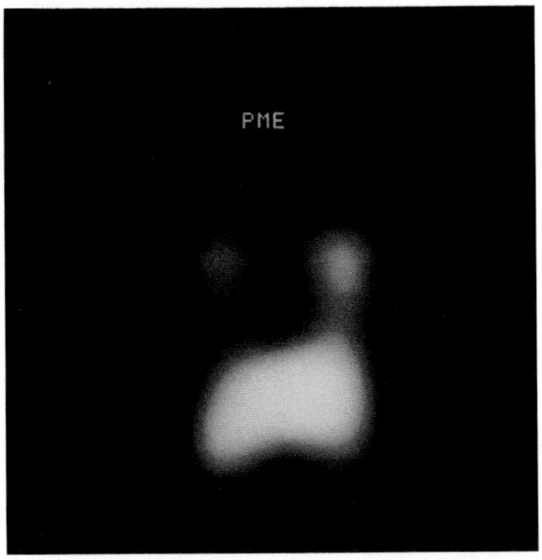

Fig. 25-5 Axial PME metabolite image.

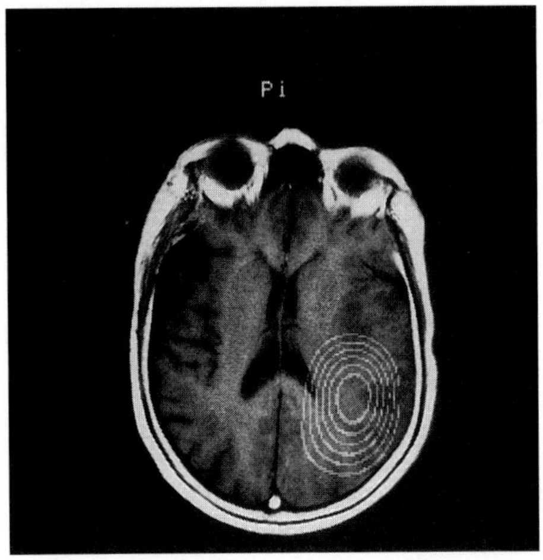

Fig. 25-6 Axial Pi contour map superimposed on T_1-weighted image (500/15).

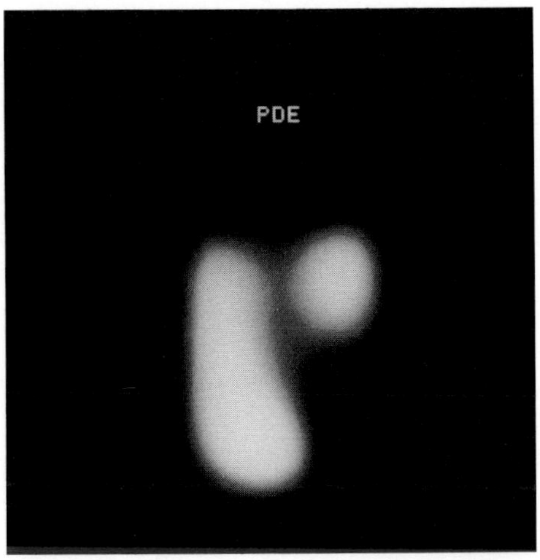

Fig. 25-7 Axial PDE metabolite image.

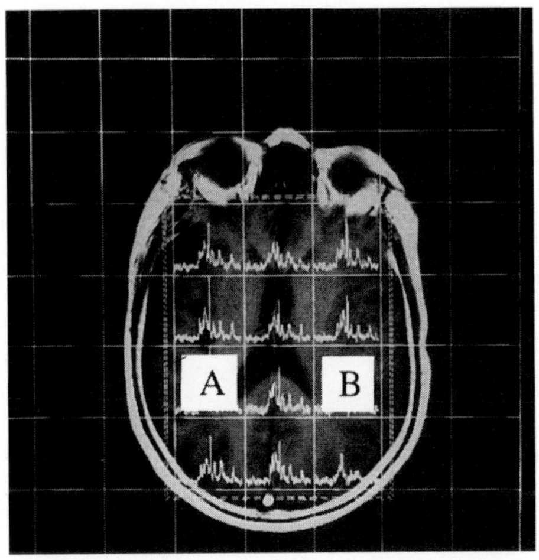

Fig. 25-8 T_1-weighted image showing the position of $3 \times 3 \times 4$ cm^3 voxels A and B.

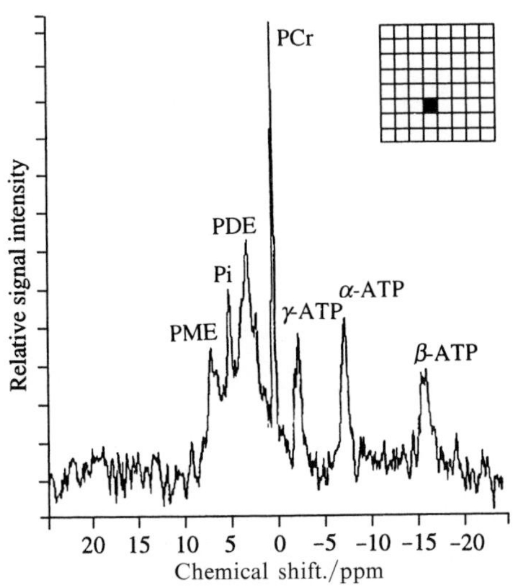

Fig. 25-9 ^{31}P spectrum of control area (voxel A).

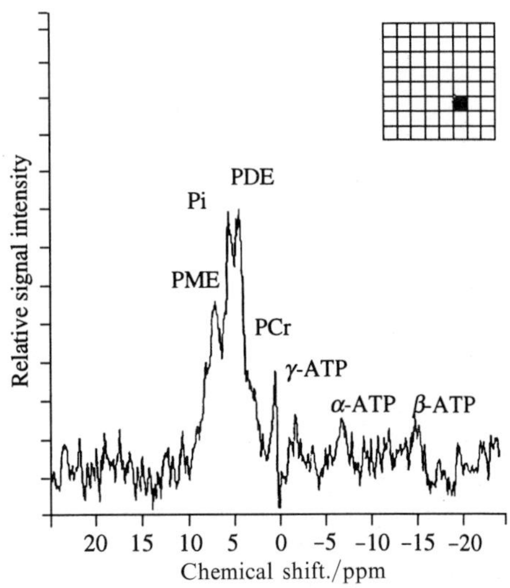

Fig. 25-10 ^{31}P spectrum of infarcted area (voxel B).

Case 25

Cerebral infarction of the right temporal and occipital lobes (7 days after the stroke)

The MRIs in Figures 25-11 and 12 show a wide area of cerebral infarction in the right temporal and occipital lobes, but little brain edema is observed. In the ^{31}P, ATP, PME, and PDE metabolite images in Figures 25-13, 14, 15, and 17, the signal intensity is reduced in the infarcted area. Although the signal intensity is increased in the infarcted area in the Pi contour map shown in Figure 25-16, the signal intensities are reduced in intensity and localization compared with the findings 2 days after the stroke (Figure 25-6). Figure 25-19 shows the ^{31}P spectrum in an area opposite the infarcted area, and Figure 25-20 shows the ^{31}P spectrum of the infarcted area. Note the overall reductions in the signal intensities in the spectrum of the infarcted area compared with 2 days after the stroke (Figure 25-10).

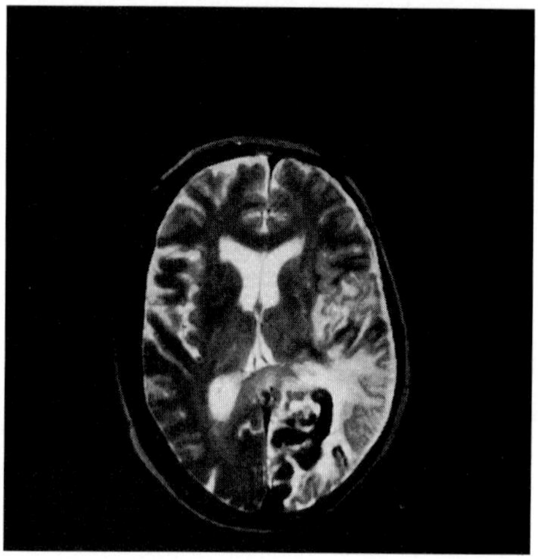

Fig. 25-11 Axial T_2-weighted image (2,200/90).

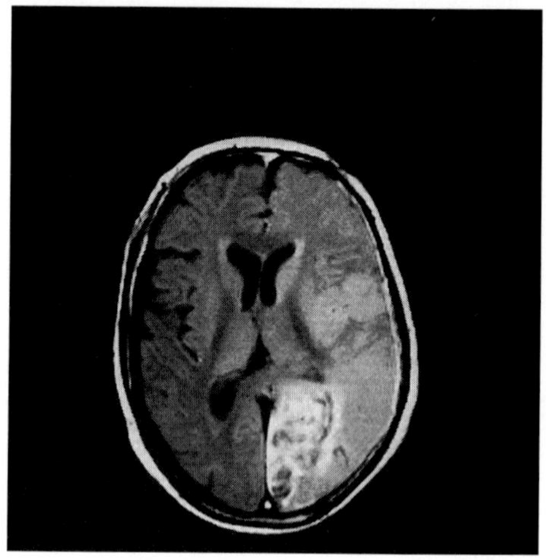

Fig. 25-12 Axial proton density-weighted image (2,200/15).

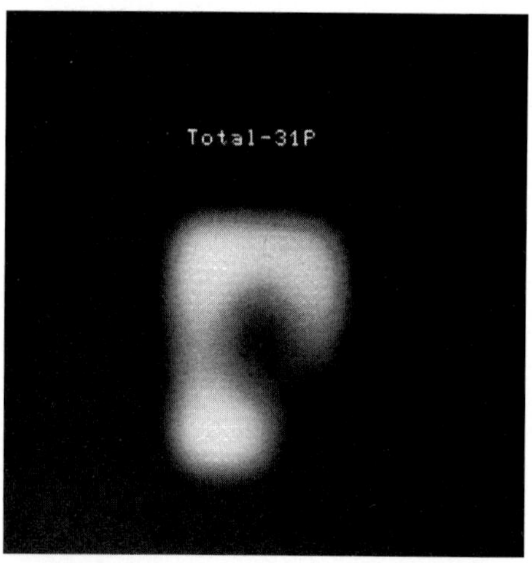

Fig. 25-13 Axial ^{31}P metabolite image.

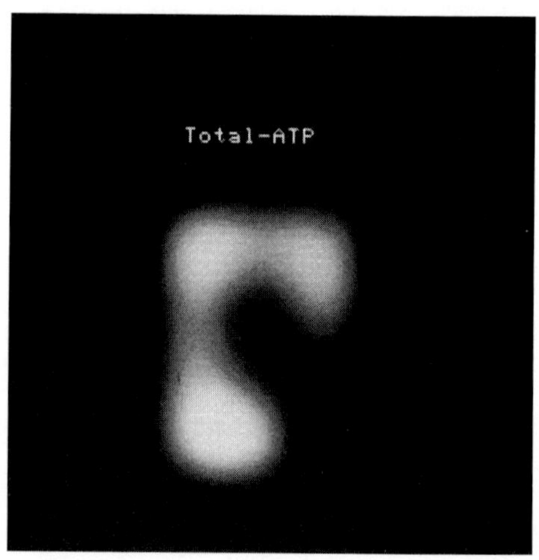

Fig. 25-14 Axial total ATP metabolite image.

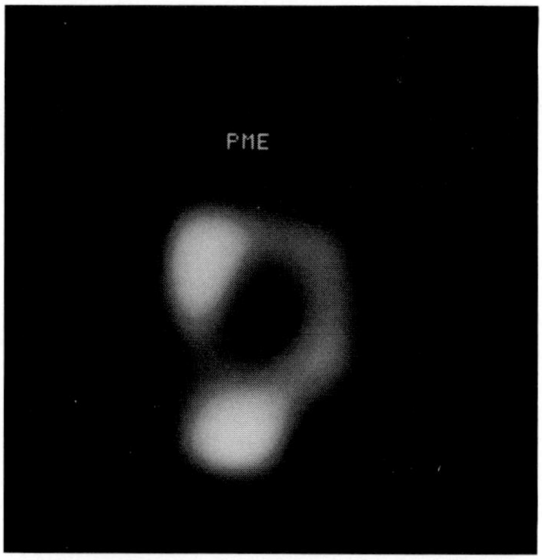

Fig. 25-15 Axial PME metabolite image.

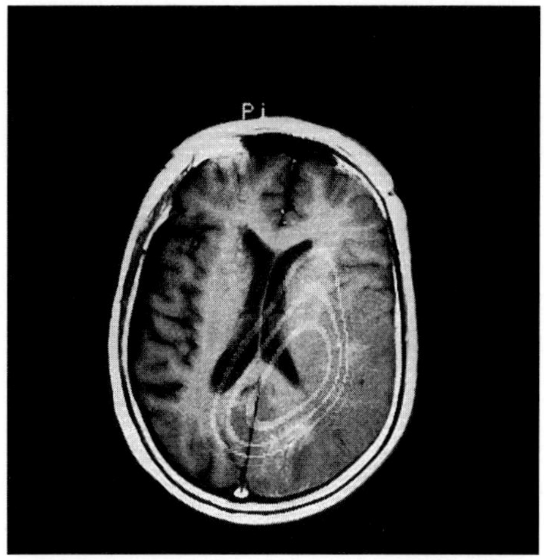

Fig. 25-16 Axial Pi contour map superimposed on T_1-weighted image (500/15).

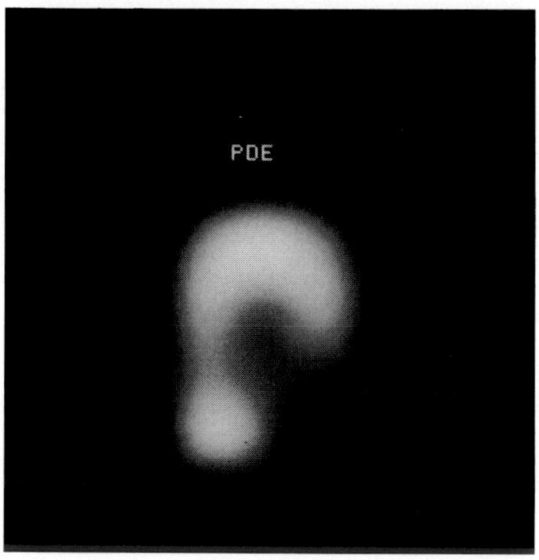

Fig. 25-17 Axial PDE metabolite image.

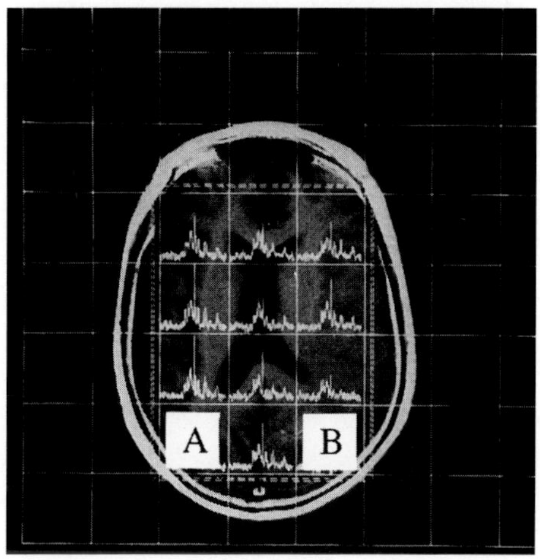

Fig. 25-18 T_1-weighted image showing the position of $3 \times 3 \times 4$ cm^3 voxels A and B.

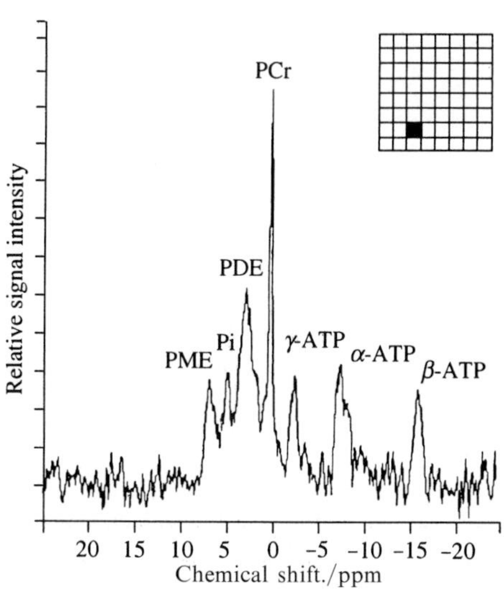

Fig. 25-19 ^{31}P spectrum of control area (voxel A).

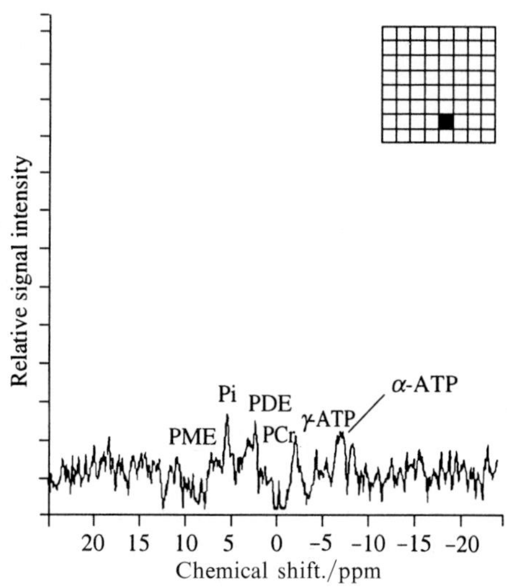

Fig. 25-20 ^{31}P spectrum of infarcted area (voxel B).

CASE 26

CASE 26: A 61-year-old male

Cerebral infarction of the right temporal lobe (2 days after the stroke)

The patient presented with sudden onset of headache, vomiting, and left hemiparesis. He gave a past history of hypertension, diabetes mellitus, and angina pectoris.

The MRIs in Figures 26-1 and 2 show cerebral infarction in the right temporal lobe. The infarction is partially hemorrhagic. The signal intensity of the infarcted area is reduced in the ^{31}P, PME, and PDE contour maps and in the ATP metabolite image in Figures 26-3, 4, 5, and 7. The signal intensity is increased in the infarcted area in the Pi contour map shown in Figure 26-6. Figures 26-9 and 26-10 show the ^{31}P spectra of an area opposite the infarcted area and the infarcted area, respectively. Note the overall low signal intensities and the relatively high Pi signal intensities in the infarcted area.

L 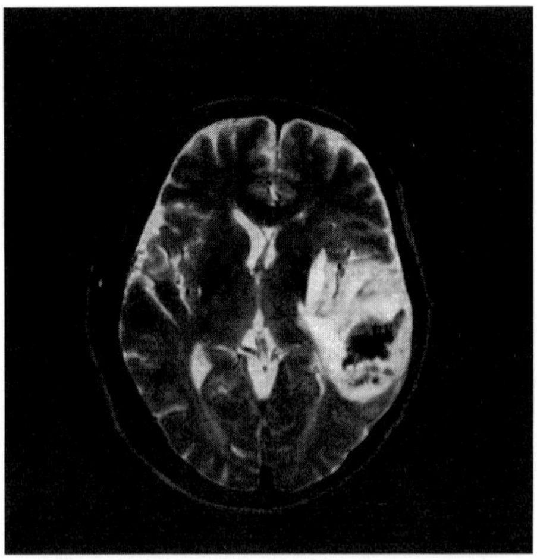 R

Fig. 26-1 Axial T_2-weighted image (2,200/90).

L 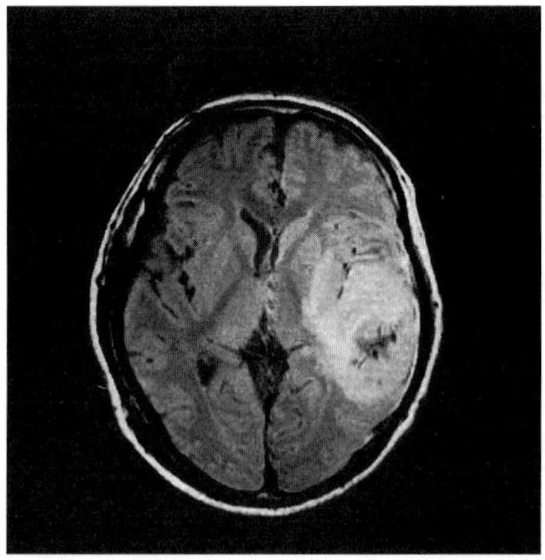 R

Fig. 26-2 Axial proton density-weighted image (2,200/15).

L 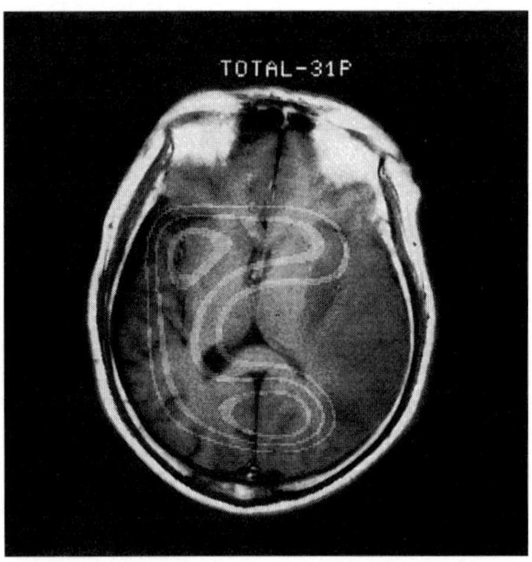 R

Fig. 26-3 Axial ^{31}P contour map superimposed on T_1-weighted image (500/15).

L 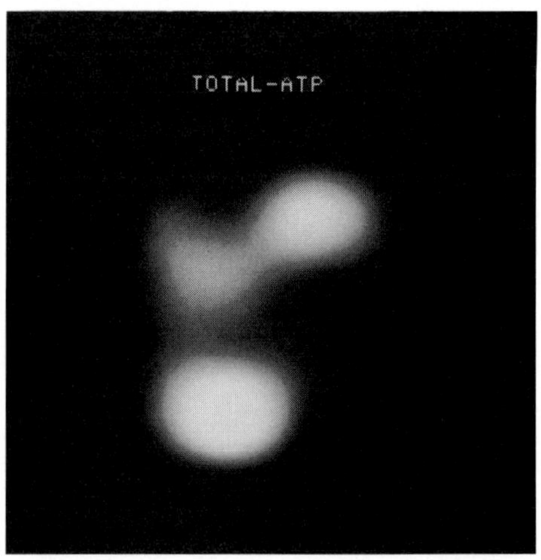 R

Fig. 26-4 Axial total ATP metabolite image.

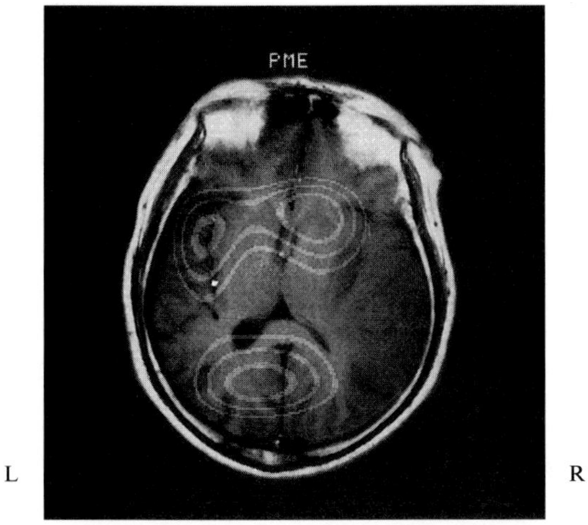

Fig. 26-5 Axial PME contour map superimposed on T_1-weighted image (500/15).

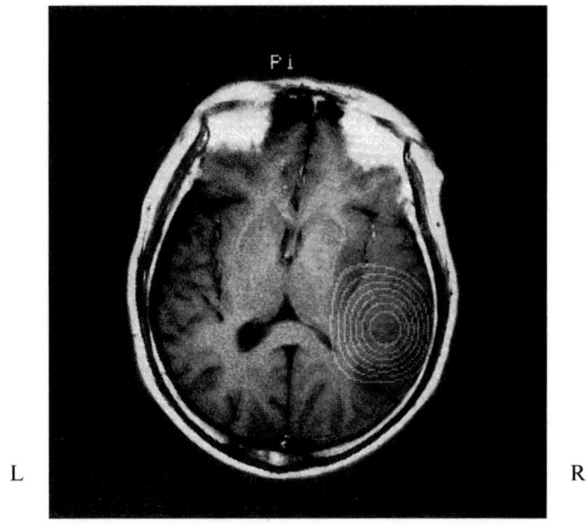

Fig. 26-6 Axial Pi contour map superimposed on T_1-weighted image (500/15).

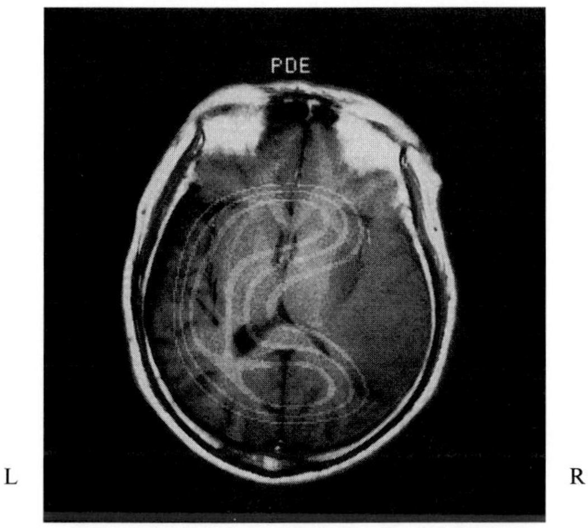

Fig. 26-7 Axial PDE contour map superimposed on T_1-weighted image (500/15).

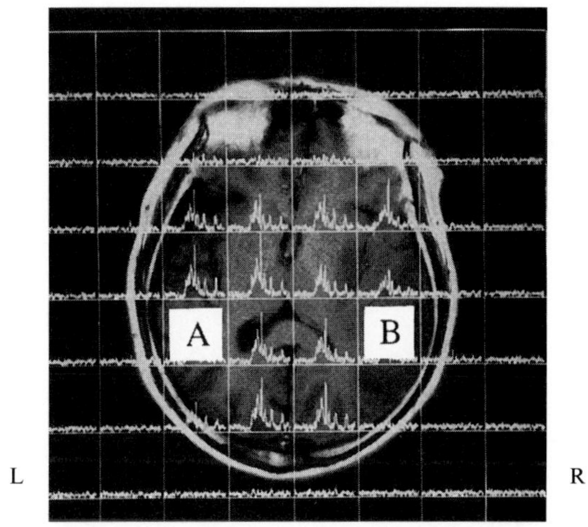

Fig. 26-8 T_1-weighted image showing the position of $3 \times 3 \times 4$ cm^3 voxels A and B.

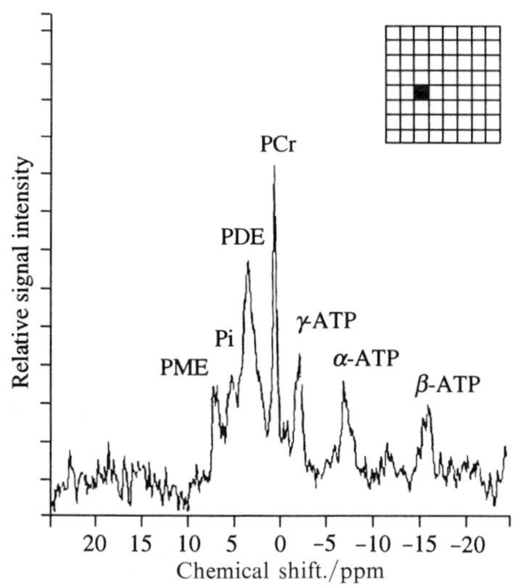

Fig. 26-9 ^{31}P spectrum of control area (voxel A).

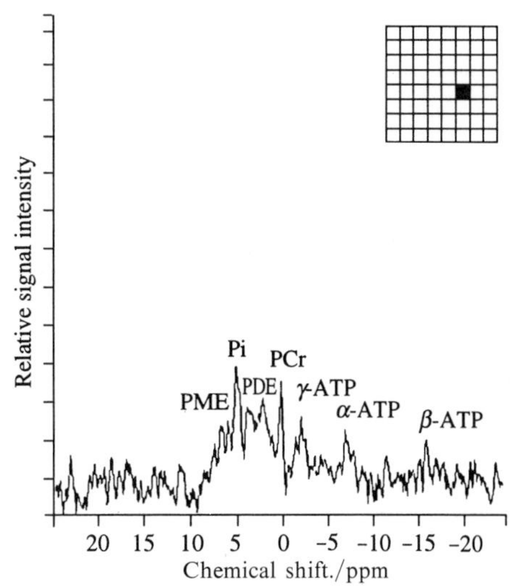

Fig. 26-10 ^{31}P spectrum of infarcted area (voxel B).

CASE 27

CASE 27: A 68-year-old female

Cerebral infarction of the left frontal and temporal lobes (2 days after the stroke)

The patient presented with sudden onset of right hemiparesis and consciousness disturbance. She gave a past history of hypertension, atrial fibrillation, and congestive cardiac failure.

The MRIs in Figures 27-1 and 2 show a wide area of cerebral infarction extending from the left frontal lobe to the temporal lobe with a midline shift due to brain edema. In the ^{31}P, ATP, PDE, and PCr metabolite images in Figures 27-3, 4, 6, and 7, the infarcted area is observed as a wide low-signal intensity area. In the Pi contour map in Figure 27-5, the signal intensity is increased in the infarcted area. Figures 27-9 and 27-10 show the ^{31}P spectra of the infarcted area and an area opposite the infarcted area, respectively. Note the strikingly high signal intensities of Pi and low signal intensities of other components in the infarcted area.

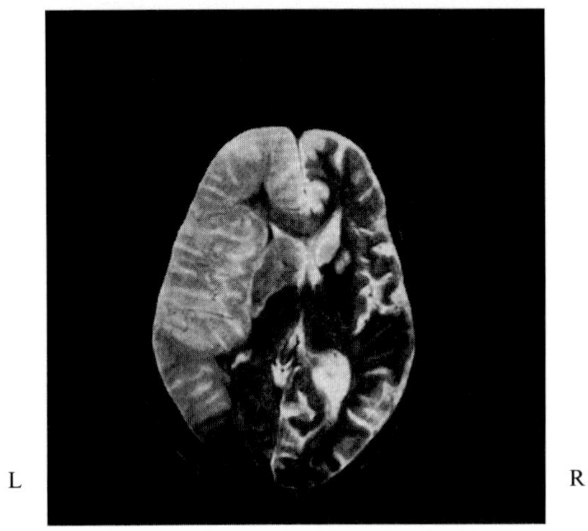

Fig. 27-1 Axial T_2-weighted image (2,200/90).

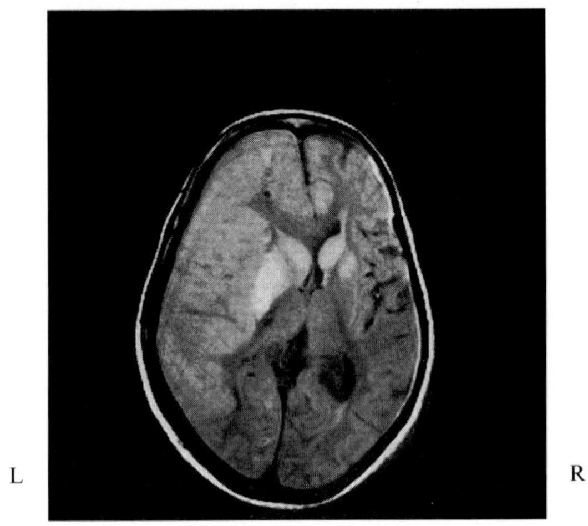

Fig. 27-2 Axial proton density-weighted image (2,200/15).

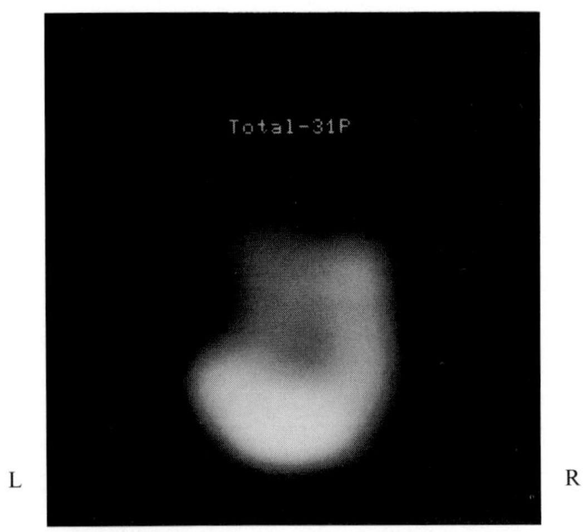

Fig. 27-3 Axial ^{31}P metabolite image.

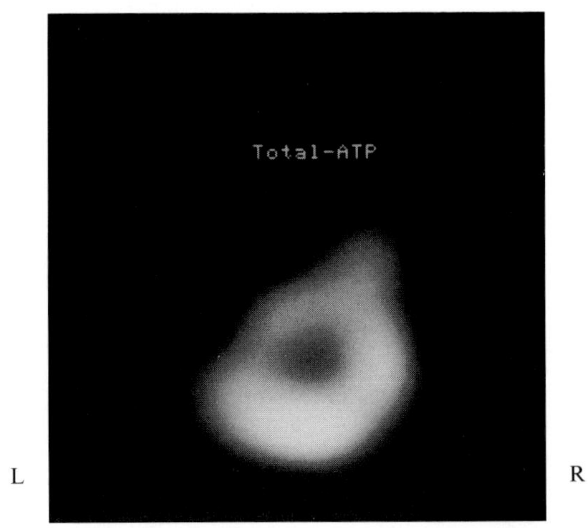

Fig. 27-4 Axial total ATP metabolite image.

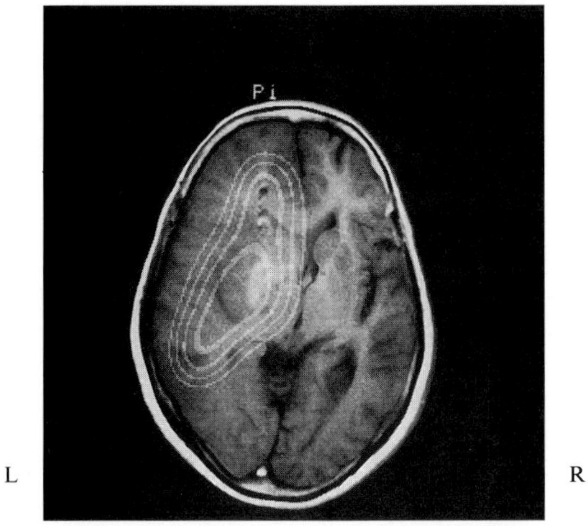

Fig. 27-5 Axial Pi contour map superimposed on T_1-weighted image (500/15).

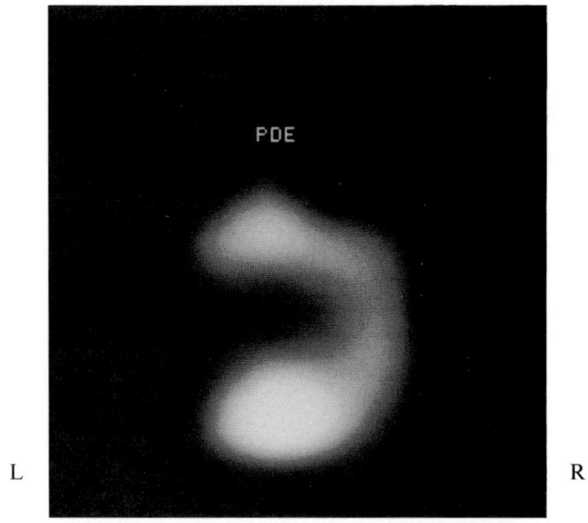

Fig. 27-6 Axial PDE metabolite image.

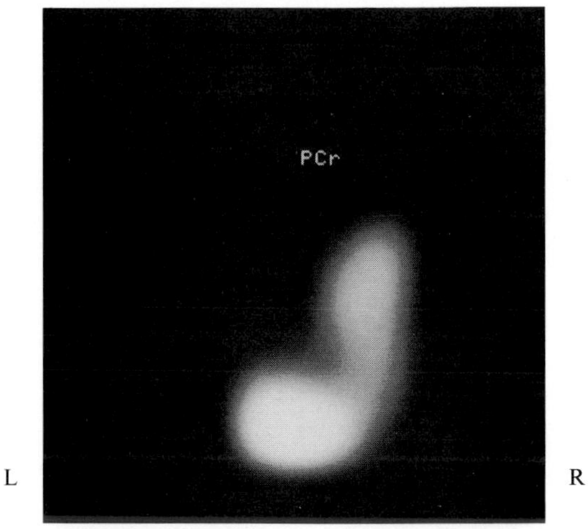

Fig. 27-7 Axial PCr metabolite image.

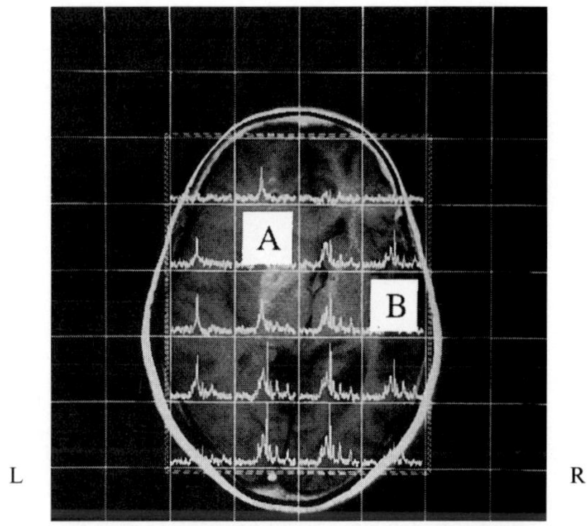

Fig. 27-8 T_1-weighted image showing the position of 3×3×4 cm^3 voxels A and B.

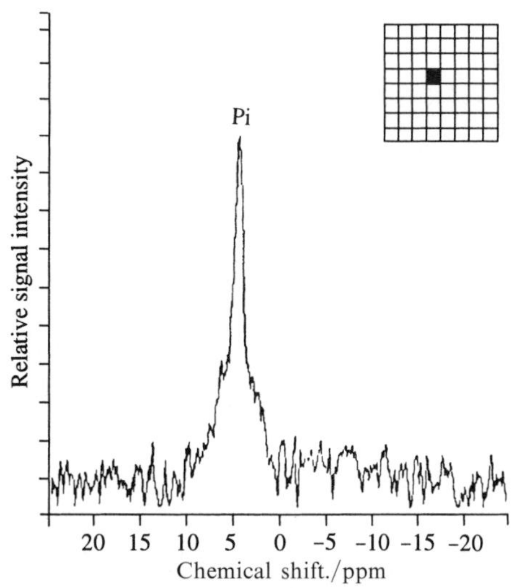

Fig. 27-9 ^{31}P spectrum of infarcted area (voxel A).

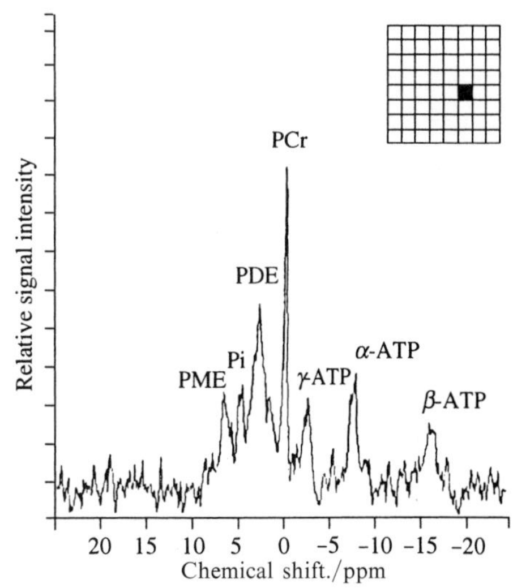

Fig. 27-10 ^{31}P spectrum of control area (voxel B).

CASE 28

CASE 28: An 80-year-old male

Cerebral infarction of the left temporal lobe (3 days after the stroke)

The patient presented with sensory aphasia and abnormal behavior upon waking in the morning.

The MRIs in Figures 28-1 and 2 show cerebral infarction in the left temporal lobe. The signal intensity of the infarcted area is reduced in the ^{31}P, ATP, Pi, PDE, and PCr metabolite images in Figures 28-3, 4, 5, 6, and 7. Figures 28-9 and 28-10 show the ^{31}P spectra of the infarcted area and an area opposite the infarcted area, respectively. Note the overall low signal intensities in the spectrum of the infarcted area.

L 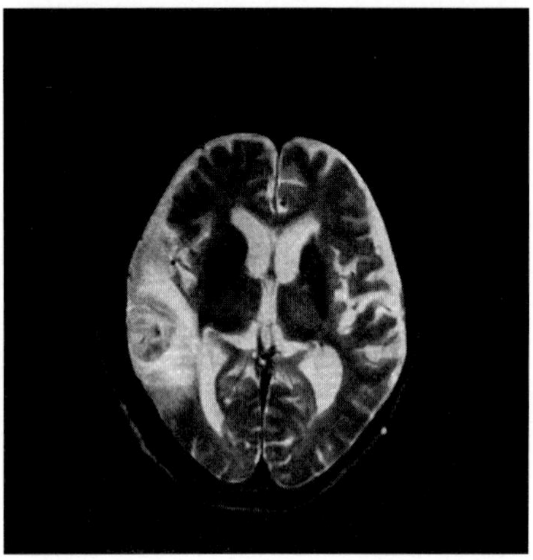 R

Fig. 28-1 Axial T_2-weighted image (2,200/90).

L 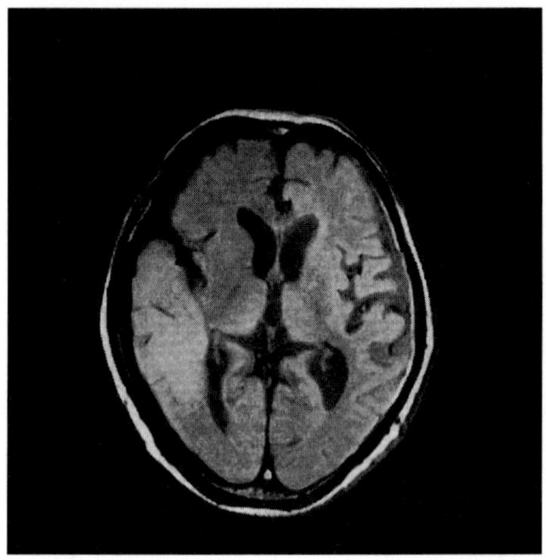 R

Fig. 28-2 Axial proton density-weighted image (2,200/15).

L 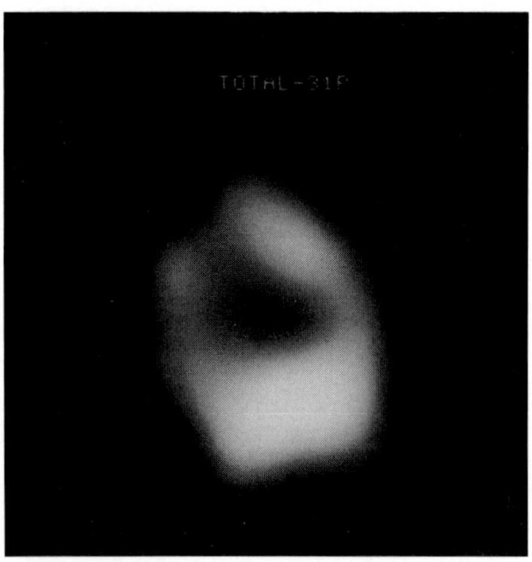 R

Fig. 28-3 Axial ^{31}P metabolite image.

L 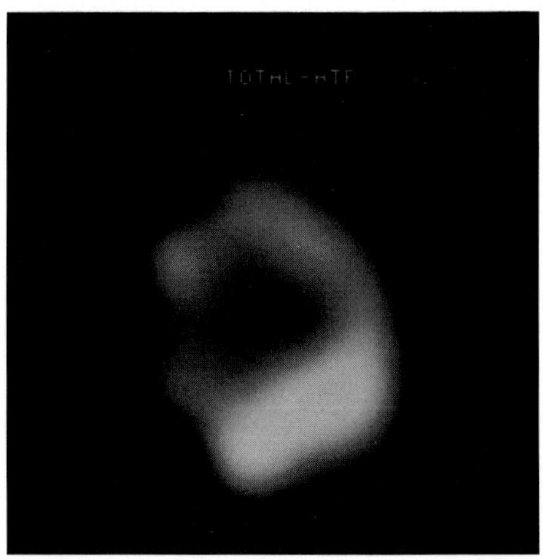 R

Fig. 28-4 Axial total ATP metabolite image.

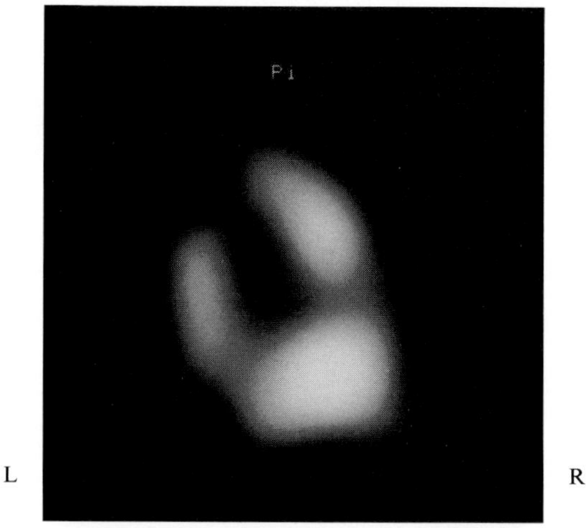

Fig. 28-5 Axial Pi metabolite image.

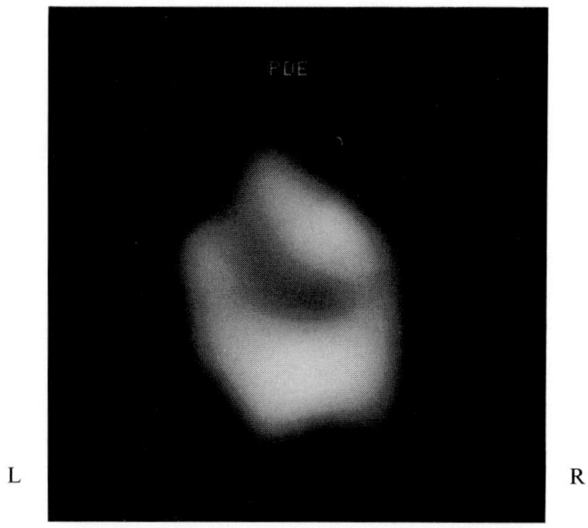

Fig. 28-6 Axial PDE metabolite image.

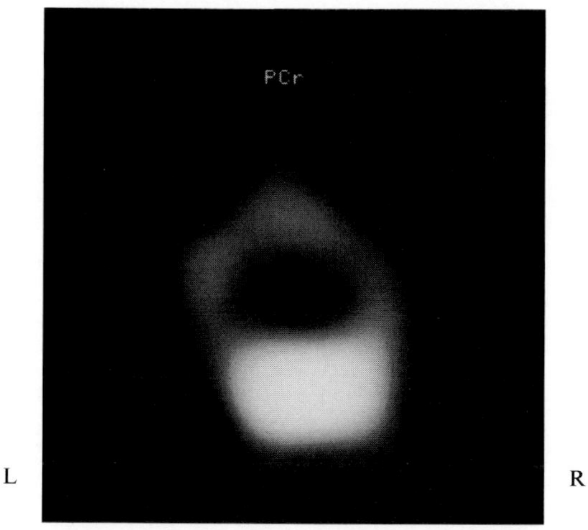

Fig. 28-7 Axial PCr metabolite image.

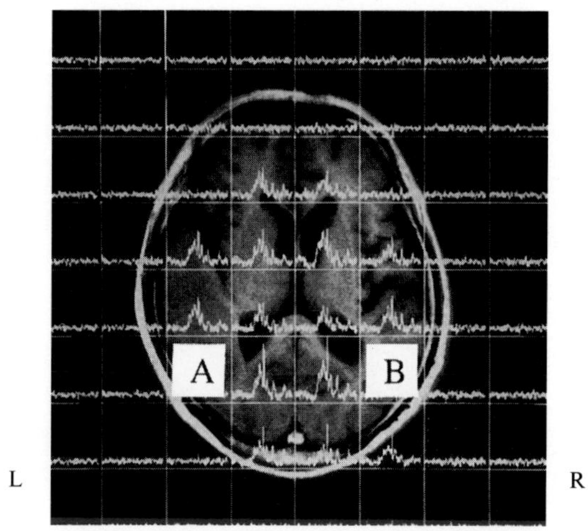

Fig. 28-8 T_1-weighted image showing the position of 3×3×4 cm^3 voxels A and B.

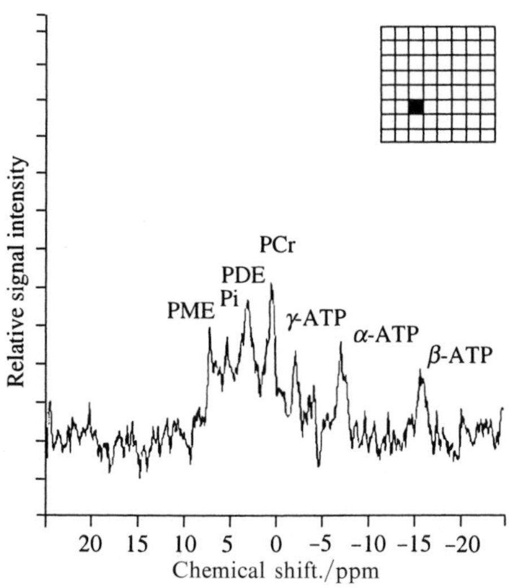

Fig. 28-9 ^{31}P spectrum of infarcted area (voxel A).

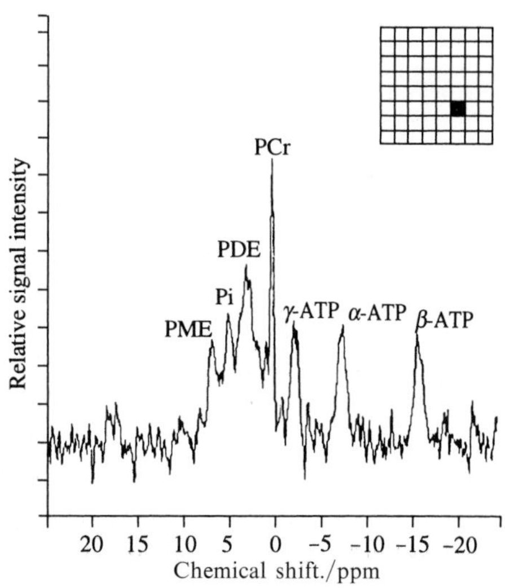

Fig. 28-10 ^{31}P spectrum of control area (voxel B).

CASE 29

CASE 29: An 85-year-old male

Cerebral infarction of the right frontal and temporal lobes (6 days after the stroke)

The patient presented with left hemiparesis and consciousness disturbance upon waking in the morning. He gave a past history of atrial fibrillation.

The MRIs in Figures 29-1 and 2 show a wide area of cerebral infarction from the right frontal lobe to the temporal lobe. The signal intensity is reduced in the infarcted area in the ^{31}P, ATP, PME, Pi, and PDE metabolite images in Figures 29-3, 4, 5, 6, and 7. Figures 29-9 and 29-10 show the ^{31}P spectra of an area opposite the infarcted area and the infarcted area, respectively. Note the generally low signal intensities in the spectrum of the infarcted area.

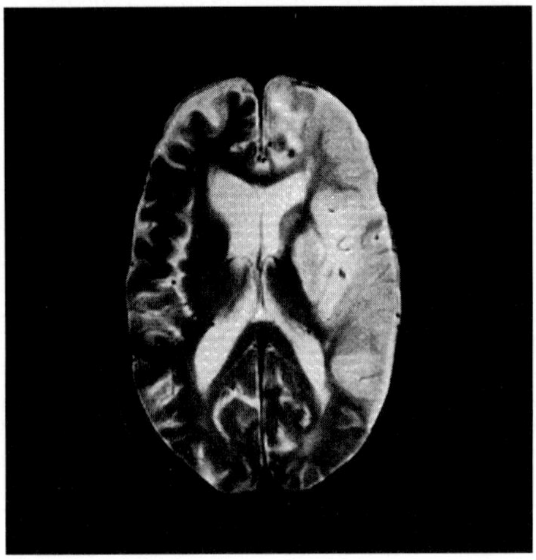

Fig. 29-1 Axial T_2-weighted image (2,200/90).

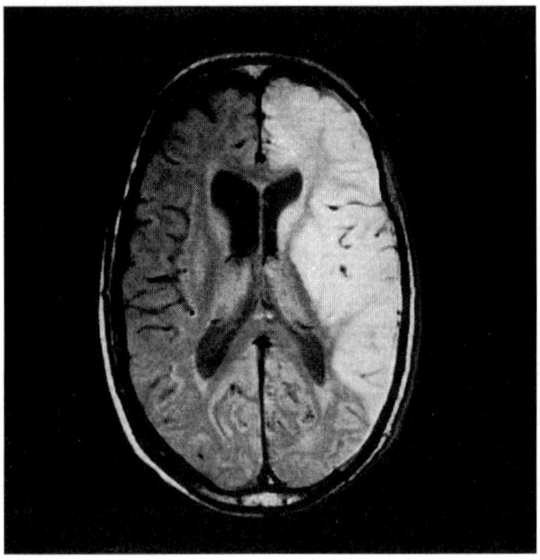

Fig. 29-2 Axial proton density-weighted image (2,200/15).

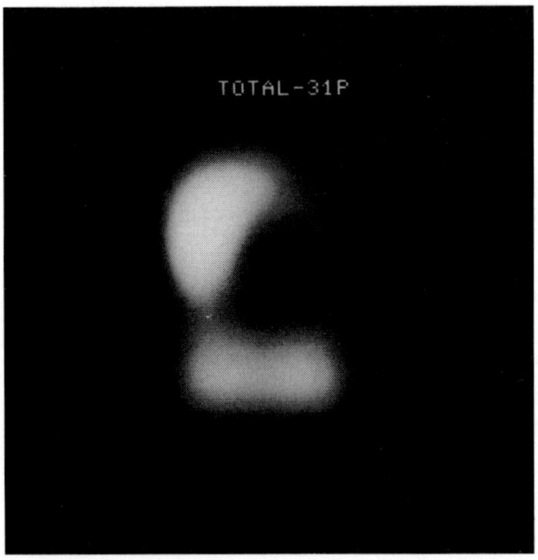

Fig. 29-3 Axial ^{31}P metabolite image.

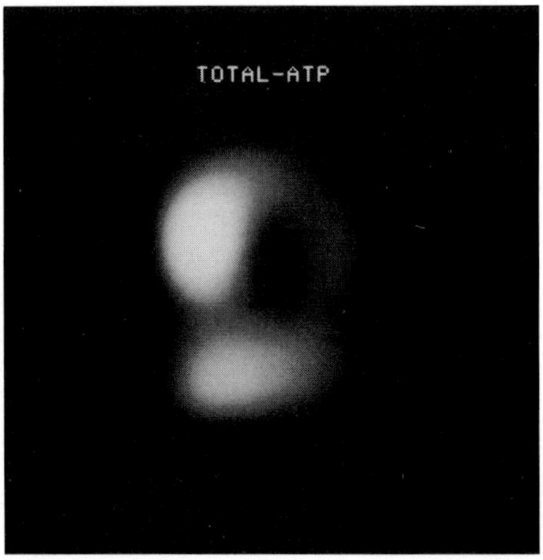

Fig. 29-4 Axial total ATP metabolite image.

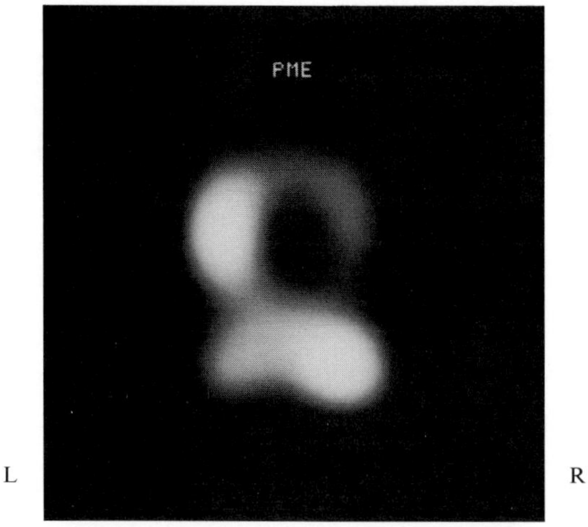

Fig. 29-5 Axial PME metabolite image.

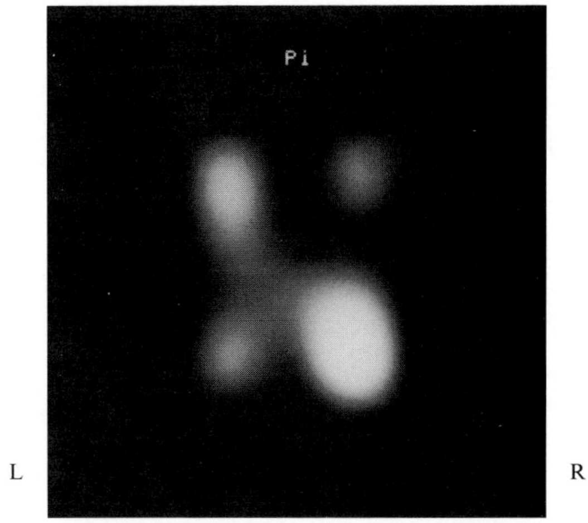

Fig. 29-6 Axial Pi metabolite image.

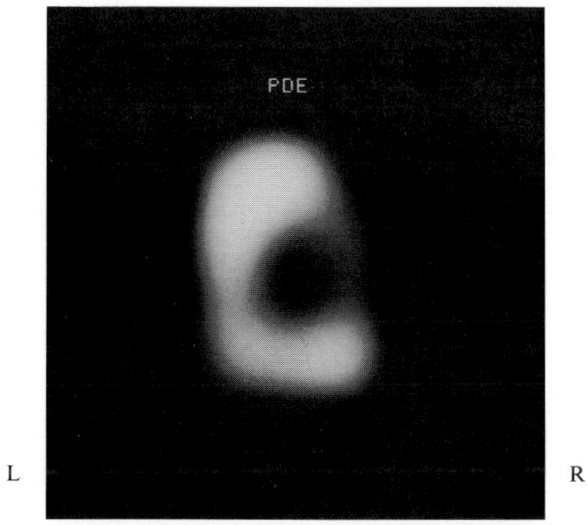

Fig. 29-7 Axial PDE metabolite image.

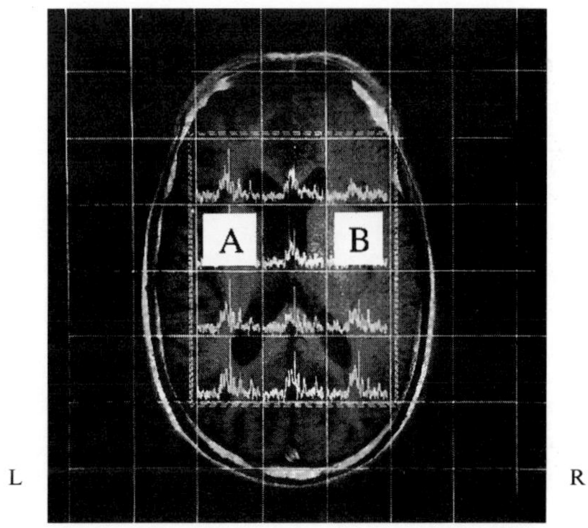

Fig. 29-8 T_1-weighted image showing the position of $3 \times 3 \times 4$ cm^3 voxels A and B.

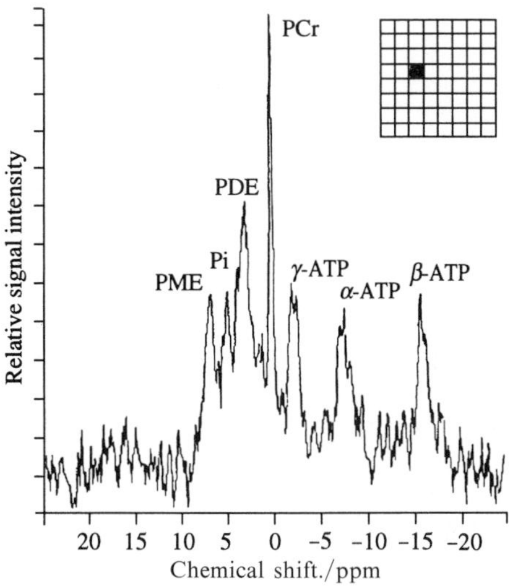

Fig. 29-9 ^{31}P spectrum of control area (voxel A).

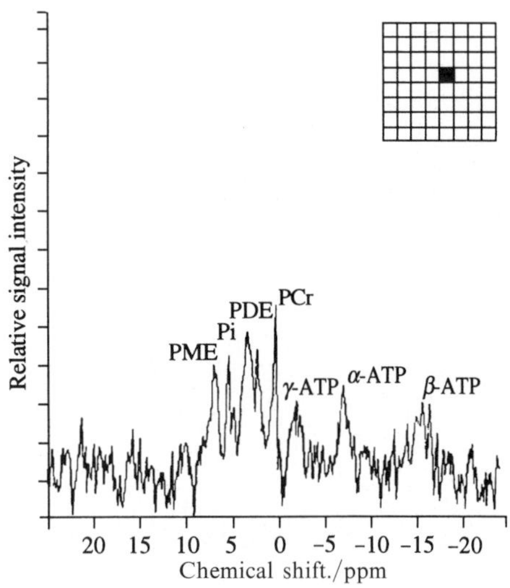

Fig. 29-10 ^{31}P spectrum of infarcted area (voxel B).

CASE 30

CASE 30: An 80-year-old female

Cerebral infarction of the right frontal lobe (7 days after the stroke)

The patient presented with sudden onset of left hemiparesis. She had a past history of hypertension and lacuna infarction that occurred several years previous.

The MRIs in Figures 30-1 and 2 show cerebral infarction in the right frontal lobe. The signal intensity of the infarcted area is reduced in the ^{31}P, ATP, PDE, and PCr contour maps in Figures 30-3, 4, 6, and 7. It is increased in the Pi contour map in Figure 30-5. Figures 30-9 and 30-10 show the ^{31}P spectra of an area opposite the infarcted area and the infarcted area, respectively. Note the generally low spectra and the relatively high Pi signal intensities in the spectrum of the infarcted area.

L 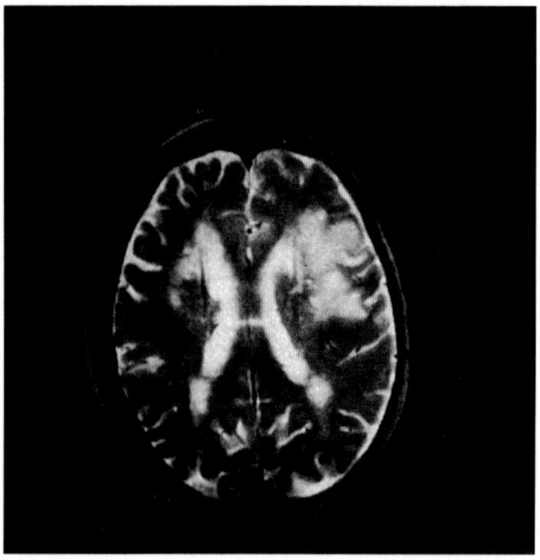 R

Fig. 30-1 Axial T_2-weighted image (2,200/90).

L 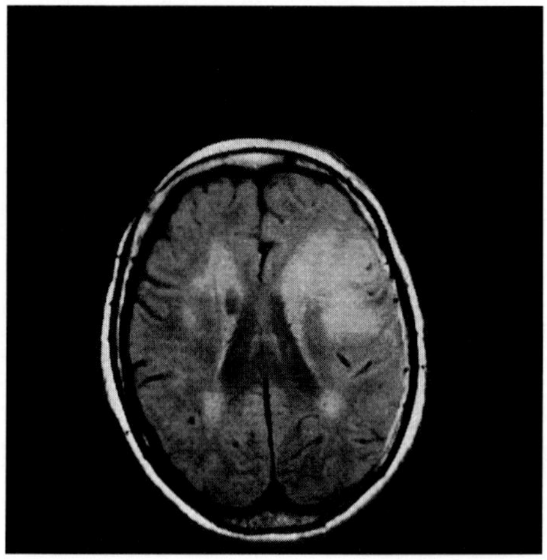 R

Fig. 30-2 Axial proton density-weighted image (2,200/15).

L 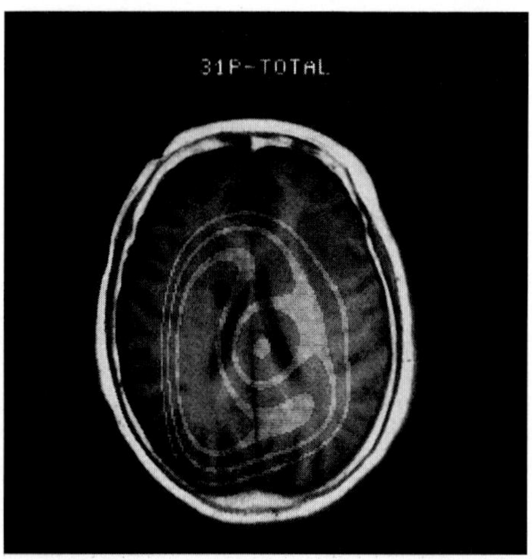 R

Fig. 30-3 Axial ^{31}P contour map superimposed on T_1-weighted image (500/15).

L 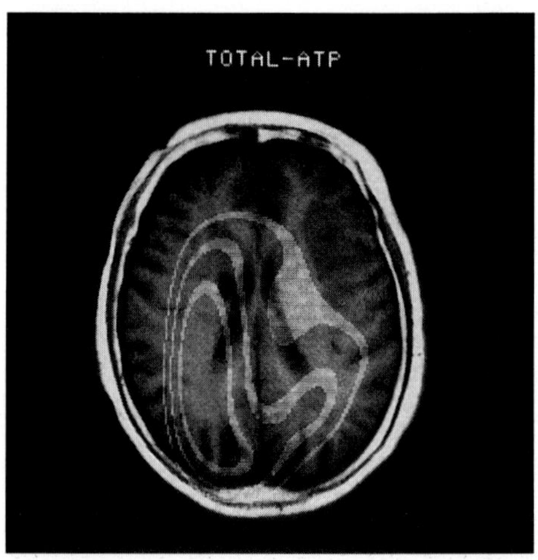 R

Fig. 30-4 Axial total ATP contour map superimposed on T_1-weighted image (500/15).

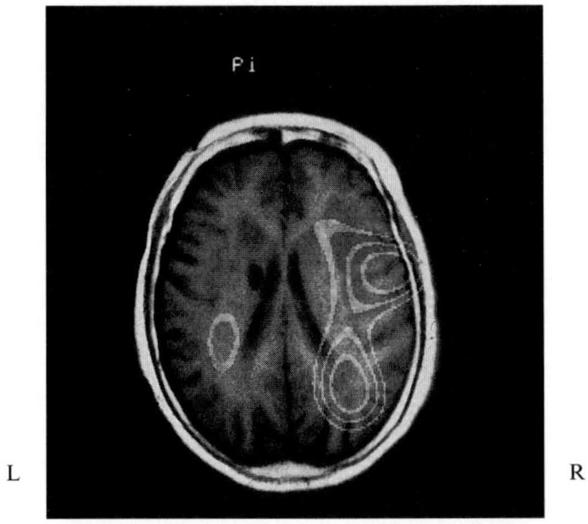

Fig. 30-5 Axial Pi contour map superimposed on T_1-weighted image (500/15).

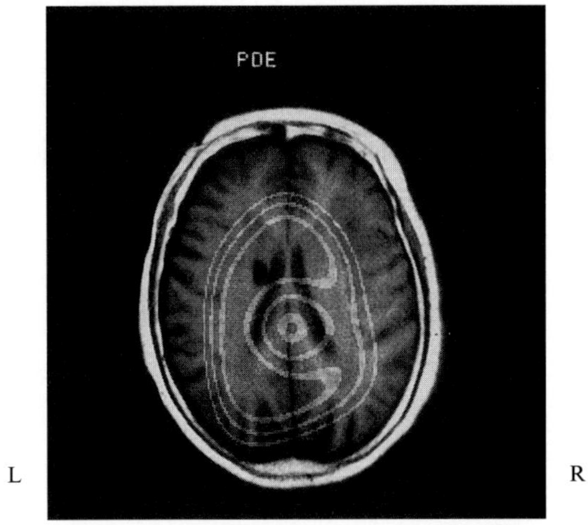

Fig. 30-6 Axial PDE contour map superimposed on T_1-weighted image (500/15).

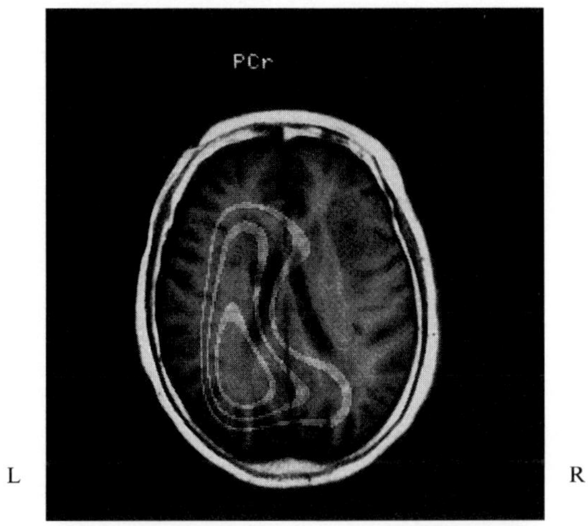

Fig. 30-7 Axial PCr contour map superimposed on T_1-weighted image (500/15).

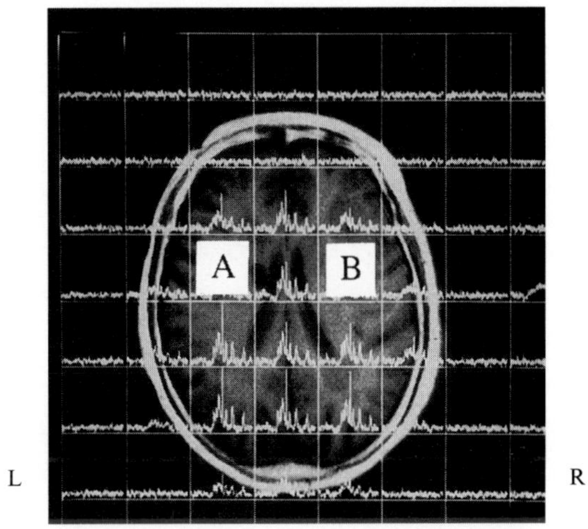

Fig. 30-8 T_1-weighted image showing the position of $3 \times 3 \times 4$ cm^3 voxels A and B.

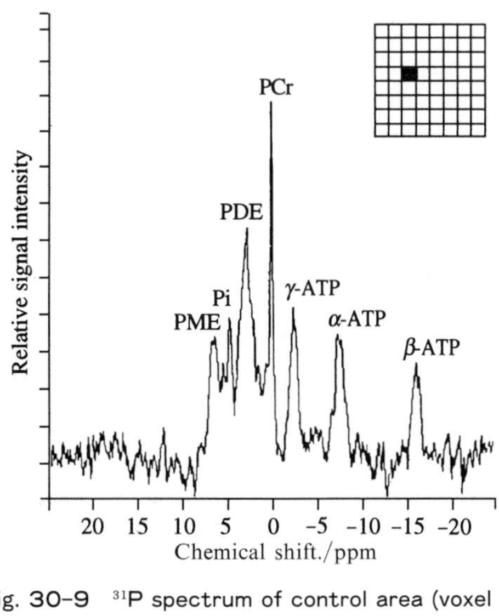

Fig. 30-9 ^{31}P spectrum of control area (voxel A).

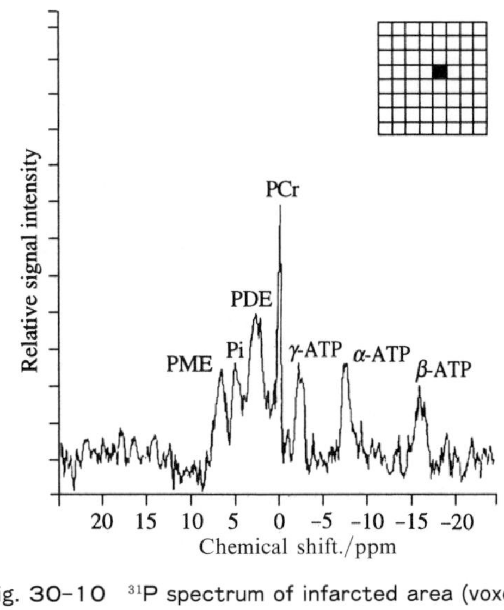

Fig. 30-10 ^{31}P spectrum of infarcted area (voxel B).

CASE 31

CASE 31: A 43-year-old male

Cerebral infarction in a medial part of the right occipital lobe (7 days after the stroke)

The patient presented with headache and left homonymous hemianopsia upon waking in the morning. He gave a past history of hypertension.

The MRIs in Figures 31-1 and 2 show cerebral infarction in a medial part of the right occipital lobe. The signal intensity is reduced in the infarcted area in the ^{31}P, ATP, and PDE metabolite images in Figures 31-3, 4, and 7. It is slightly increased in the infarcted area in the PME and Pi metabolite images in Figures 31-5 and 6. Figures 31-9 and 31-10 show the ^{31}P spectra of an area opposite the infarcted area and the infarcted area, respectively. Note the generally low signal intensities in the spectrum of the infarcted area.

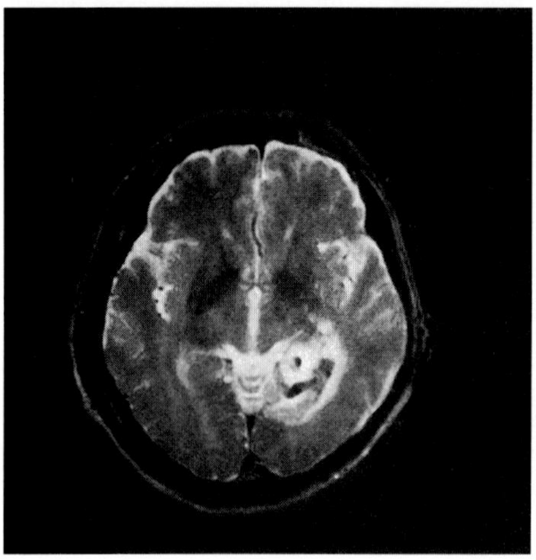

Fig. 31-1 Axial T_2-weighted image (2,200/90).

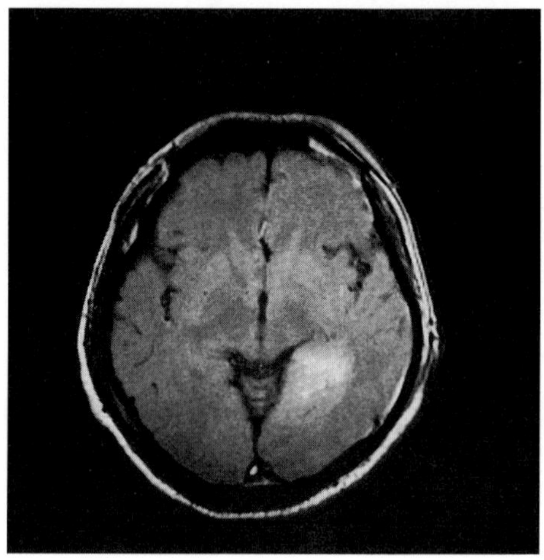

Fig. 31-2 Axial proton density-weighted image (2,200/15).

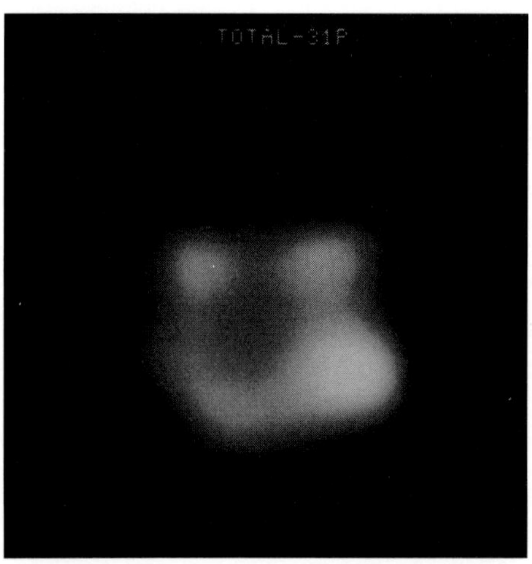

Fig. 31-3 Axial ^{31}P metabolite image.

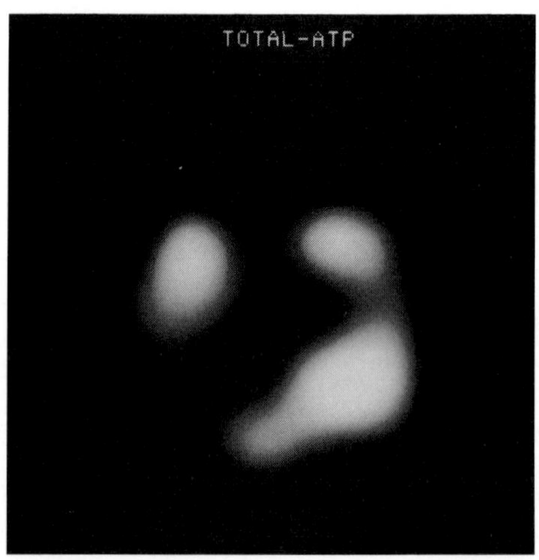

Fig. 31-4 Axial total ATP metabolite image.

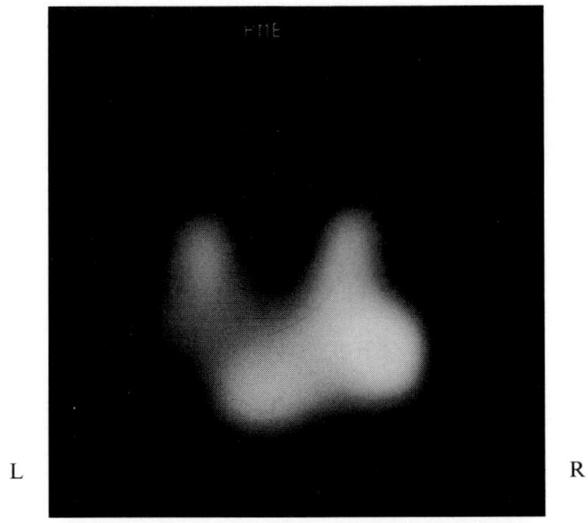

Fig. 31-5 Axial PME metabolite image.

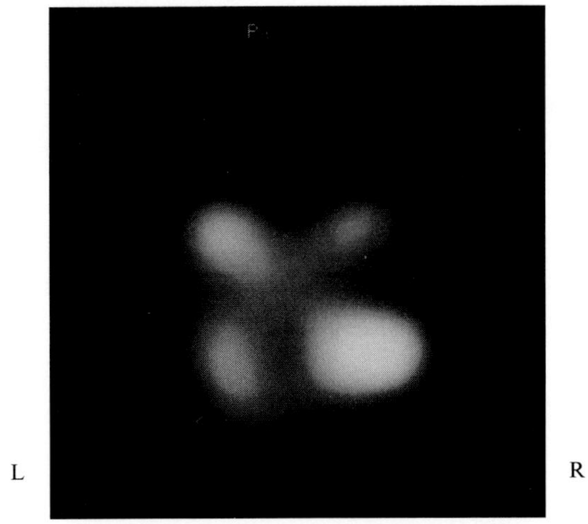

Fig. 31-6 Axial Pi metabolite image.

Fig. 31-7 Axial PDE metabolite image.

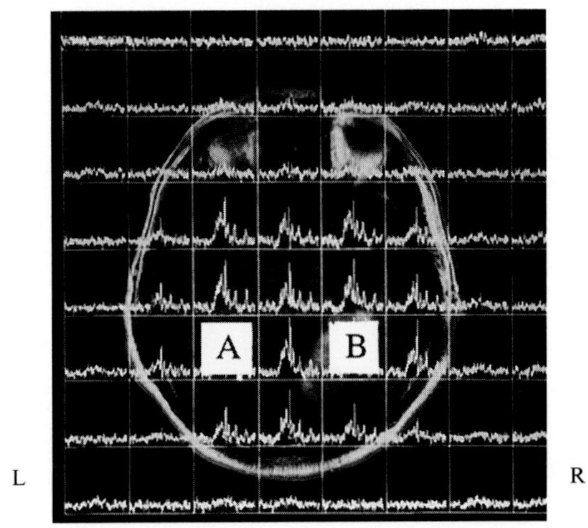

Fig. 31-8 T_1-weighted image showing the position of $3 \times 3 \times 4$ cm^3 voxels A and B.

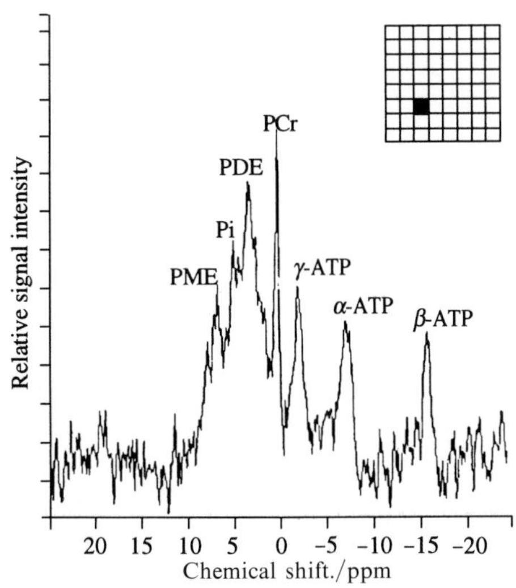

Fig. 31-9 ^{31}P spectrum of control area (voxel A).

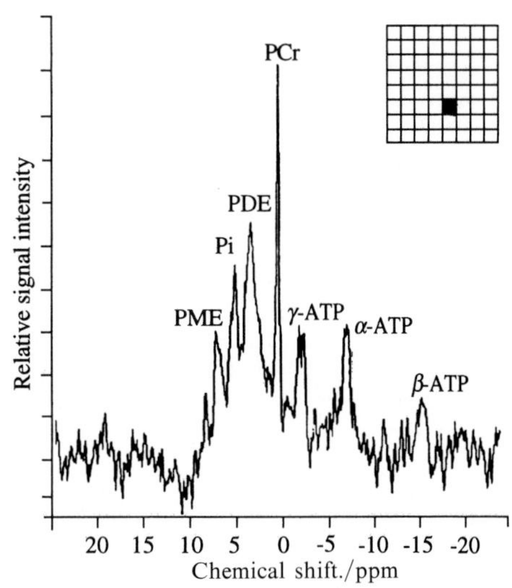

Fig. 31-10 ^{31}P spectrum of infarcted area (voxel B).

CASE 32

CASE 32: A 67-year-old female

Cerebral infarction of the right temporal lobe

(11 weeks after the stroke)

The patient presented with sudden onset of dysarthria and left hemiparesis. She gave a past history of atrial fibrillation and diabetes mellitus.

The MRIs in Figures 32-1 and 2 show cerebral infarction in the right temporal lobe. The signal intensity is reduced in the infarcted area in the ^{31}P, PME, and PDE contour maps and metabolite image in Figures 32-3, 5, and 7. No laterality is observed in the ATP contour map in Figure 32-4. The signal intensity of the infarcted area is slightly increased in the Pi metabolite image in Figure 32-6. Figures 32-9 and 32-10 show the ^{31}P spectra of an area opposite the infarcted area and the infarcted area, respectively. Note the generally low signal intensities in the spectrum of the infarcted area.

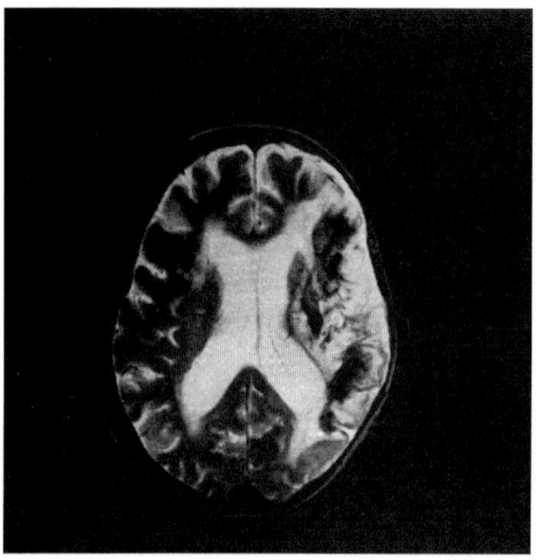

Fig. 32-1 Axial T_2-weighted image (2,200/90).

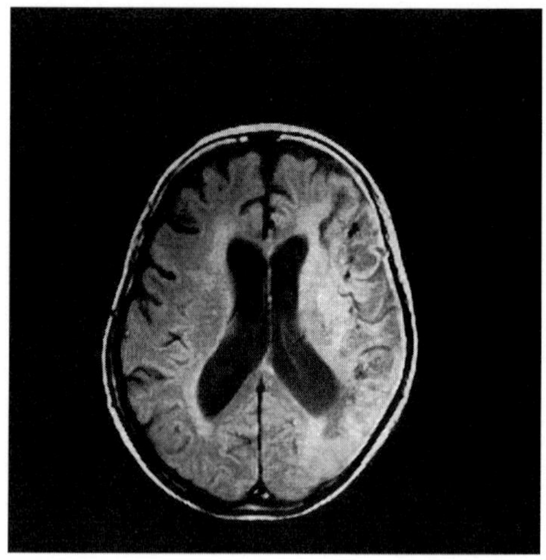

Fig. 32-2 Axial proton density-weighted image (2,200/15).

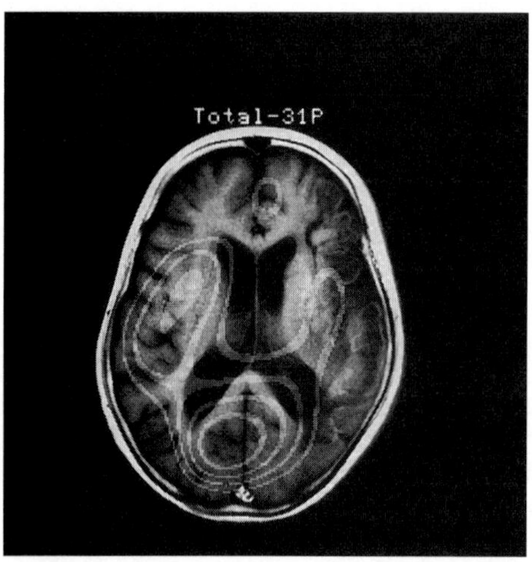

Fig. 32-3 Axial ^{31}P contour map superimposed on T_1-weighted image (500/15).

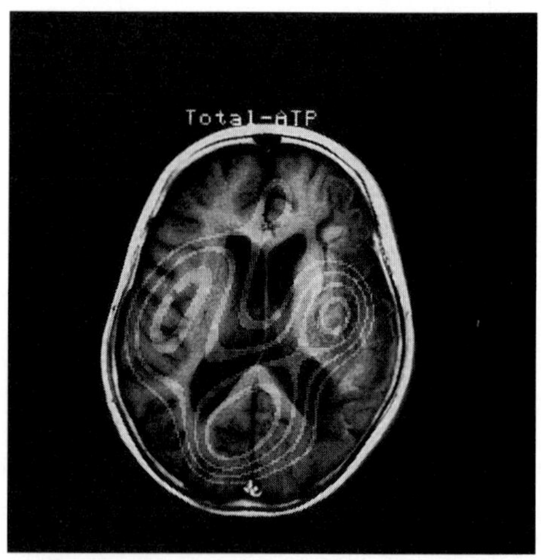

Fig. 32-4 Axial total ATP contour map superimposed on T_1-weighted image (500/15).

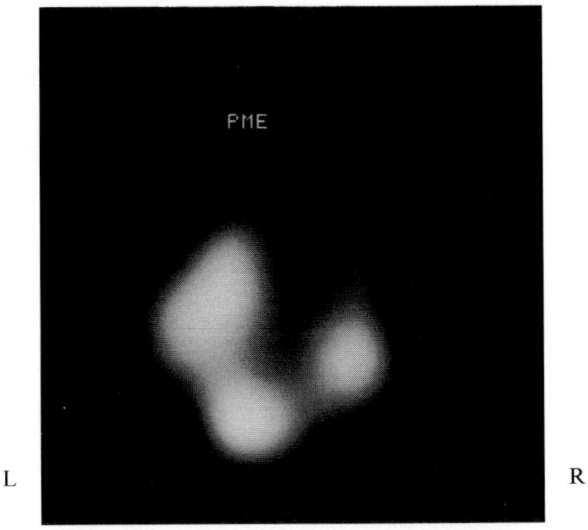

Fig. 32-5 Axial PME metabolite image.

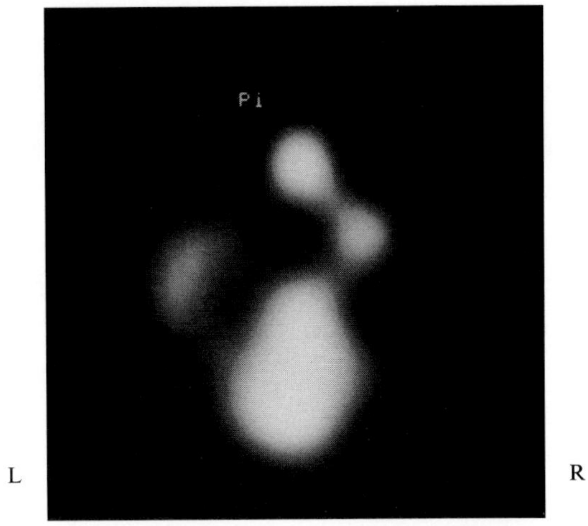

Fig. 32-6 Axial Pi metabolite image.

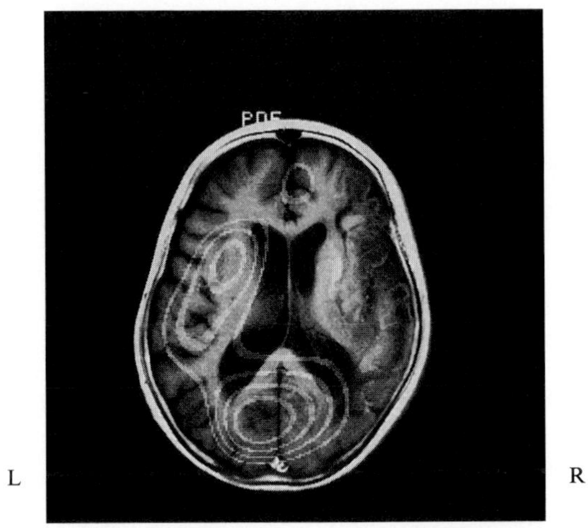

Fig. 32-7 Axial PDE contour map superimposed on T_1-weighted image (500/15).

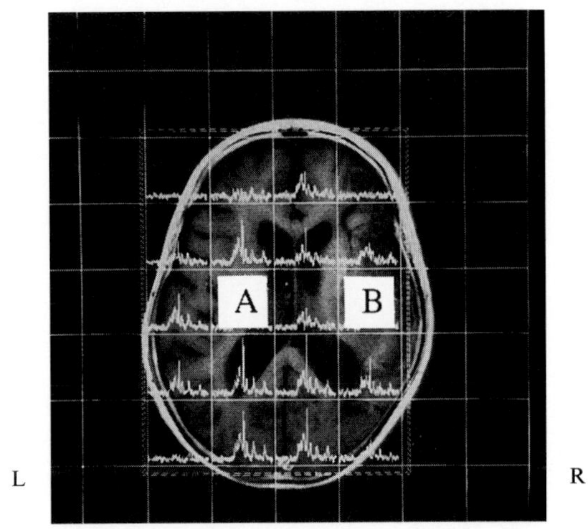

Fig. 32-8 T_1-weighted image showing the position of 3×3×4 cm^3 voxels A and B.

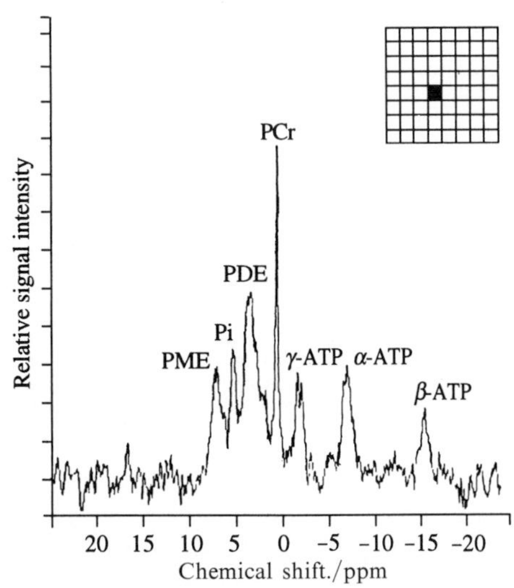

Fig. 32-9 ^{31}P spectrum of control area (voxel A).

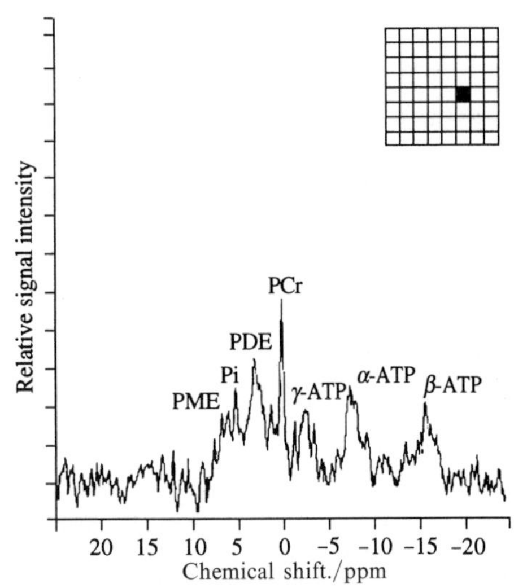

Fig. 32-10 ^{31}P spectrum of infarcted area (voxel B).

CASE 33

CASE 33: A 75-year-old male

Cerebral infarction of the left temporal lobe (17 months after the stroke)

The patient presented with left hemiparesis 17 months previous. He gave a past history of hyperlipidemia and hyperuricemia.

The MRIs in Figures 33-1 and 2 show cerebral infarction in the left temporal lobe. The signal intensity of the infarcted area is reduced in the ^{31}P, ATP, PME, Pi, and PDE metabolite images in Figures 33-3, 4, 5, 6, and 7. Figures 33-9 and 33-10 show the ^{31}P spectra of the infarcted area and an area opposite the infarcted area, respectively. Note the generally low signal intensities in the spectrum of the infarcted area.

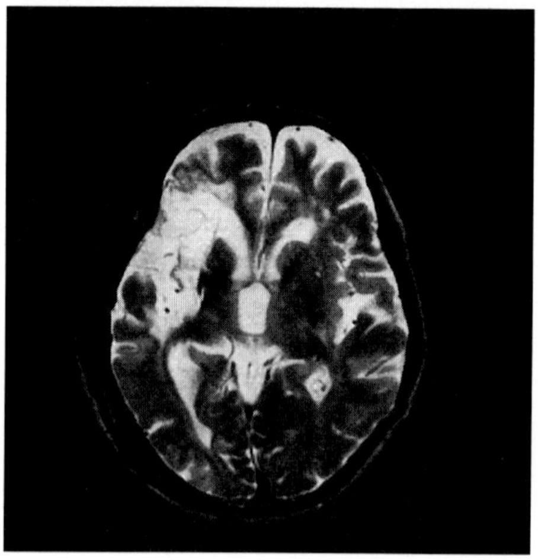

Fig. 33-1 Axial T_2-weighted image (2,200/90).

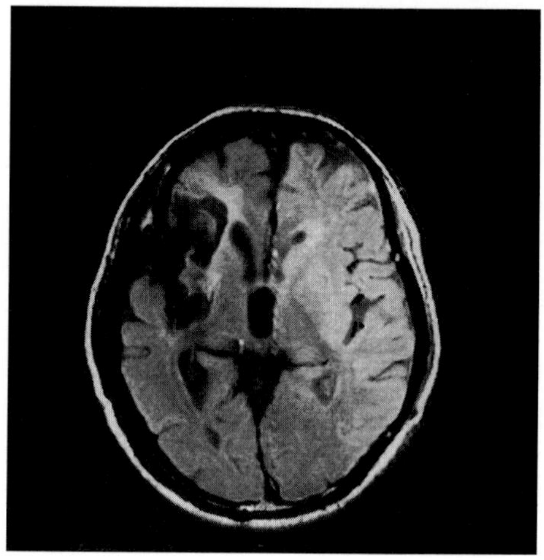

Fig. 33-2 Axial proton density-weighted image (2,200/15).

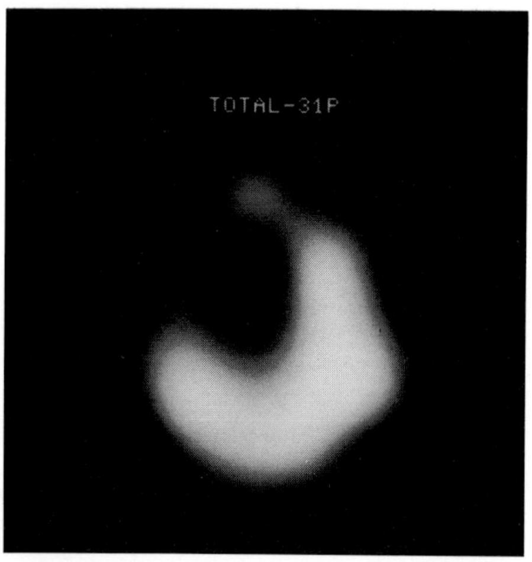

Fig. 33-3 Axial ^{31}P metabolite image.

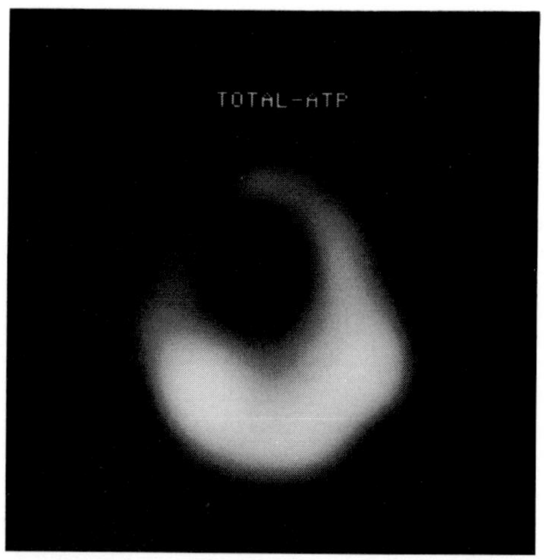

Fig. 33-4 Axial total ATP metabolite image.

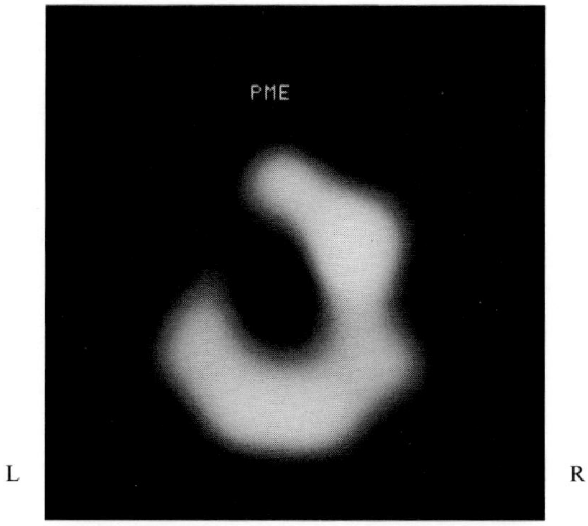

Fig. 33-5 Axial PME metabolite image.

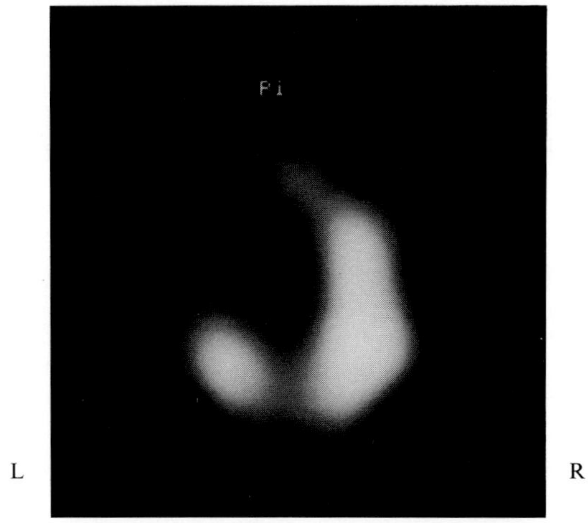

Fig. 33-6 Axial Pi metabolite image.

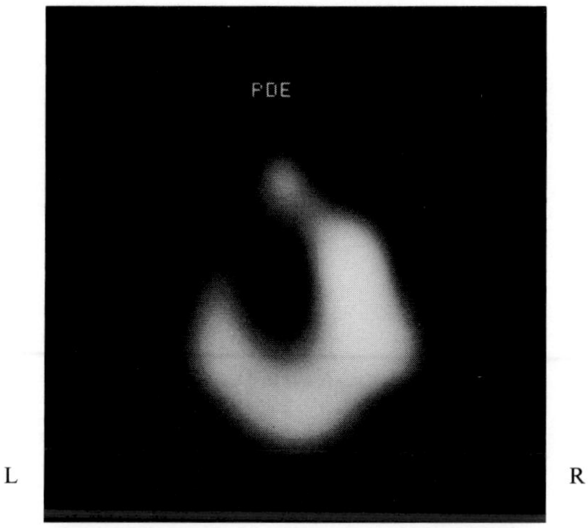

Fig. 33-7 Axial PDE metabolite image.

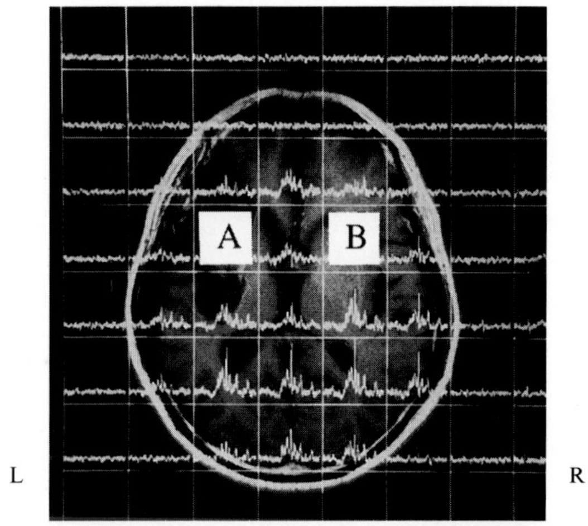

Fig. 33-8 T_1-weighted image showing the position of $3 \times 3 \times 4$ cm^3 voxels A and B.

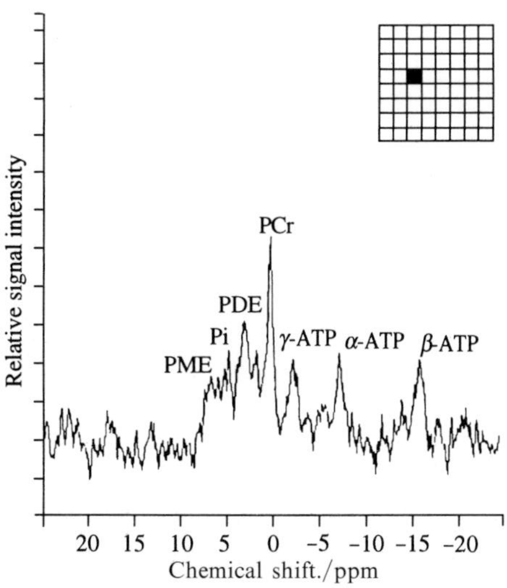

Fig. 33-9 ^{31}P spectrum of infarcted area (voxel A).

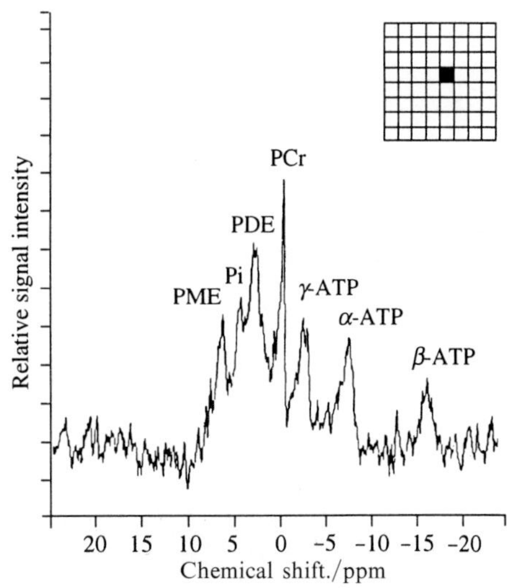

Fig. 33-10 ^{31}P spectrum of control area (voxel B).

CASE 34

CASE 34: A 72-year-old male

Cerebral infarction of the left temporal lobe (6 years after the stroke)

The patient presented with right hemiparesis and sensory aphasia 6 years previous. He gave a past history of atrial fibrillation.

The MRIs in Figures 34-1 and 2 show cerebral infarction in the left temporal lobe. The signal intensity is reduced in the infarcted area in the ^{31}P, ATP, and PDE metabolite images in Figures 34-3, 4, and 7. It is slightly increased in the PME and Pi metabolite images in Figures 34-5 and 6. Figures 34-9 and 34-10 show the ^{31}P spectra of the infarcted area and an area opposite the infarcted area, respectively. No clear differences can be observed between the two areas.

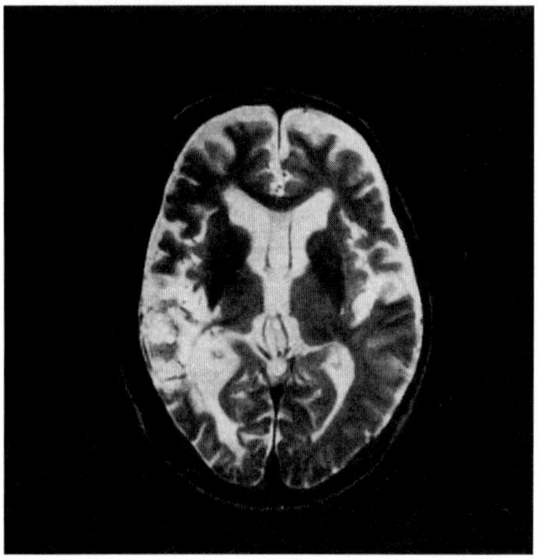

Fig. 34-1 Axial T_2-weighted image (2,200/90).

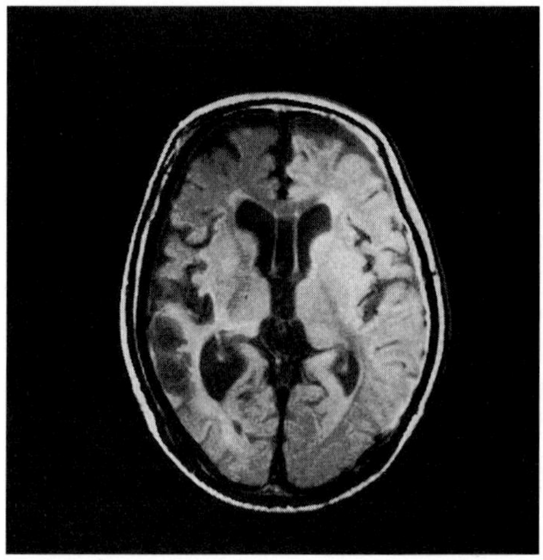

Fig. 34-2 Axial proton density-weighted image (2,200/15).

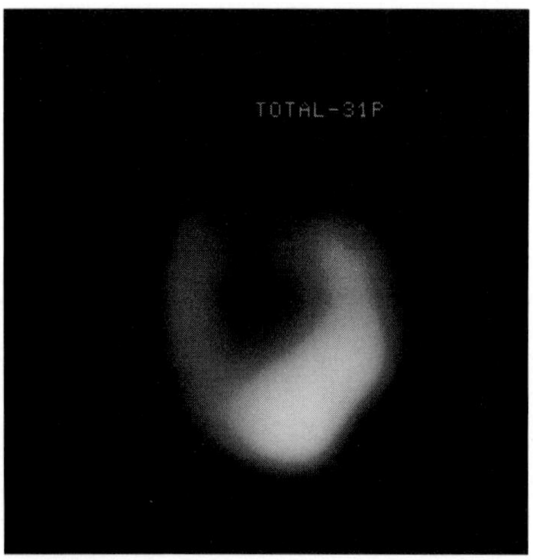

Fig. 34-3 Axial ^{31}P metabolite image.

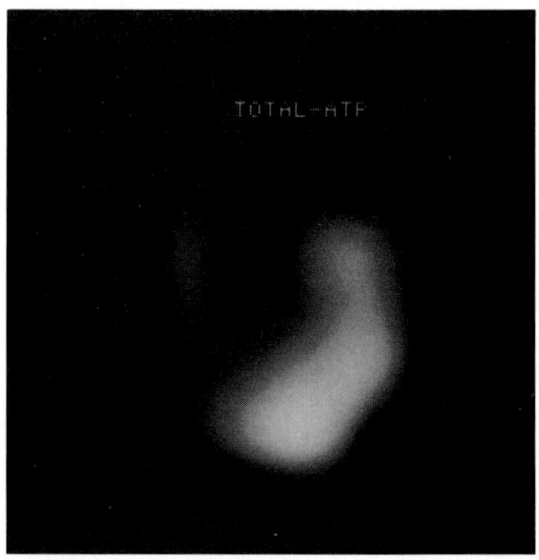

Fig. 34-4 Axial total ATP metabolite image.

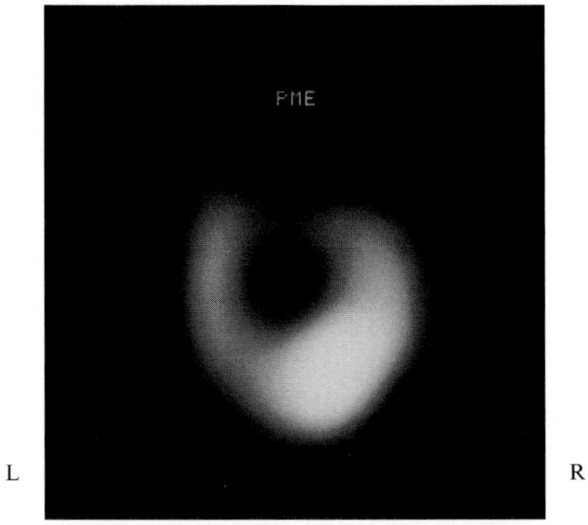

Fig. 34-5 Axial PME metabolite image.

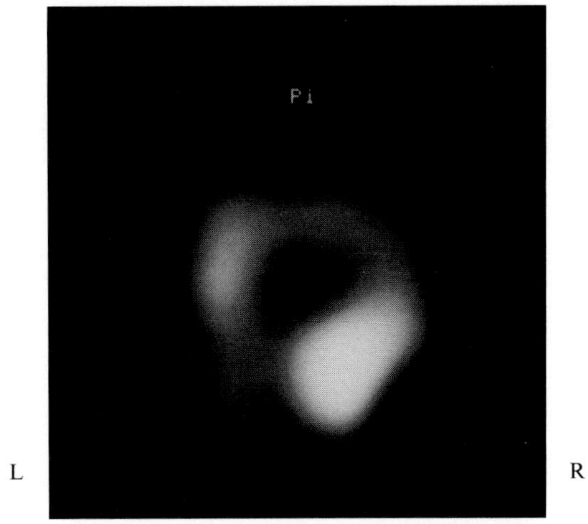

Fig. 34-6 Axial Pi metabolite image.

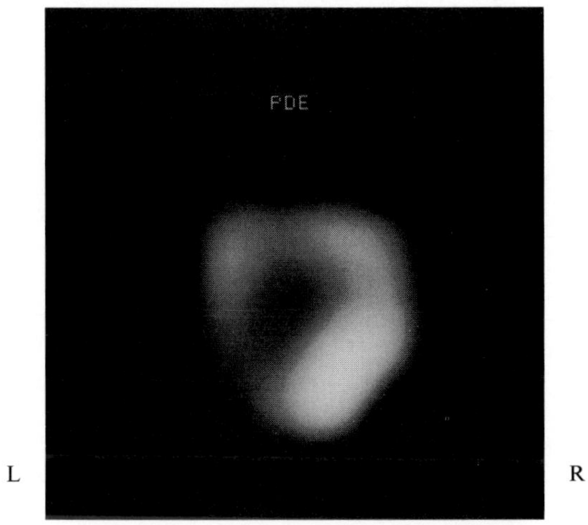

Fig. 34-7 Axial PDE metabolite image.

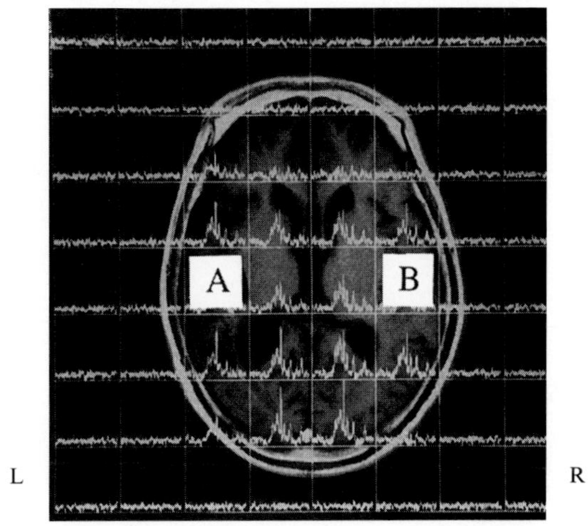

Fig. 34-8 T_1-weighted image showing the position of 3×3×4 cm^3 voxels A and B.

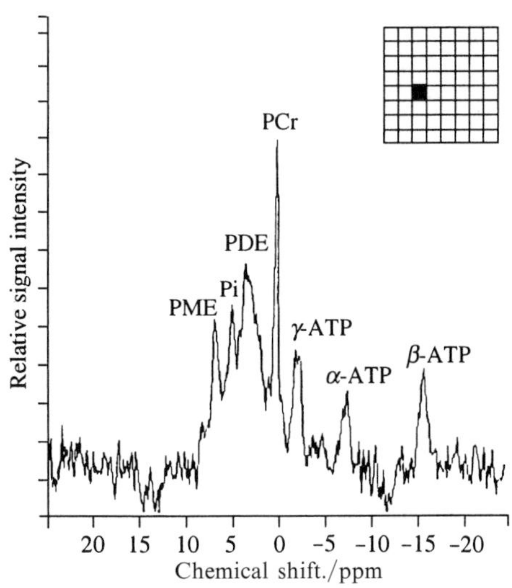

Fig. 34-9 ^{31}P spectrum of infarcted area (voxel A).

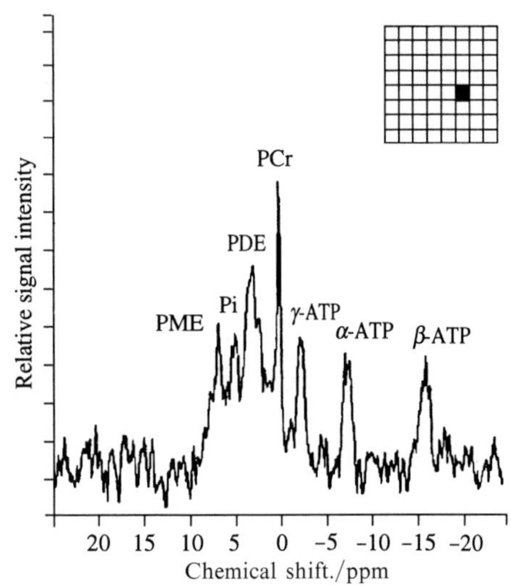

Fig. 34-10 ^{31}P spectrum of control area (voxel B).

35. Course of ^{31}P MRS of cerebral infarction: A summary of 12 cases

Figures 35-1 to 5 are graphs showing serial changes in PCr, Pi, PME, PDE, and β-ATP signal intensities in the infarcted areas of 12 patients relative to normal brain tissue. Only Pi increased immediately after the stroke and returned gradually to the normal range, but other components remained reduced immediately after the stroke. Figure 35-6 is a graph of serial changes in the intracellular pH (pHi) in the infarcted area. The intracellular pH was acidotic immediately after the stroke but became alkalotic after 3-4 days and remained shifted to alkalosis over a long period even after normalization of Pi.

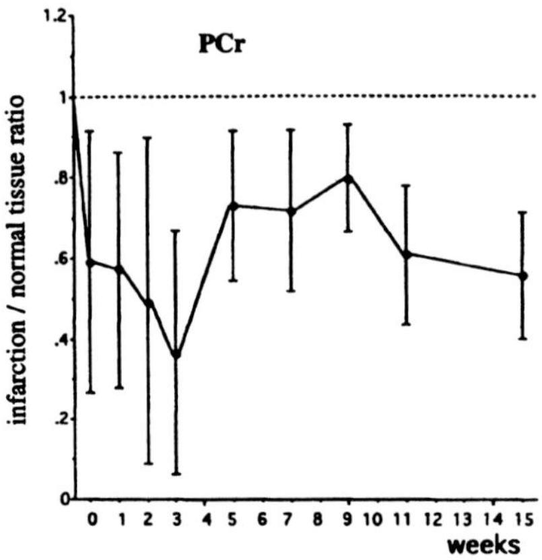

Fig. 35-1 Changes of infarction to normal tissues ratio of PCr due to time course of disease.

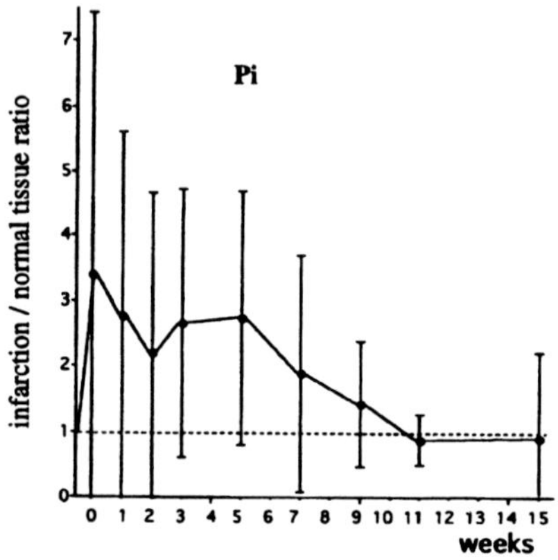

Fig. 35-2 Changes of infarction to normal tissues ratio of Pi due to time course of disease.

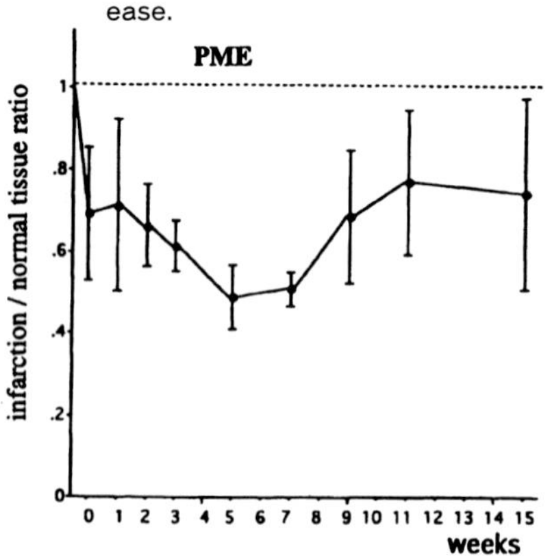

Fig. 35-3 Changes of infarction to normal tissues ratio of PME due to time couse of disease.

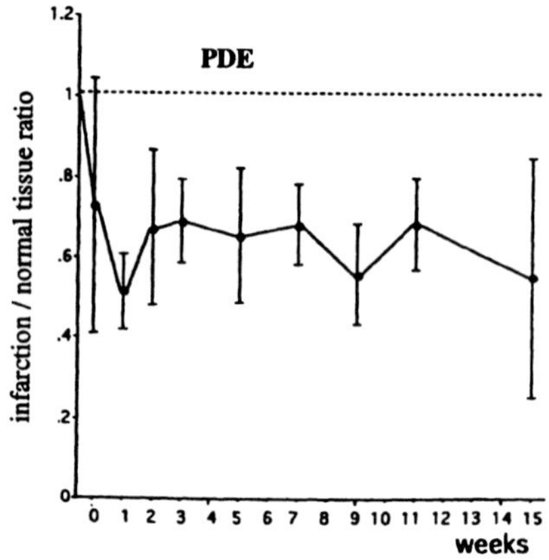

Fig. 35-4 Changes of infarction to normal tissues ratio of PDE due to time couse of disease.

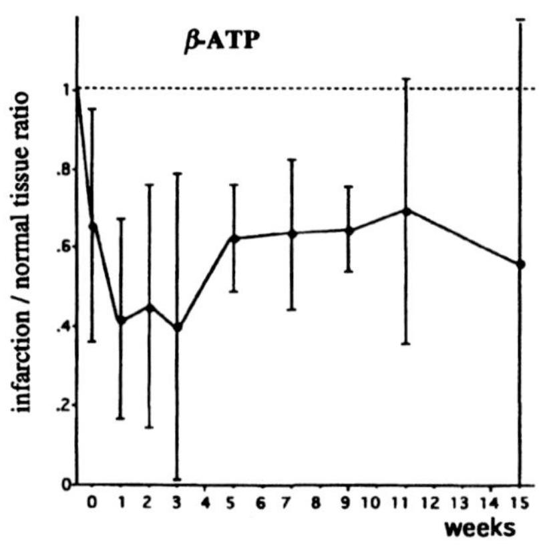

Fig. 35-5 Changes of infarction to normal tissues ratio of β-ATP due to time course of disease.

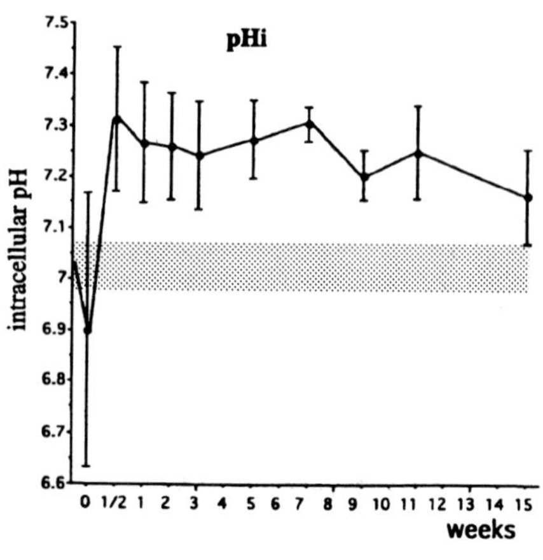

Fig. 35-6 Changes of pHi due to time course of disease.

Chapter 7 Cerebral Arteriovenous Malformation (AVM), Moya Moya Disease

Kousaku Terada

7.1 CHARACTERISTICS OF THE SPECTRUM

According to reports concerning the circulatory dynamics in cerebral arteriovenous malformation (AVM), findings on single photon emission computed tomography (SPECT) and positron emission tomography (PET) suggest that rCBF is reduced and rCBV is increased in a state of misery perfusion around the nidus, and that this condition is caused by the steal associated with an AV shunt.[1] According to findings on ^{31}P–MRS, Pi was increased and PCr and ATP were reduced in the AVM and surrounding tissues, indicating chronic cerebral ischemia, similar to results obtained by SPECT and PET. Therefore, ^{31}P–MRS may be applicable to the evaluation of cerebral ischemia associated with the steal in tissues around AVM and, further, to the prediction of postoperative normal perfusion pressure breakthrough.

Moya Moya disease is a condition in which an abnormal vascular network develops in the basal ganglia as collateral circulation as a result of an obstruction of the carotid bifurcation of the internal carotid artery. The disease causes chronic cerebral ischemia in many patients. ^{31}P–MRS findings in the ischemic area were similar to those in cerebral infarction, i.e., an increase in Pi, decreases in PCr and ATP, and mild alkalosis,[2] in patients who were suspected to have a reduced cerebral blood flow on SPECT and a reduced reserve of the cerebral circulation by SPECT with acetazolamide loading even when no large cerebral infarction was demonstrated by CT or MRI.

These findings suggest that ^{31}P–MRS is useful for the pathogenetic analysis of chronic cerebral ischemia and warrants further evaluation in this respect.

REFERENCES

1) Sasahira, M.; Uchimura, K.; Nagayama, T. et al. Evaluation of cerebral blood flow and cerebral phosphorus metabolism in arteriovenous malformations by ^{123}I IMP SPECT and ^{31}P chemical shift imaging. *Progress in CT* 12: 641–649; 1990. [Japanese]

2) Terada, K.; Moriya, N.; Fujimoto, T. et al. ^{31}P chemical shift imaging in cerebral ischemic disorders. *Abstracts of 51st Annual Meeting of the Japan Neurosurgical Society. Book 2. Kagoshima* p. 198; 1992.

7.2 CASES (36-40)

CASE 36

CASE 36: A 28-year-old male
AVM of the right parietal lobe

The patient presented with generalized convulsions.

The MRA and MRIs in Figures 36-1, 2, and 3 show AVM in the right parietal lobe. The laterality is unclear in the ^{31}P and ATP metabolite images in Figures 36-4 and 5. The signal intensity is increased on the vertical side of the AVM in the Pi metabolite image in Figure 36-6, but is decreased in the AVM area in the PME and PCr metabolite images shown in Figures 36-7 and 8. Figures 36-10 and 36-11 show the ^{31}P spectra of an area superior to the AVM and an area opposite the AVM, respectively. Note the generally low signal intensities and the relatively high Pi signal intensities in the spectrum of the AVM area.

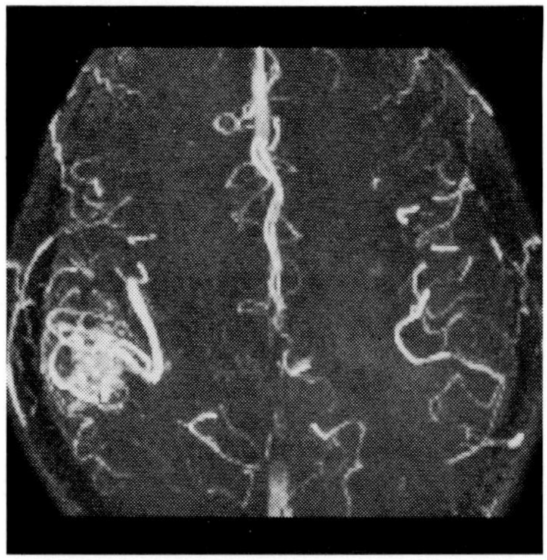
R L

Fig. 36-1 Magnetic Resonance Angiography.

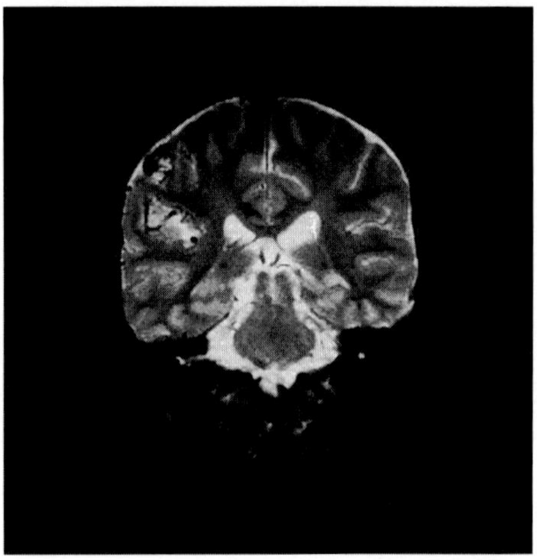
R L

Fig. 36-2 Coronal T_2-weighted image (2,200/90).

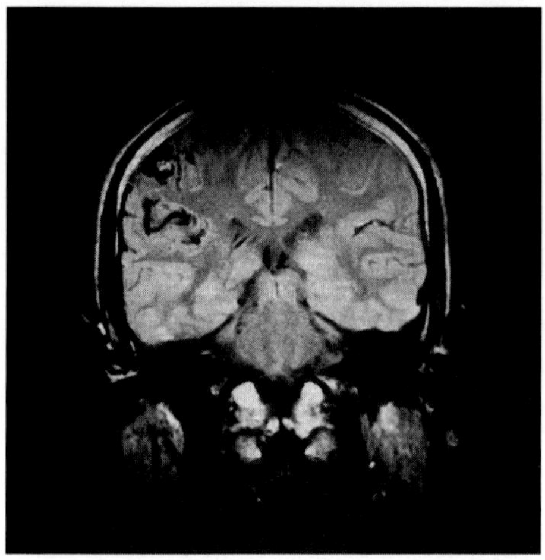
R L

Fig. 36-3 Coronal proton density-weighted image (2,200/15).

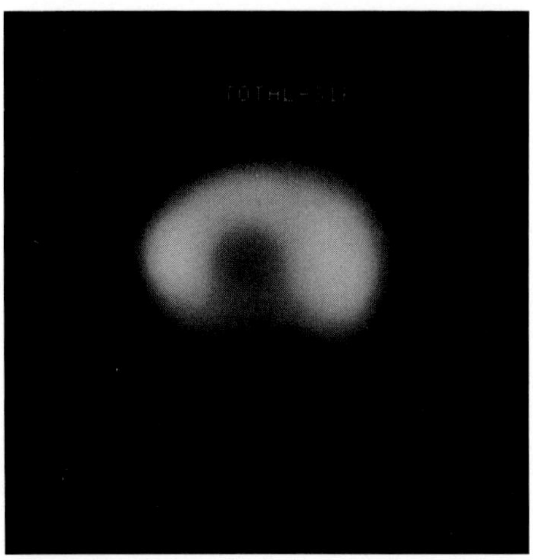
R L

Fig. 36-4 Coronal ^{31}P metabolite image.

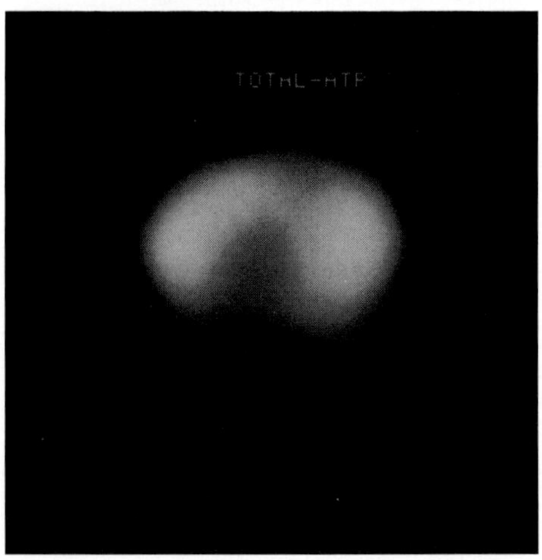
R L

Fig. 36-5 Coronal total ATP metabolite image.

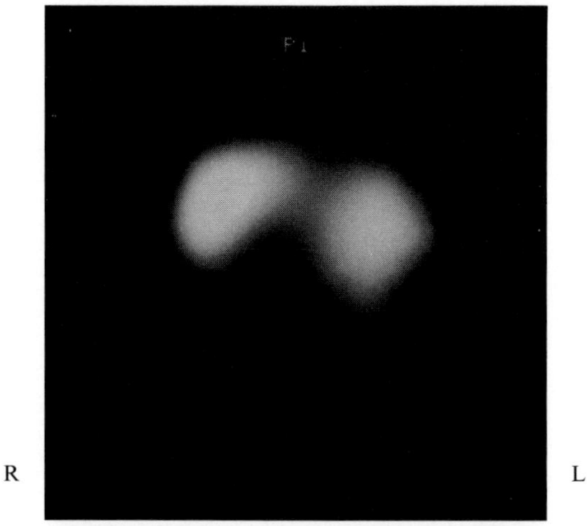

Fig. 36-6 Coronal Pi metabolite image.

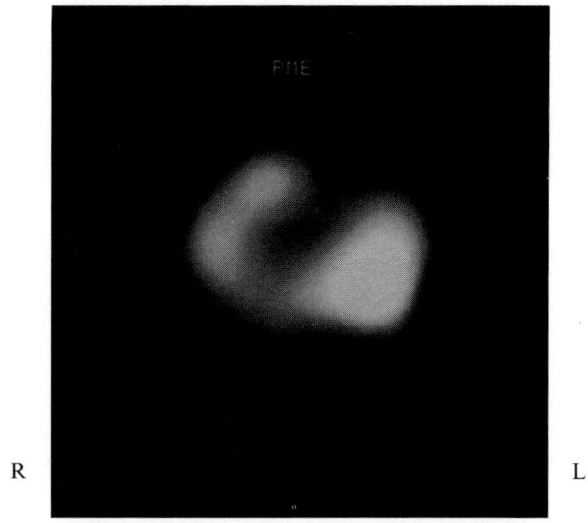

Fig. 36-7 Coronal PME metabolite image.

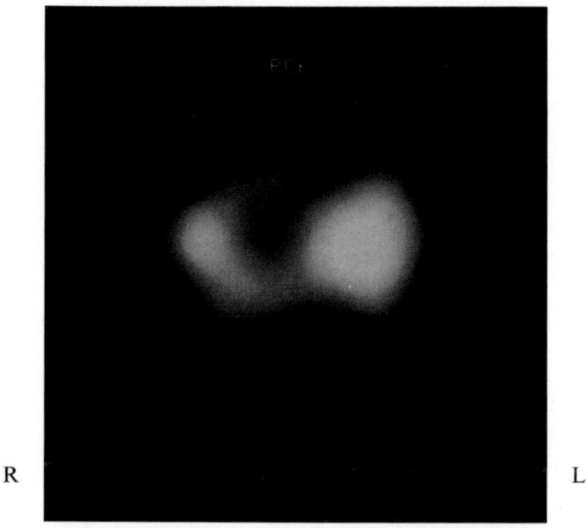

Fig. 36-8 Coronal PCr metabolite image.

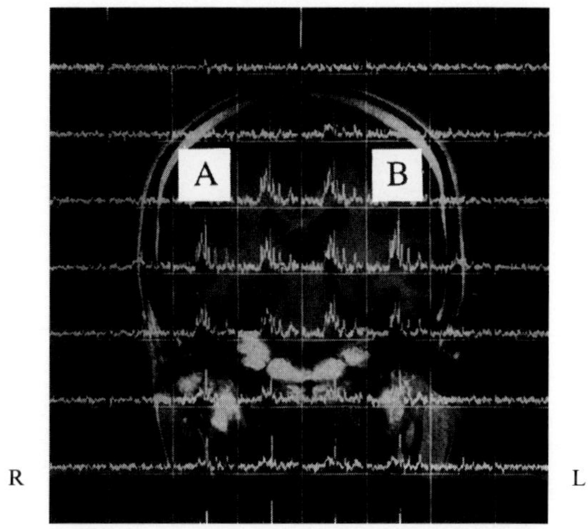

Fig. 36-9 T_1-weighted image showing the position of $3 \times 3 \times 4$ cm^3 voxels A and B.

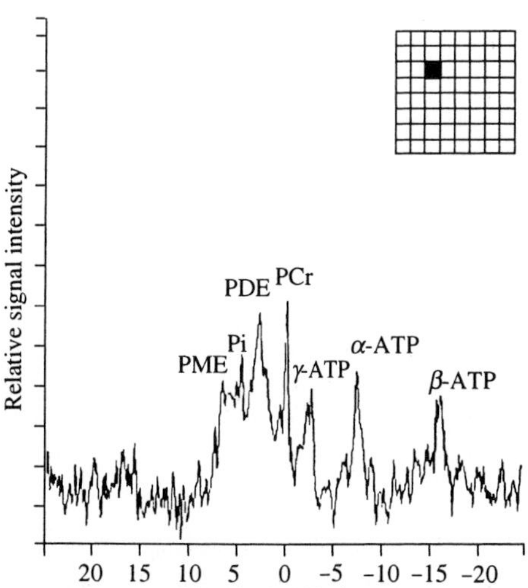

Fig. 36-10 ^{31}P spectrum of AVM area (voxel A).

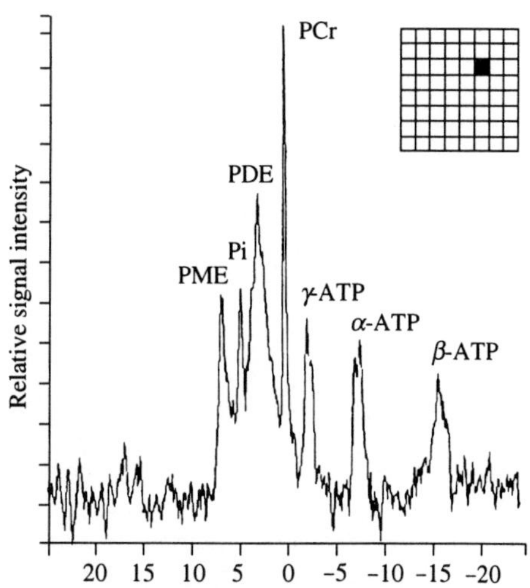

Fig. 36-11 ^{31}P sepctrum of control area (voxel B).

CASE 37

CASE 37: A 31-year-old male

AVM of the right frontal lobe

The patient presented with psychomotor seizure.

The MRA and MRIs in Figures 37-1, 2, and 3 show a large AVM in the right frontal lobe. A low signal intensity area is observed widely near the AVM in the ^{31}P, ATP, PME, Pi, and PDE metabolite images in Figures 37-4, 5, 6, 7, and 8. Figures 37- 10 and 37-11 show the ^{31}P spectra of an area opposite the AVM and the AVM area, respectively. Note the generally low signal intensities and relatively high Pi signal intensities in the AVM area.

R 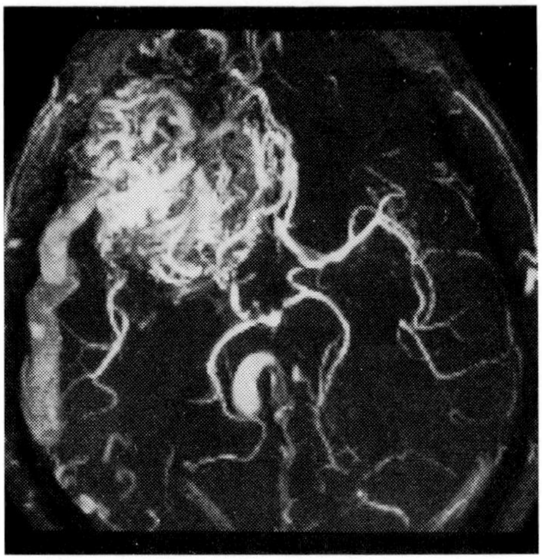 L

Fig. 37-1 Magnetic Resonance Angiography.

L 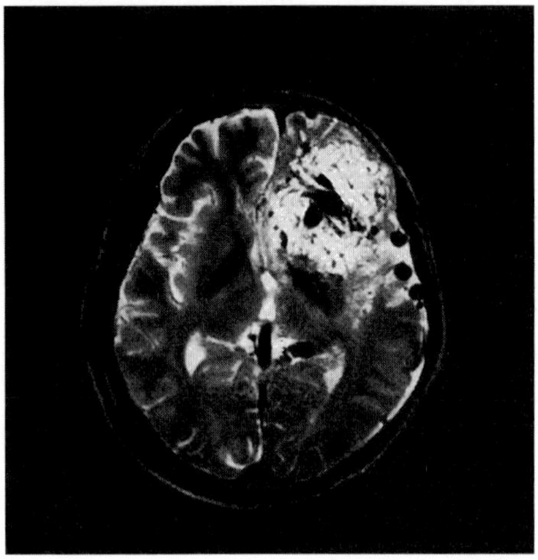 R

Fig. 37-2 Axial T_2-weighted image (2,200/90).

L 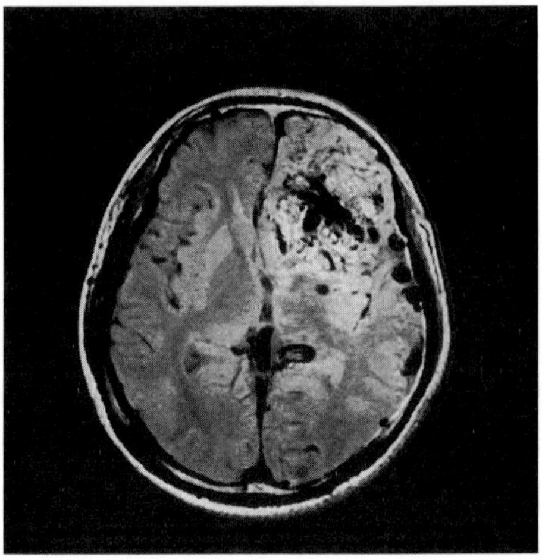 R

Fig. 37-3 Axial proton density-weighted image (2,200/15).

L 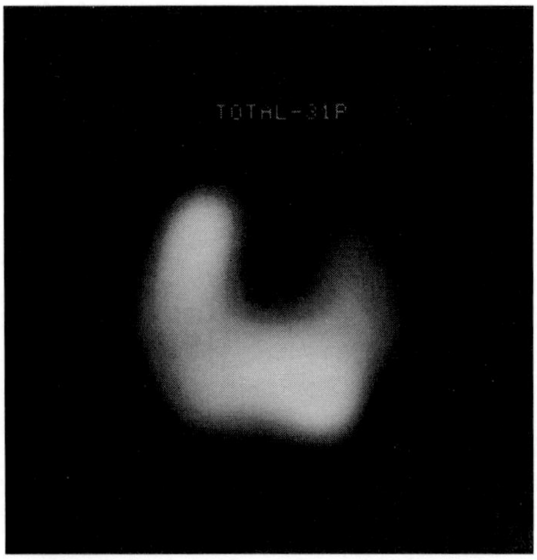 R

Fig. 37-4 Axial ^{31}P metabolite image.

L 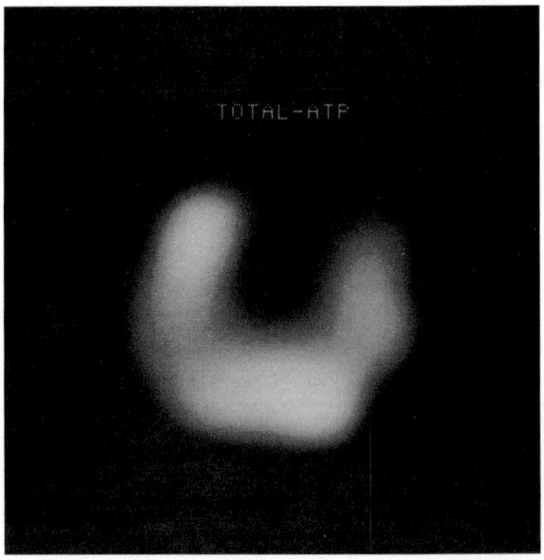 R

Fig. 37-5 Axial total ATP metabolite image.

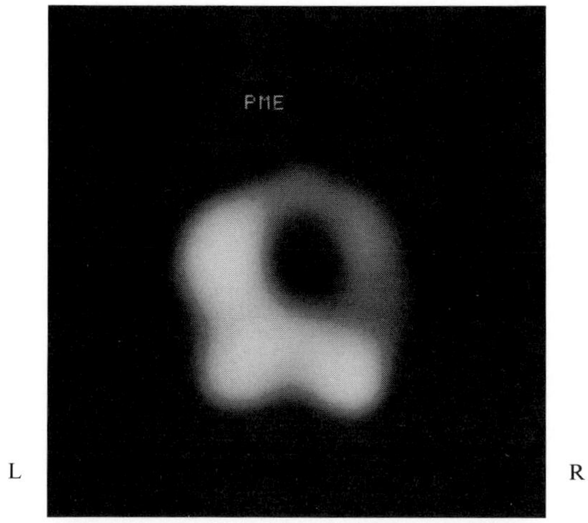

Fig. 37-6 Axial PME metabolite image.

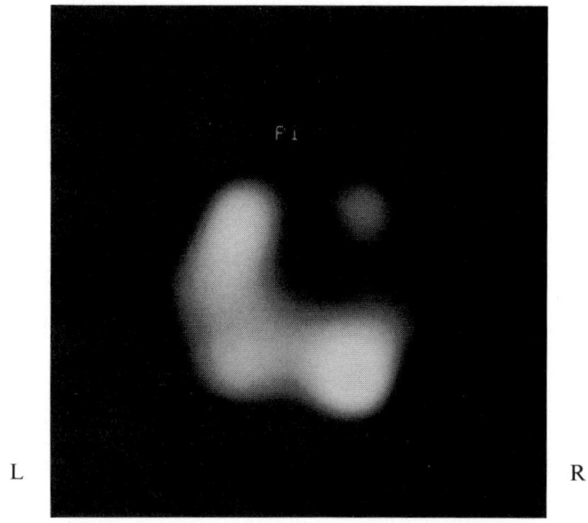

Fig. 37-7 Axial Pi metabolite image.

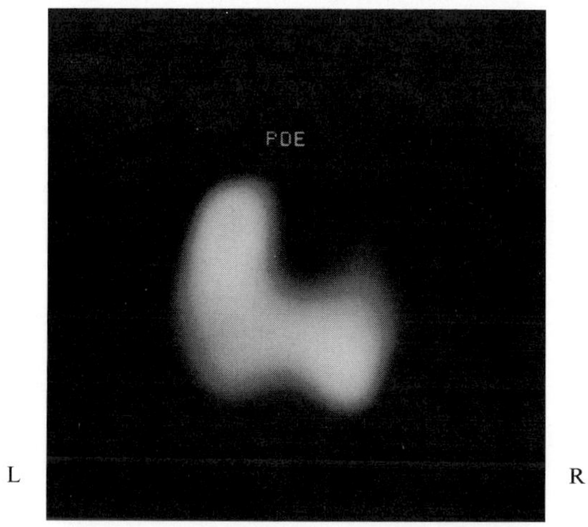

Fig. 37-8 Axial PDE metabolite image.

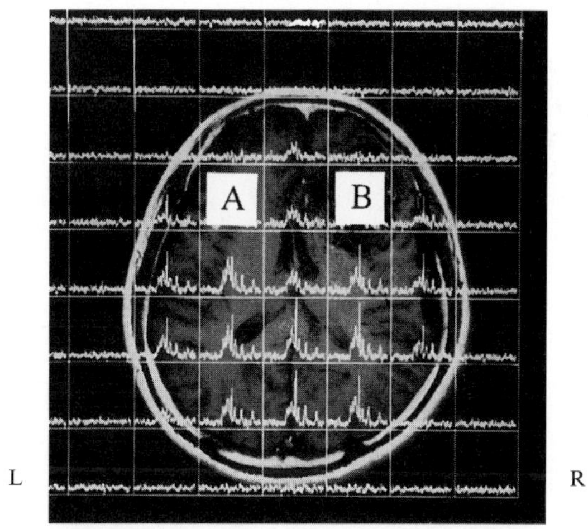

Fig. 37-9 T_1-weighted image showing the position of 3×3×4 cm^3 voxels A and B.

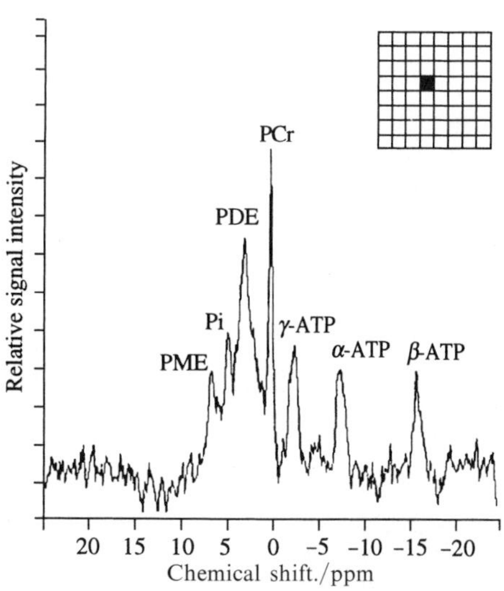

Fig. 37-10 ^{31}P spectrum of control area (voxel A).

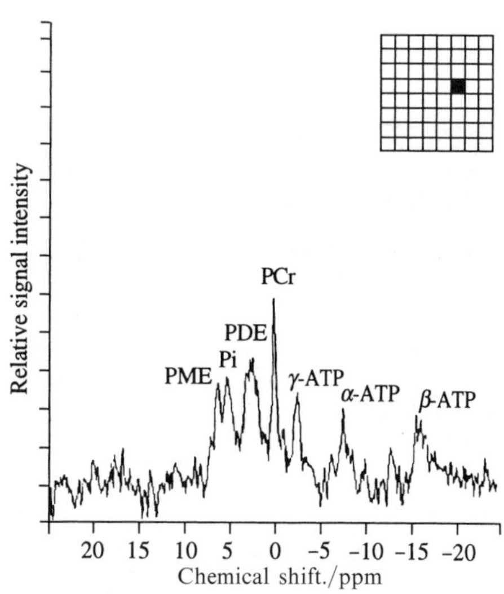

Fig. 37-11 ^{31}P spectrum of AVM area (voxel B).

CASE 38

CASE 38: A 60-year-old male

AVM of the left frontal lobe

The patient presented with slowly progressive dementia.

The MRA and MRIs in Figures 38-1, 2, and 3 show a huge AVM in the left frontal lobe. A low signal intensity area is observed widely near the AVM in the ^{31}P, ATP, and PCr metabolite images shown in Figures 38-4, 5, and 8. PME signal intensities are increased, and Pi signal intensities are slightly increased, in the PME and Pi metabolite images in Figures 38-6 and 7. Figures 38-10 and 38-11 show the ^{31}P spectra of the AVM area and an area opposite the AVM area. Note the generally low signal intensities and relatively high PME and Pi signal intensities in the AVM area.

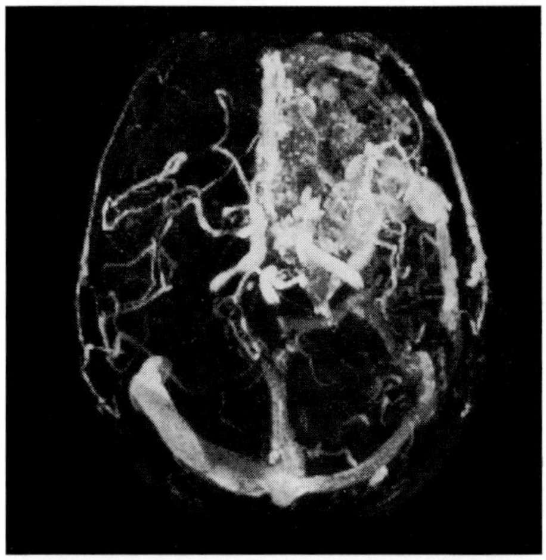

Fig. 38-1 Magnetic Resonance Angiography.

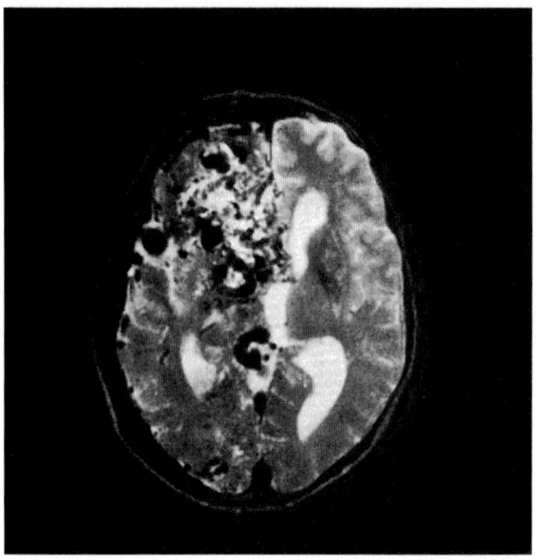

Fig. 38-2 Axial T_2-weighted image (2,200/90).

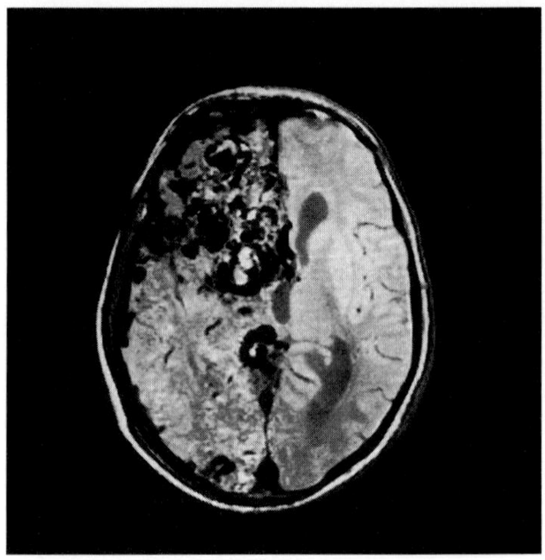

Fig. 38-3 Axial proton density-weighted image (2,200/15).

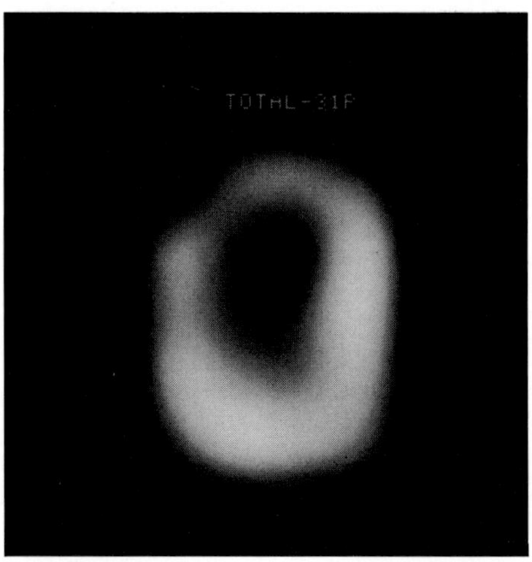

Fig. 38-4 Axial ^{31}P metabolite image.

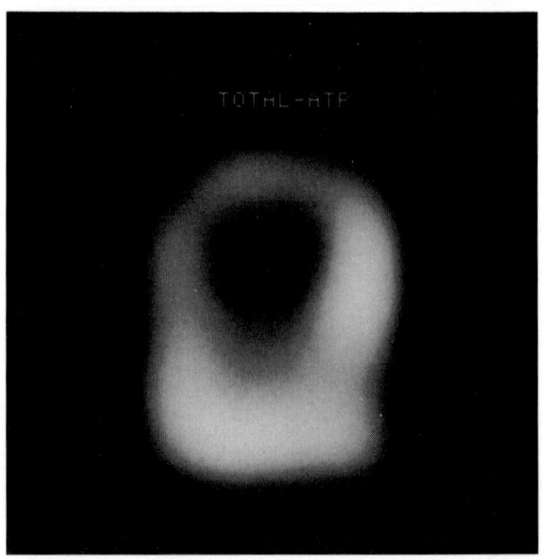

Fig. 38-5 Axial total ATP metabolite image.

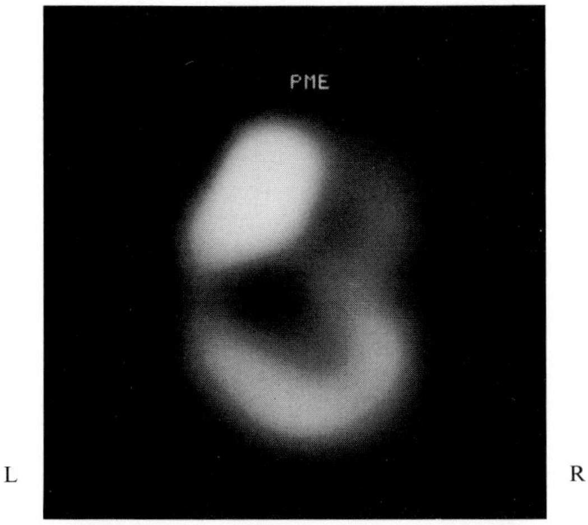

Fig. 38-6 Axial PME metabolite image.

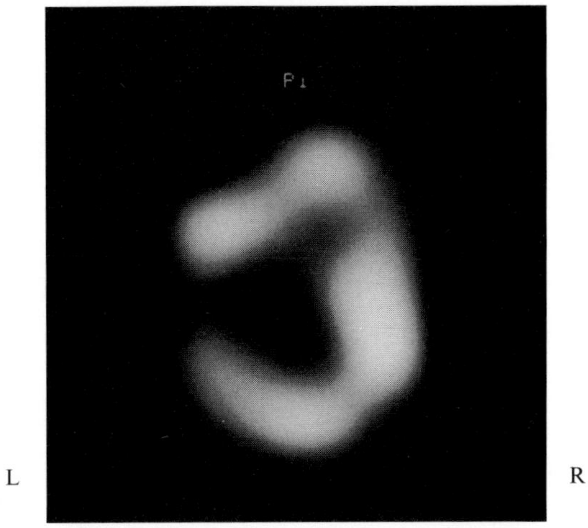

Fig. 38-7 Axial Pi metabolite image.

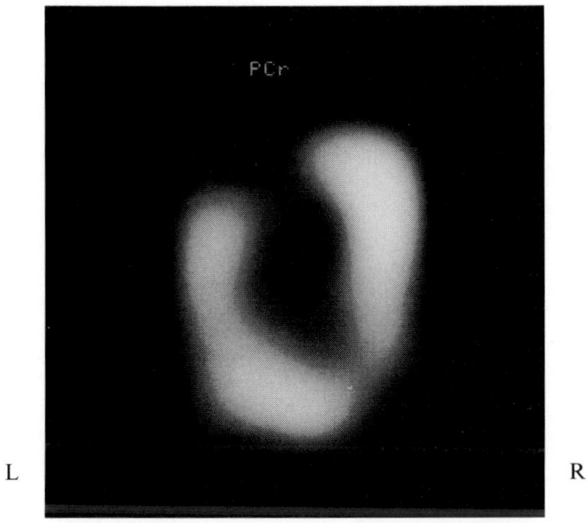

Fig. 38-8 Axial PCr metabolite image.

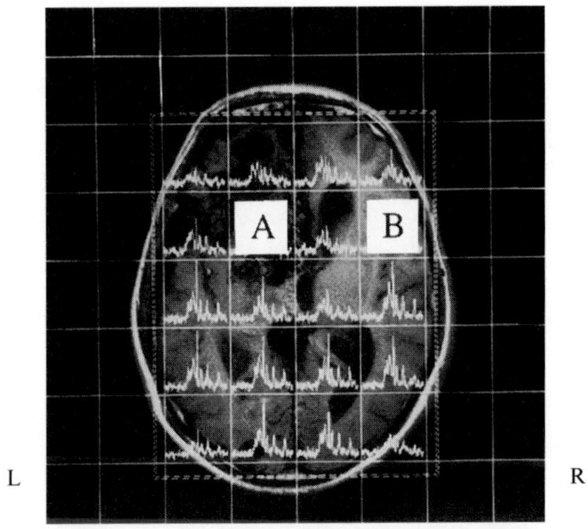

Fig. 38-9 T_1-weighted image showing the position of $3 \times 3 \times 4$ cm^3 voxels A and B.

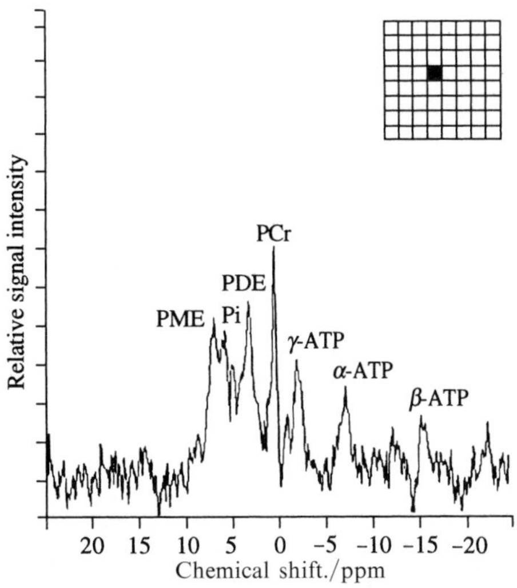

Fig. 38-10 ^{31}P spectrum of AVM area (voxel A).

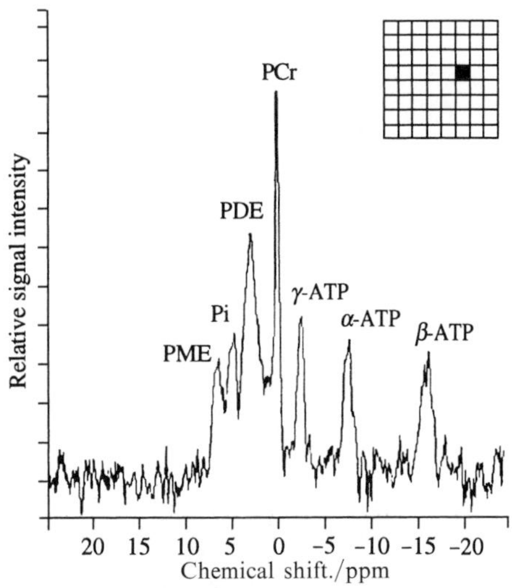

Fig. 38-11 ^{31}P spectrum of control area (voxel B).

CASE 39

CASE 39: A 16-year-old female

Moya Moya disease (the blood flow on the right side is maintained due to a bypass operation)

The patient presented with transient ischemic attack: right hemiparesis. She gave a past history of right STA-MCA anastomosis that was performed 7 years previous.

The MRIs in Figures 39-1 and 2 show old cerebral infarction in the bilateral occipital lobes. A flow void of Moya Moya vessels is noted in the left basal ganglia. The signal intensity is lower in the left hemisphere than in the right hemisphere in the ^{31}P, ATP, and PCr contour maps in Figures 39-3, 4, and 7. PME signal intensities are slightly increased in the left frontal lobe, and Pi signal intensities are increased from the left frontal lobe to the temporal lobe in the PME and Pi metabolite images in Figures 39-5 and 6. Figures 39-9 and 39-10 show the ^{31}P spectra of the left temporal lobe and right temporal lobe, respectively. Note the generally low signal intensities, relatively high Pi and PME signal intensities and relatively low PCr signal intensities in the left temporal lobe, where no clear findings suggestive of cerebral infarction are observed on MRI.

L 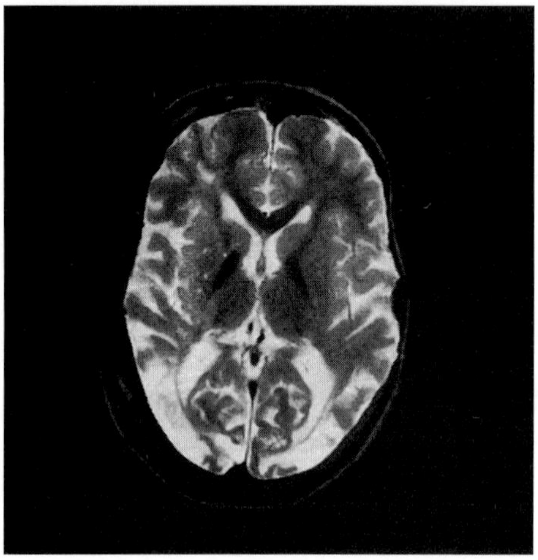 R

Fig. 39-1 Axial T_2-weighted image (2,200/90).

L 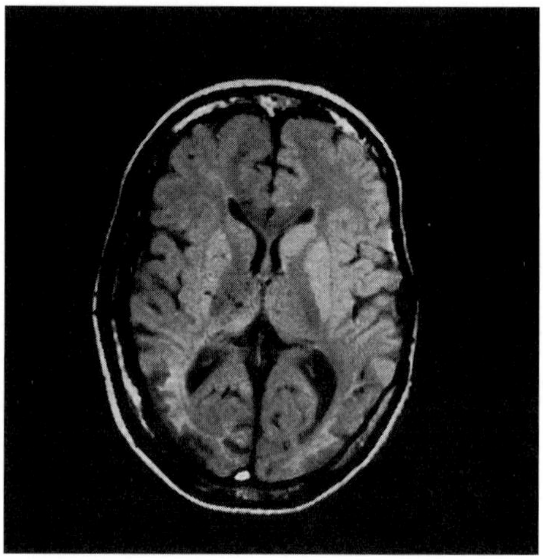 R

Fig. 39-2 Axial proton density-weighted image (2,200/15).

L 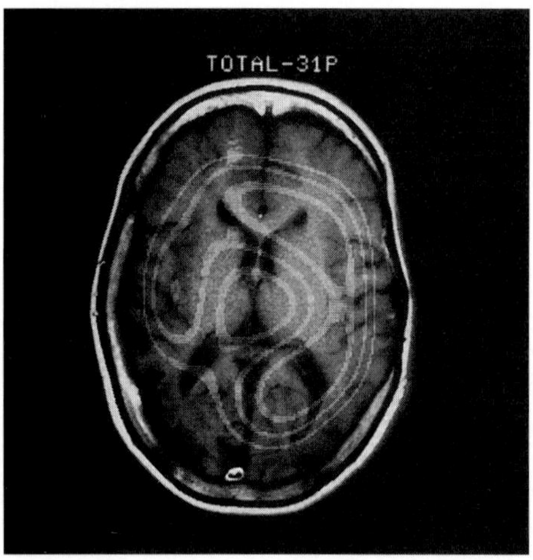 R

Fig. 39-3 Axial ^{31}P contour map superimposed on T_1-weighted image (500/15).

L 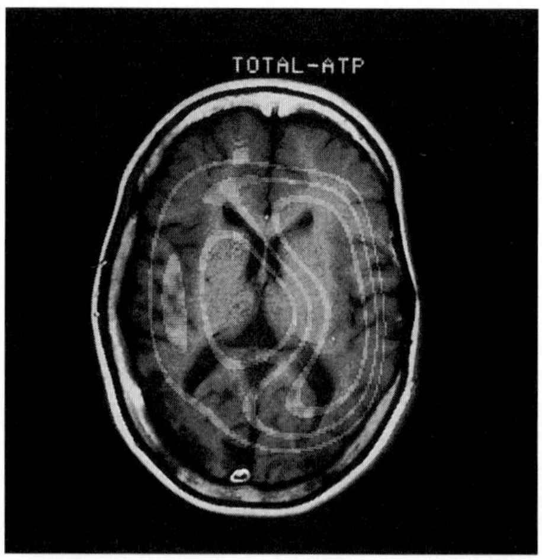 R

Fig. 39-4 Axial total ATP contour map superimposed on T_1-weighted image (500/15).

L R
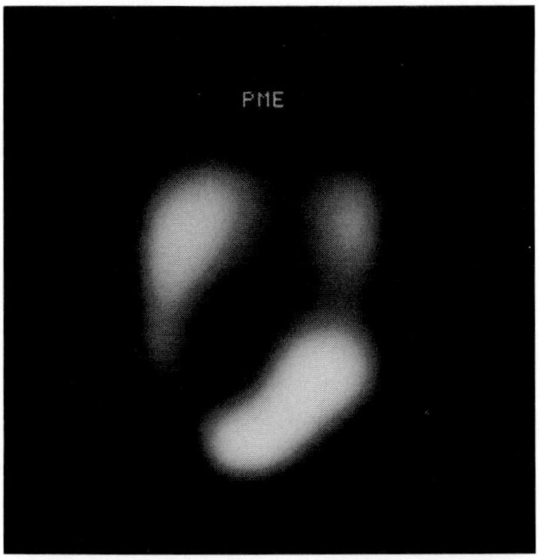

Fig. 39-5 Axial PME metabolite image.

L R
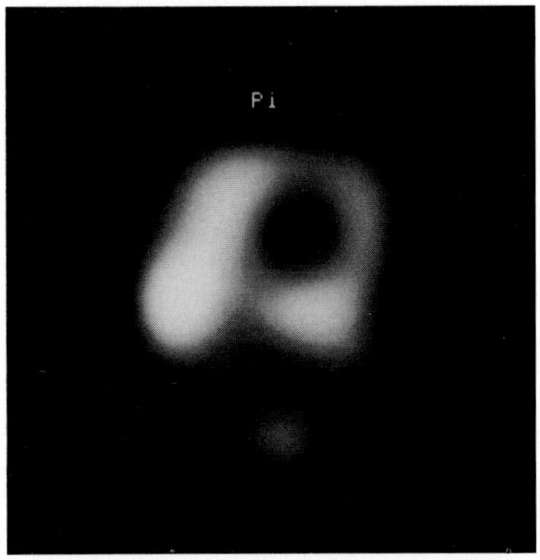

Fig. 39-6 Axial Pi metabolite image.

L R
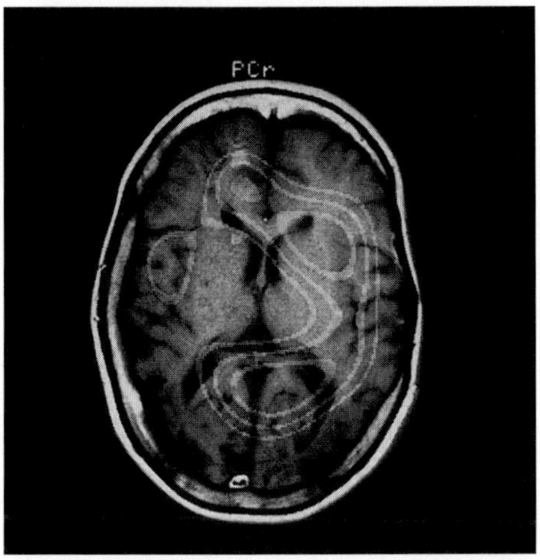

Fig. 39-7 Axial PCr contour map superimposed on T_1 weighted image (500/15).

L R
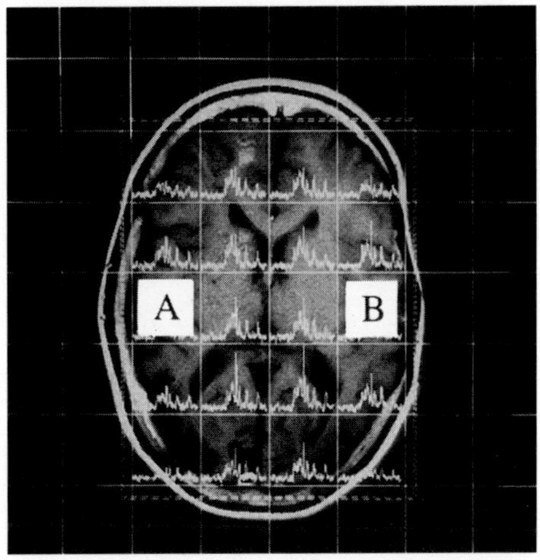

Fig. 39-8 T_1-weighted image showing the position of 3×3×4 cm^3 voxels A and B.

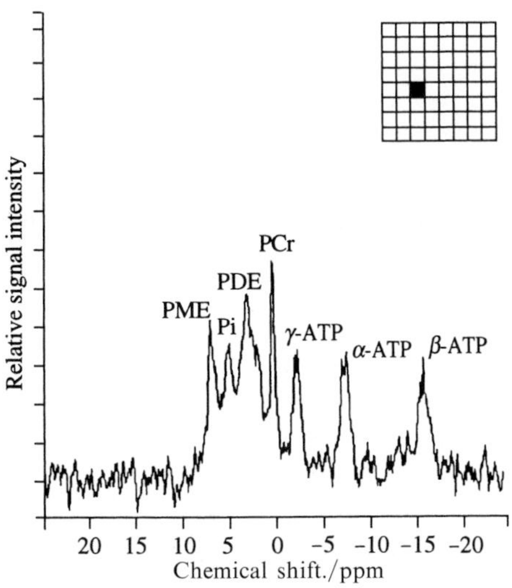

Fig. 39-9 ^{31}P spectrum of left temporal area (voxel A).

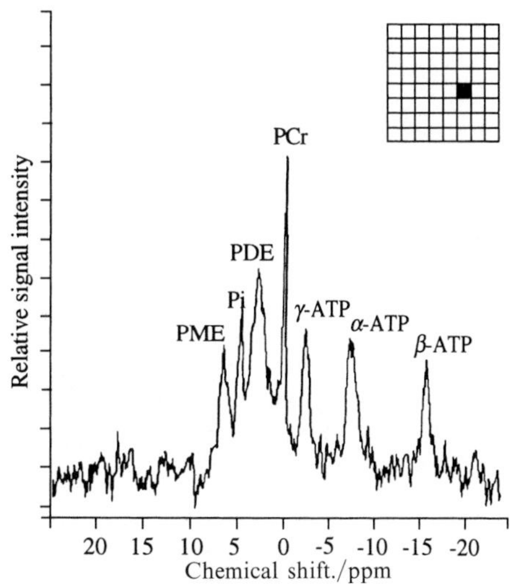

Fig. 39-10 ^{31}P spectrum of right temporal area (voxel B).

CASE 40

CASE 40: A 43-year-old female

Moya Moya disease

The patient presented with no symptoms: incidental case.

The MRI and MRA in Figures 40-1 and 2 show a flow void of Moya Moya vessels in the bilateral basal ganglia. No laterality is observed in the ^{31}P, ATP, β-ATP, α-ATP, and PDE contour maps or metabolite images in Figures 40-3, 4, 5, 6, and 7. Figures 40-9 and 40-10 show the ^{31}P spectra of the right basal ganglia and left basal ganglia, respectively. No laterality is observed.

L 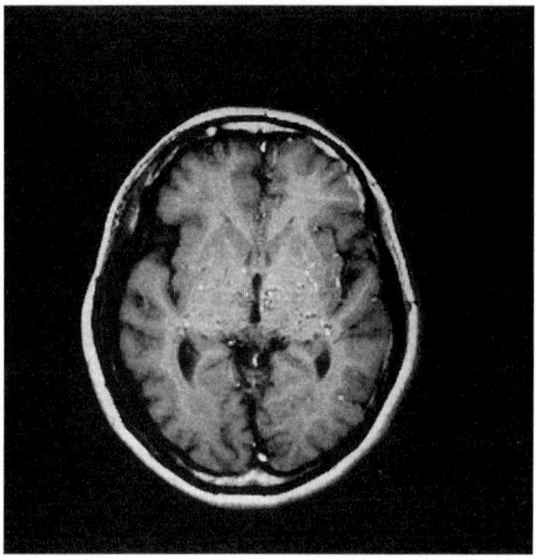 R

Fig. 40-1 Axial T_1-weighted image (500/15).

R 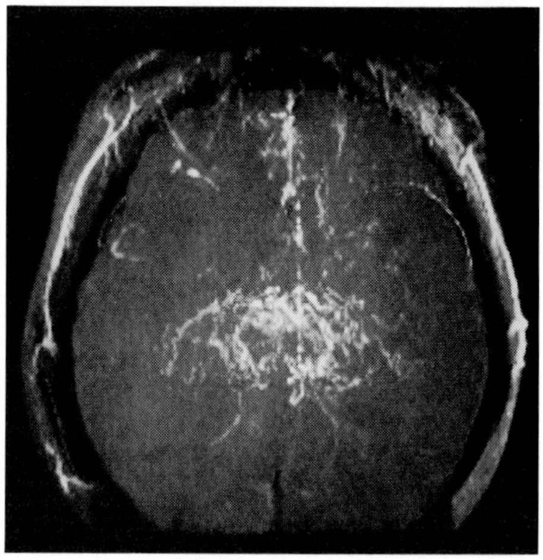 L

Fig. 40-2 Magnetic Resonance Angiography.

R 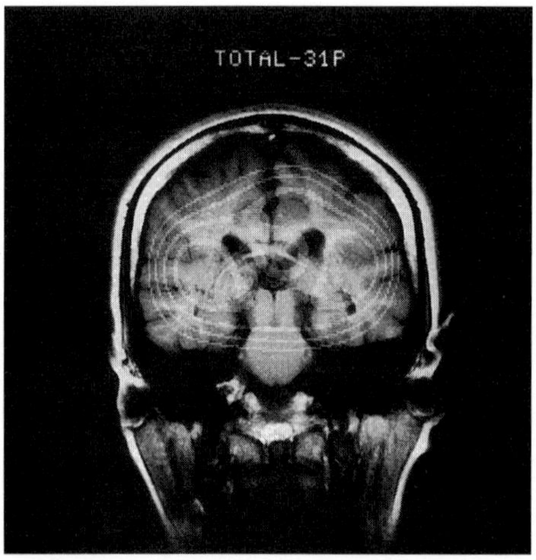 L

Fig. 40-3 Coronal ^{31}P contour map superimposed on T_1-weighted image (500/15).

R 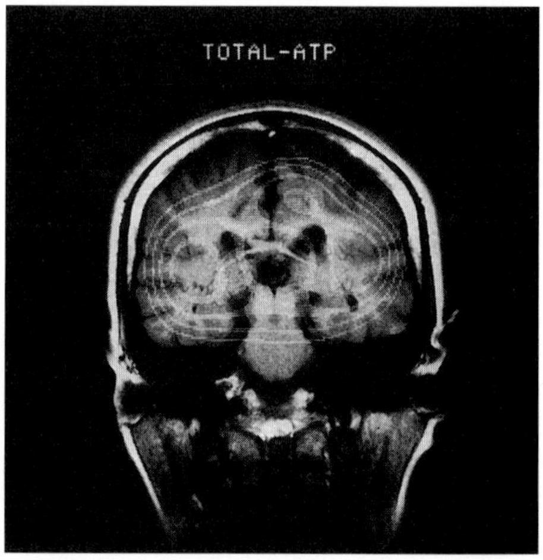 L

Fig. 40-4 Coronal total ATP contour map superimposed on T_1-weighted image (500/15).

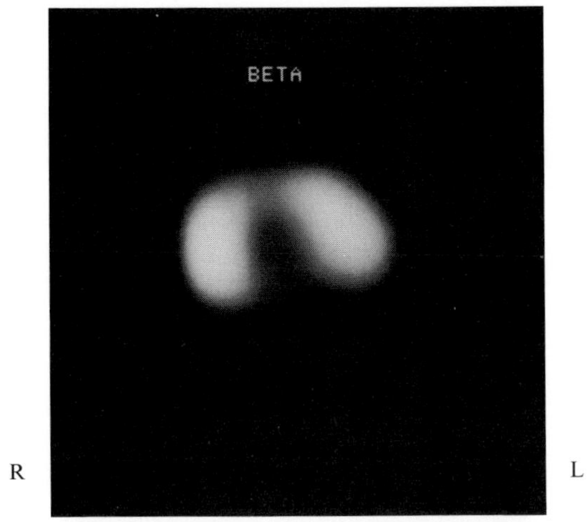

Fig. 40-5 Coronal β-ATP metabolite image.

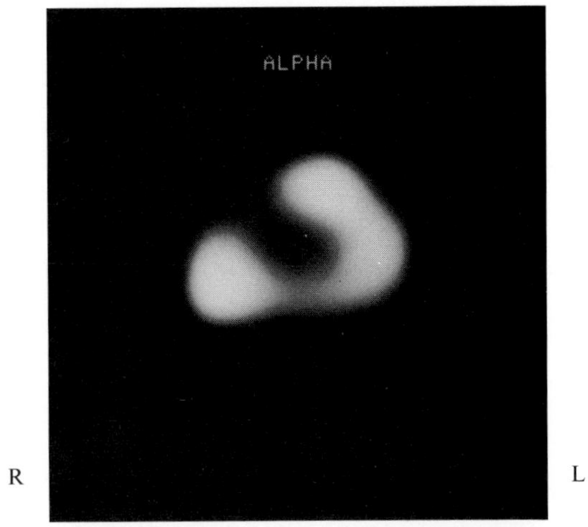

Fig. 40-6 Coronal α-ATP metabolite image.

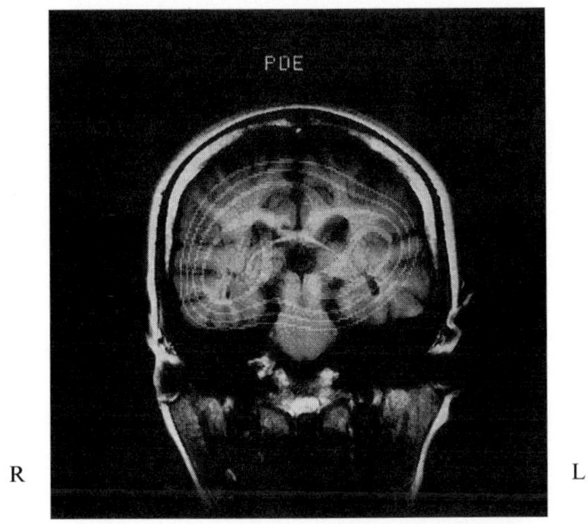

Fig. 40-7 Coronal PDE contour map superimposed on T_1-weighted image (500/15).

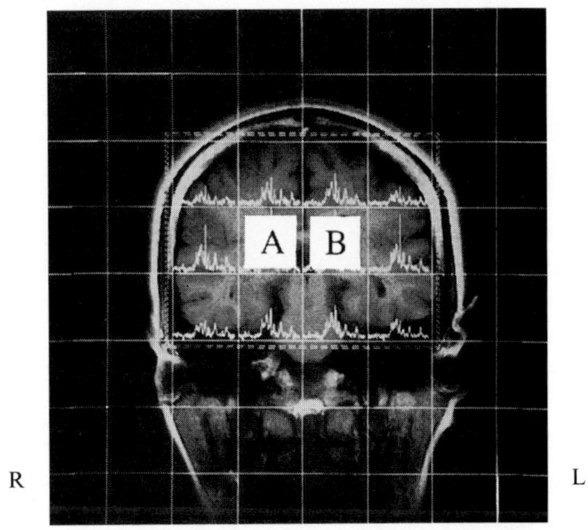

Fig. 40-8 T_1-weighted image showing the position of $3 \times 3 \times 4$ cm^3 voxels A and B.

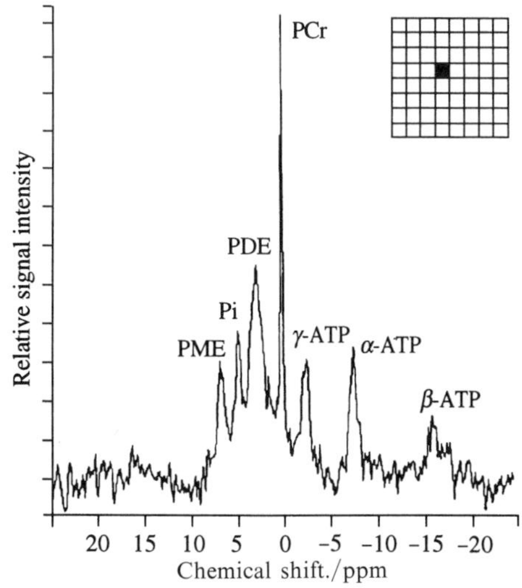

Fig. 40-9 ^{31}P spectrum of right basal ganglia (voxel A).

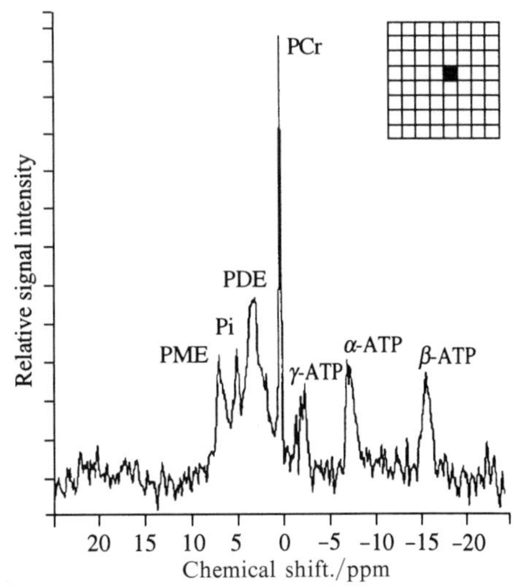

Fig. 40-10 ^{31}P spectrum of left basal ganglia (voxel B).

Chapter 8 Intracerebral Hemorrhage

Kousaku Terada

8.1 CHARACTERISTICS OF THE SPECTRUM

^{31}P-MRS in patients with hypertensive intracerebral hemorrhage showed an increase in Pi localized in the hematoma, and decreases in PCr and ATP in the area including the tissues around the hematoma in the acute stage. These changes during the acute stage are considered to reflect primarily ischemic changes in brain tissues around the hematoma caused by compression.[1] However, these changes include signal intensities derived from anaerobic glycolysis of extravasated erythrocytes in the hematoma. Moreover, as oxyhemoglobin in erythrocytes changes to methemoglobin and hemosiderin, which are paramagnetic substances, the homogeneity of the regional magnetic field is considered to be disturbed, and signal losses and effects on T_1 and T_2 may result in changes in the spectrum.[2] Therefore, caution is essential in the evaluation of energy metabolism of the brain with cerebral hemorrhage. It is considered more reasonable to interpret areas showing reductions in PCr and ATP rather than those showing increases in Pi as areas with impairment of energy metabolism associated with hematoma. ^{31}P-MRS is considered to be applicable also to the evaluation of impairment of the cerebral circulation and metabolism in distant areas associated with nerve fiber communication such as transneural depression and crossed cerebellar diaschisis due to hematoma.

REFERENCES

1) Asakura, T.; Sasahira, M. Magnetic resonance spectroscopy and chemical shift imaging of the brain. *Neurosciences* 20: 83-101; 1994.

2) Uchimura, K.; Asakura, T.; Sasahira, M.; Terada, K. et al. Magnetic resonance spectroscopy (MRS) and chemical shift imaging (CSI) studies on cerebral metabolism in cerebrovascular disease. *Nippon Rinsho* 51 (suppl): 132-139; 1993. [Japanese]

8.2 CASES (41-53)

CASE 41

CASE 41: A 58-year-old male

Hypertensive intracerebral hemorrhage (left thalamic hemorrhage) on the day of the stroke

The patient presented with sudden onset of right hemiparesis and consciousness disturbance. He gave a past history of hypertension.

The MRIs in Figures 41-1 and 2 show a moderate amount of hematoma in the left thalamus. The signal intensity is reduced around the hematoma in the ^{31}P, ATP, PME, Pi, and PCr metabolite images in Figures 41-3, 4, 5, 6, and 7. Figures 41-9 and 41- 10 show the ^{31}P spectra of the hematoma area and an area opposite the hematoma. Note the general reduction in the signal intensities in the hematoma area.

L 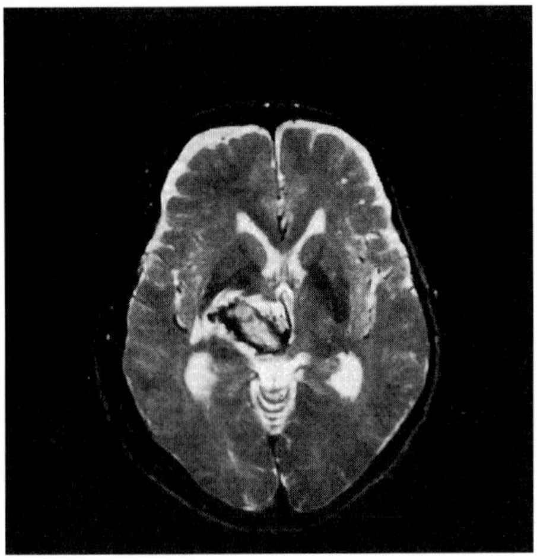 R

Fig. 41-1 Axial T_2-weighted image (2,200/90).

L 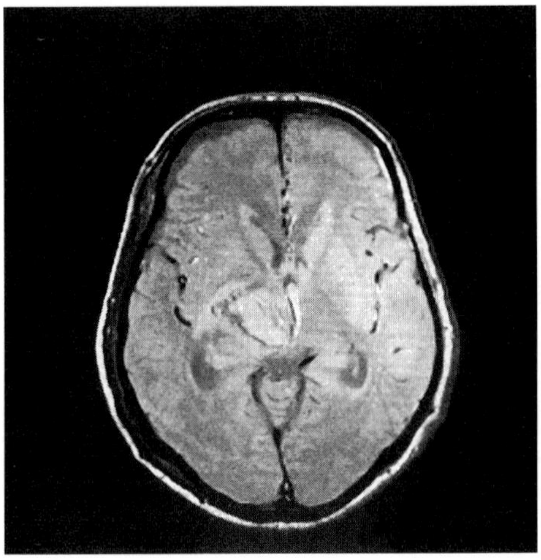 R

Fig. 41-2 Axial proton density-weighted image (2,200/15).

L 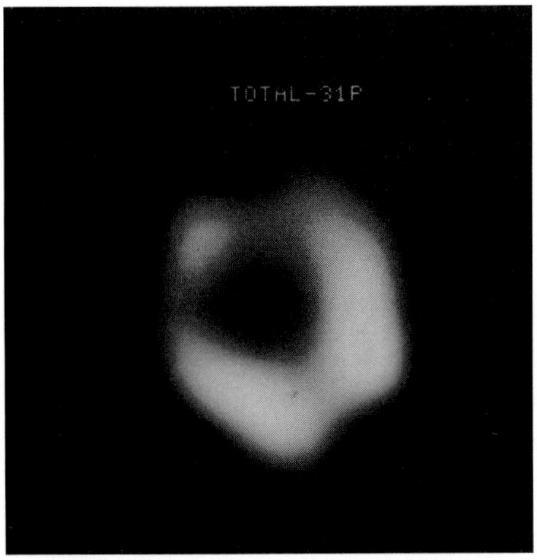 R

Fig. 41-3 Axial ^{31}P metabolite image.

L 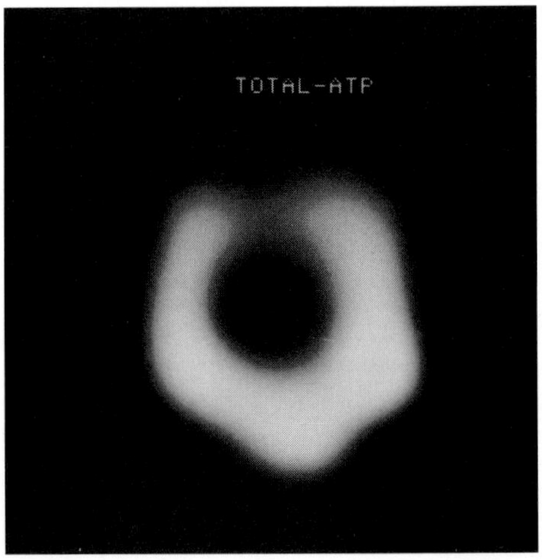 R

Fig. 41-4 Axial total ATP metabolite image.

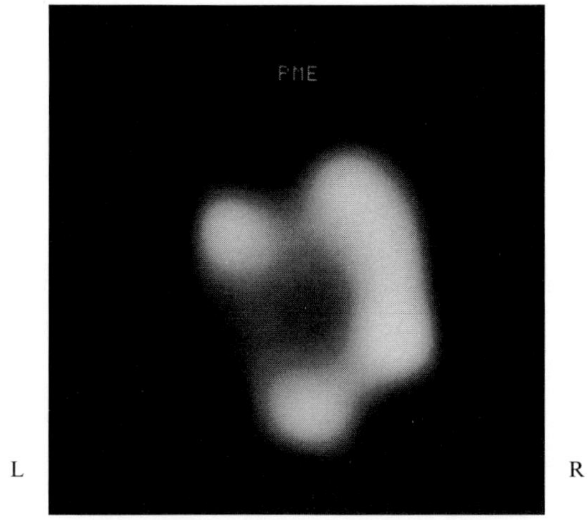

Fig. 41-5 Axial PME metabolite image.

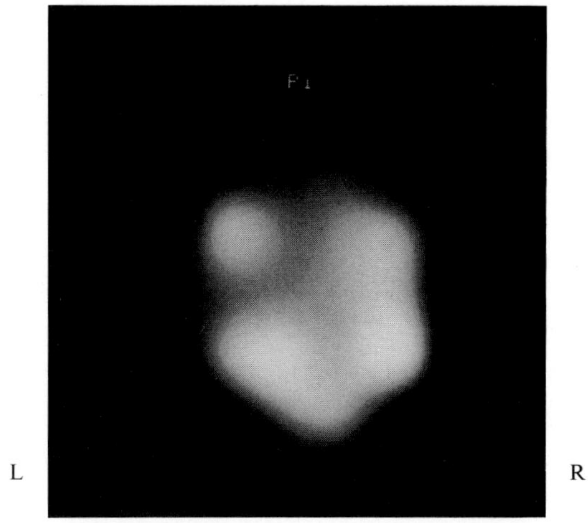

Fig. 41-6 Axial Pi metabolite image.

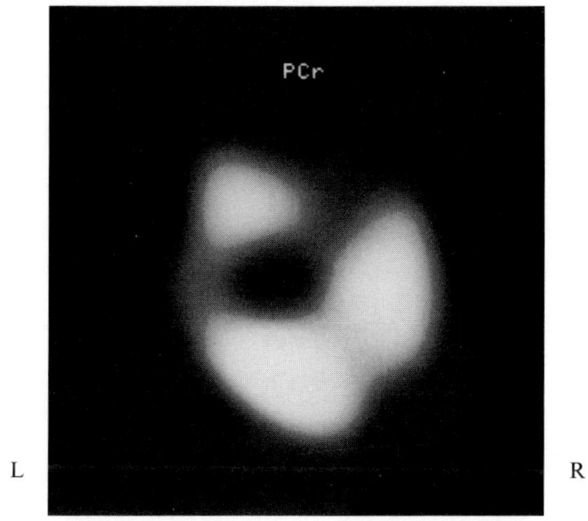

Fig. 41-7 Axial PCr metabolite image.

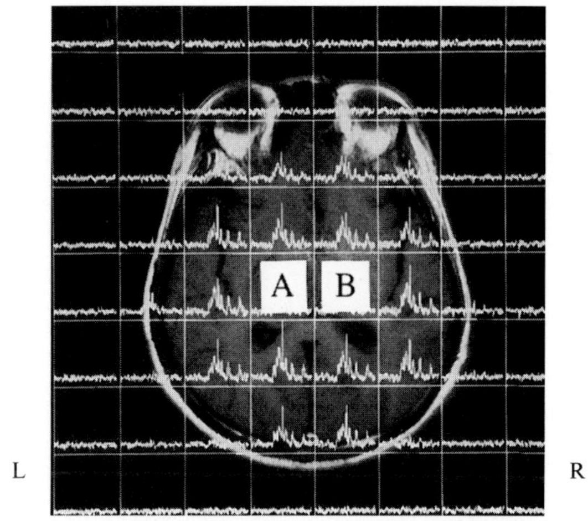

Fig. 41-8 T_1-weighted image showing the position of 3×3×4 cm^3 voxels A and B.

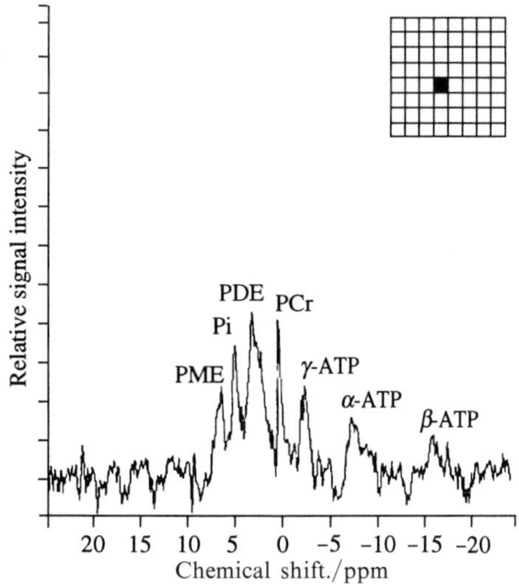

Fig. 41-9 ^{31}P spectrum of hematoma area (voxel A).

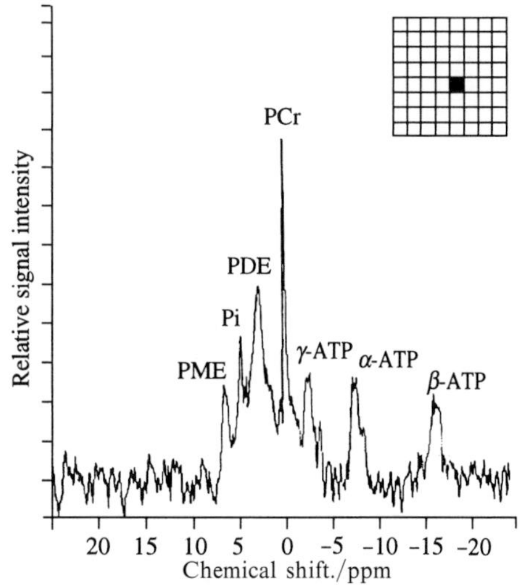

Fig. 41-10 ^{31}P spectrum of control area (voxel B).

CASE 42

CASE 42: A 57-year-old male

Hypertensive intracerebral hemorrhage (right thalamic hemorrhage) 1 day after the stroke

The patient presented with sudden onset of vomiting, left hemiparesis, and consciousness disturbance. He gave a past history of hypertension and left putaminal hemorrhage which occurred several years previous.

The MRIs in Figures 42-1 and 2 show a moderate amount of hematoma in the right thalamus. The signal intensity is reduced around the hematoma in the ^{31}P, ATP, and PCr metabolite images in Figures 42-3, 4, and 7. A high signal intensity area is observed around the hematoma in the Pi metabolite image and the contour map in Figures 42-5 and 6. Figures 42-9 and 42-10 show the ^{31}P spectra of an area opposite the hematoma and the hematoma area, respectively. Note the general reduction in the signal intensities and high Pi signal intensities near the hematoma.

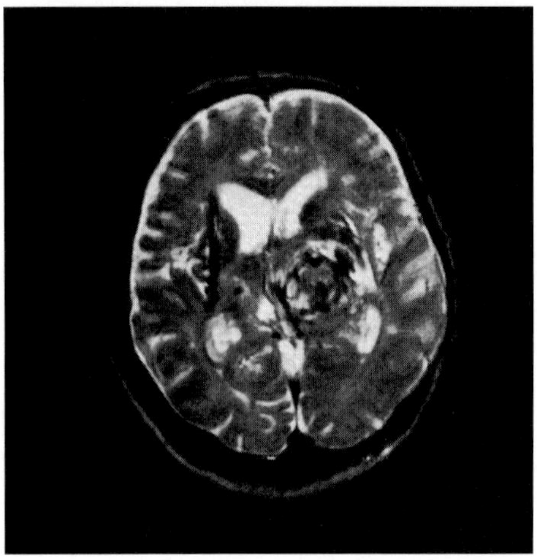

Fig. 42-1 Axial T_2-weighted image (2,200/90).

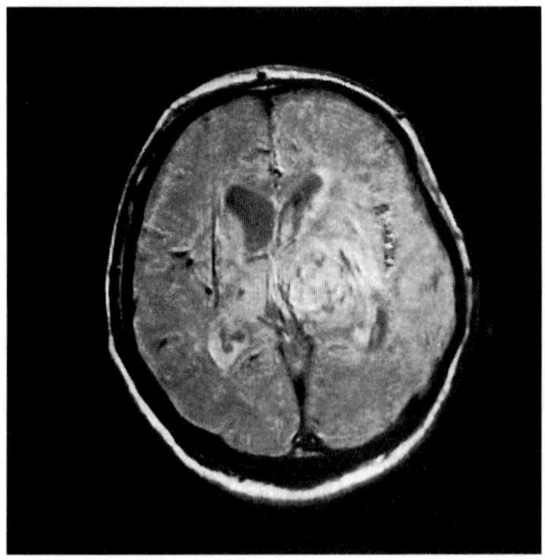

Fig. 42-2 Axial proton density-weighted image (2,200/15).

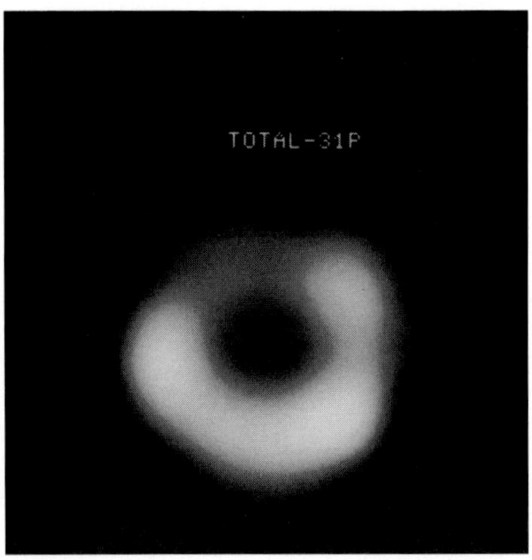

Fig. 42-3 Axial ^{31}P metabolite image.

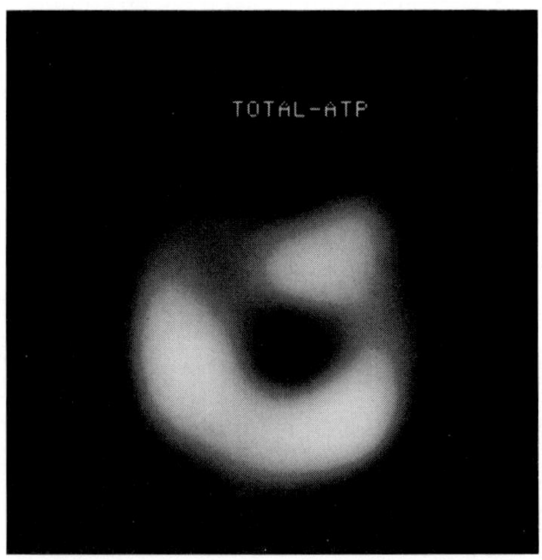

Fig. 42-4 Axial total ATP metabolite image.

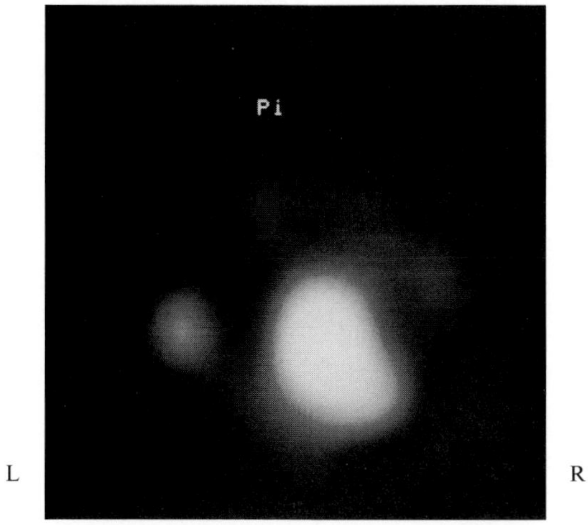

Fig. 42-5 Axial Pi metabolite image.

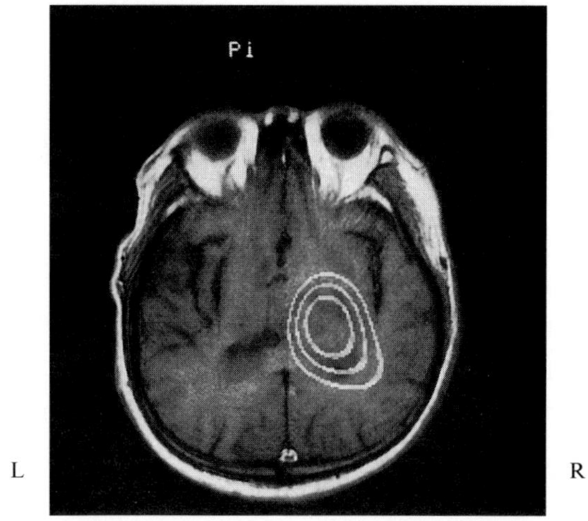

Fig. 42-6 Axial Pi contour map superimposed on T_1-weighted image (500/15).

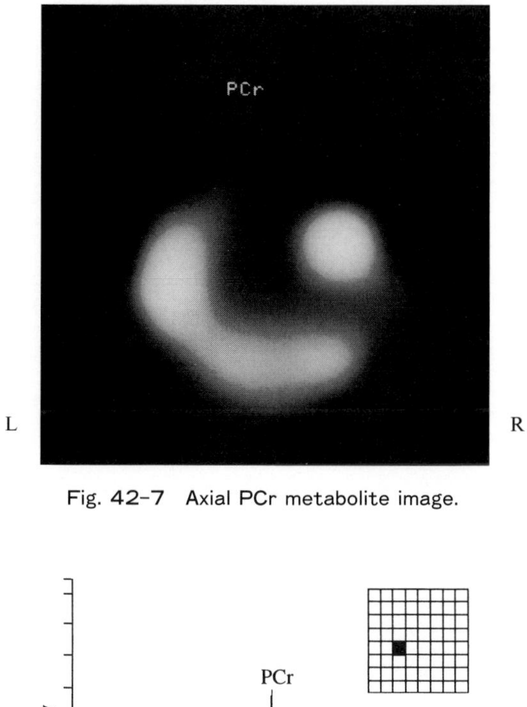

Fig. 42-7 Axial PCr metabolite image.

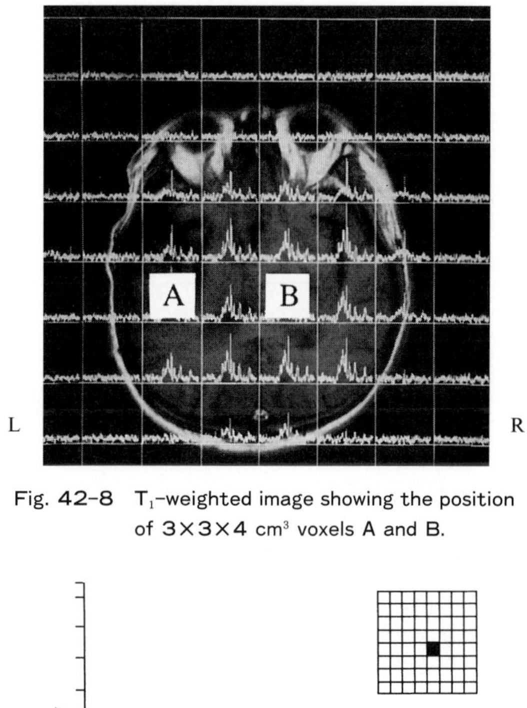

Fig. 42-8 T_1-weighted image showing the position of $3 \times 3 \times 4$ cm^3 voxels A and B.

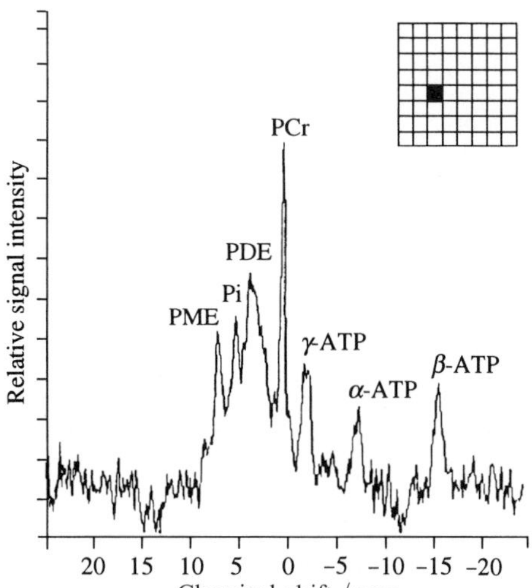

Fig. 42-9 ^{31}P spectrum of control area (voxel A).

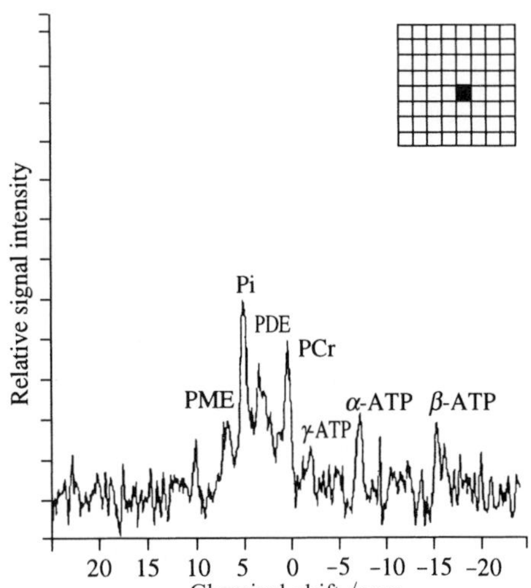

Fig. 42-10 ^{31}P spectrum of hematoma area (voxel B).

CASE 43

CASE 43: A 56-year-old female

Hypertensive intracerebral hemorrhage (left thalamic hemorrhage) 1 day after the stroke

The patient presented with sudden onset of vomiting, right hemiparesis, and consciousness disturbance. She gave a past history of hypertension.

The MRIs in Figures 43-1 and 2 show a moderate amount of hematoma in the left thalamus. The signal intensity is reduced around the hematoma in the ^{31}P, ATP, and PCr contour maps in Figures 43-3, 4, and 6. Figure 43-7 is a contour map of Pi/PCr. Pi/PCr, which is an index of ischemia, is increased and centering around the hematoma. Figures 43-9 and 43-10 show the ^{31}P spectra of the hematoma area and an area opposite the hematoma. Note the high Pi signal intensities and low PCr signal intensities in the hematoma area.

L 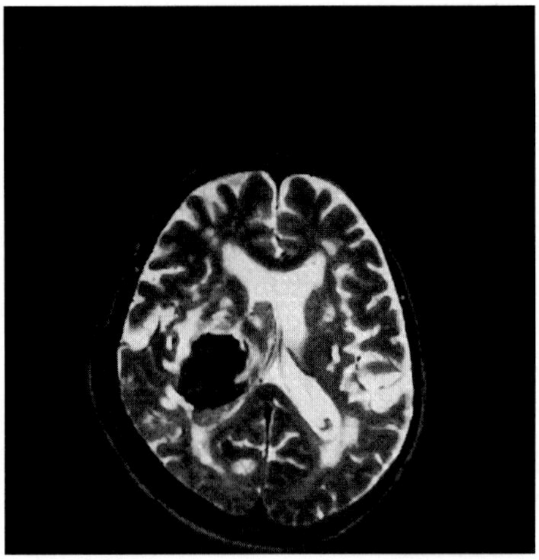 R

Fig. 43-1 Axial T_2-weighted image (2,200/90).

L 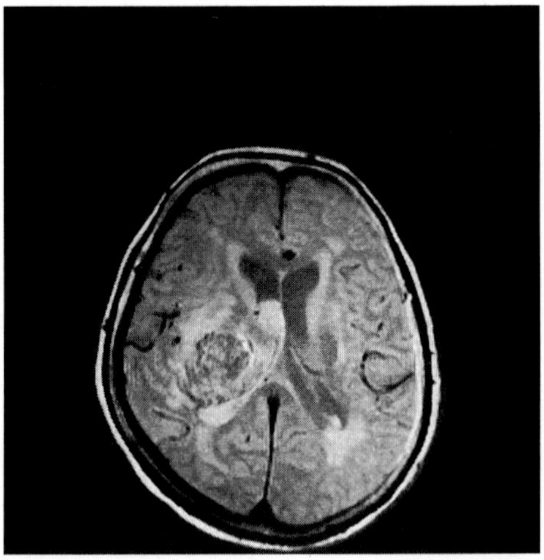 R

Fig. 43-2 Axial proton density-weighted image (2,200/15).

L 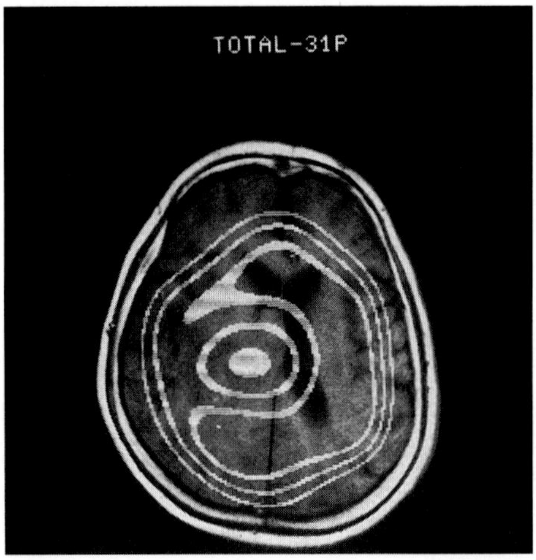 R

Fig. 43-3 Axial ^{31}P contour map superimposed on T_1-weighted image (500/15).

L 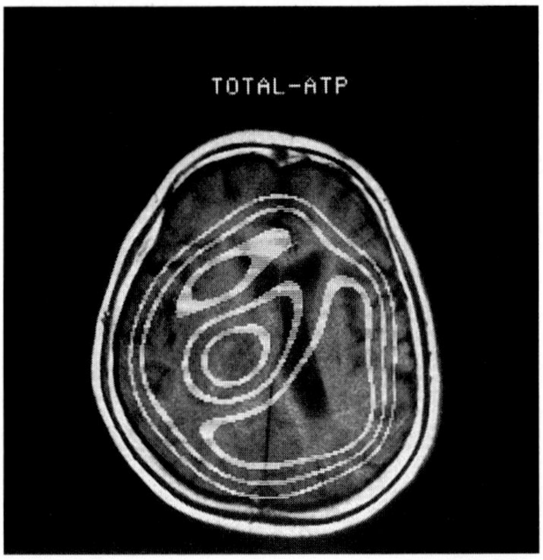 R

Fig. 43-4 Axial total ATP contour map superimposed on T_1-weighted image (500/15).

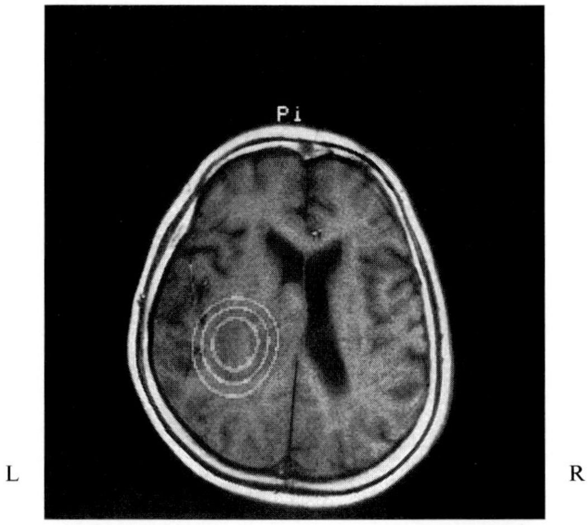

Fig. 43-5 Axial Pi contour map superimposed on T_1-weighted image (500/15).

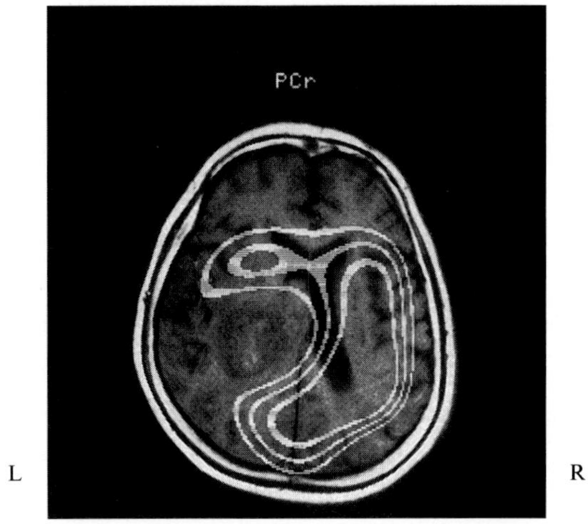

Fig. 43-6 Axial PCr contour map superimposed on T_1-weighte image (500/15).

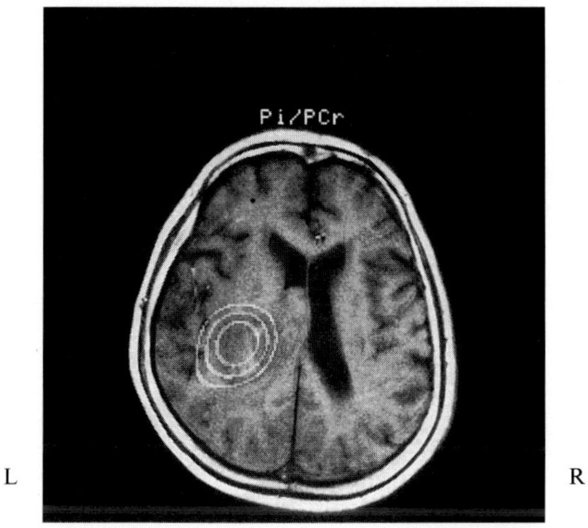

Fig. 43-7 Axial Pi/PCr contour map superimposed on T_1-weighted image (500/15).

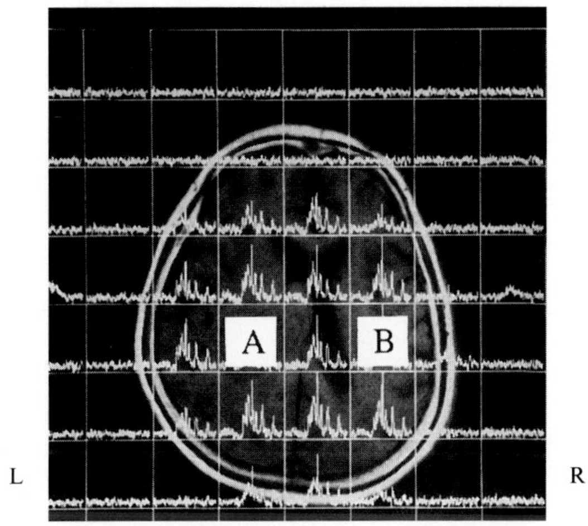

Fig. 43-8 T_1-weighted image showing the position of 3×3×4 cm^3 voxels A and B.

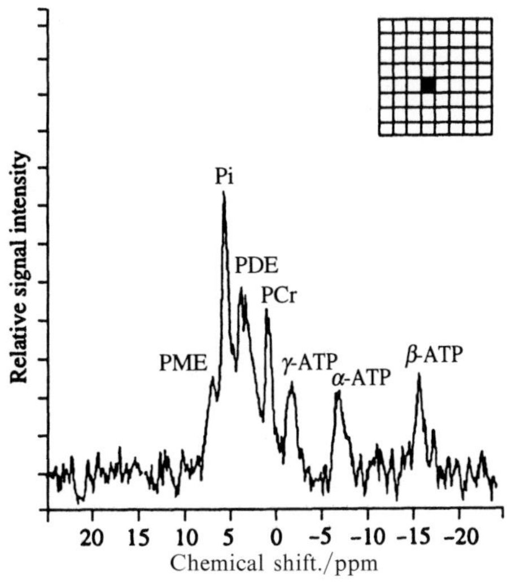

Fig. 43-9 ^{31}P spectrum of hematoma area (voxel A).

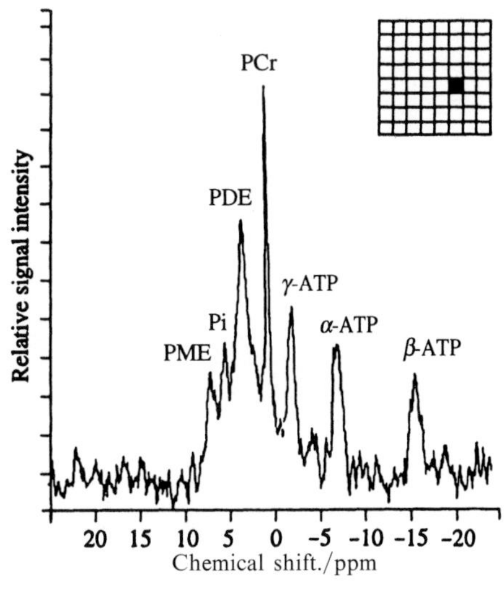

Fig. 43-10 ^{31}P spectrum of control area (voxel B).

CASE 44

CASE 44: A 68-year-old female

Hypertensive intracerebral hemorrhage (subcortical hemorrhage of the left frontal lobe) 2 days after the stroke

The patient presented with sudden onset of right hemiparesis, motor aphasia, and conjugate deviation to the left. She gave a past history of hypertension.

The MRIs in Figures 44-1 and 2 show a moderate amount of hematoma accompanied by edema of the surrounding tissues under the cortex of the left frontal lobe. The signal intensity is reduced in the left frontal lobe around the hematoma in the ^{31}P, ATP, and PCr contour maps in Figures 44-3, 4, and 6. It is increased from the hematoma to the subcortical tissue in the Pi contour map in Figure 44-5. Figure 44-7 is a contour map of Pi/PCr. Pi/PCr, which is an index of ischemia, is increased and centering around the hematoma. Figure 44-8 shows a 16×16 matrix derived from the data of a 8×8 matrix by interpolation. Figures 44-9 and 44-10 show the ^{31}P spectra of an area opposite the hematoma and the hematoma area, respectively. Note the general reduction in the signal intensities and the relative increase in Pi signal intensities around the hematoma.

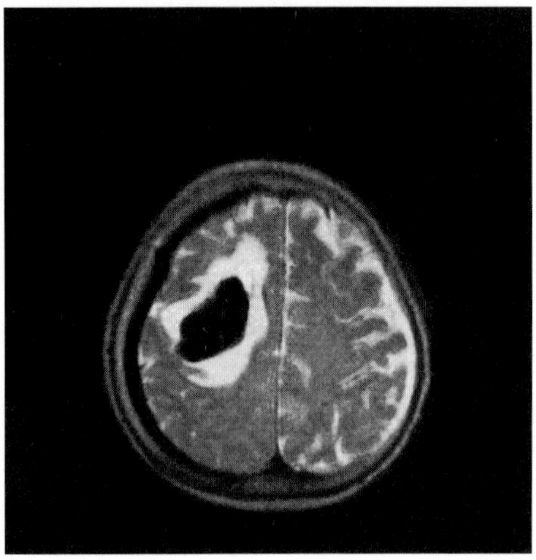

Fig. 44-1 Axial T_2-weighted image (2,200/90).

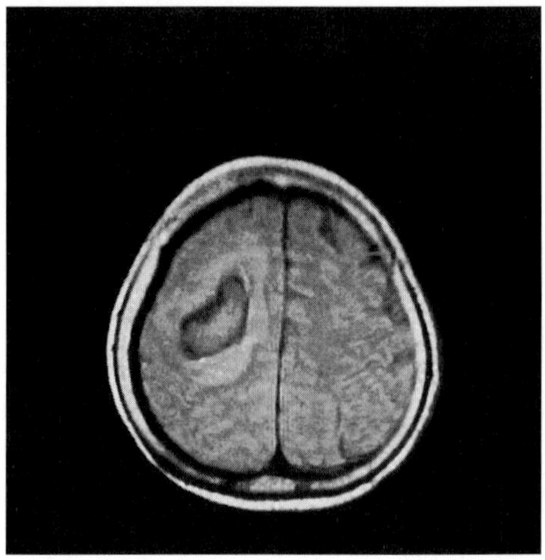

Fig. 44-2 Axial proton density-weighted image (2,200/15).

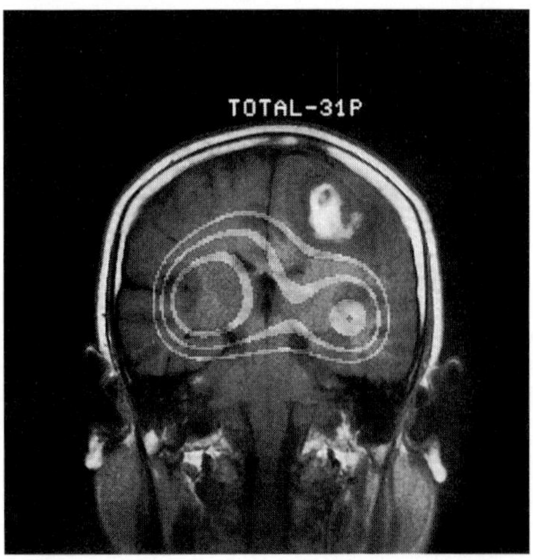

Fig. 44-3 Coronal ^{31}P contour map superimposed on T_1-weighted image (500/15).

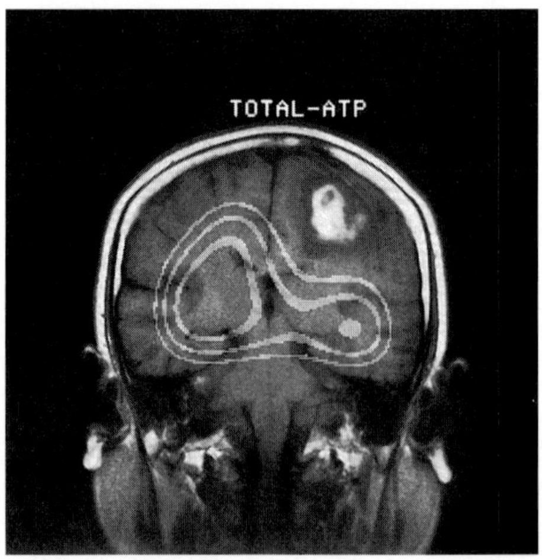

Fig. 44-4 Coronal total ATP contour map superimposed on T_1-weighted image (500/15).

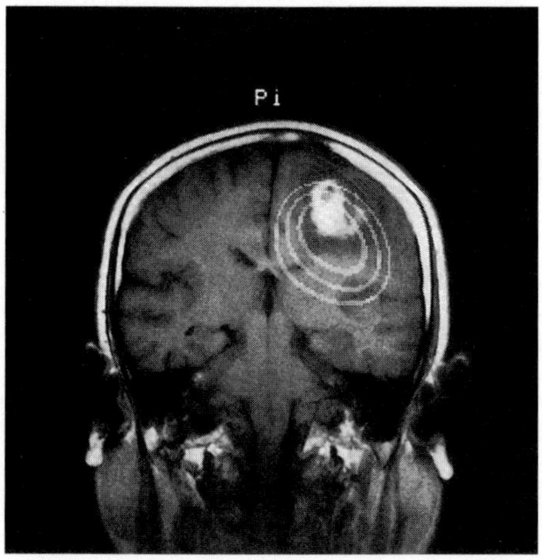

Fig. 44-5 Coronal Pi contour map superimposed on T_1-weighted image (500/15).

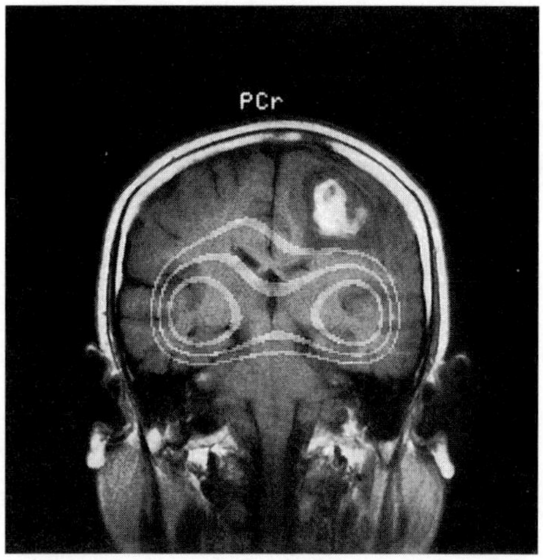

Fig. 44-6 Coronal PCr contour map superimposed on T_1-weighted image (500/15).

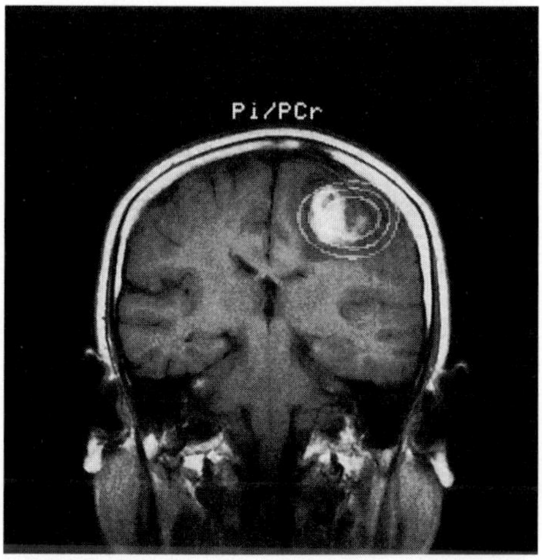

Fig. 44-7 Coronal Pi/PCr contour map superimposed on T_1-weighted image (500/15).

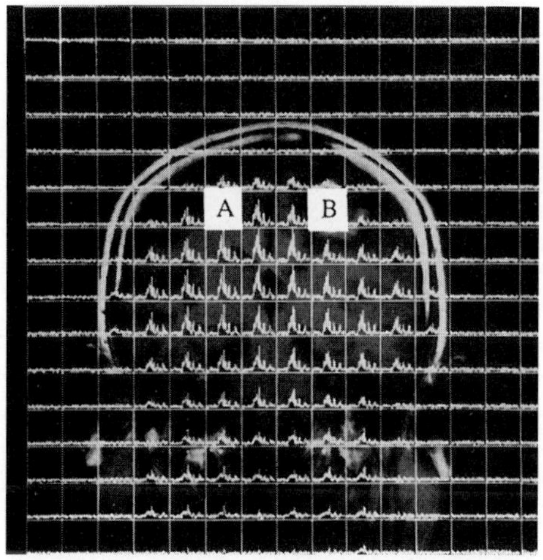

Fig. 44-8 T_1-weighted image showing the position of $1.5\times1.5\times4$ cm^3 voxels A and B.

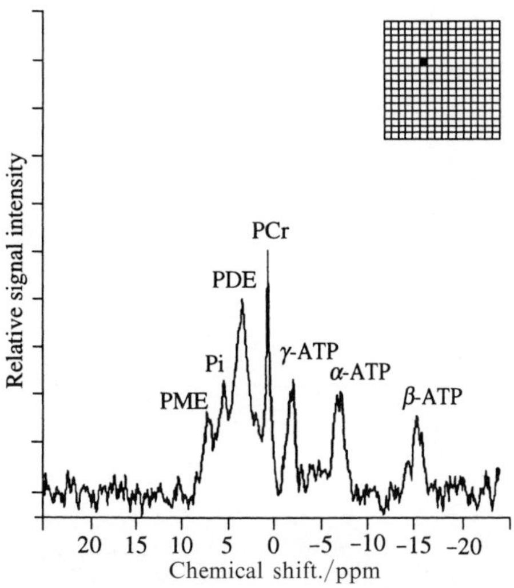

Fig. 44-9 ^{31}P spectrum of control area (voxel A).

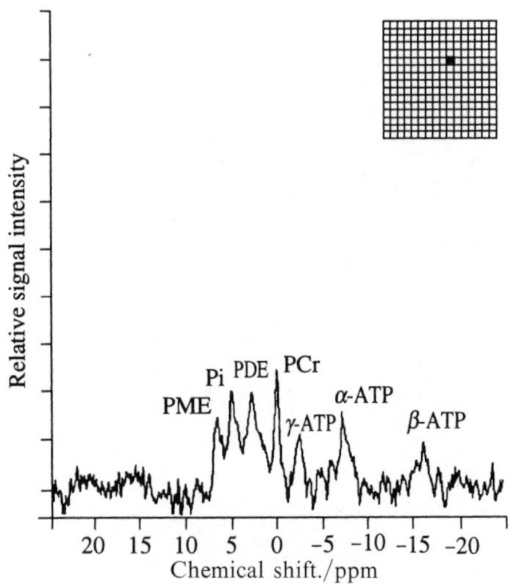

Fig. 44-10 ^{31}P spectrum of hematoma area (voxel B).

CASE 45

CASE 45: A 67-year-old male

Intracerebral hemorrhage (subcortical hemorrhage of the right temporal and parietal lobes) 2 days after the stroke

The patient presented with sudden onset of vertigo, vomiting, and left homonymous hemianopsia.

The MRIs in Figures 45-1 and 2 show a large amount of hematoma under the cortex of the right temporal and parietal lobes. The signal intensity is reduced around the hematoma in the ^{31}P, ATP, and PCr metabolite images in Figures 45-3, 4, and 7. A high-signal intensity area centering around the hematoma is observed in the Pi metabolite image and contour map in Figures 45-5 and 6. Figures 45-9 and 45- 10 show the ^{31}P spectra of an area opposite the hematoma and the hematoma area, respectively. Note the general reduction in the signal intensities and high Pi signal intensities in the hematoma area.

L 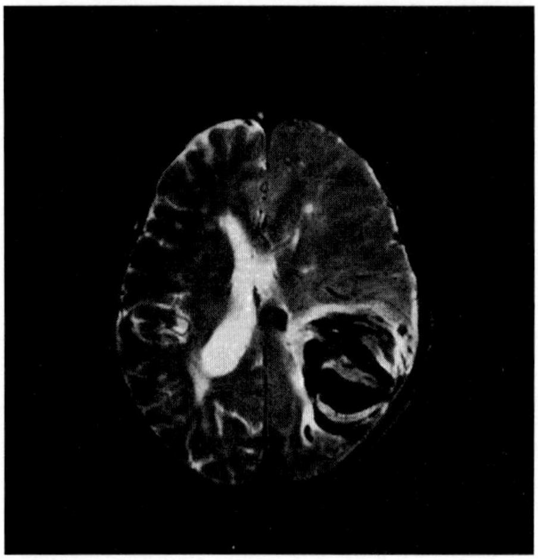 R

Fig. 45-1 Axial T_2-weighted image (2,200/90).

L 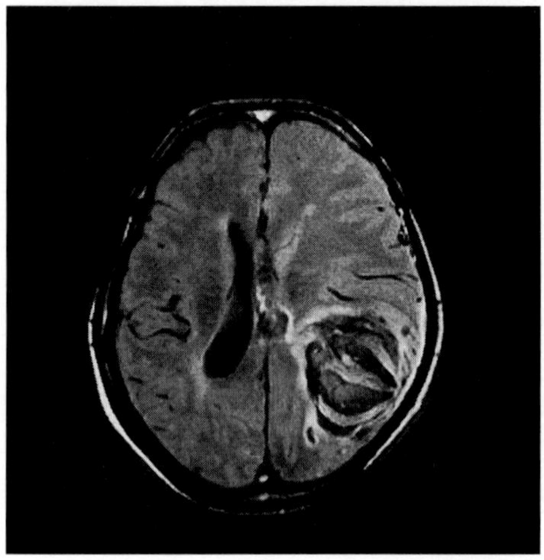 R

Fig. 45-2 Axial proton density-weighted image (2,200/15).

L 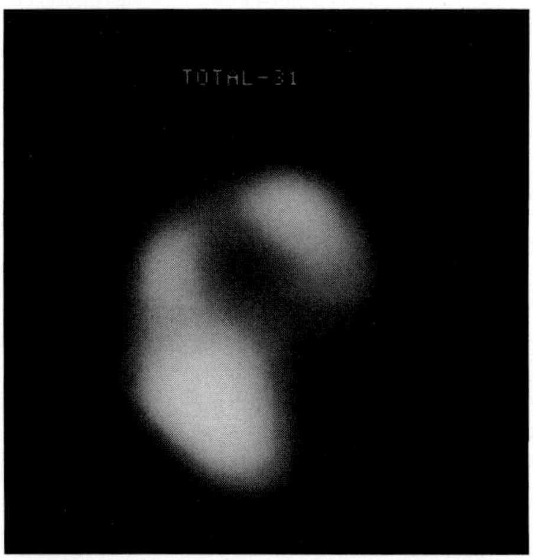 R

Fig. 45-3 Axial ^{31}P metabolite image.

L 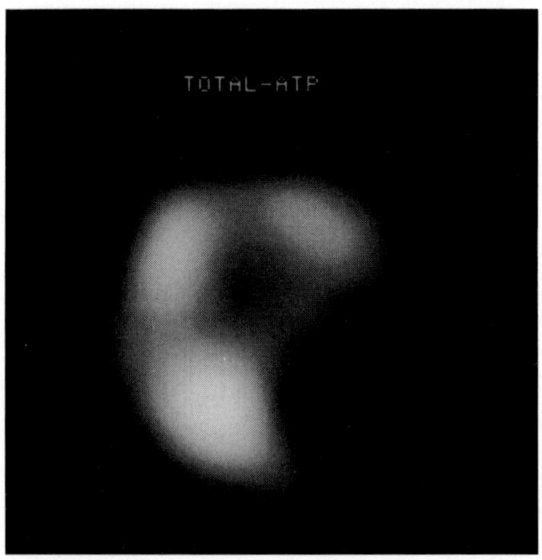 R

Fig. 45-4 Axial total ATP metabolite image.

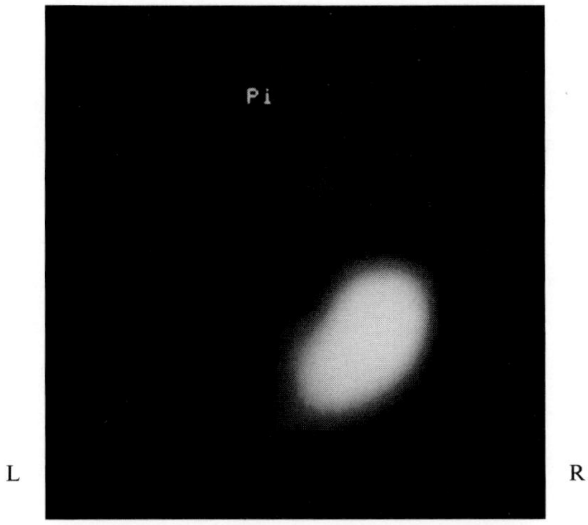

Fig. 45-5 Axial Pi metabolite image.

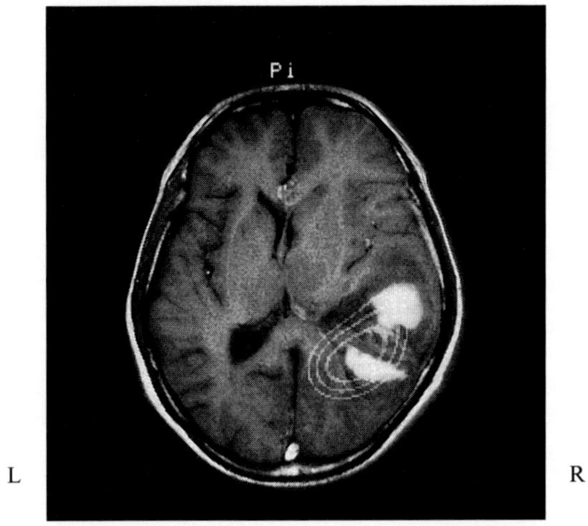

Fig. 45-6 Axial Pi contour map superimposed on T_1-weighted image (500/15).

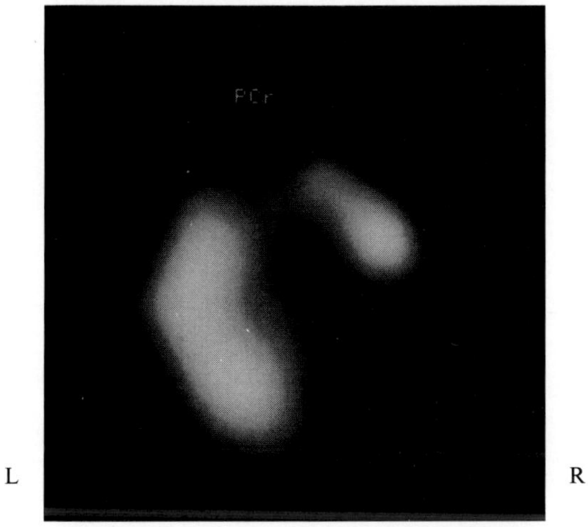

Fig. 45-7 Axial PCr metabolite image.

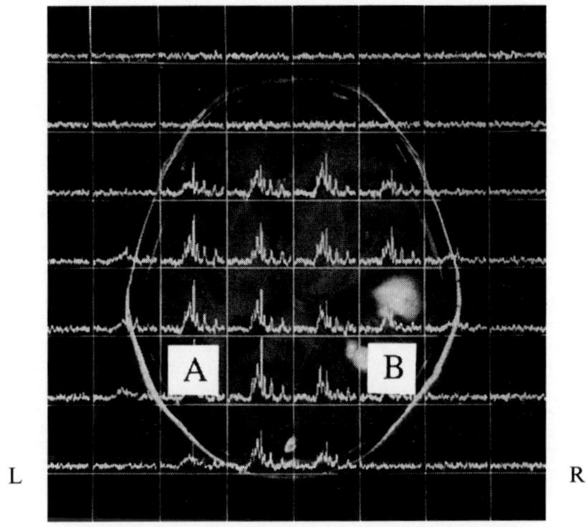

Fig. 45-8 T_1-weighted image showing the position of 3×3×4 cm^3 voxels A and B.

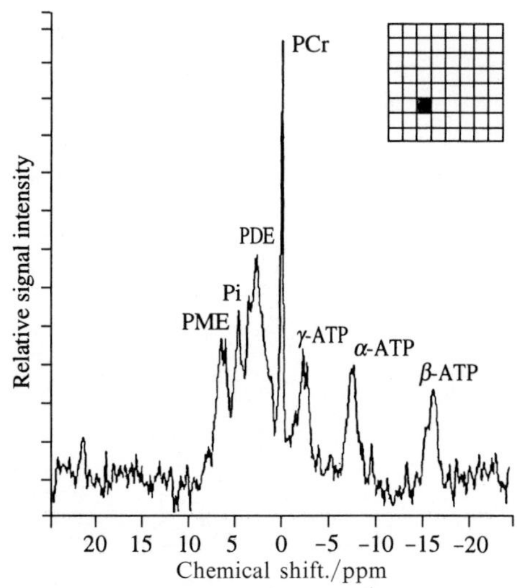

Fig. 45-9 ^{31}P spectrum of control area (voxel A).

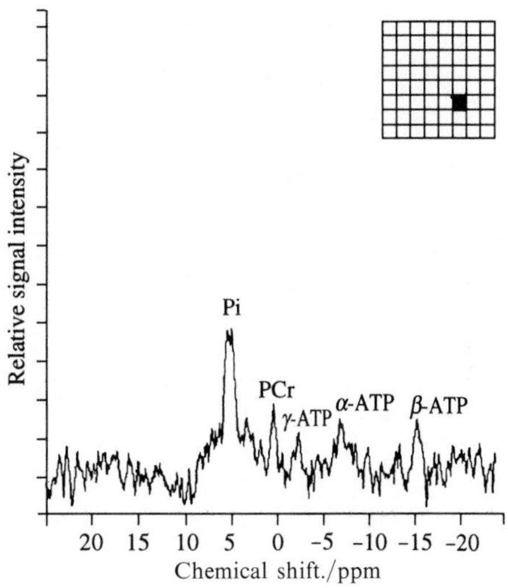

Fig. 45-10 ^{31}P spectrum of hematoma area (voxel B).

CASE 46

CASE 46: A 58-year-old male

Hypertensive intracerebral hemorrhage (right putaminal hemorrhage) 3 days after the stroke

The patient presented with sudden onset of headache and left hemiparesis. He gave a past history of hypertension.

The MRIs in Figures 46-1 and 2 show a moderate amount of hematoma in the right putamen. The signal intensity is reduced around the hematoma in the ^{31}P, ATP, and PCr metabolite images and contour maps in Figures 46-3, 4, 5, and 7. A high signal intensity area centering around the hematoma is observed in the Pi contour map in Figure 46-6. Figures 46-9 and 46-10 show the ^{31}P spectra of an area opposite the hematoma and the hematoma area, respectively. Note the general decrease in the signal intensities and relatively high Pi signal intensities in the hematoma area.

L 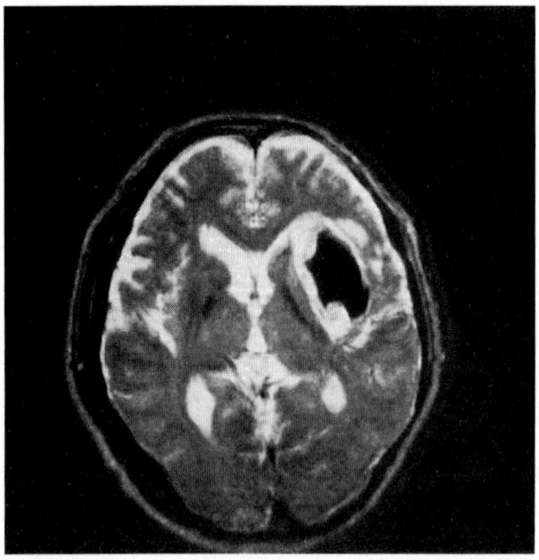 R

Fig. 46-1 Axial T_2-weighted image (2,200/90).

L 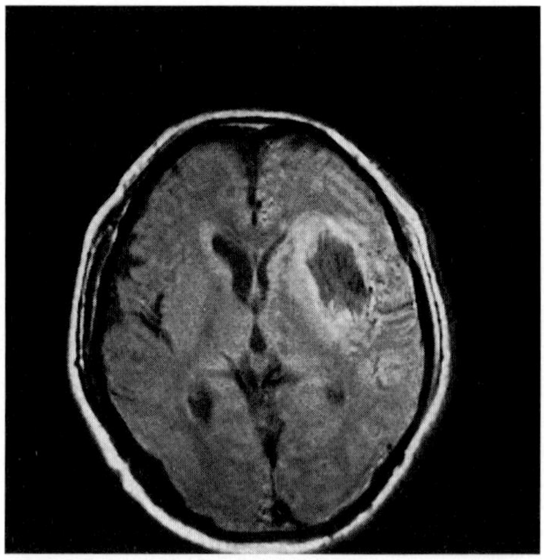 R

Fig. 46-2 Axial proton density-weighted image (2,200/15).

L 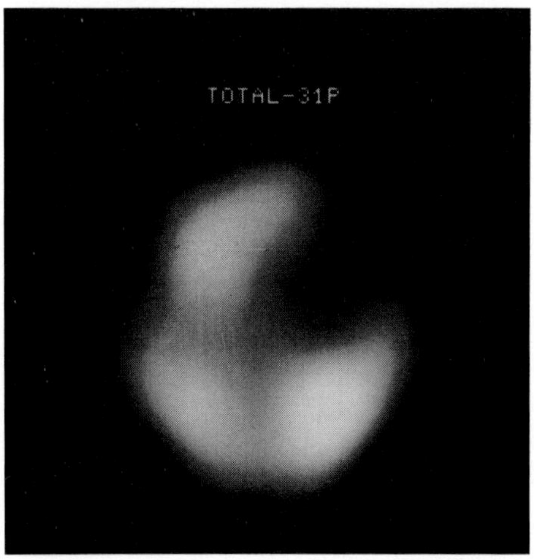 R

Fig. 46-3 Axial ^{31}P metabolite image.

L 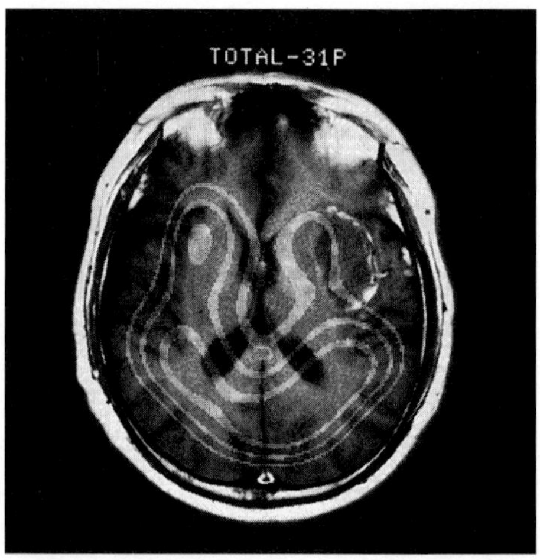 R

Fig. 46-4 Axial ^{31}P contour map superimposed on T_1-weighted image (500/15).

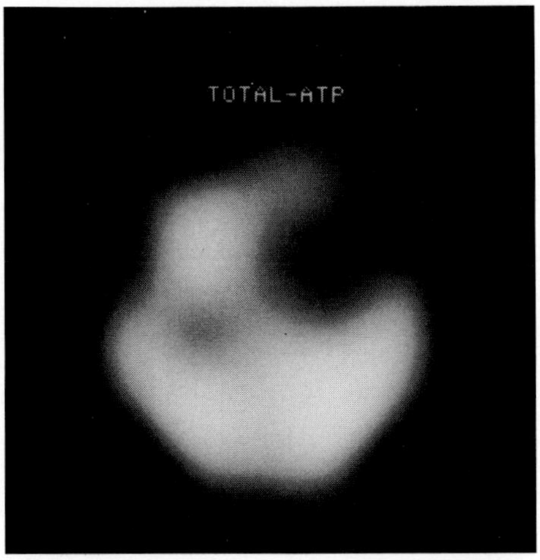

Fig. 46-5 Axial total ATP metabolite image.

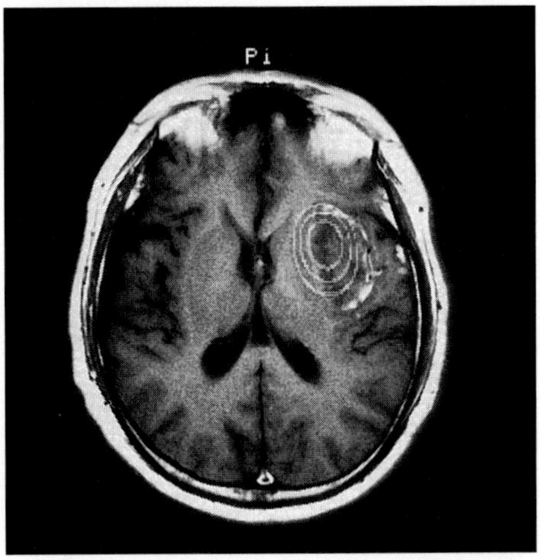

Fig. 46-6 Axial Pi contour map superimposed on T_1-weighted image (500/15).

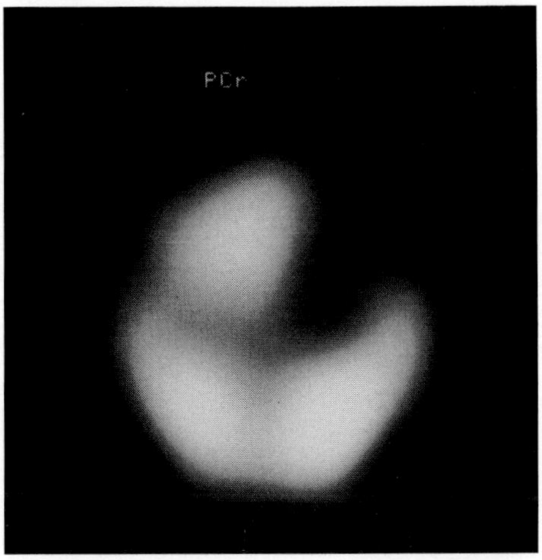

Fig. 46-7 Axial PCr metabolite image.

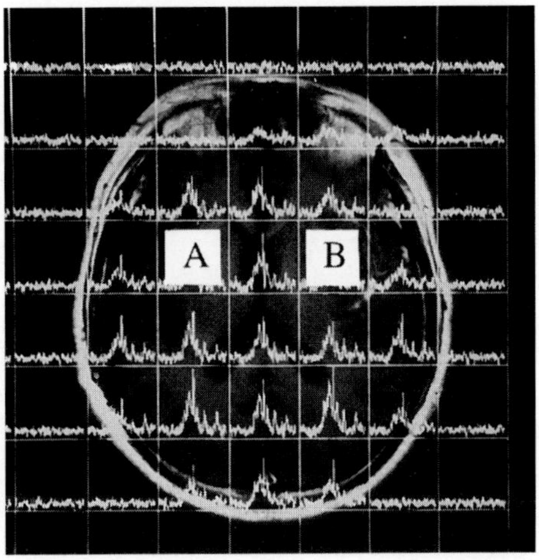

Fig. 46-8 T_1-weighted image showing the position of $3 \times 3 \times 4$ cm^3 voxels A and B.

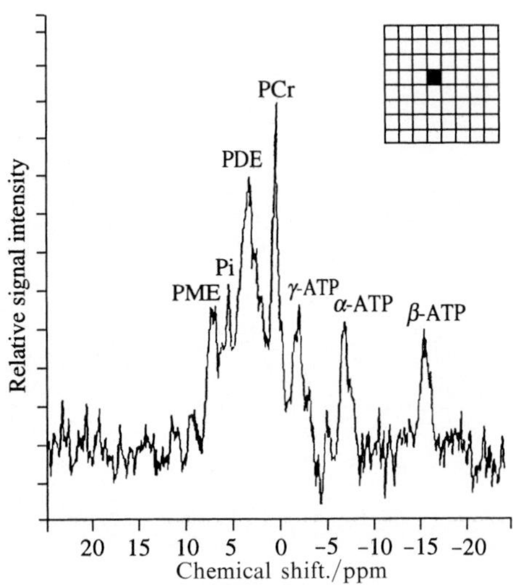

Fig. 46-9 ^{31}P spectrum of control area (voxel A).

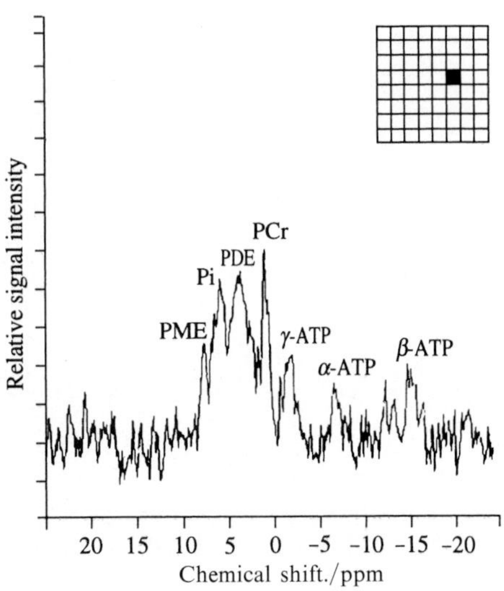

Fig. 46-10 ^{31}P spectrum of hematoma area (voxel B).

CASE 47

CASE 47: A 40-year-old female

Hypertensive intracerebral hemorrhage (right putaminal hemorrhage) 3 days after the stroke

The patient presented with sudden onset of left hemiparesis. She gave a past history of hypertension.

The MRIs in Figures 47-1 and 2 show a moderate amount of hematoma in the right putamen and brain edema in the surrounding tissue. The signal intensity is reduced around the hematoma in the ^{31}P, ATP, and PCr contour maps in Figures 47-3, 4, and 5. A high-signal intensity area around the hematoma is observed in the Pi contour map shown in Figure 47-6. The Pi/PCr contour map in Figure 47-7 shows an increase centering around the hematoma area. Figures 47-9 and 47-10 show the ^{31}P spectra of an area opposite the hematoma and the hematoma area, respectively. Note the general decrease in the signal intensities and relatively high Pi signal intensities in the hematoma.

L 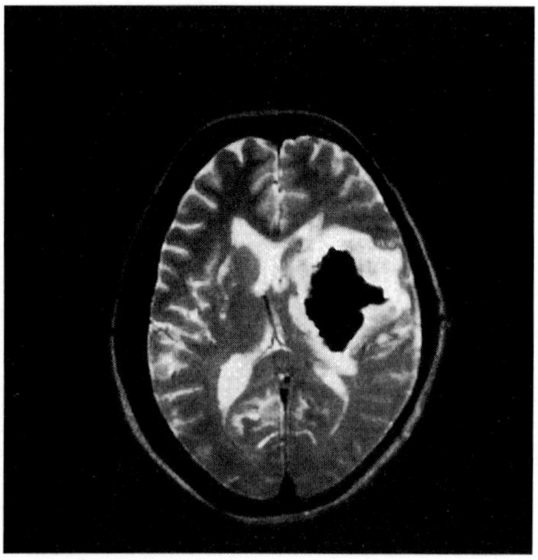 R

Fig. 47-1 Axial T_2-weighted imaged (2,200/90).

L 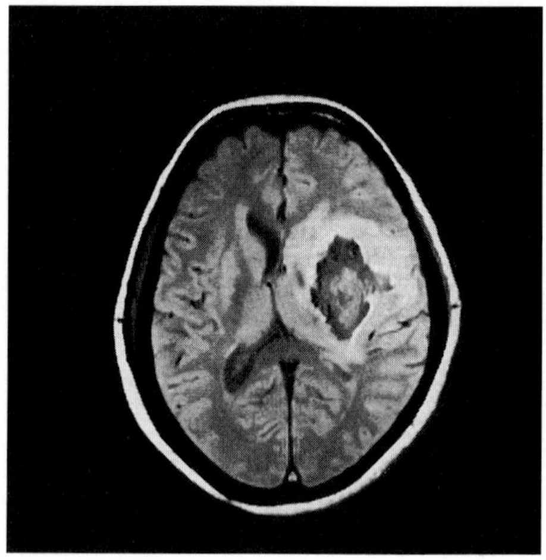 R

Fig. 47-2 Axial proton density-weighted image (2,200/15).

L 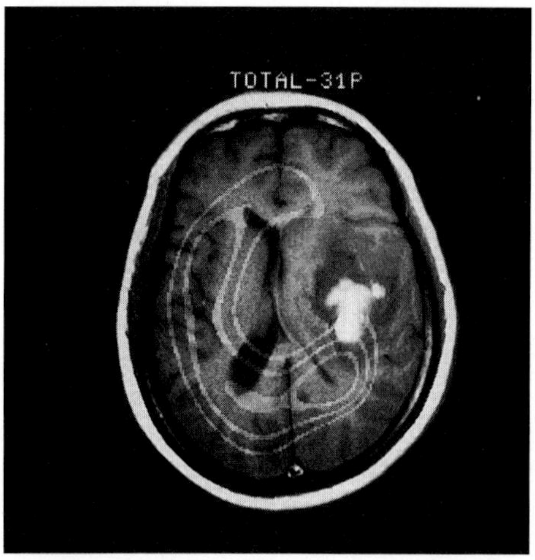 R

Fig. 47-3 Axial ^{31}P contour map superimposed on T_1-weighted image (500/15).

L 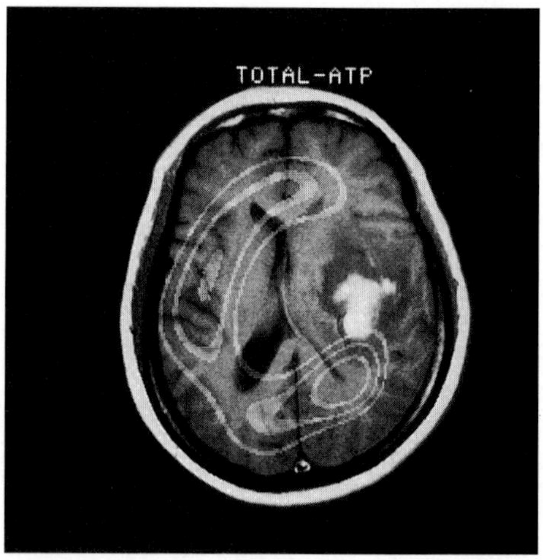 R

Fig. 47-4 Axial total ATP contour map superimposed on T_1-weighted image (500/15).

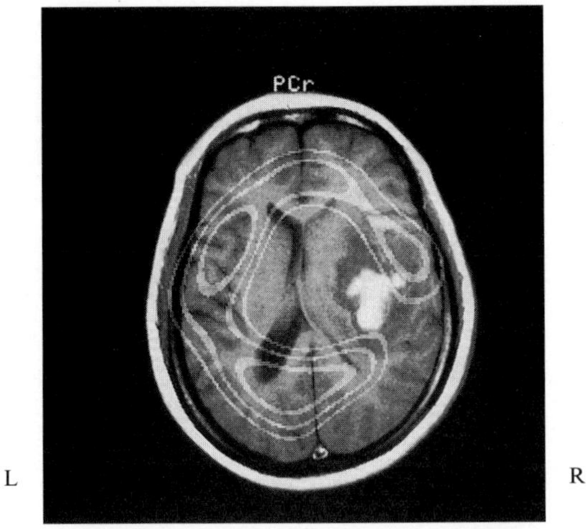

Fig. 47-5 Axial PCr contour map superimposed on T_1-weighted image (500/15).

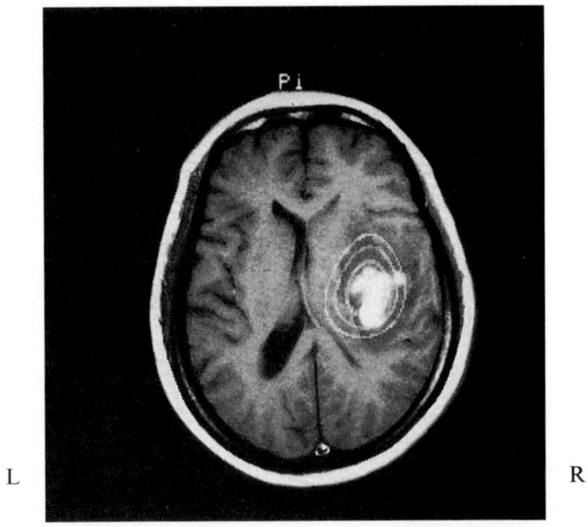

Fig. 47-6 Axial Pi contour map superimposed on T_1-weighted image (500/15).

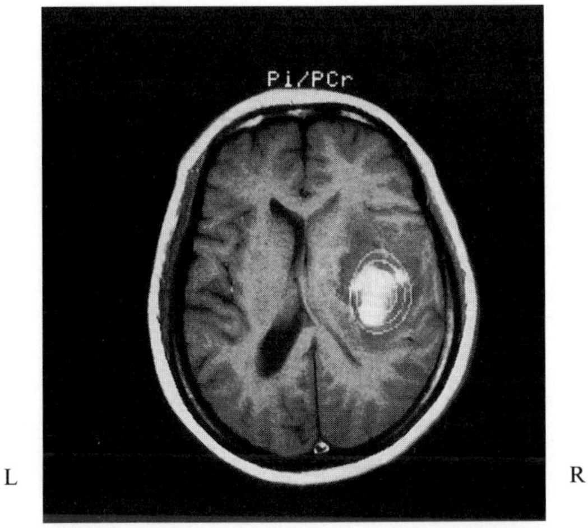

Fig. 47-7 Axial Pi/PCr contour map superimposed on T_1-weighted image (500/15).

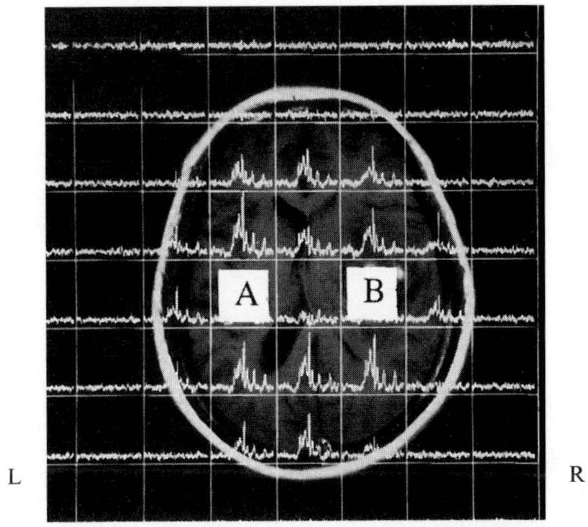

Fig. 47-8 T_1-weighted image showing the position of 3×3×4 cm^3 voxels A and B.

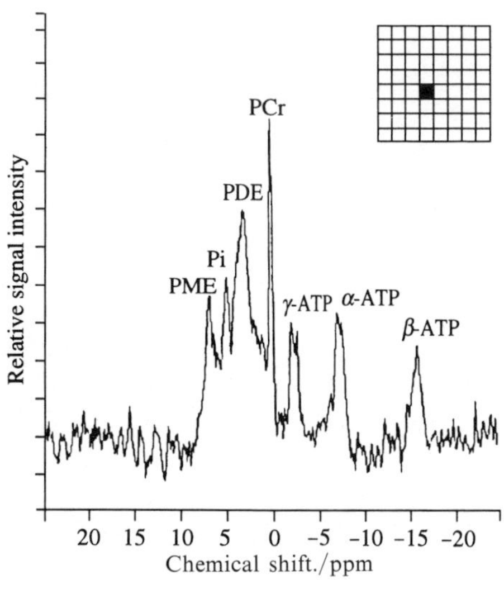

Fig. 47-9 ^{31}P spectrum of control area (voxel A).

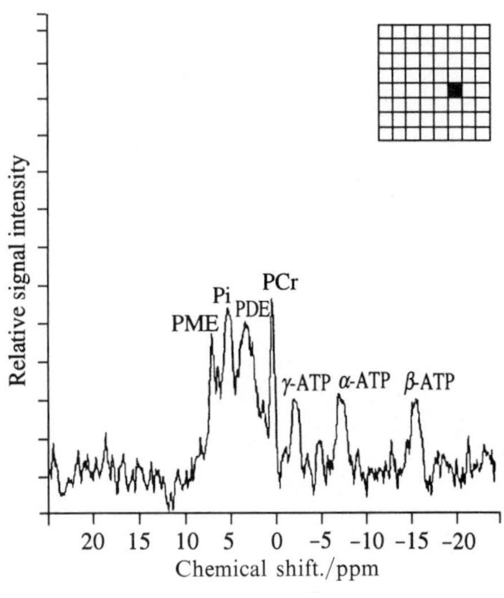

Fig. 47-10 ^{31}P spectrum of hematoma area (voxel B).

CASE 48

CASE 48: A 77-year-old male

Hypertensive intracerebral hemorrhage (left putaminal hemorrhage) 4 days after the stroke

The patient presented with sudden onset of right hemiparesis and consciousness disturbance. He gave a past history of hypertension.

The MRIs in Figures 48-1 and 2 show a moderate amount of hematoma in the left putamen. The signal intensity is reduced around the hematoma in the ^{31}P metabolite image and contour map in Figures 48-3 and 4. A high-signal intensity area is observed medially to the hematoma in the Pi metabolite image and contour map in Figures 48-5 and 6. A high-signal intensity area is also observed medially to the hematoma in the PME metabolite image in Figure 48-7. Figures 48-9 and 48-10 show the ^{31}P spectra of an area opposite the hematoma and the hematoma area, respectively. Note the general decrease in the signal intensities and relatively high Pi signal intensities in the hematoma area.

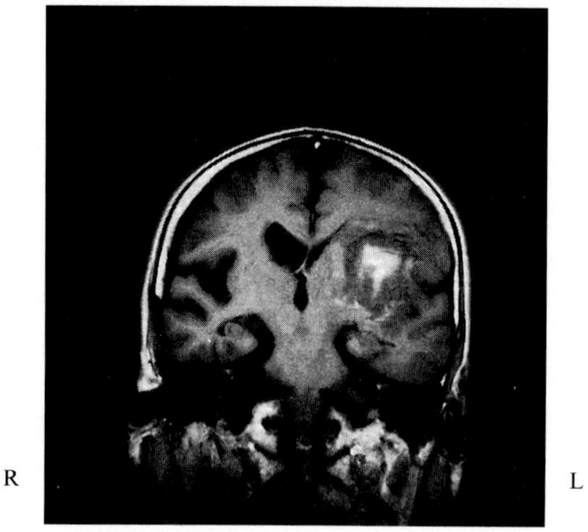

Fig. 48-1 Coronal T_1-weighted image (500/15).

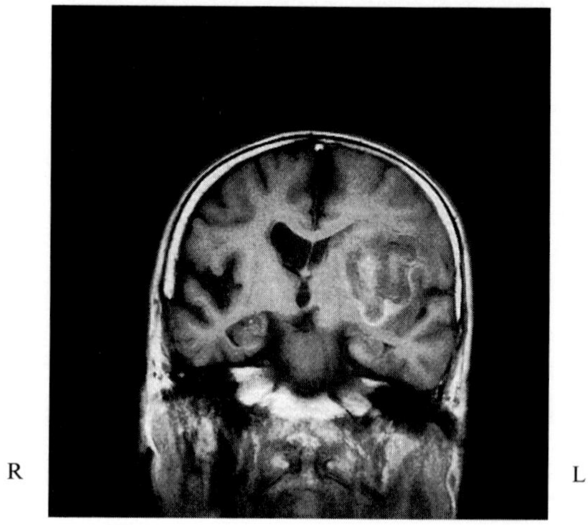

Fig. 48-2 Coronal T_1-weighted image (500/15).

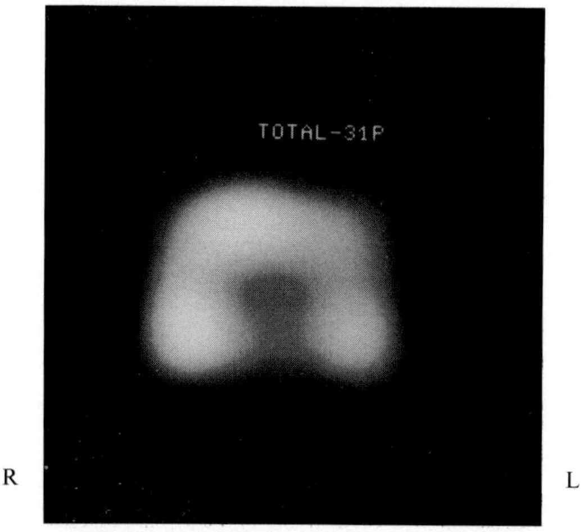

Fig. 48-3 Coronal ^{31}P metabolite image.

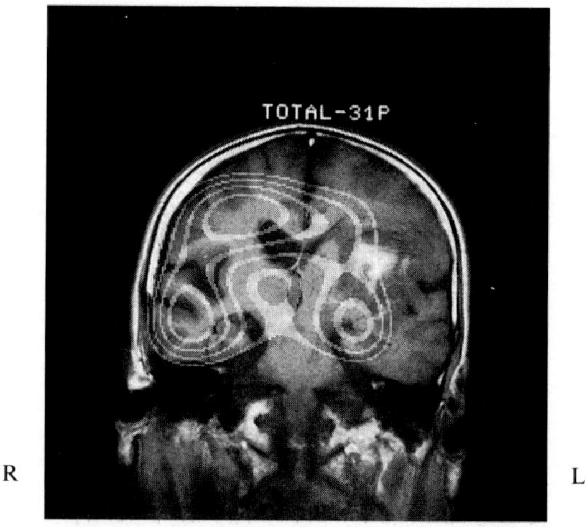

Fig. 48-4 Coronal ^{31}P contour map superimposed on T_1-weighted image (500/15).

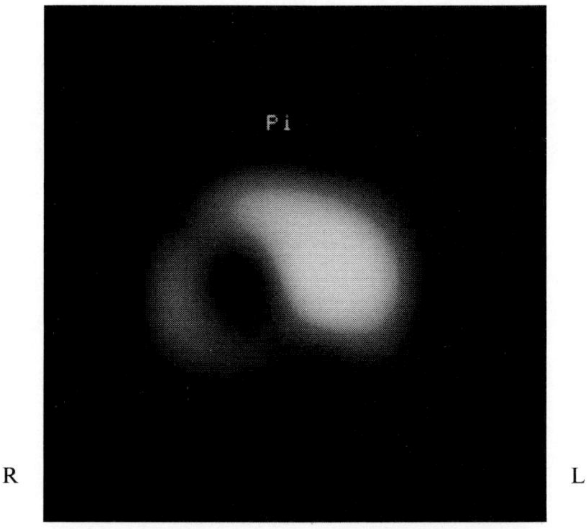

Fig. 48-5 Coronal Pi metabolite image.

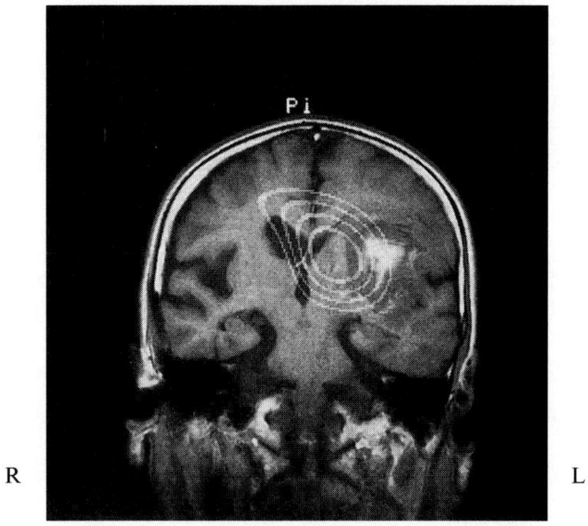

Fig. 48-6 Coronal Pi contour map superimposed on T_1-weighted image (500/15).

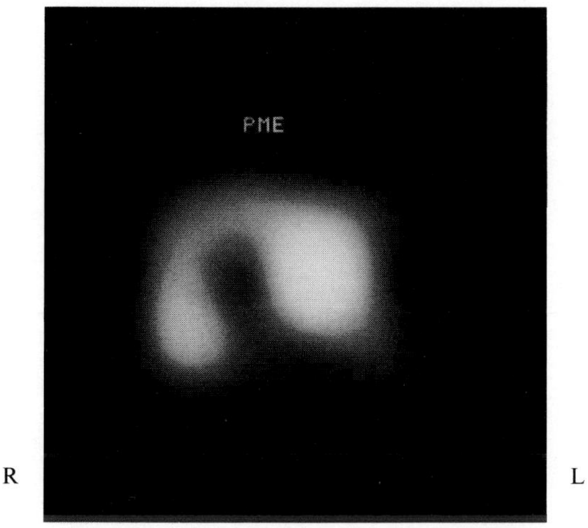

Fig. 48-7 Coronal PME metabolite image.

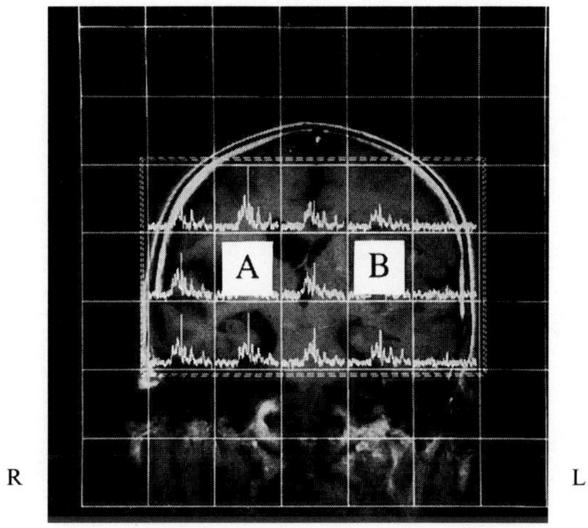

Fig. 48-8 T_1-weighted image showing the position of 3×3×4 cm^3 voxels A and B.

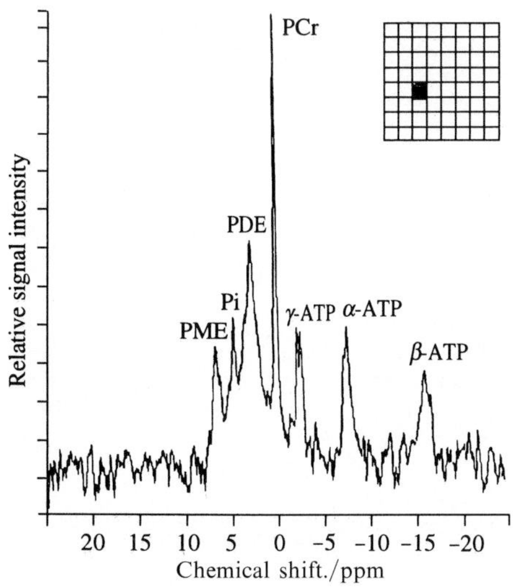

Fig. 48-9 ^{31}P spectrum of control area (voxel A).

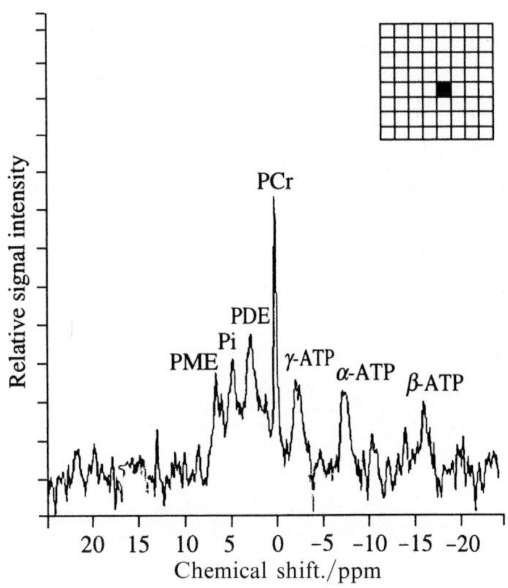

Fig. 48-10 ^{31}P spectrum of hematoma area (voxel B).

CASE 49

CASE 49: A 74-year-old male

Hypertensive intracerebral hemorrhage (left putaminal hemorrhage) 6 days after the stroke

The patient presented with sudden onset of right hemiparesis and consciousness disturbance. He gave a past history of hypertension.

The MRIs in Figures 49-1 and 2 show a moderate amount of hematoma in the left putamen. The signal intensity is reduced around the hematoma in the ^{31}P and PCr metabolite images and contour maps in Figures 49-3, 4, 5, and 6. It is slightly increased in the hematoma area in the Pi contour map in Figure 49- 7. Figures 49-9 and 49-10 show the ^{31}P spectra of an area opposite the hematoma and the hematoma area, respectively. Note the general decrease in the signal intensities in the hematoma area.

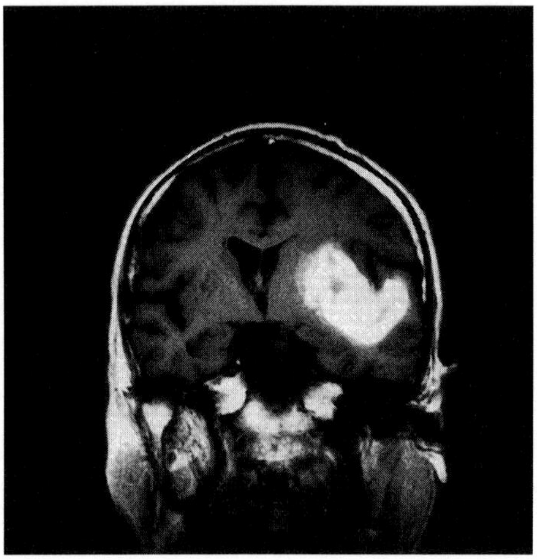

Fig. 49-1 Coronal T_1-weighted image (500/15).

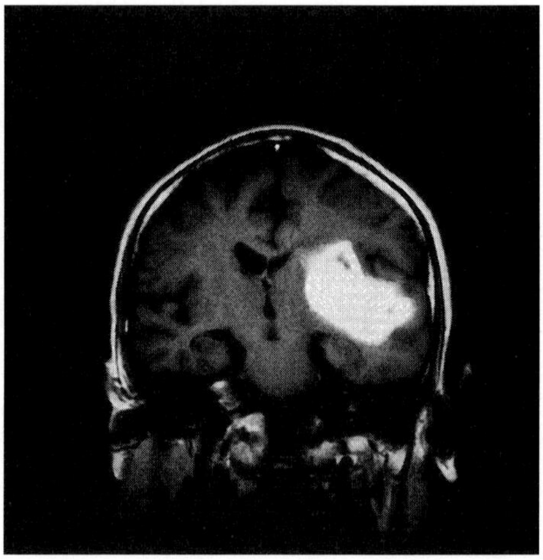

Fig. 49-2 Coronal T_1-weighted image (500/15).

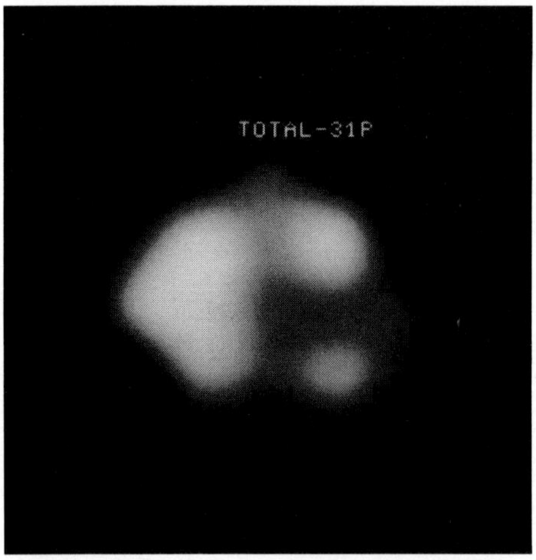

Fig. 49-3 Coronal ^{31}P metabolite image.

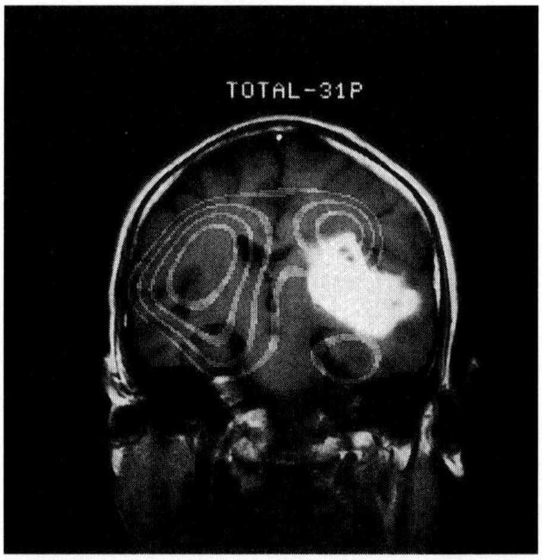

Fig. 49-4 Coronal ^{31}P contour map superimposed on T_1-weighted image (500/15).

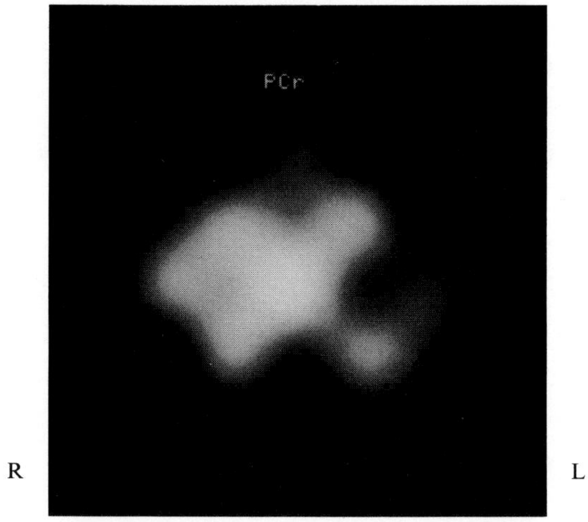

Fig. 49-5 Coronal PCr metabolite image.

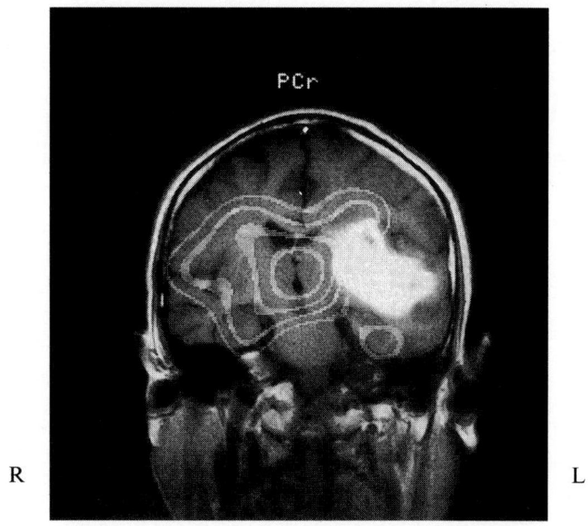

Fig. 49-6 Coronal PCr contour map superimposed on T_1-weighted image (500/15).

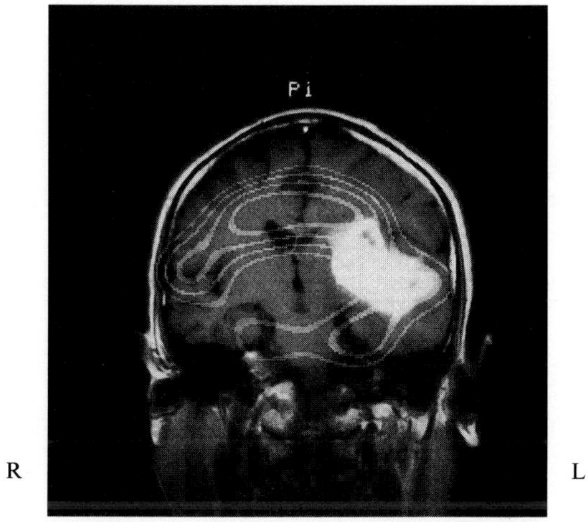

Fig. 49-7 Coronal Pi contour map superimposed on T_1-weighted image (500/15).

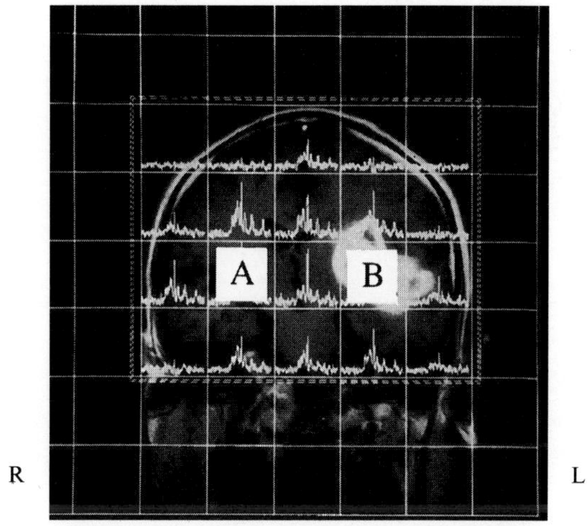

Fig. 49-8 T_1-weighted image showing the position of $3 \times 3 \times 4$ cm^3 voxels A and B.

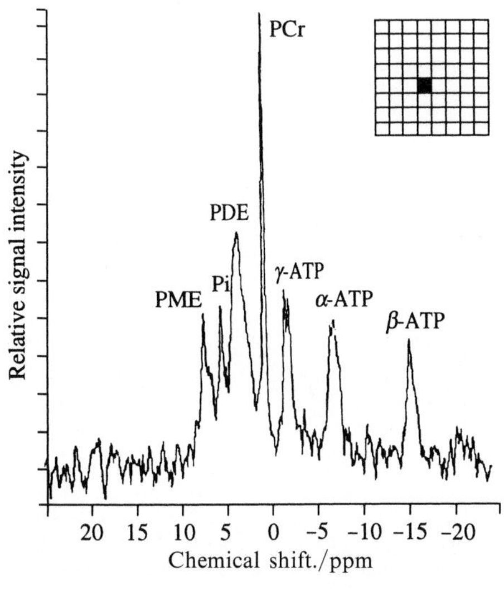

Fig. 49-9 ^{31}P spectrum of control area (voxel A).

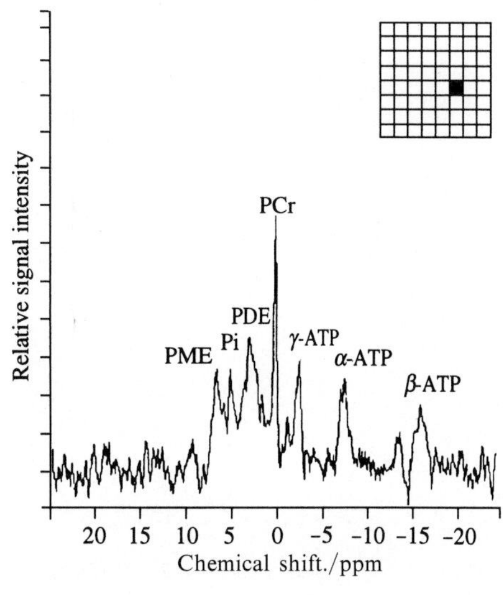

Fig. 49-10 ^{31}P spectrum of hematoma area (voxel B).

CASE 50

CASE 50: A 54-year-old male

Hypertensive intracerebral hemorrhage (right thalamic hemorrhage) 7 days after the stroke

The patient presented with sudden onset of vomiting, left hemiparesis, and consciousness disturbance. He gave a past history of hypertension.

The MRIs in Figures 50-1 and 2 show a moderate amount of hematoma in the right thalamus. The signal intensity is reduced around the hematoma in the ^{31}P, ATP, PCr, and PME metabolite images in Figures 50-3, 4, 6, and 7. It is increased in the hematoma area in the Pi metabolite image in Figure 50-5. During this period, localization of energy metabolism is not as prominent as in the acute period. Figures 50-9 and 50-10 show the ^{31}P spectra of an area opposite the hematoma and the hematoma area, respectively. Note the general decrease in the signal intensities and relative high Pi signal intensities in the hematoma area.

L 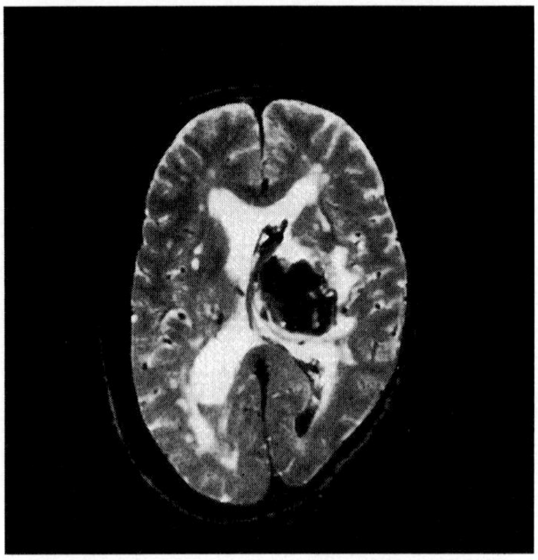 R

Fig. 50-1 Axial T_2-weighted image (2,200/90).

L 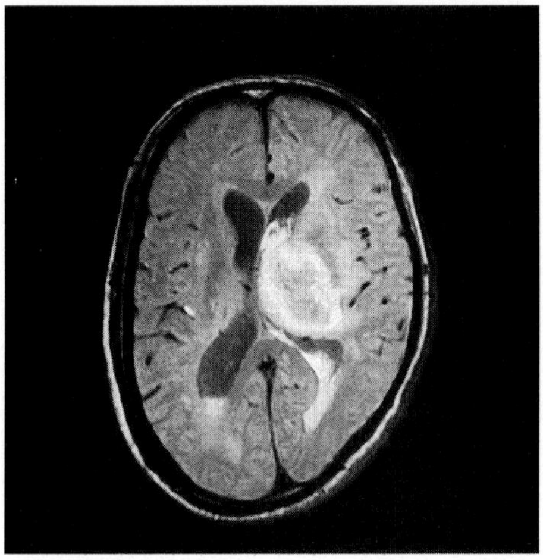 R

Fig. 50-2 Axial proton density-weighted image (2,200/15).

L 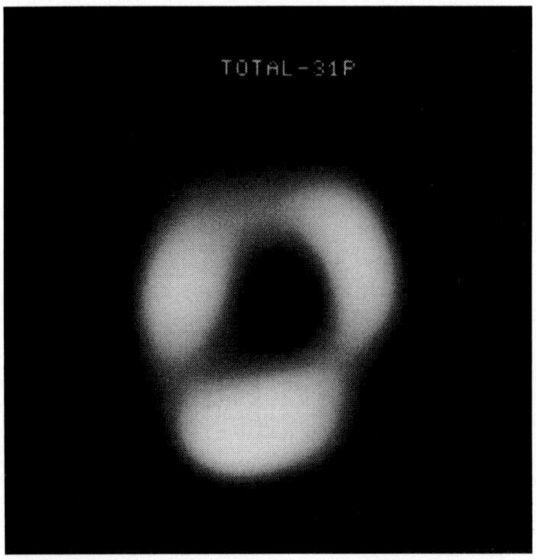 R

Fig. 50-3 Axial ^{31}P metabolite image.

L 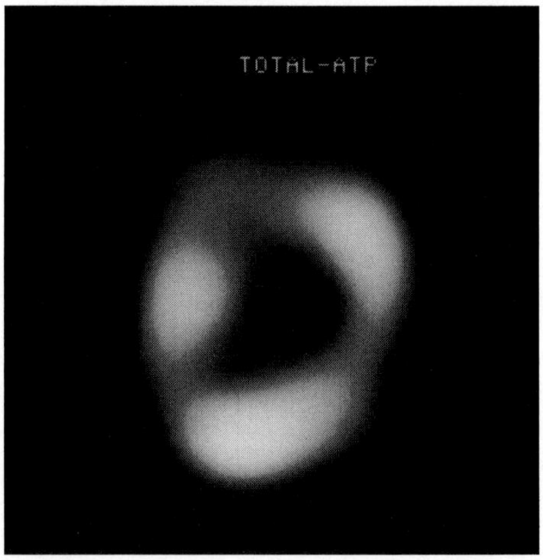 R

Fig. 50-4 Axial total ATP metabolite image.

Fig. 51-5 Axial Pi

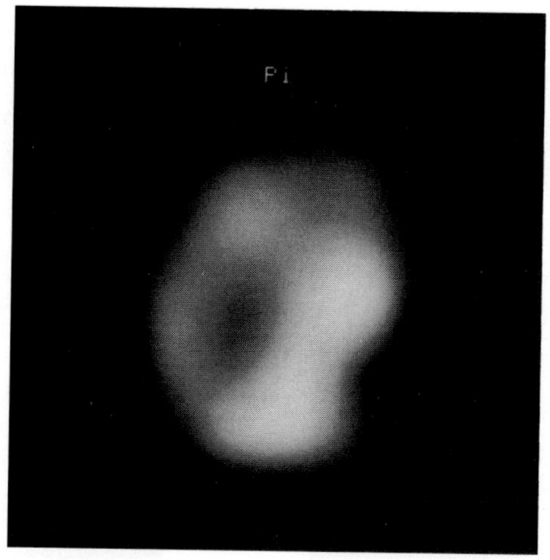

Fig. 50-5 Axial Pi metabolite image.

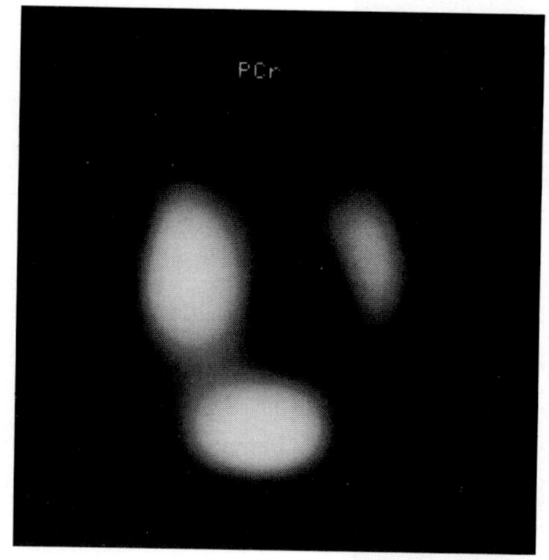

Fig. 50-6 Axial PCr metabolite image.

Fig. 51-7 Axial β-AT

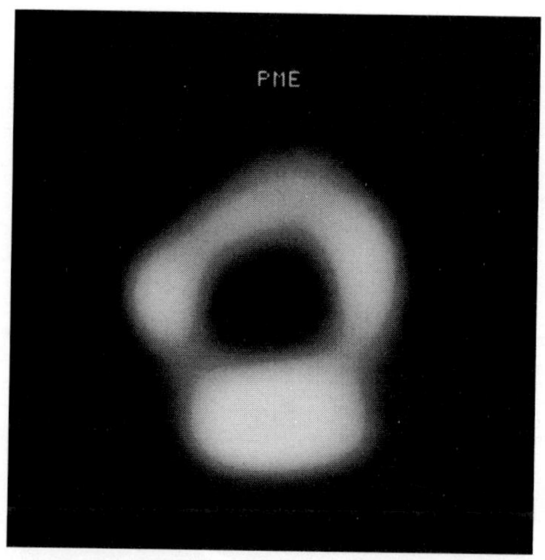

Fig. 50-7 Axial PME metabolite image.

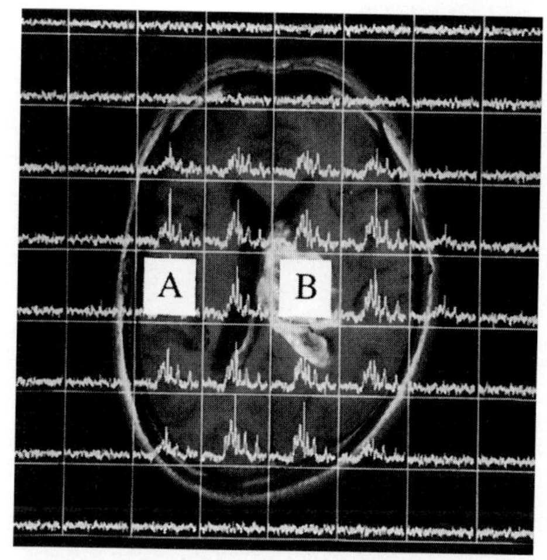

Fig. 50-8 T_1-weighted image showing the position of $3 \times 3 \times 4$ cm^3 voxels A and B.

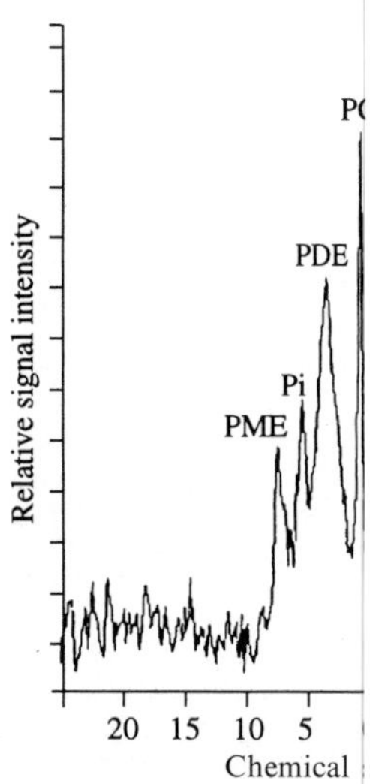

Fig. 51-9 ^{31}P spectrum

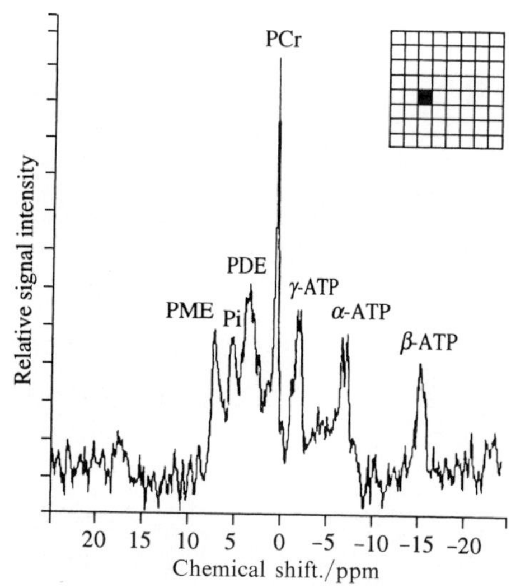

Fig. 50-9 ^{31}P spectrum of control area (voxel A).

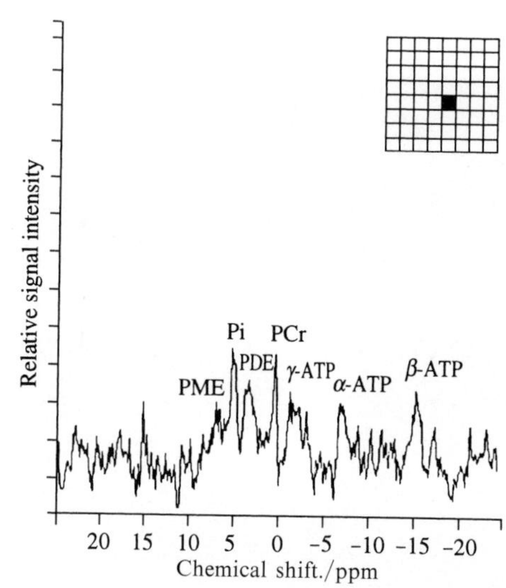

Fig. 50-10 ^{31}P spectrum of hematoma area (voxel B).

CASE 52

CASE 52: A 72-year-old male

Hypertensive intracerebral hemorrhage (left thalamic hemorrhage) 11 days after the stroke

The patient presented with sudden onset of right hemiparesis and motor aphasia. He gave a past history of hypertension, diabetes mellitus, and liver dysfunction.

The MRIs in Figures 52-1 and 2 show a small amount of hematoma in the left thalamus. The signal intensity is reduced around the hematoma in the ^{31}P, Pi, PCr, PDE, and α-ATP metabolite images in Figures 52-3, 4, 5, 6, and 7. Figures 52-9 and 52-10 show the ^{31}P spectra of the hematoma area and an area opposite the hematoma. Note the general decrease in the signal intensities in the hematoma area.

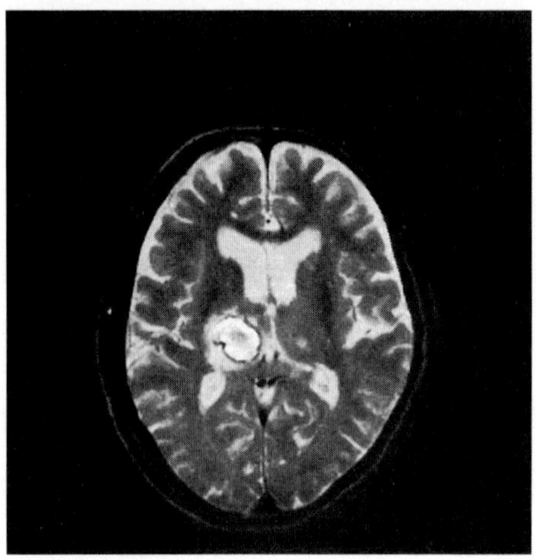

Fig. 52-1 Axial T_2-weighted image (2,200/90).

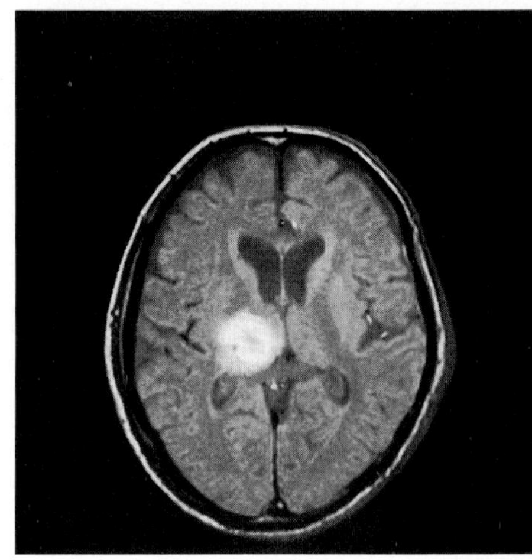

Fig. 52-2 Axial proton density-weighted image (2,200/15).

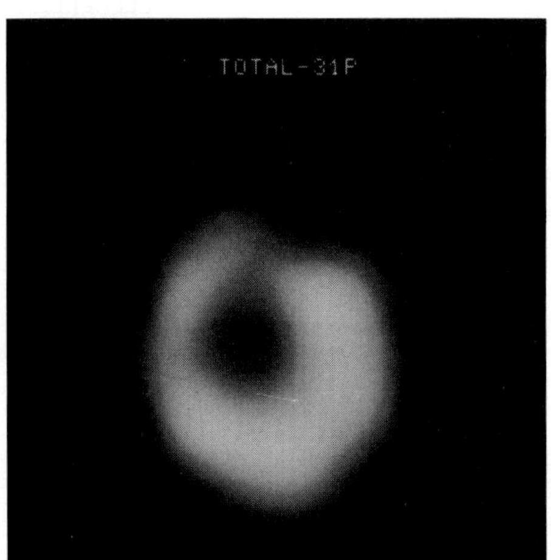

Fig. 52-3 Axial ^{31}P metabolite image.

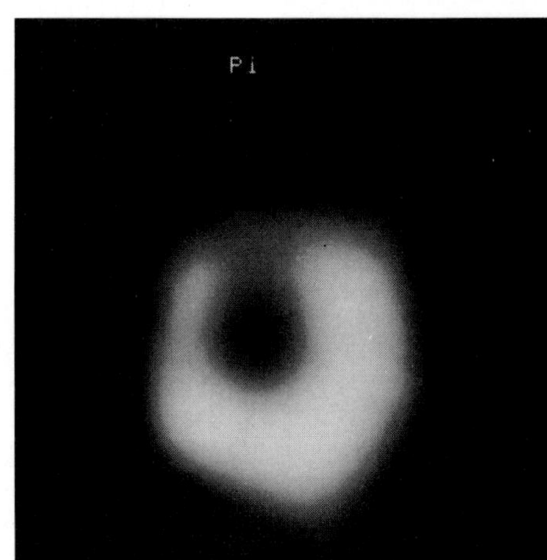

Fig. 52-4 Axial Pi metabolite image.

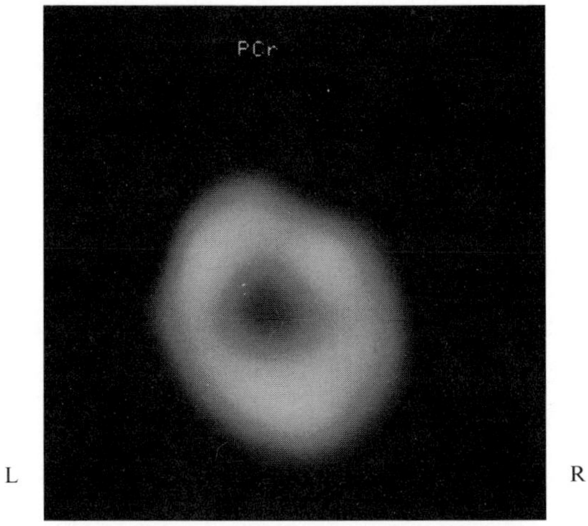

Fig. 52-5 Axial PCr metabolite image.

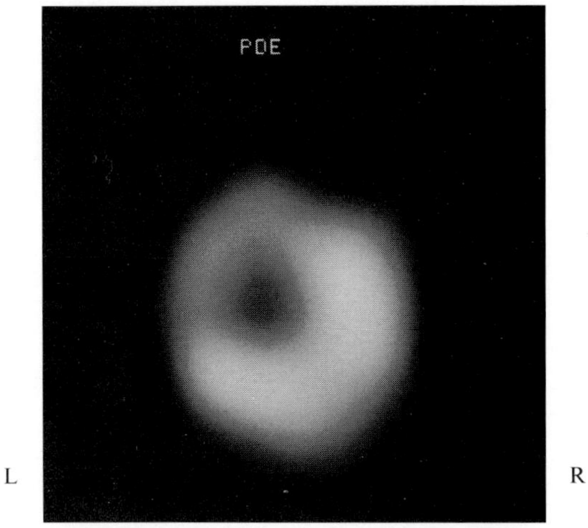

Fig. 52-6 Axial PDE metabolite image.

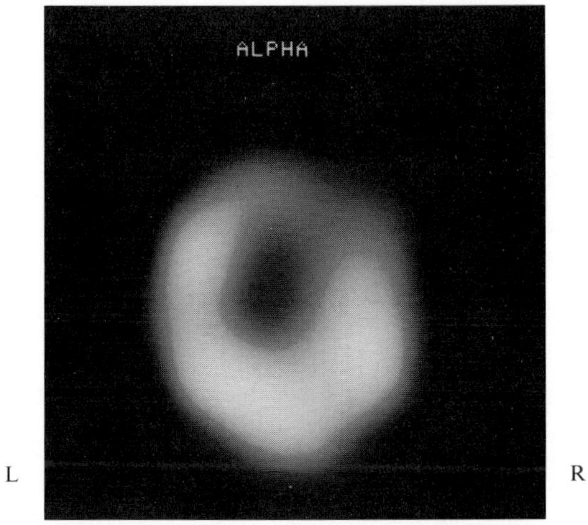

Fig. 52-7 Axial α-ATP metabolite image.

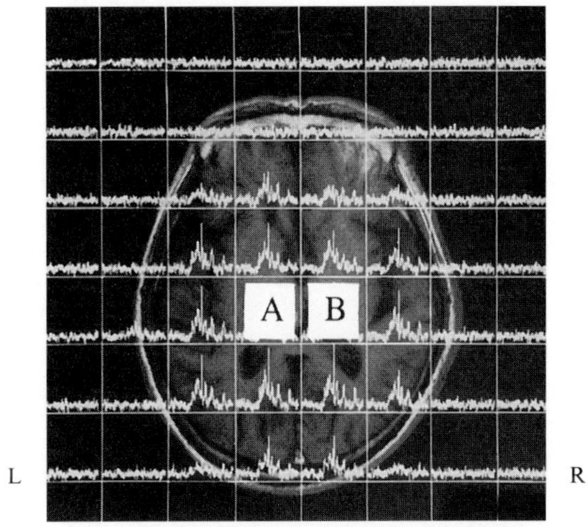

Fig. 52-8 T_1-weighted image showing the position of 3×3×4 cm^3 voxels A and B.

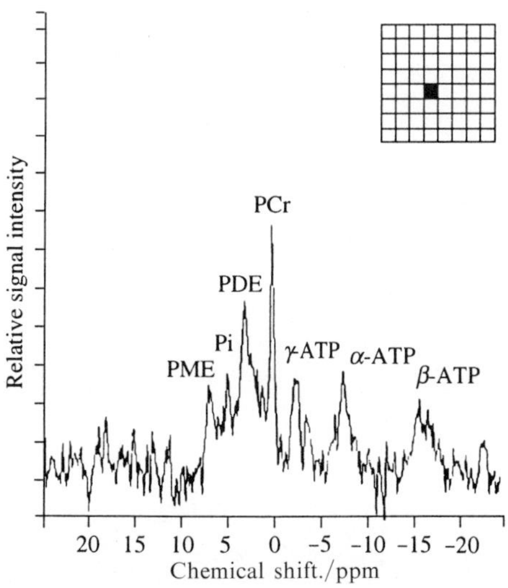

Fig. 52-9 ^{31}P spectrum of hematoma area (voxel A).

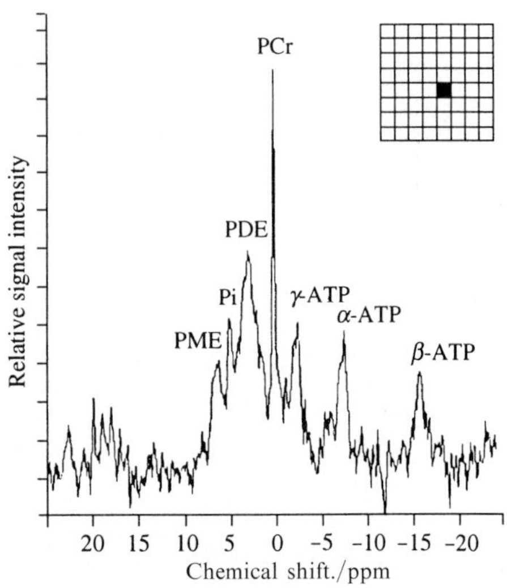

Fig. 52-10 ^{31}P spectrum of control area (voxel B).

CASE 53

CASE 53: A 55-year-old male

Hypertensive intracerebral hemorrhage (right putaminal hemorrhage) 14 days after the stroke

The patient presented with sudden onset of left hemiparesis and consciousness disturbance. He gave a past history of hypertension and left putaminal hemorrhage which occurred several years previous.

The MRIs in Figures 53-1 and 2 show a moderate amount of hematoma in the right putamen. The signal intensity is reduced around the hematoma in the ^{31}P, PME, Pi, PCr, and α-ATP metabolite images in Figures 53-3, 4, 5, 6, and 7. Figures 53-9 and 53-10 show the ^{31}P spectra in an area opposite the hematoma and the hematoma area, respectively. Note the general decrease in the signal intensities in the hematoma area.

L 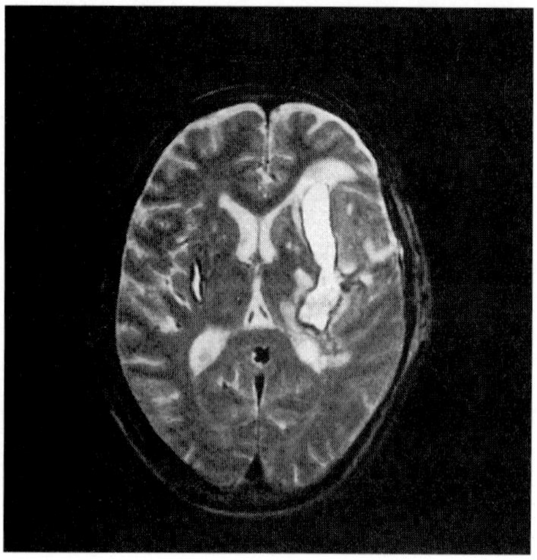 R

Fig. 53-1 Axial T_2-weighted image (2,200/90).

L 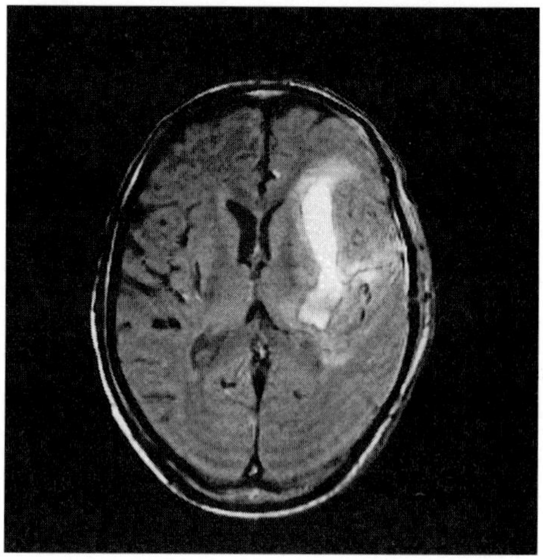 R

Fig. 53-2 Axial proton density-weighted image (2,200/15).

L 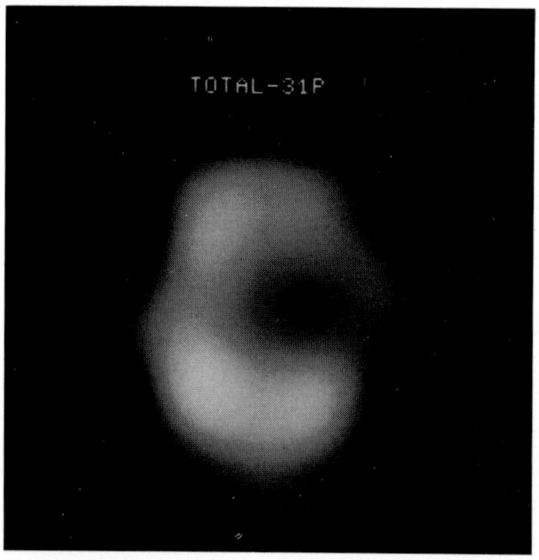 R

Fig. 53-3 Axial ^{31}P metabolite image.

L 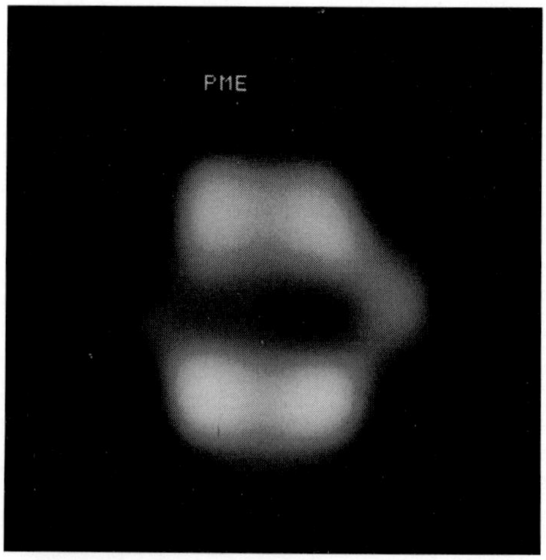 R

Fig. 53-4 Axial PME metabolite image.

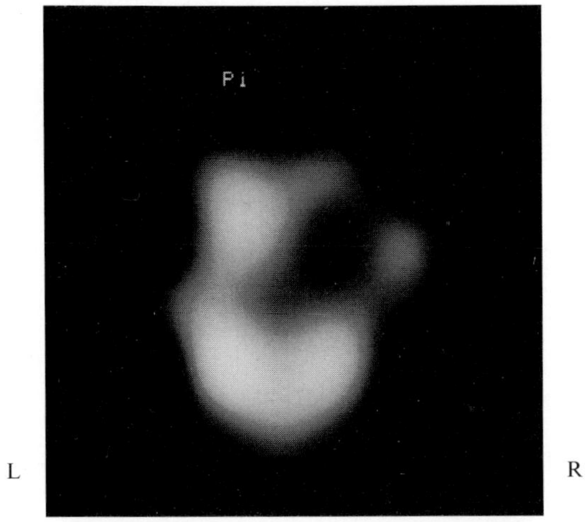

Fig. 53-5 Axial Pi metabolite image.

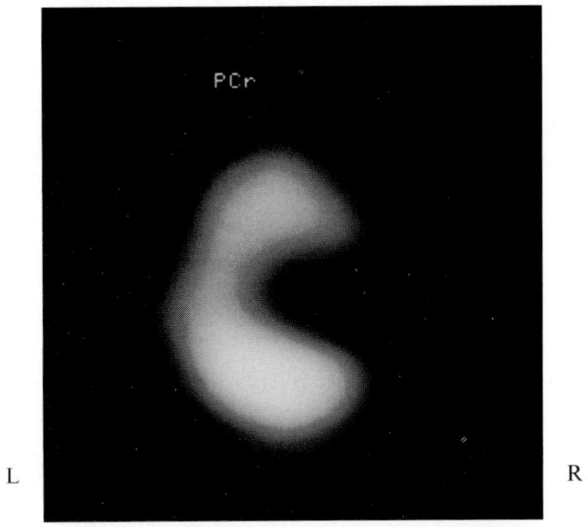

Fig. 53-6 Axial PCr metabolite image.

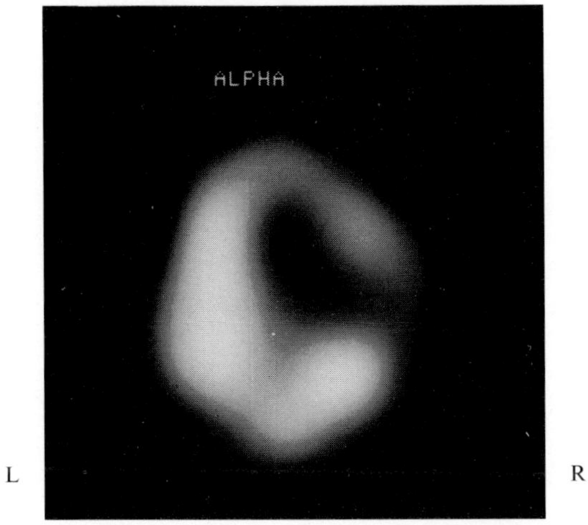

Fig. 53-7 Axial α-ATP metabolite image.

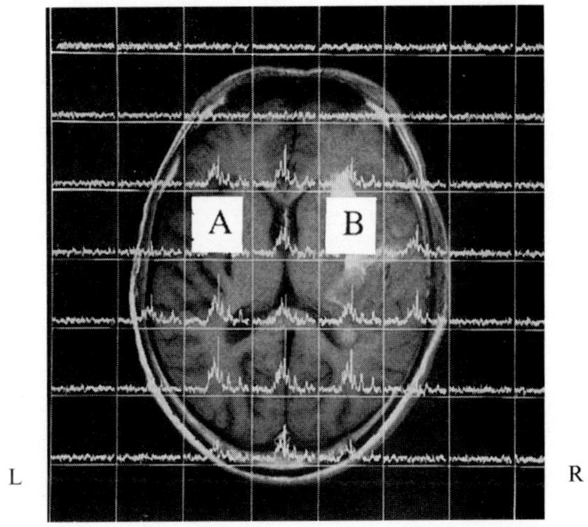

Fig. 53-8 T_1-weighted image showing the position of $3 \times 3 \times 4$ cm^3 voxels A and B.

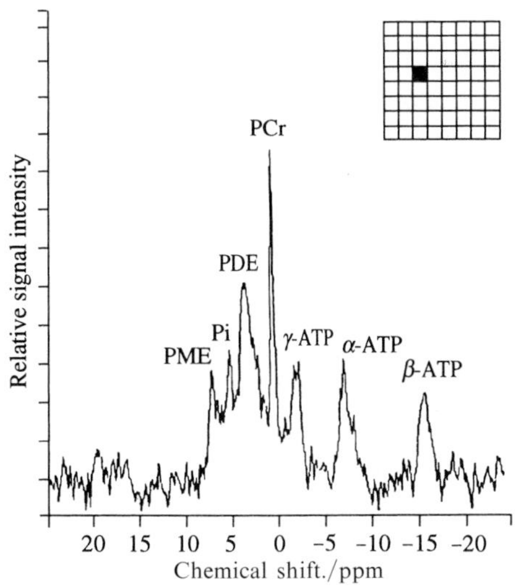

Fig. 53-9 ^{31}P spectrum of control area (voxel A).

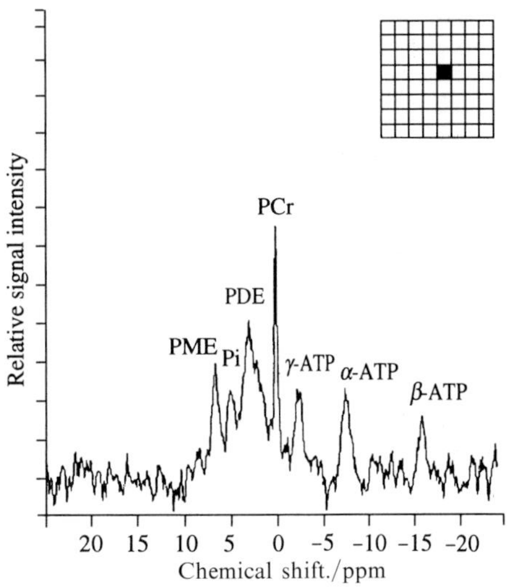

Fig. 53-10 ^{31}P spectrum of hematoma area (voxel B).

Chapter 9 Dementia

Toshiro Fujimoto and Yasuhiko Utatsu

9.1 CHARACTERISTICS OF SPECTRUM

9.1.1 Dementia of Alzheimer type (AD)

(1) ^{31}***P MRS***

There have been many reports on ^{31}P MRS concerning dementia of Alzheimer type (AD), however, these are mostly inconsistent. Possible reasons for such discrepancies are that AD is a progressive disorder and the metabolism of the brain may differ according to the time after the onset of the disease and the anatomical region of the brain affected. In addition, the symptoms of dementia exhibit individual differences and a close relationship with aging so that the stage of the disease is difficult to determine with the one-dimensional scale at initial examination. Technical differences produce different spectra. In addition, sensitivity of ^{31}P MRS is relatively low, and the voxel size of ^{31}P MRS cannot be reduced sufficiently because of technical limitations.

In the studies of brain samples obtained at autopsies of AD patients by NMR, Bărâny et al.[1] found increased grycerol-3-phosphorylcholine (GPC), and Miatto et al.[2,3] reported decreased levels of PME and increased levels of PDE with no alteration of Pi levels in the frontal and parietal regions. Pettegrew et al.[4–6] showed increases in PME and PDE levels in autopsied samples acquired from the middle frontal and the superotemporal gyri of AD patients. These *in vitro* studies suggested abnormalities in phospholipids metabolism in the brain of AD.

In an *in vivo* study of AD patients, Brown et al.[7] reported elevation in PME and in the PME/PDE ratio in the temporoparietal region, and elavation in the Pi level in the frontal and temporoparietal regions. The PME levels increased in mildly demented patients and declined as the disease progressed. The increased PME level was explained as either increased synthesis of membrane phospholipids or a relative metabolic block in the catabolic pathway, or both.[8] The level of PDE being the breakdown products of membrane phospholipids, increased as the stage of dementia progressed, and the increased level in PDE reflected the degeneration of the membrane phospholipids.[4] Bueri et al.[9] reported a trend in reduced PCr/β-ATP, PME/β-ATP, and PDE/β-ATP in AD. In early onset AD patients, Fujimoto et al.[10–12] observed increased ratios of PME+Pi/α-ATP and PDE/α-ATP in the temporoparietal regions, in contrast to a later study[11] that showed increased PME/PDE ratio and reduced level of PDE in the frontoparietal region.[13]

Bottomley et al.[14], however, noted inconsistencies in the PME levels in literatures, and showed that there were no significant alterations in the concentration and relative ratios of PCr, ATP, Pi, PME, and PDE in whole sections through the lateral ventricles of the brain of AD patients. Reported differences in ratio may be due to the prevalence of atrophy or differences in metabolite T_1 values between AD patients and control subjects, and they concluded that ^{31}P MRS appears to be of limited value in the examination of AD. Murphy et al.[15] confirmed the observations of Bottomley et al. and noted that it is not possible to state any antemortem association between PME or PDE and severity of dementia. Using proton decoupled ^{31}P MRS, an advanced technology,

Bluml et al.[16] found no abnormality in the peak of glycerophosphocholine (GPC) in the parietal region. Sappey-Marinier et al.[17] reported that ^{31}P MRS with a voxel size of $8 \times 3 \times 3 cm^3$ did not detect any metabolic difference between AD and normal aging.

In a later study, Bonmartin et al.[18] described decreased PME/ATP and PDE/ATP ratios in the left and right hippocampal formations, that suggested a decrease in phospholipids metabolism of AD, using ^{31}P MRS with a voxel size of $1 \times 1 \times 1 cm^3$. These findings suggested that alteration in phospholipids metabolism may be detectable with a smaller voxel size in ^{31}P MRS. Fujimoto et al.[19] reported that disturbances in phospholipids and high energy phosphate metabolism worsen as AD progresses. The chemical shift imagings from Cases 54 to 56 in this book demonstrate the reduction of PDE in the mesial temporal regions. Laterality of PDE and PME levels are observed in temporal regions, indicating that changes in phospholipids with the progress of AD are not symmetrical.

(2) ^{1}***H MRS***

Miller et al.,[20] Longo et al.[21] and Renshaw et al.[22] reported the reduced level of NAA in the brain of AD patients with *in vivo* ^{1}H MRS. The NAA levels decreased in the center of the temporal lobe (Frederick et al.[23]), the supraventricular region (Meyerhoff et al.[24]), occipital gray matter (Moats et al.[25], Shonk et al.[26]), the midline of the brain (MacKay et al.[27]), and the hippocampus (Block et al.[28]). Schuff et al.[29] noted that changes of NAA in AD are more prominent in the hippocampus than in the cortical gray matter. Klunk et al.[30] reported a decreased level of NAA in autopsy brain samples of AD. Decreased NAA levels may reflect the neuronal loss associated with AD.[20,30] Christiansen et al.[31] showed no significant differences in T_1 and T_2 relaxation time of NAA in AD patients. NAA levels also decreased in all brain regions with normal aging, reflecting the loss of neurons.[32]

In addition, Miller et al.[20] found increased levels of *myo*-inositol, but this elevation was not observed in any other dementia.[26] Increased levels of *myo*-inositol may reflect the inhibition of the enzymes responsible for conversion of *myo*-inositol to phosphatidylinositol.[20] Shonk et al.[36] found increases in the *myo*-inositol level and decreases in the NAA level in Down's syndrome, suggesting the striking similarity to AD, and commented that elevation of *myo*-inositol level may precede loss of NAA in both AD and Down's syndrome.

Reduced GABA levels were observed in *in vitro* MRS studies of AD (Klunk et al.[30] and Mohanakrishnan et al.[33]). The Cho/Cr ratio has been reported to increase in the temporal lobe gray matter, reflecting changes in the membrane or temporal lobe atrophy.[23] Fujimoto et al.[34] have demonstrated that white matter signal high intensities were also occasionally observed in AD, and Constans et al.[35] showed that large white matter signal high intensities of AD were associated with decreases in the NAA level and increases in the Cho level.

9.1.2 Pick's disease

(1) ^{31}***P MRS***

Case 57-1, 2, 3, and 4 show changes in ^{31}P chemical shift imagings of a patient with probable Pick's disease. The PCr signal was decreased in the frontal lobe at the first stage and was reduced in the right and left mesial temporal lobes with progression of the disease. ATP signals were also reduced in the frontal lobe followed by the mesial temporal lobes as the disease progressed. The PCr and ATP signals showed marked decreases at the severe stage of the dementia. These findings suggest that Pick's disease may begin with mild disturbance of the high-energy phosphate metabolism, which worsens with progression of the disease. Decreases in high-energy phosphate metabolism may have a close relation with psychiatric disturbance. The decrease in PCr level in the frontal lobe in Pick's disease could be detected earlier than the atrophy of the frontal lobe detected by MRI or CT. Further study is required to clarify the disturbance of the high-energy phosphate metabolism in Pick's disease. Decreases in the PME and PDE signals in the CSI also progressed, reflecting alterations in phospholipids as the disease worsened. The ^{31}P signal (Case 57-4-1) was decreased in the frontal lobe and the mesial temporal lobes at the severe stage of dementia which reflected severe atrophy of those regions. Smith et al.[37] demonstrated elevated levels of PME and PDE in postmortem brain extracts of Pick's disease. The microscopic findings in Pick's disease show Pick's bodies, collections of the components of the normal cell disarray, and, in most cases, absence of plaque and tangles.[38] Chemical shift imagings of Pick's disease are different from those of cases of AD in this book, reflecting neuropathological differences between these diseases.

(2) ^{1}***H MRS***

^{1}H spectra of the left mesial temporal lobe in Case 57-5 shows a decreased level of NAA, suggesting neuronal loss in Pick's disease. The increased level of Cho/Cr ratio reflects changes in the membrane.

9.1.3 Multi-infarct dementia (MID)

(1) ^{31}***P MRS***

In Cases 58 and 59, signal intensities of ^{31}P images are reduced in lesions corresponding to cerebral infarctions, indicating the reduction of ^{31}P metabolism. ATP, Pi, and PCr signals are decreased in corresponding lesions to multiple cerebral infarcts shown by MRI. This suggests a decreased high-energy phosphate metabolism in multi-infarct lesions. The areas of decreased high-energy phosphate metabolism appear not only to overlap the areas of multiple infarction, but also to extend beyond the area of infarction indicated by MRI. ^{31}P MRS has very high sensitivity to vascular damage. Sappey-Marinier et al.[39] found reduced phosphorus metabolite concentration and a higher intracellular pH in infarcted regions, while Pi and PCr concentrations showed smaller, insignificant decreases. Sappey-Marinier et al.[40] also reported that areas of high-intensity in the white matter show reductions in metabolite concentrations and disturbance of cellular energy metabolism. Brown et al.[7] demonstrated elevations in the PCr/Pi ratio of multiple subcortical infarct dementia implying disturbance of high-energy phosphate metabolism. Kamei et al.[41] demonstrated decreased levels in PME and PDE in cerebrovascular dementia. The PME and PDE levels are also reduced in Cases 58 and 59, indicating abnormalities of phospholipids or phospholipids metabolism. These findings demonstrate that ^{31}P MRS studies provide information such as decreased high-energy phosphate metabolism which is useful for the diagnosis of MID.

(2) ^{1}***H MRS***

MacKay et al.[27,42] found reduction of the NAA/Cr ratio in the frontal white matter in patients of subcortical ischemic vascular dementia. White matter signal hyperintensity (WMSH) areas are known to be observed on T_2-weighted MRI images of patients with multi-infarct dementia and Alzheimer's disease.[34] In patients with ischemic vascular dementia, Constans et al.[35] reported that the WMSH were secondary to ischemia and/or infarction, and that the Cho/Cr level was higher in WMSH areas than in contralateral normal-appearing white matter, and the NAA/Cr level was reduced in WMSH areas. Oppenheimer et al.[43] observed a decreased level of NAA, indicating neuronal/axonal loss, and no changes in Cho level in asymptomatic white matter hyperintensity lesions and lactate signals in these lesions in some patients.

9.1.4 Binswanger's disease

(1) ^{31}***P MRS***

In Case 60, the white matter signal hyperintensity (WMSH) is observed in the frontal and temporal lobes in the T_2-weighted image, and enlargement of cerebral ventricles is also shown. Reductions in ^{31}P signals of the CSI suggest overall metabolic dysfunction. Decreased ATP signals indicate disturbances in high-energy phosphate metabolism in the frontal and temporal lobes corresponding to WMSH. Decreases in the PME and PDE levels are observed in the frontal and temporal lobes, and reflect abnormality in phospholipid metabolism.

(2) ***^1H MRS***

Brooks et al.[44] reported reduction in NAA levels in Binswanger's disease, indicating axonal dropout, and the trend of elevation in the Cho level, suggesting disruption of the membrane.

References

1) Bárány, M.; Chang, Y-C.; Arús, C. et al. Increased glycerol-3-phosphorylcholine in post-mortem Alzheimer's brain. *Lancet* 2: 517; 1985.

2) Miatto, O.; Gonzalez, R. G.; Buonanno, F. et al. *In vitro* ^{31}P NMR spectroscopy detects altered phospholipid metabolism in Alzheimer's disease. *Can. J. Neurol. Sci*. 13: 535-539; 1986.

3) Miatto, O.; Gonzalez, G.; Buonanno, F. S. et al. 31-Phosphorus nuclear magnetic resonance studies in dementia. *Neurology* 36 (Suppl 1): 105; 1986.

4) Pettegrew, J. W.; Panchalingam, K.; Moossy, J. et al. Correlation of phosphorus-31 magnetic resonance spectroscopy and morphologic findings in Alzheimer's disease. *Arch. Neurol*. 45: 1093-1096; 1988.

5) Pettegrew, J. W.; Moossy, J.; Withers, G. et al. ^{31}P Nuclear magnetic resonance study of the brain in Alzheimer's disease. *J. Neuropathol. Exp. Neurol*. 47: 235-248; 1988.

6) Pettegrew, J. W. Molecular insights into Alzheimer's disease. *Ann. NY. Acad. Sci*. 568: 5-28; 1989.

7) Brown, G. G.; Levine, S. R.; Gorell, J. M. et al. In vivo ^{31}P NMR profiles of Alzheimer's disease and multiple subcortical infarct dementia. *Neurology* 39: 1423-1427; 1989.

8) Pettegrew, J. W.; Panchalingam, K.; Klunk, W. E. et al. Alterations of cerebral metabolism in probable Alzheimer's disease: A preliminary study. *Neurobiol. Aging* 15: 117-132; 1994.

9) Bueri, J. A.; Gorell, J. M.; Levine, S. R. et al. Cerebral phosphate metabolism in Alzheimer and Parkinson dementia measured by ^{31}P NMR spectroscopy. *Neurology* 37 (Suppl. 1): 160; 1987.

10) Fujimoto, T.; Nakano, T.; Noguchi, S. et al. In-vivo ^{31}P multivoxel spectroscopy in Alzheimer's disease. *Progress in CT* 11: 435-441; 1989. [Japanese]

11) Fujimoto, T.; Nakano, T.; Noguchi, S. et al. Study of dementia of Alzheimer type using ^{31}P chemical shift imaging and ^{31}P-NMR spectroscopy. *Japanese Journal of Psychiatric Treatment* 4: 1249-1257; 1989. [Japanese]

12) Fujimoto, T.; Noguchi, S.; Nakano, T. et al. In vivo phosphorous-31 NMR spectroscopy in Alzheimer's disease. In: T. Nagatsu, A. Fisher, M. Yoshida (Eds). Basic, Clinical, and Therapeutic Aspects of Alzheimer's and Parkinson's Diseases Volume 2. Advances in Behavioral Biology Volume 38B, New York: Plenum Press, 1990: pp. 67-72.

13) Fujimoto, T.; Nakano, T.; Noguchi, S. et al. Study of dementia of the Alzheimer type (presenile onset) using in vivo ^{31}P NMR chemical shift imaging. *Japanese Journal of Psychiatric Treatment* 7: 531-540; 1992. [Japanese]

14) Bottomley, P. A.; Cousins, J. P.; Pendrey, D. L. et al. Alzheimer dementia: Quantification of energy metabolism and mobile phosphoesters with P-31 NMR spectroscopy. *Radiology* 183: 695-699; 1992.

15) Murphy, D. G. M.; Bottomley, P. A.; Salerno, J. A. et al. An in vivo study of phosphorus and glucose metabolism in Alzheimer's disease using magnetic resonance spectroscopy and PET. *Arch. Gen. Psychiatry* 50: 341-349; 1993.

16) Bluml, S.; Danielsen, E. R.; Ross, B. D. Proton decoupled ^{31}P MRS in Alzheimer disease. *In: Proceedings: Fourth Scientific Meeting and Exhibition of the International Society for Magnetic Resonance in Medicine, Vol. 1. New York, USA: ISMRM* ; 1996: 304.

17) Sappey-Marinier, D.; Bonmartin, A.; Angelié, E. et al. ^1H MRSI and ^{31}P MRS did not detect any metabolic difference between Alzheimer's disease and normal aging. *In: Proceedings: Third Scientific Meeting and Exhibition of the Society of Magnetic Resonance, Vol. 3. Nice, France: SMR* ; 1995: 1811.

18) Bonmartin, A.; Sappey-Marinier, D.; Barbier, E. et al. Comparative morphometric and metabolic study between Alzheimer's disease and normal aging using 3D-MRI and ^{31}P MRS. *In: Proceedings: Fourth Scientific Meeting and Exhibition of the International Society for Magnetic Resonance in Medicine, Vol. 2. New York, USA: ISMRM*; 1996: 927.

19) Fujimoto, T.; Matsumoto, T.; Takano, T. et al.

Changes of ^{31}P spectra in hippocampal regions in patients with Alzheimer disease due to the progress of the disease. *In: Proceedings: Fifth Scientific Meeting and Exhibition of the International Society for Magnetic Resonance in Medicine, Vol. 2. Vancouver, Canada: ISMRM*; 1997: 1180.

20) Miller, B. L.; Moats, R. A.; Shonk, T. et al. Alzheimer disease: Depiction of increased cerebral *myo*-inositol with proton MR spectroscopy. *Radiology* 187: 433-437; 1993.

21) Longo, R.; Giorgini, A.; Magnaldi, S. et al. Alzheimer's disease histologically proven studied by MRI and MRS: Two cases. *Magn. Reson. Imaging* 11: 1209-1215; 1993.

22) Renshaw, P. F.; Satlin, A.; Johnson, K. A. Parietal lobe proton MRS in patients with Alzheimer's disease. *In: Proceedings: Twelfth Annual Scientific Meeting of the Society of Magnetic Resonance in Medicine, Vol. 1. New York, USA: SMRM*; 1993: 232.

23) Frederick, B. deB.; Satlin, A.; Yurgelun-Todd, D. et al. *In vivo* proton MRS of Alzheimer's disease in the parietal and temporal lobes. *In: Proceedings: Third Scientific Meeting and Exhibition of the Society of Magnetic Resonance, Vol. 3. Nice, France: SMR*; 1995: 1810.

24) Meyerhoff, D. J.; MacKay, S.; Constans, J. -M. et al. Axonal injury and membrane alterations in Alzheimer's disease suggested by in vivo proton magnetic resonance spectroscopic imaging. *Ann. Neurol.* 36: 40-47; 1994.

25) Moats, R. A.; Ernst, T.; Shonk, T. K. et al. Abnormal cerebral metabolite concentrations in patients with probable Alzheimer disease. *Magn. Reson. Med.* 32: 110-115; 1994.

26) Shonk, T. K.; Moats, R. A.; Gifford, P. et al. Probable Alzheimer disease: Diagnosis with proton MR spectroscopy. *Radiology* 195: 65-72; 1995.

27) MacKay, S.; Ezekiel, F.; Sclafani, V. D. et al. Alzheimer disease and subcortical ischemic vascular dementia: Evaluation by combining MR imaging segmentation and H-1 MR spectroscopic imaging. *Radiology* 198: 537-545; 1996.

28) Block, W.; Träber, F.; Horn, R. et al. Metabolic changes detected by ^{1}H-MR-spectroscopic imaging of the hippocampus in patients with Alzheimer's disease. *In: Proceedings: Third Scientific Meeting and Exhibition of the Society of Magnetic Resonance, Vol. 3. Nice, France: SMR*; 1995: 1813.

29) Schuff, N.; Knowlton, R.; Amend, D. L. et al. Changes of NAA in Alzheimer's disease are more prominent in hippocampus than in cortical gray matter: A ^{1}H MR spectroscopic imaging study. *In: Proceedings: Fourth Scientific Meeting and Exhibition of the International Society for Magnetic Resonance in Medicine, Vol. 1. New York, USA: ISMRM*; 1996: 308.

30) Klunk, W. E.; Panchalingam, K; Moossy, J. et al. *N*-acetyl-$_{L}$-aspartate and other amino acid metabolites in Alzheimer's disease brain: A preliminary proton nuclear magnetic resonance study. *Neurology* 42: 1578-1585; 1992.

31) Christiansen, P.; Schlosser, A.; Henriksen, O. Reduced *N*-acetylaspartate content in the frontal part of the brain in patients with probable Alzheimer's disease. *Magn. Reson. Imaging* 13: 457-462; 1995.

32) Sappey-Marinier, D.; Angelié, E.; Meltz, P. et al. Brain metabolic changes during normal aging detected by proton MR spectroscopic imaging. *In: Proceedings: Fourth Scientific Meeting and Exhibition of the International Society for Magnetic Resonance in Medicine, Vol. 2. New York, USA: ISMRM*; 1996: 926.

33) Mohanakrishnan, P.; Vonsattel, J. P.; Husain, M. M. et al. Regional metabolic changes in Alzheimer's disease using high resolution proton NMR. *In: Proceedings: Third Scientific Meeting and Exhibition of the Society of Magnetic Resonance, Vol. 3. Nice, France: SMR*; 1995: 1815.

34) Fujimoto, T.; Noguchi, S.; Tsuji, T. et al. Study of dementia in the elderly using magnetic resonance (MR). Part II. —Application of high field MRI. *Japanese Journal of Psychiatric Treatment* 3: 909-917; 1988. [Japanese]

35) Constans, J. M.; Meyerhoff, D. J.; Gerson, J. et al. H-1 MR spectroscopic imaging of white matter signal hyperintensities: Alzheimer disease and ischemic vascular dementia. *Radiology* 197: 517-523; 1995.

36) Shonk, T.; Ross, B. D. Role of increased cerebral *myo*-inositol in the dementia of down syndrome. *Magn. Reson. Med.* 33: 858-861; 1995.

37) Smith, C. D.; Gallenstein III, L. G.; Markesbery, W. R. ^{31}P spectroscopy in Alzheimer's and Pick's disease using post-mortem perchloric acid brain extracts. *In: Book of Abstracts: Seventh Annual Meeting and Exhibition of the Society of Magnetic Resonance in Medicine, Vol. 1. San Francisco, California USA: SMRM*; 1988: 444.

38) Lishman, W. A. Organic Psychiatry. The Psychological Consequences of Cerebral Disorder, Second Edition. Oxford: Blackwell Scientific Publications, 1987: pp. 392-393.

39) Sappey-Marinier, D.; Hubesch, B.; Matson, G. B. et al. Decreased phosphorus metabolite concentrations and alkalosis in chronic cerebral infarction. *Radiology* 182: 29-34; 1992.

40) Sappey-Marinier, D.; Deicken, R. F.; Fein, G. et al.

Alterations in brain phosphorus metabolite concentrations associated with areas of high signal intensity in white matter at MR imaging. *Radiology* 183: 247–256; 1992.

41) Kamei, S.; Oishi, M.; Takasu, T. Evaluation of fasudil hydrochloride treatment for wandering symptoms in cerebrovascular dementia with ^{31}P–magnetic resonance spectroscopy and Xe–Computed tomography. *Clin. Neuropharmacol.* 19: 428–438; 1996.

42) MacKay, S.; Meyerhoff, D. J.; Constans, J. M. et al. Effects of subcortical ischemic vascular dementia on cerebral ^{1}H metabolites. *In: Proceedings: Second Meeting of the Society of Magnetic Resonance, Vol. 2. San Francisco, California USA: SMR*; 1994: 597.

43) Oppenheimer, S. M.; Bryan, R. N.; Conturo, T. E. et al. Proton magnetic resonance spectroscopy and gadolinium–DTPA perfusion imaging of asymptomatic MRI white matter lesions. *Magn. Reson. Med.* 33: 61–68; 1995.

44) Brooks, W. M.; Wesley, M. H.; Kodituwakku, P. et al. ^{1}H–MRS in Binswanger's disease and leukoencephalopathy of normal aging. *In: Proceedings: Third Scientific Meeting and Exhibition of the Society of Magnetic Resonance, Vol. 1. Nice, France: SMR*; 1995: 386.

9.2 CASES (54-60)

CASE 54

CASE 54: A 66-year-old female
Dementia of Alzheimer type
Age at onset : 62 years.

The patient had severe dementia showing deterioration of personality and intellect with incontinence and wandering. The proton density image in Figure 54-1 shows severe brain atrophy. Figure 54-2 illustrates voxels from which ^{1}H MR spectra are obtained in the mesial temporal lobes. In Figure 54-3, a reduction of NAA/Cr ratio and an elevated Cho/Cr ratio are observed in the right mesial temporal lobe. Figure 54-4 also demonstrates a reduction of NAA/Cr ratio and an elevated Cho/Cr ratio in the left mesial temporal lobe. The ^{31}P contour map and metabolite image in Figures 54-5 and 6 show symmetrical signal intensities in the temporal regions. The PME metabolite image shows an elevated signal intensity in the right mesial temporal lobe (Figure 54-7). Figure 54-8 illustrates voxels for ^{31}P spectra placed in mesial temporal lobes. The %PME and the %β-ATP are elevated, but %Pi and %PDE are almost in the normal range in voxel 11 placed in the right mesial temporal lobe (Figure 54-9). The pHi is in the normal range. In the left mesial temporal lobe (voxel 13), the %Pi, the %PDE and the %PCr are reduced, and the %α-ATP is increased, but the %PME and the %β-ATP are in the normal ranges (Figure 54-10). The pHi is increased. The ^{31}P and ^{1}H MR spectra suggest abnormalities in the phospholipids and high-energy phosphate metabolism, alkalosis, and neuronal loss in the mesial temporal lobes.

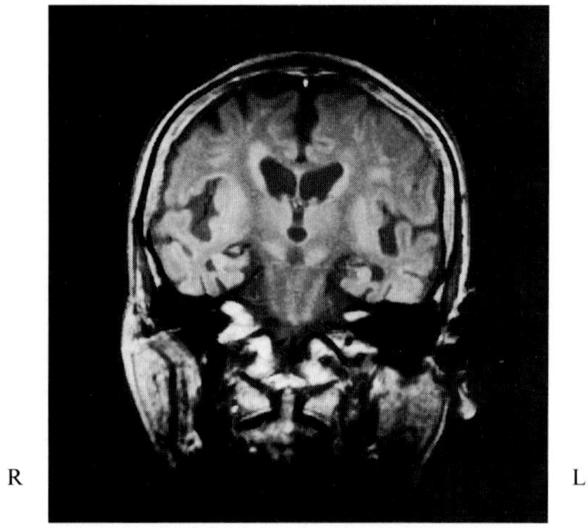

Fig. 54-1 Coronal proton density-weighted image (2,200/15).

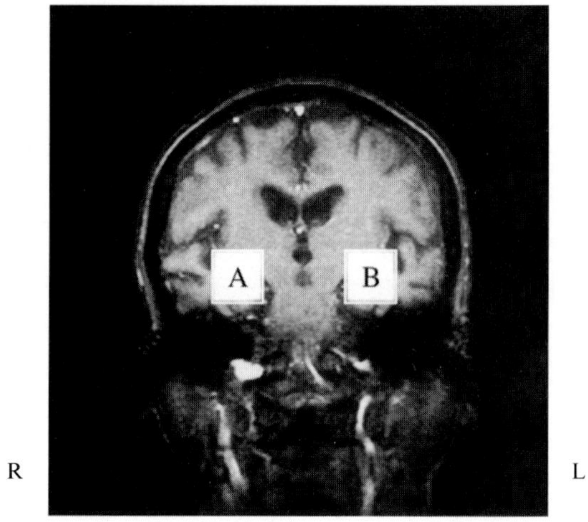

Fig. 54-2 T_1-weighted image showing the position of 2.5×2.5×2.5cm^3 voxels A and B.

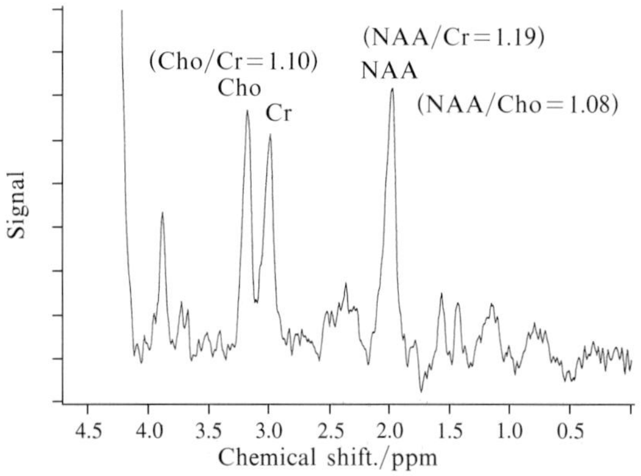

Fig. 54-3 ^{1}H spectrum of right mesial temporal lobe (voxel A). STEAM (2,000/60)

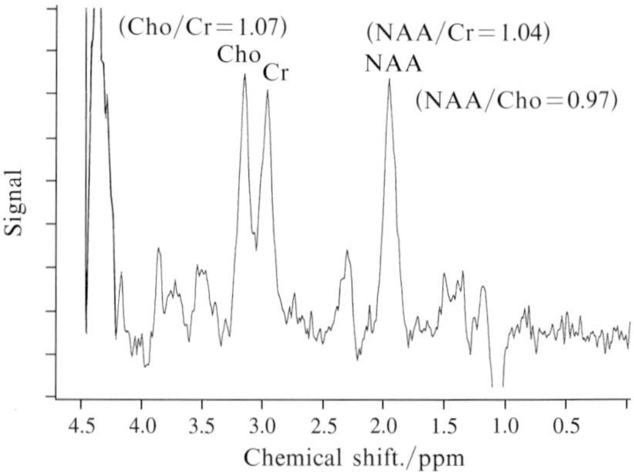

Fig. 54-4 ^{1}H spectrum of left mesial temporal lobe (voxel B). STEAM (2,000/60)

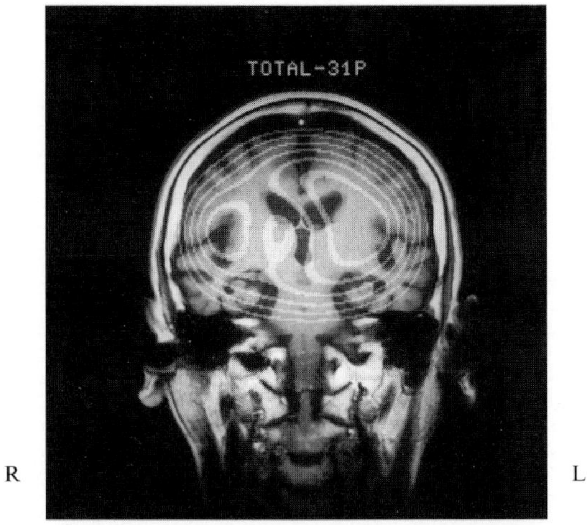

Fig. 54-5 Coronal ^{31}P contour map superimposed on T_1-weighted image (500/15)

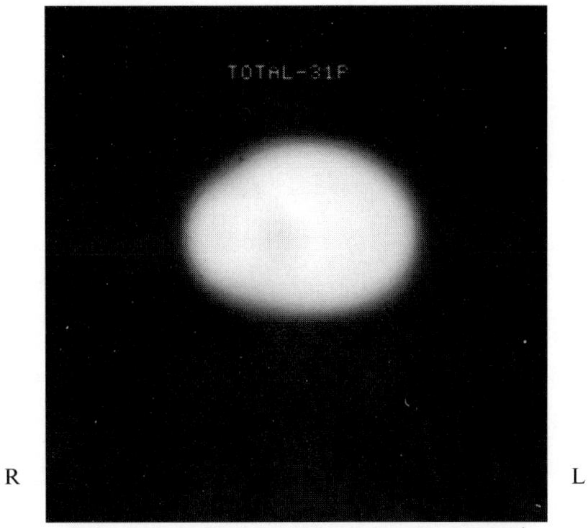

Fig. 54-6 Coronal ^{31}P metabolite image.

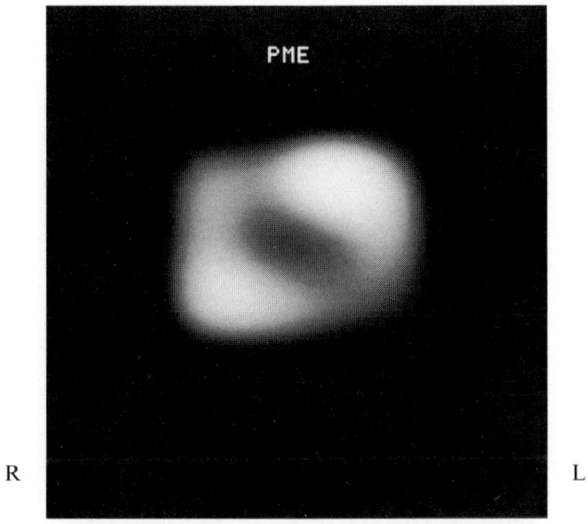

Fig. 54-7 Coronal PME metabolite image.

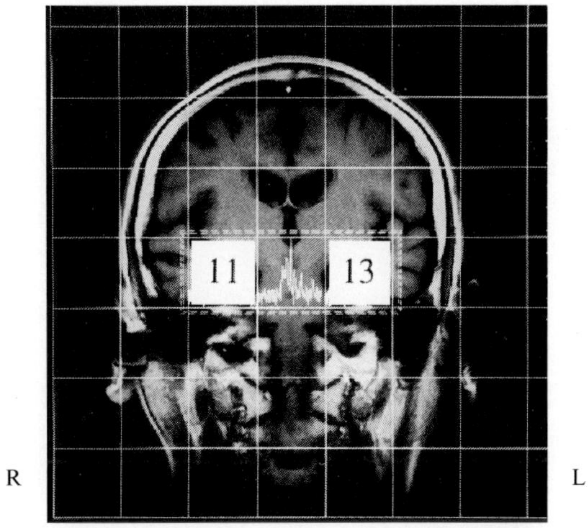

Fig. 54-8 T_1-weighted image showing the position of $3 \times 3 \times 4 cm^3$ voxels 11 and 13.

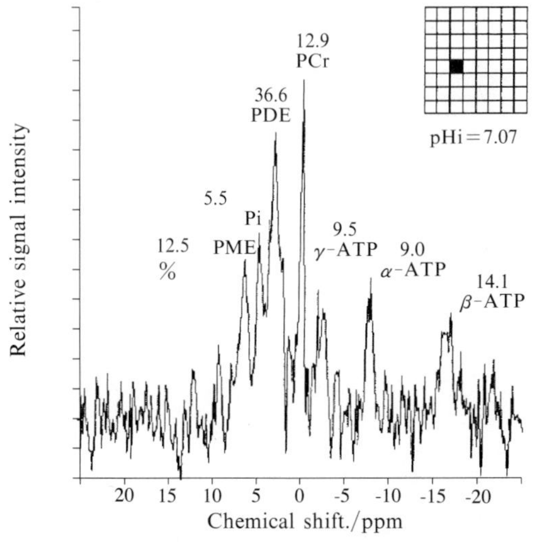

Fig. 54-9 ^{31}P spectrum of right mesial temporal lobe (voxel 11).

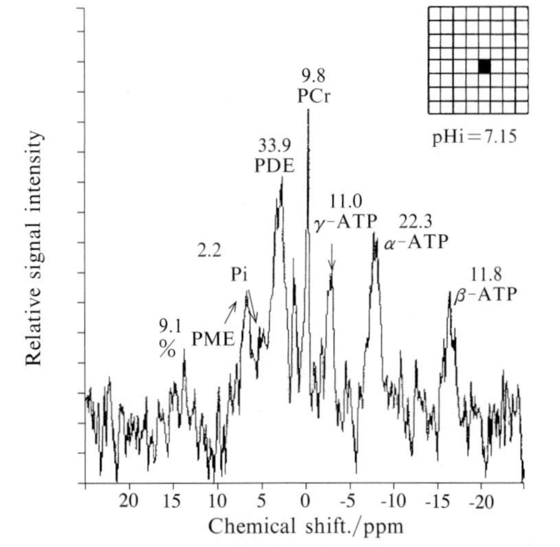

Fig. 54-10 ^{31}P spectrum of left mesial temporal lobe (voxel 13).

CASE 55

CASE 55: A 69-year-old female
Dementia of Alzheimer type
Age at onset: about 57 years.

The patient had severe dementia showing intellectual and personality disturbance with wandering and incontinence. The X-CT in Figure 55-1 shows marked brain atrophy. In the ^{31}P and total ATP metabolite images in Figures 55-2 and 3, signal intensities are distributed nearly symmetrically. The PME signal intensities are elevated in the right temporal lobe and left frontal lobe in the metabolite image, (Figure 55-4). In the PDE contour map and metabolite image in Figures 55-5 and 6, signal intensities of PDE are increased in the left mesial temporal lobe. In the PCr contour map in Figure 55-7, the signal intensity of PCr is elevated in the frontal lobe and the right temporal lobe. Figure 55-8 shows voxels placed in the mesial temporal lobes. In Figure 55-9 a ^{31}P spectrum of the right mesial temporal lobe obtained from voxel 11 is shown. The %PCr and the pHi are increased, and the %PME and the % PDE are mildly reduced. In the ^{31}P spectrum of the left mesial temporal lobe (voxel 13 in Figure 55-10), decreases in %PME and increased pHi are observed. The ^{31}P spectra demonstrate abnormalities in phospholipids and high-energy phosphate metabolism, and alkalosis in the mesial temporal lobes.

L 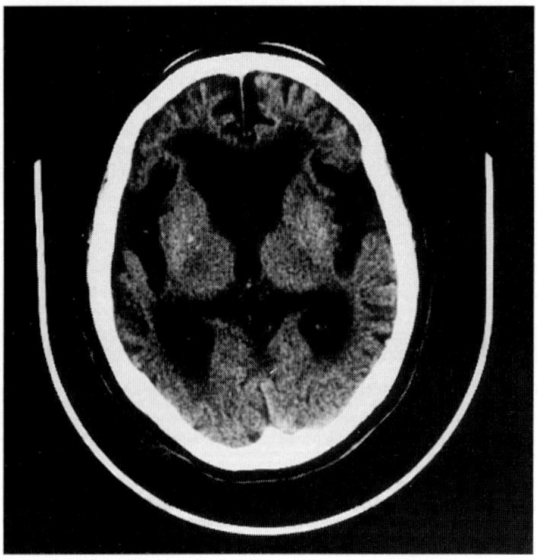 R

Fig. 55-1 Axial X-CT image.

R 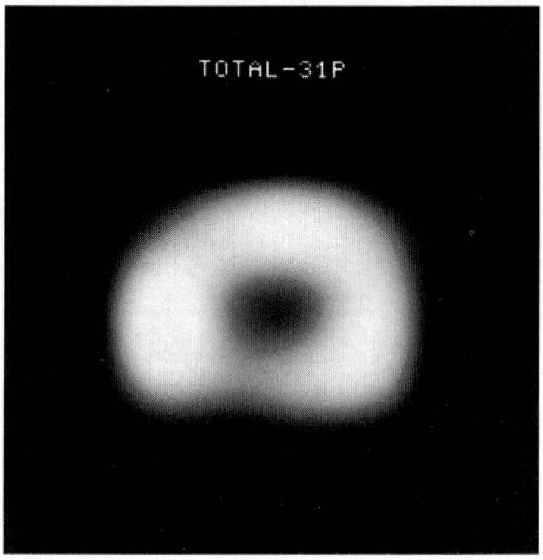 L

Fig. 55-2 Coronal ^{31}P metabolite image.

R 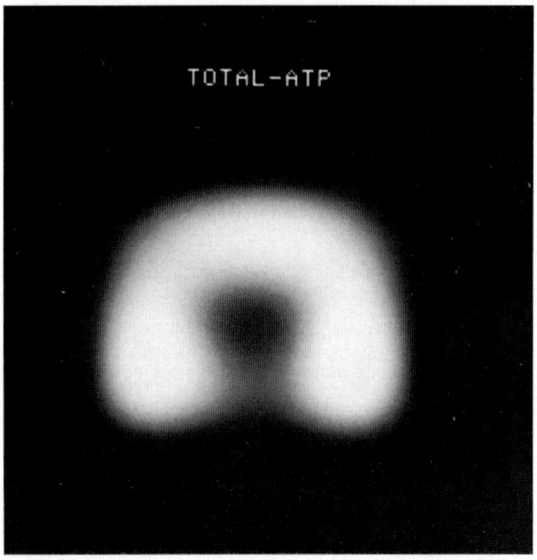 L

Fig. 55-3 Coronal total ATP metabolite image.

R 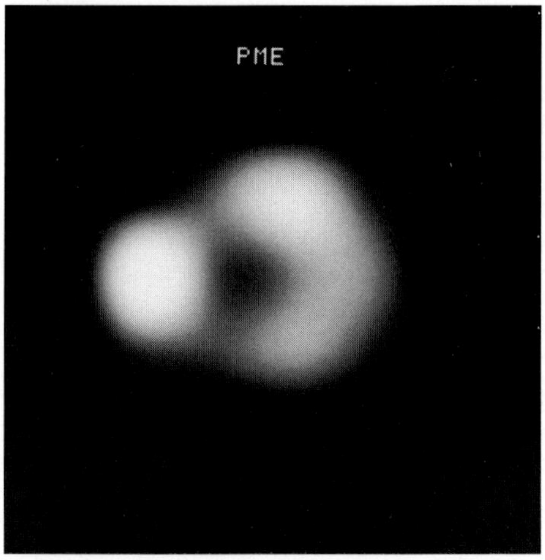 L

Fig. 55-4 Coronal PME metabolite image.

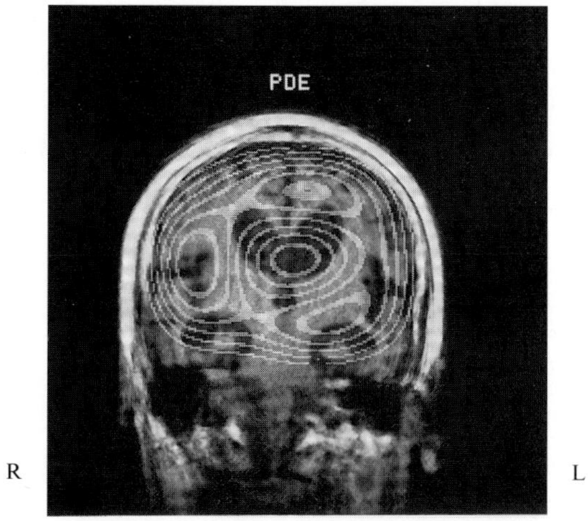

Fig. 55-5 Coronal PDE contour map superimposed on T_1-weighted image (500/15).

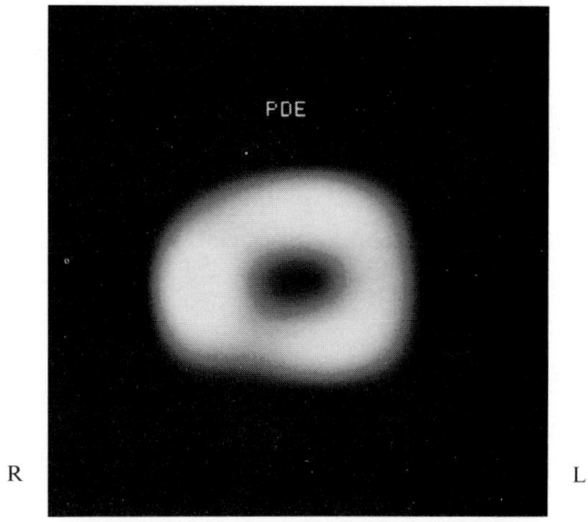

Fig. 55-6 Coronal PDE metabolite image.

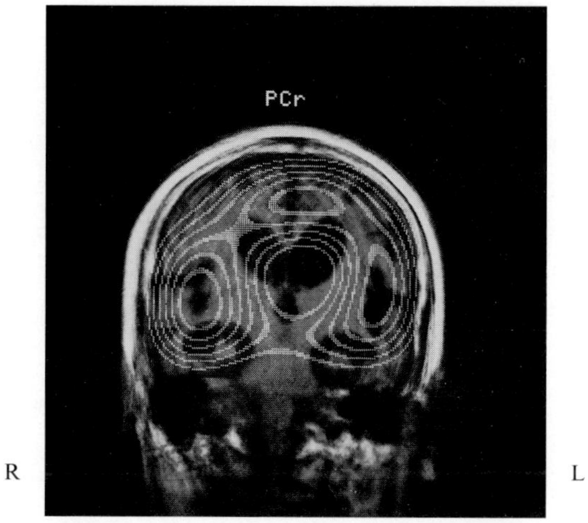

Fig. 55-7 Coronal PCr contour map superimposed on T_1-weighted image (500/15).

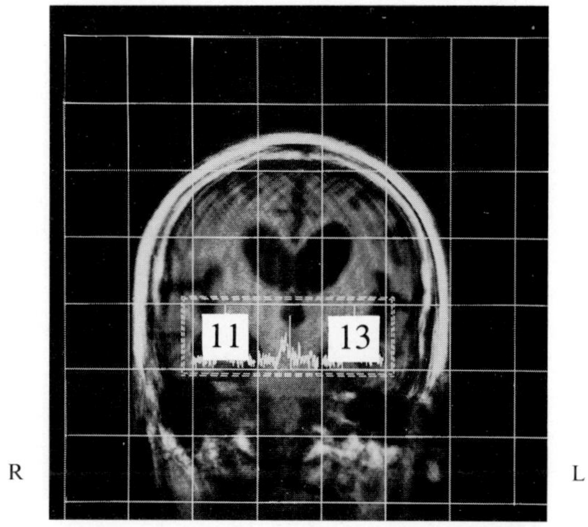

Fig. 55-8 T_1-weighted image showing the position of $3 \times 3 \times 4 cm^3$ voxels 11 and 13.

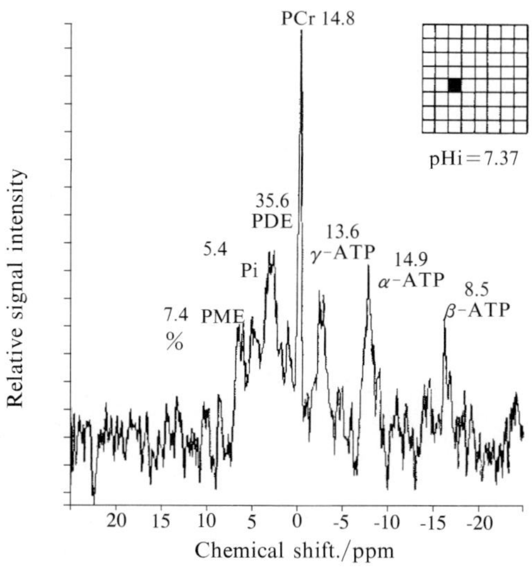

Fig. 55-9 ^{31}P spectrum of right mesial temporal lobe (voxel 11).

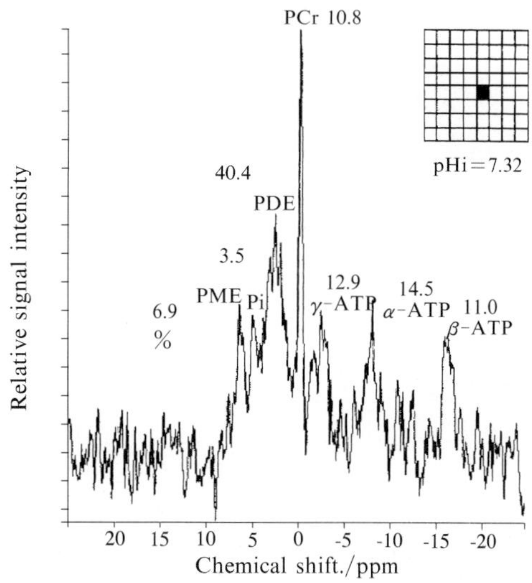

Fig. 55-10 ^{31}P spectrum of left mesial temporal lobe (voxel 13).

CASE 56

CASE 56: A 63-year-old female

Dementia of Alzheimer type

Age at onset: about 61 years.

Moderate dementia with memory disturbance, impairment of language such as paraphasia, and personality changes were present. The signal intensity is almost symmetric in the ^{31}P contour map and metabolite image in Figures 56-1 and 2. The signal intensities in the right temporal lobe are reduced in the total ATP contour map and metabolite image in Figures 56-3 and 4. The PME contour map and metabolite image in Figures 56-5 and 6 show reduced signal intensities in the left frontal lobe. In the PDE contour map and metabolite image in Figures 56-7 and 8, signal intensities are reduced in the mesial temporal lobes. In Figure 56-10 a ^{31}P spectrum from the voxel 13 (Figure 56-9) in the left mesial temporal lobe, the %PDE is decreased. The decreases in % PDE suggests disturbances in the phospholipids, and changes in the distribution of ATP signal intensity indicates alterations in high-energy phosphate metabolism.

R 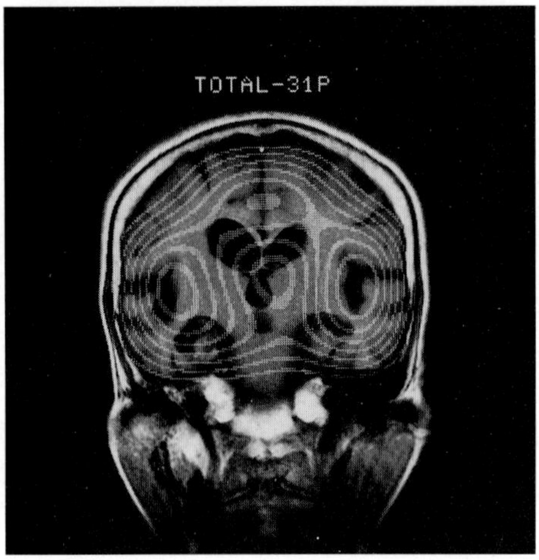 L

Fig. 56-1 Coronal ^{31}P contour map superimposed on T_1-weighted image (500/15).

R 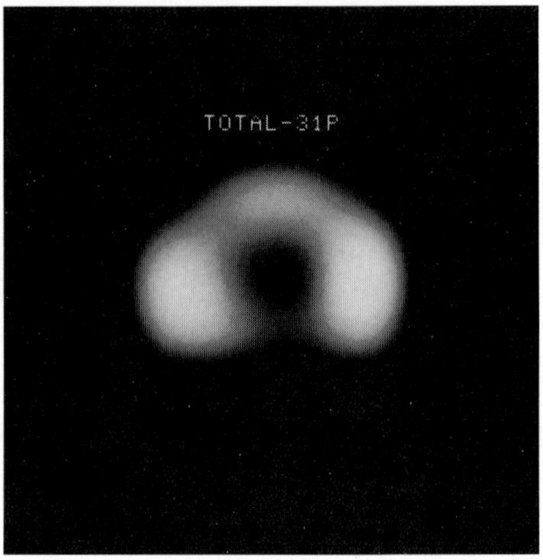 L

Fig. 56-2 Coronal ^{31}P metabolite image.

R 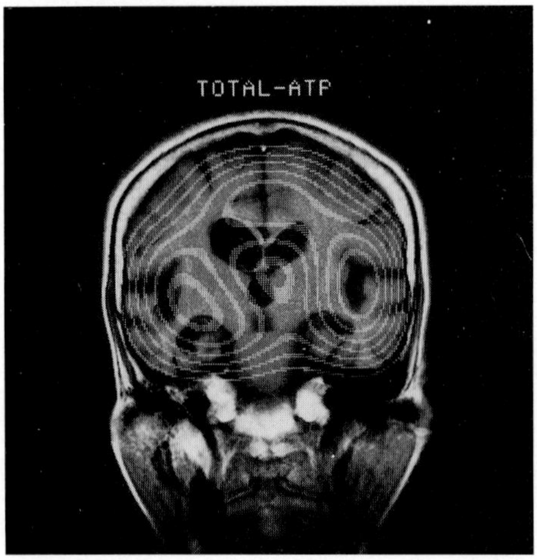 L

Fig. 56-3 Coronal total ATP contour map superimposed on T_1-weighted image (500/15).

R 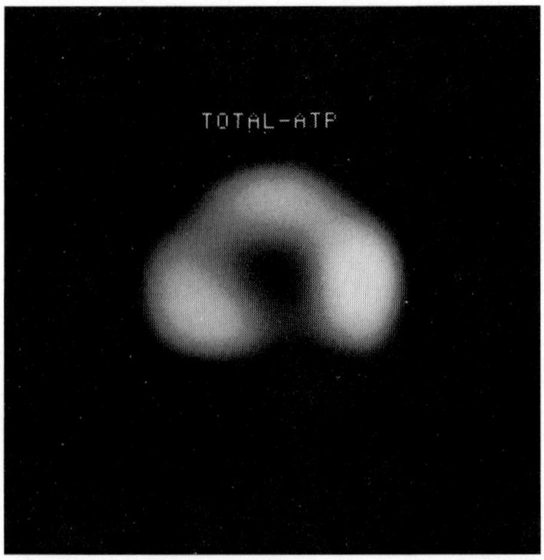 L

Fig. 56-4 Coronal total ATP metabolite image.

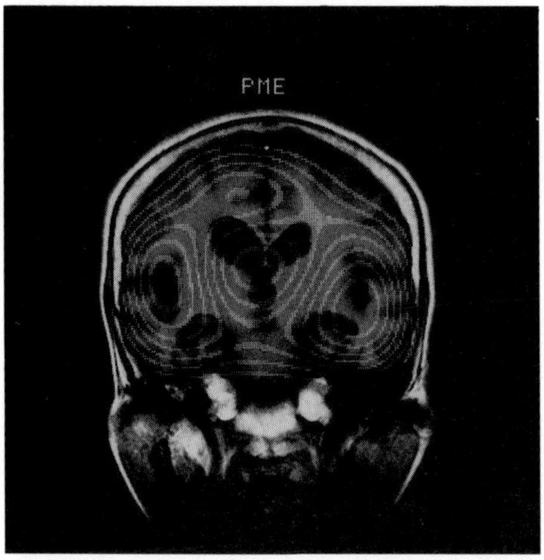

Fig. 56-5 Coronal PME contour map superimposed on T_1-weighted image (500/15).

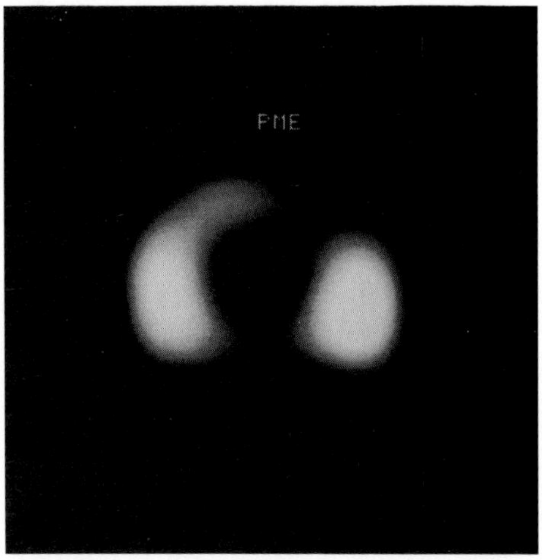

Fig. 56-6 Coronal PME metabolite image.

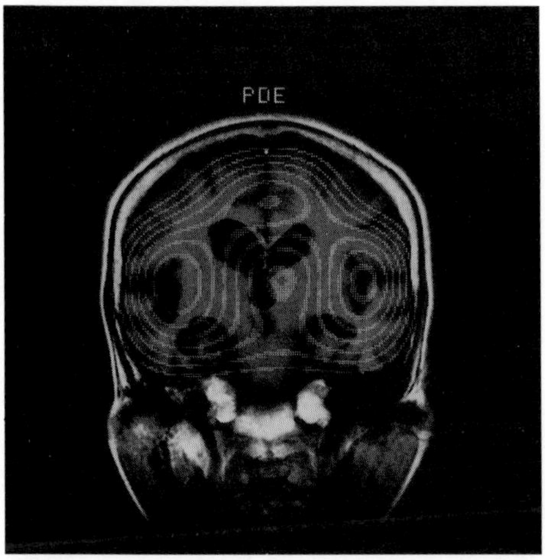

Fig. 56-7 Coronal PDE contour map superimposed on T_1-weighted image (500/15).

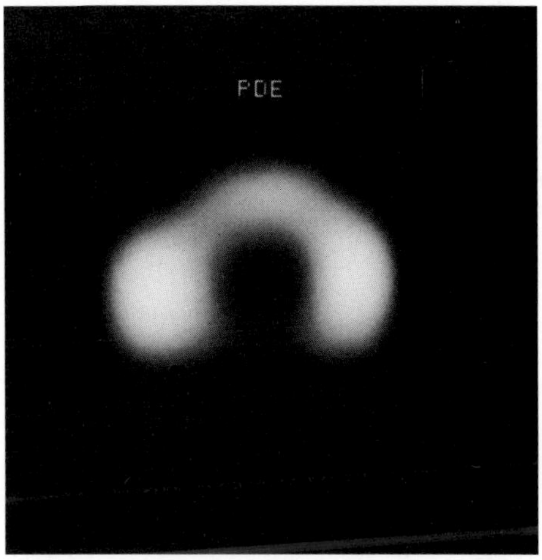

Fig. 56-8 Coronal PDE metabolite image.

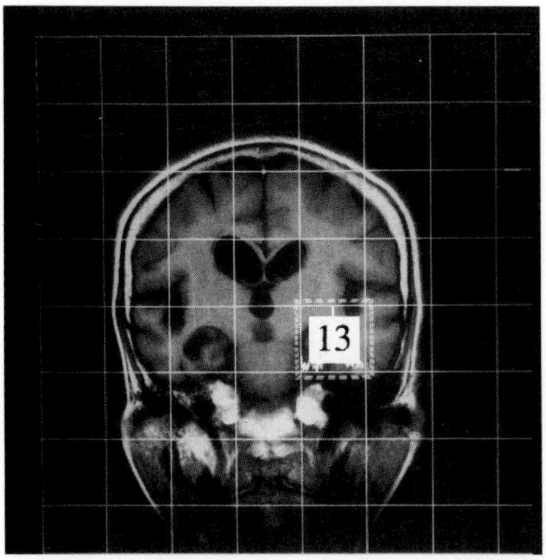

Fig. 56-9 T_1-weighted image showing the position of 3×3×4cm^3 voxel 13.

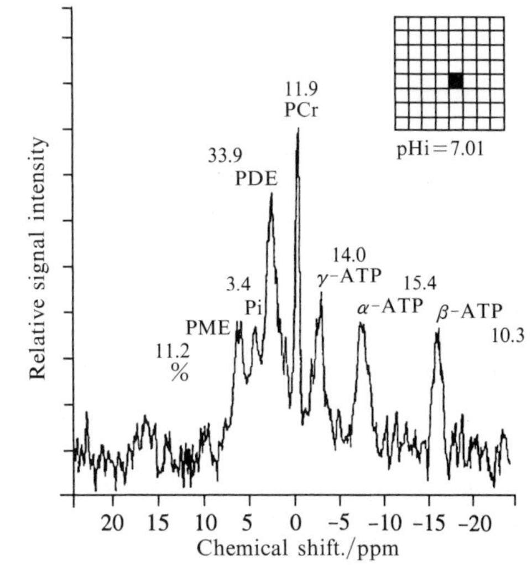

Fig. 56-10 ^{31}P spectrum of left mesial temporal lobe (voxel 13).

CASE 57-1

CASE 57-1: **Probable Pick's disease**

Age at onset : 43 years.

1. First ^{31}P MRS study at 44 years

Early stage of Pick's disease. The patient was an excellent technical expert. One year prior to this examination, a mild decrease in attention span and deterioration of interpersonal relationships were noticed in his workplace, causing him to resign from his job. Although changes in character and episodes of tactless and insensitive behaviors were observed, the Wechsler Adult Intelligence Scale (WAIS) was in the normal range (verbal score, 85; performance score 89; full scale IQ, 86). The standard neurological examination was also normal. In Figures 57-1-1 and 2, the contour map and the metabolite image of ^{31}P are almost symmetrical and in the normal range. A small decrease in signal intensities is observed in the frontal lobe in the total ATP images (Figures 57-1-3 and 4). The PDE signal intensity is decreased in the left frontal lobe (Figures 57-1-7 and 8), suggesting disturbance of the phospholipids. The PCr image shows decreased signal intensities in the frontal lobe and the left basal ganglia region (Figures 57-1-9 and 10). The decrease in the PCr signal intensities suggests a disturbance in high-energy phosphate metabolism, which can be detected in the early stage of Pick's disease by MRS. Reduction in high-energy phosphate metabolism and the disturbance of phospholipids in the frontal lobe may be associated with psychological changes.

R 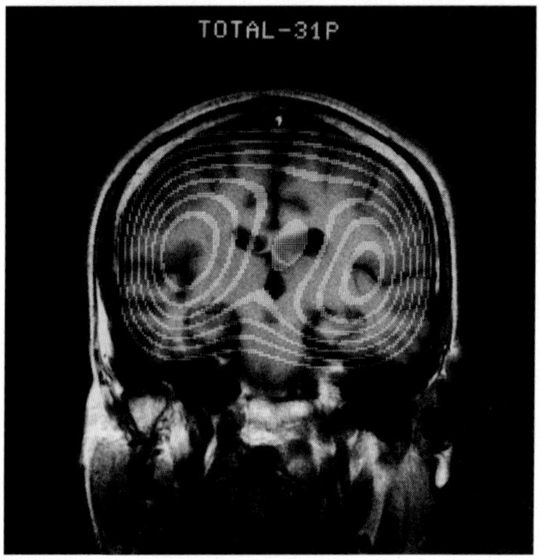 L

Fig. 57-1-1 Coronal ^{31}P contour map superimposed on T_1-weighted image (500/15).

R 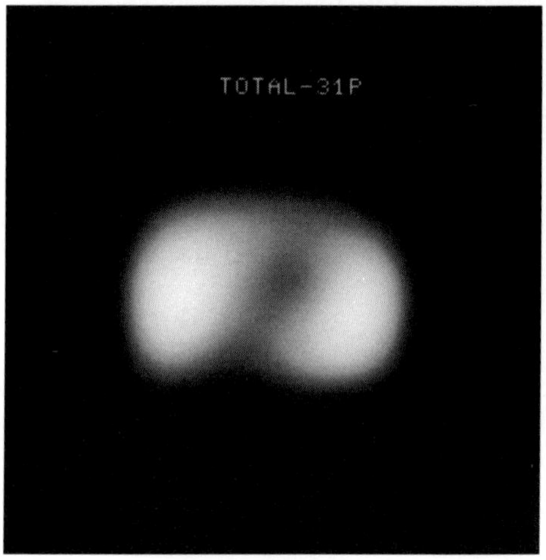 L

Fig. 57-1-2 Coronal ^{31}P metabolite image.

R 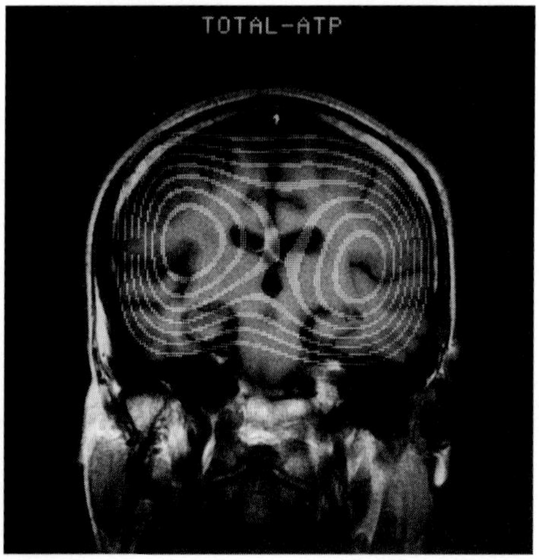 L

Fig. 57-1-3 Coronal total ATP contour map superimposed on T_1-weighted image(500/15).

R 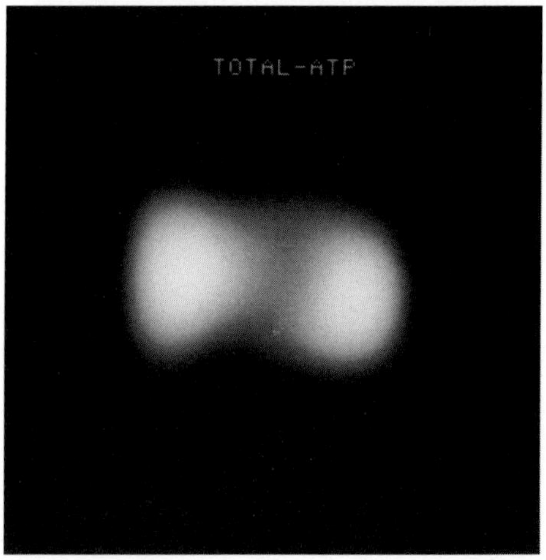 L

Fig. 57-1-4 Coronal total ATP metabolite image.

R 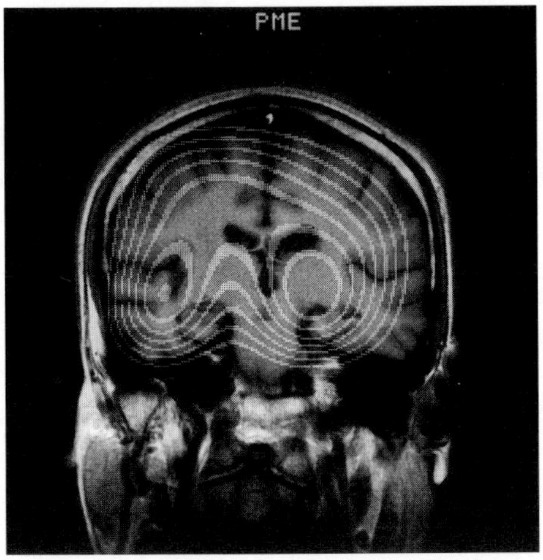 L

Fig. 57-1-5 Coronal PME contour map superimposed on T_1-weighted image (500/15).

R 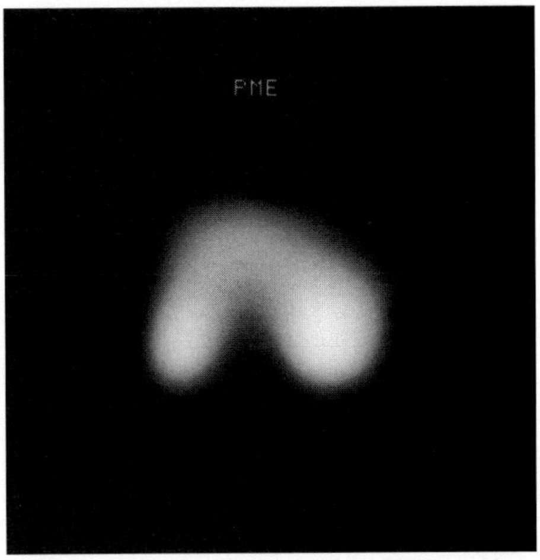 L

Fig. 57-1-6 Coronal PME metabolite image.

R 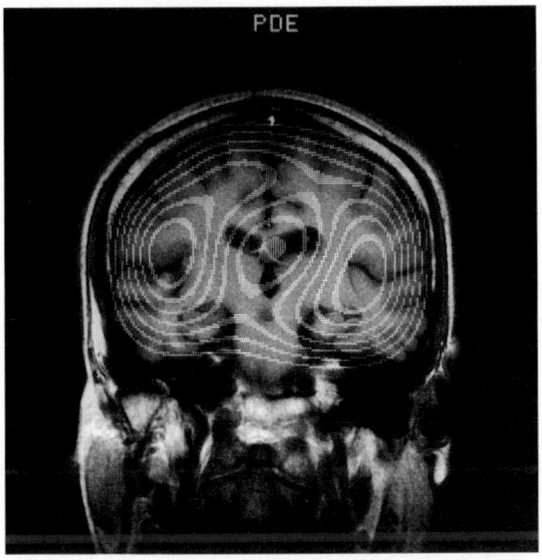 L

Fig. 57-1-7 Coronal PDE contour map superimposed on T_1-weighted image (500/15).

R 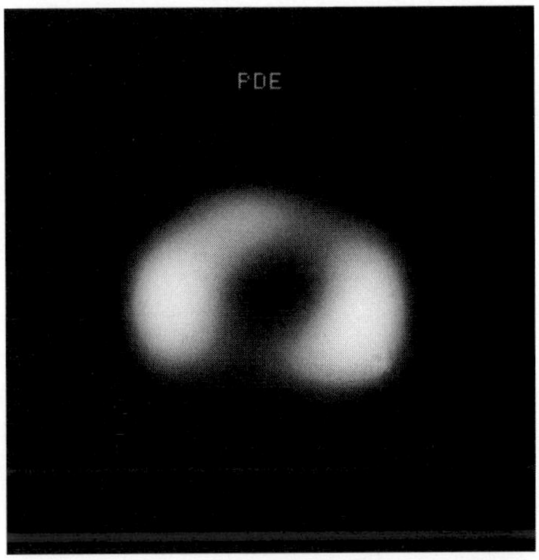 L

Fig. 57-1-8 Coronal PDE metabolite image.

R 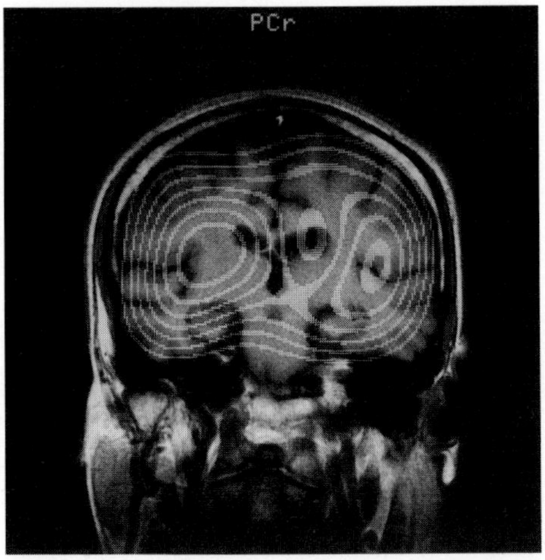 L

Fig. 57-1-9 Coronal PCr contour map superimposed on T_1-weighted image (500/15).

R 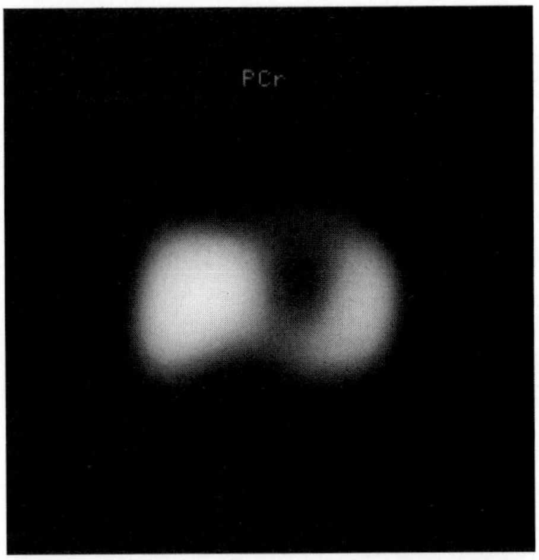 L

Fig. 57-1-10 Coronal PCr metabolite image.

CASE 57-2

CASE 57-2: **Probable Pick's disease**

Age at onset : 43 years.

2. Second ^{31}P MRS study at 44 years (4 months after the first examination)

Pick's disease early middle stage. The patient was divorced and living with his parents in a relaxed, stress-free environment. He began to show mild euphoria and a tendency toward emotional lability. The results of the Wechsler Adult Intelligence Scale showed improvement over the first examination (verbal score, 94 ; performance score, 93 ; full scale IQ, 93). The standard neurological examination was also normal. In Figures 57-2-1 and 2, the contour map and the metabolite image of ^{31}P show a decreased signal intensity in the mesial temporal lobe. The total ATP images also illustrate a reduction of signal intensity in the mesial temporal lobe (Figures 57-2-3 and 4). The signal intensites of PME are markedly increased in the middle region of the frontal lobe and the left temporal lobe, and reduced in the right temporal lobe (Figures 57-2-5 and 6). The signal intensities of PDE are decreased in the mesial temporal lobes (Figures 57-2-7 and 8). Changes in PME and PDE suggest that alterations in phospholipids extended from the frontal lobe to the temporal lobe over a 4 month period. In Figures 57-2-9 and 10, the PCr signal intensities are elevated in the right basal ganglia region and reduced in the mesial temporal lobe, suggesting the spread in disturbance of high-energy phosphate metabolism from the frontal lobe to the mesial temporal lobe, as well. The second ^{31}P MRS study demonstrates the acceleration of Pick's disease over 4 months.

R 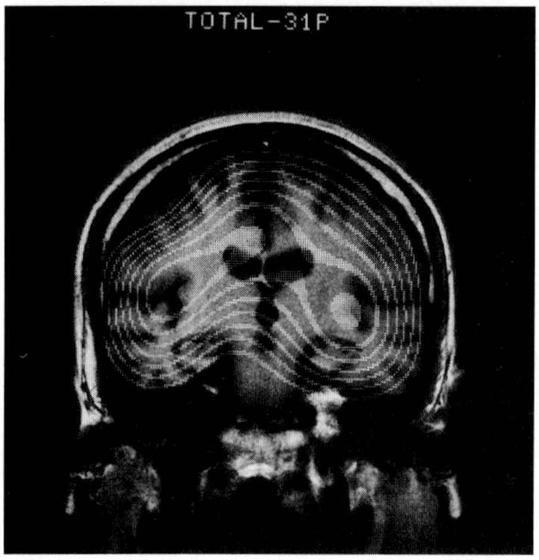 L

Fig. 57-2-1 Coronal ^{31}P contour map superimposed on T_1-weighted image (500/15).

R 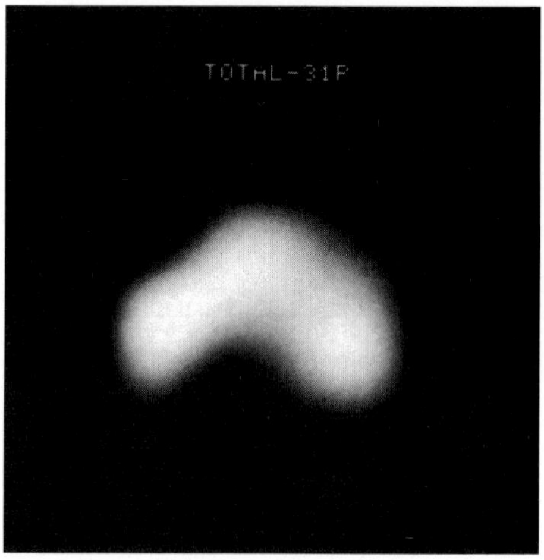 L

Fig. 57-2-2 Coronal ^{31}P metabolite image.

R 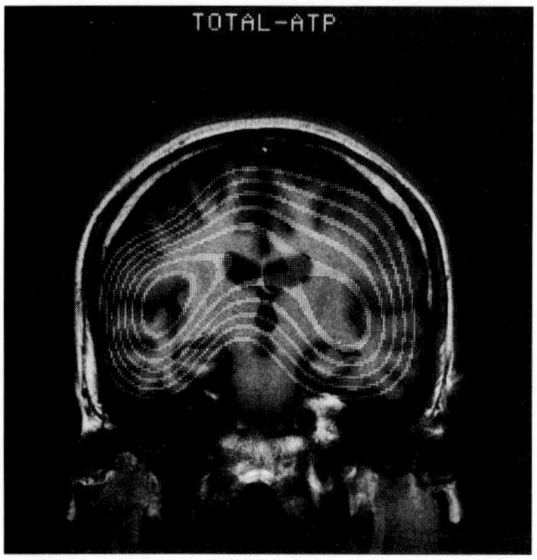 L

Fig. 57-2-3 Coronal total ATP contour map superimposed on T_1-weighted image (500/15).

R 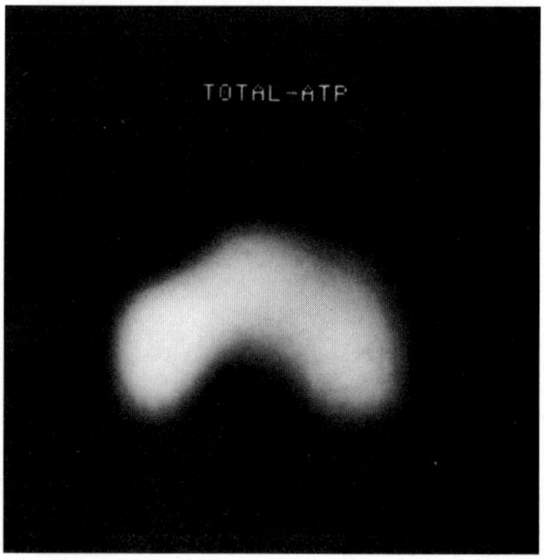 L

Fig. 57-2-4 Coronal total ATP metabolite image.

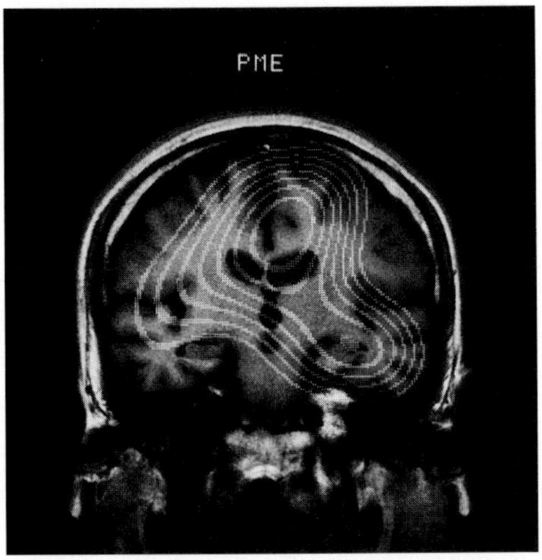

Fig. 57-2-5 Coronal PME contour map superimposed on T_1-weighted image (500/15).

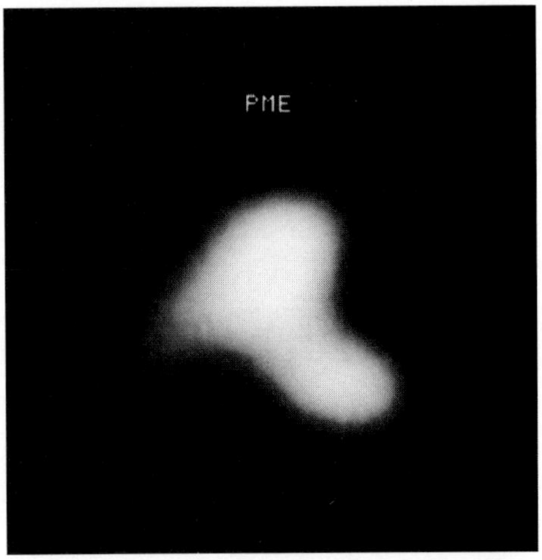

Fig. 57-2-6 Coronal PME metabolite image.

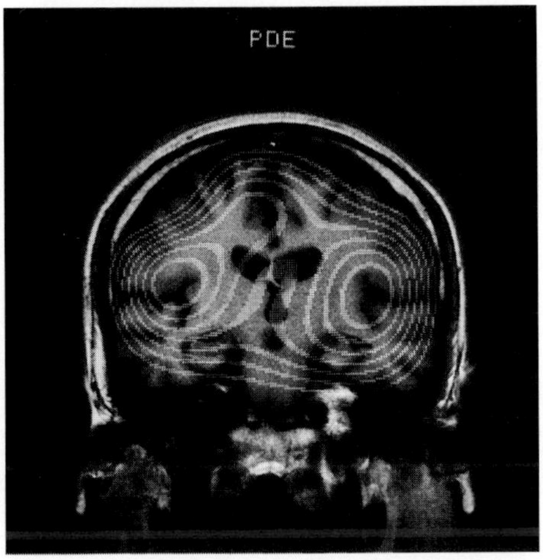

Fig. 57-2-7 Coronal PDE contour map superimposed on T_1-weighted image (500/15).

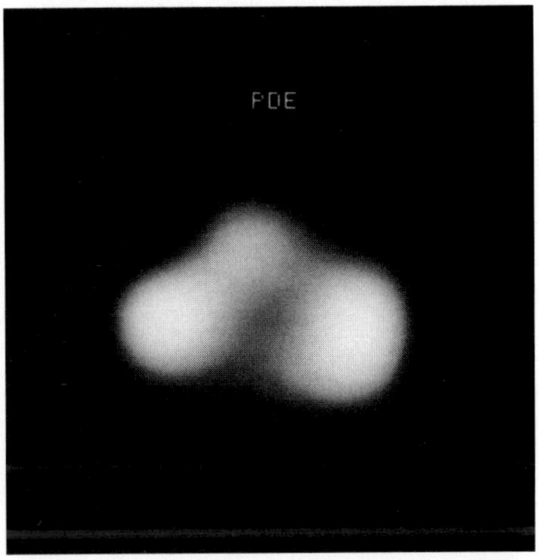

Fig. 57-2-8 Coronal PDE metabolite image.

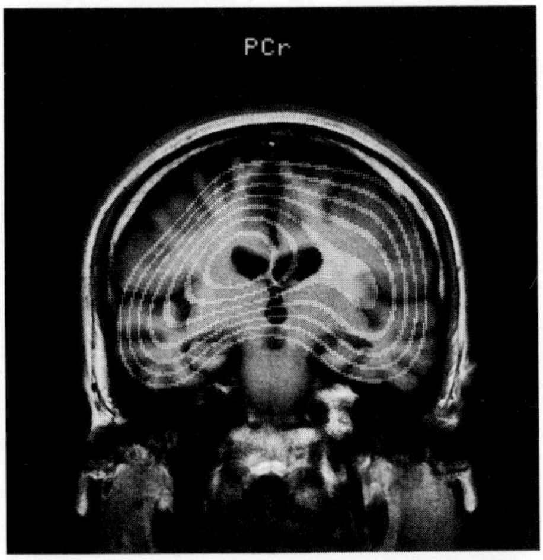

Fig. 57-2-9 Coronal PCr contour map superimposed on T_1-weighted image (500/15).

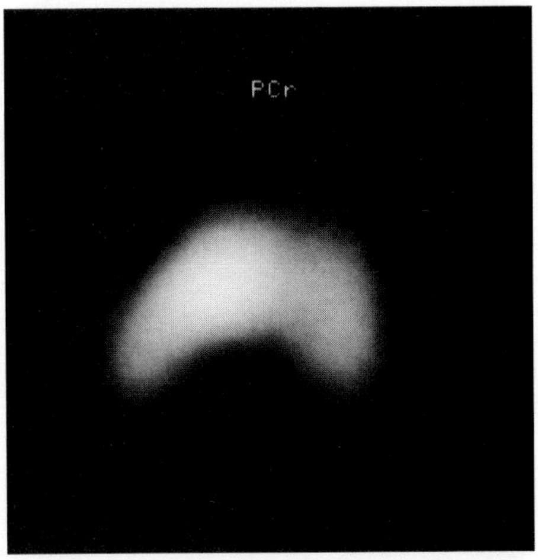

Fig. 57-2-10 Coronal PCr metabolite image.

CASE 57-3

CASE 57-3: **Probable Pick's disease**

Age at onset : 43 years.

3. Third ^{31}P MRS study at 45 years (10 months after the first examination)

Middle stage of Pick's disease. Changes in character, tactless and insensitive behavior, and euphoria had progressed. Distractability, memory disturbance with some hypermnesia, restlessness, and poor judgment with occasional disinhibited behaviour were also observed. The Wechsler Adult Intelligence Scale had worsened (verbal score, 68; performance score could not be tested because of the patient's refusal at examination), when compared to the first and second examinations. In Figures 57-3-1 and 2, the contour map and the metabolite image of ^{31}P shows mildly decreased signal intensities in the frontal lobe and the mesial temporal lobe. The total ATP images also illustrate reduced signal intensities in the frontal lobe and the mesial temporal lobe (Figures 57-3-3 and 4). The signal intensites of PME are reduced in the frontal lobe and the left temporal lobe (Figures 57-3-5 and 6). The signal intensities of PDE are also decreased in the frontal lobe and the temporal lobe (Figures 57-3-7 and 8). Decreased signal intensities of PDE and PME reflect abnormalities in phospholipids. In Figures 57-3-9 and 10, the PCr signal intensities are reduced in the frontal lobe and the mesial temporal lobe, suggesting disturbance in high-energy phosphate metabolism. The third ^{31}P MRS study demonstrates the progress of alterations in phospholipids and high-energy phosphate metabolism in the frontal lobe and the temporal lobe.

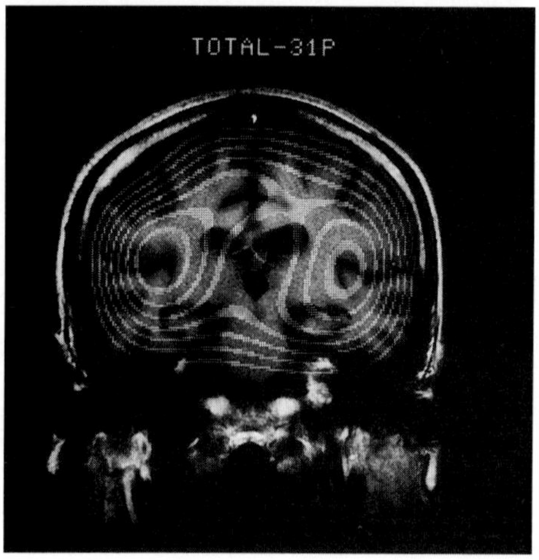

Fig. 57-3-1 Coronal ^{31}P contour map superimposed on T_1-weighted image (500/15).

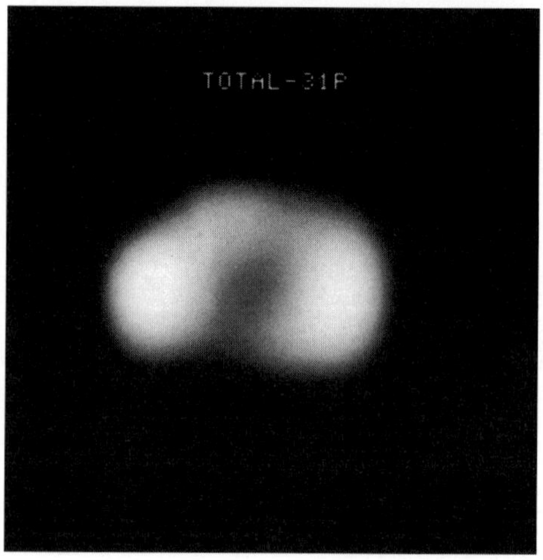

Fig. 57-3-2 Coronal ^{31}P metabolite image.

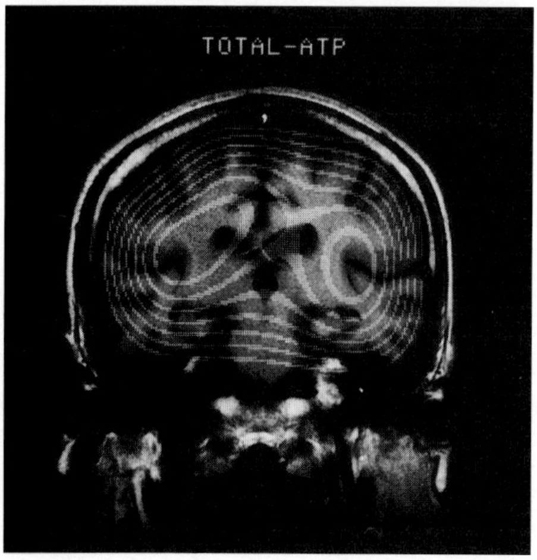

Fig. 57-3-3 Coronal total ATP contour map superimposed on T_1-weighted image (500/15).

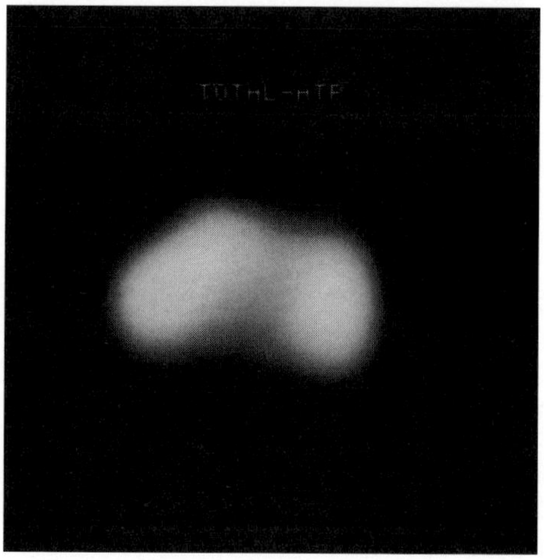

Fig. 57-3-4 Coronal total ATP metabolite image.

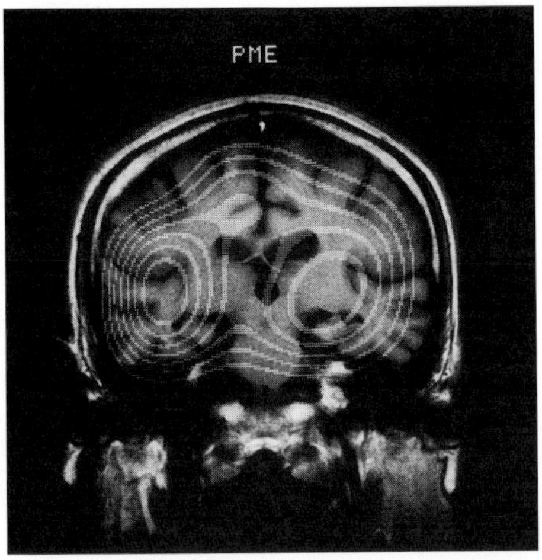

Fig. 57-3-5 Coronal PME contour map superimposed on T_1-weighted image (500/15).

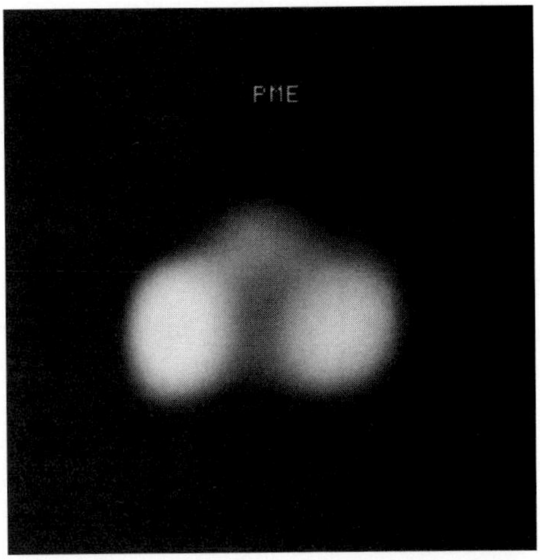

Fig. 57-3-6 Coronal PME metabolite image.

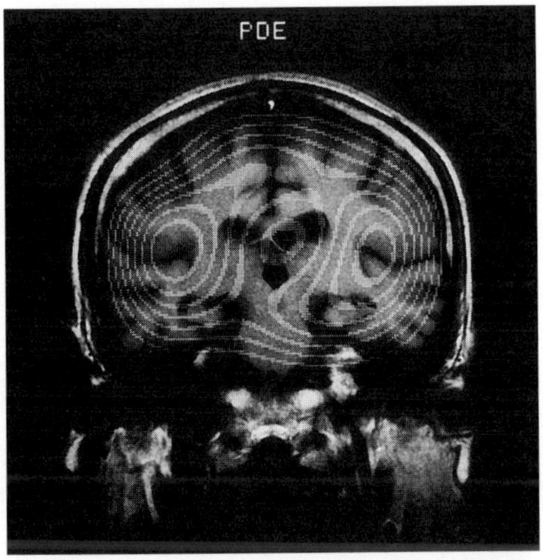

Fig. 57-3-7 Coronal PDE contour map superimposed on T_1-weighted image (500/15).

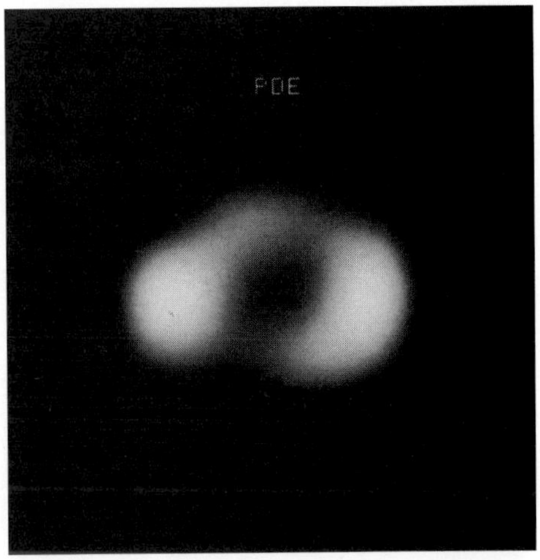

Fig. 57-3-8 Coronal PDE metabolite image.

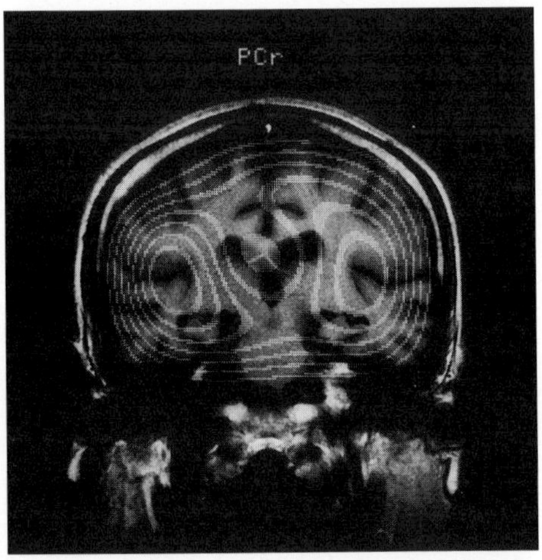

Fig. 57-3-9 Coronal PCr contour map superimposed on T_1-weighted image (500/15).

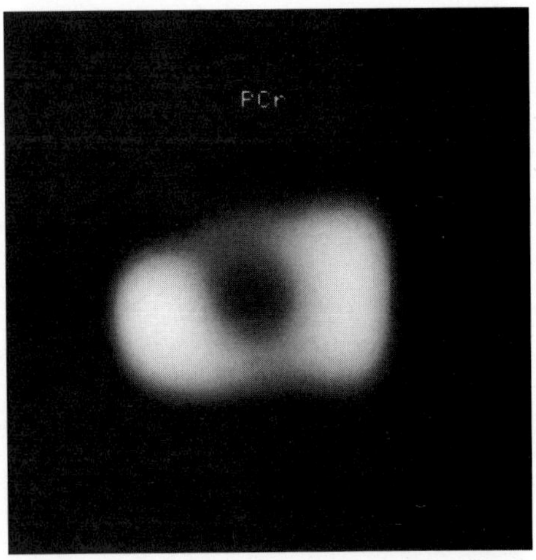

Fig. 57-3-10 Coronal PCr metabolite image.

CASE 57-4

CASE 57-4: **Probable Pick's disease**

Age at onset : 43 years.

4. Fourth ^{31}P MRS study at 45 years (2 years after the first examination)

Late stage of Pick's disease. The general disintegration of personality and intellect had progressed. Loss of speech, affective blunting with indifference, restlessness, wandering, and aimless behaviour were observed. Extrapyramidal signs were present. In Figures 57-4-1 and 2, the contour map and the metabolite image of ^{31}P show marked decreases of signal intensities in the frontal lobe and the mesial temporal lobe. The total ATP images also illustrate marked reductions of signal intensities in the frontal lobe and the mesial temporal lobe (Figures 57-4-3 and 4). The signal intensities of PME have disappeared in the frontal lobe, and are decreased in the mesial temporal lobe (Figures 57-4-5 and 6). The signal intensities of PDE are also decreased in the frontal lobe and the mesial temporal lobe (Figures 57-4-7 and 8). Reduced signal intensities of PDE and PME reflect abnormalities in phospholipids. In Figures 57-4-9 and 10, the PCr signal intensities are severely reduced in the frontal lobe and the mesial temporal lobe, suggesting disturbance in high-energy phosphate metabolism. The fourth ^{31}P MRS study demonstrates severe alterations in phospholipids and high-energy phosphate metabolism in the frontal lobe, the temporal lobe, and the basal ganglia region reflecting advanced dementia at the late stage of Pick's disease.

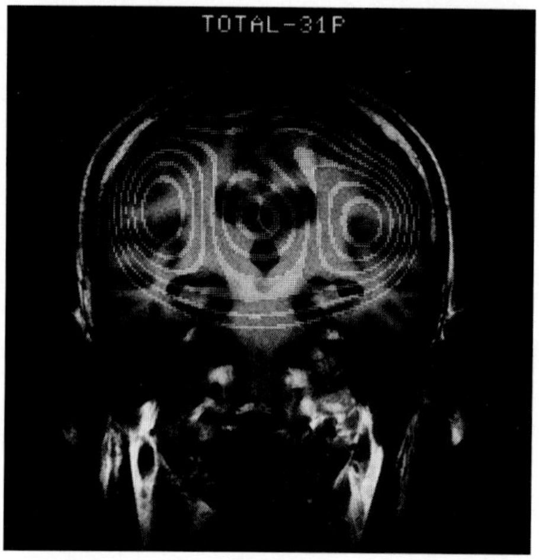

Fig. 57-4-1 Coronal ^{31}P contour map superimposed on T_1-weighted image (500/15).

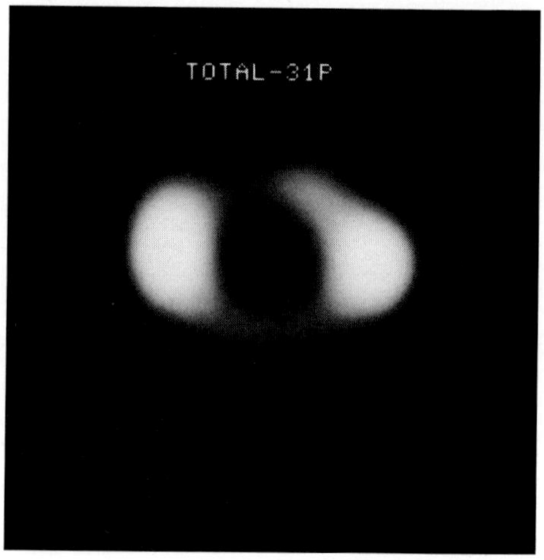

Fig. 57-4-2 Coronal ^{31}P metabolite image.

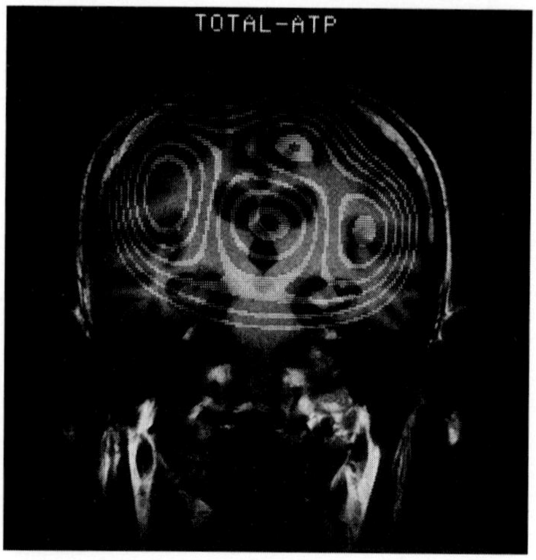

Fig. 57-4-3 Coronal total ATP contour map superimposed on T_1-weighted image (500/15).

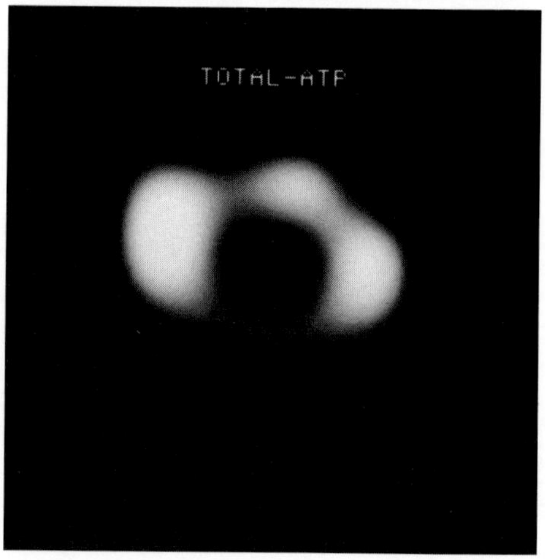

Fig. 57-4-4 Coronal total ATP metabolite image.

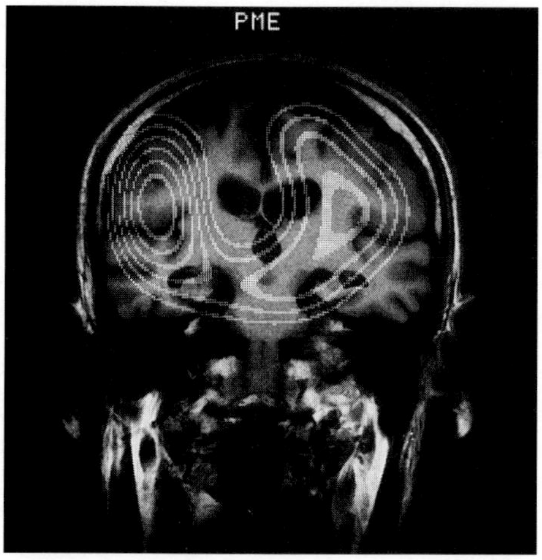

Fig. 57-4-5 Coronal PME contour map superimposed on T_1-weighted image (500/15).

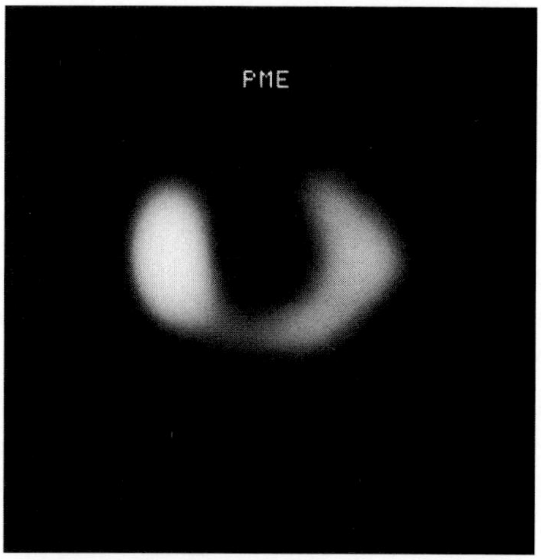

Fig. 57-4-6 Coronal PME metabolite image.

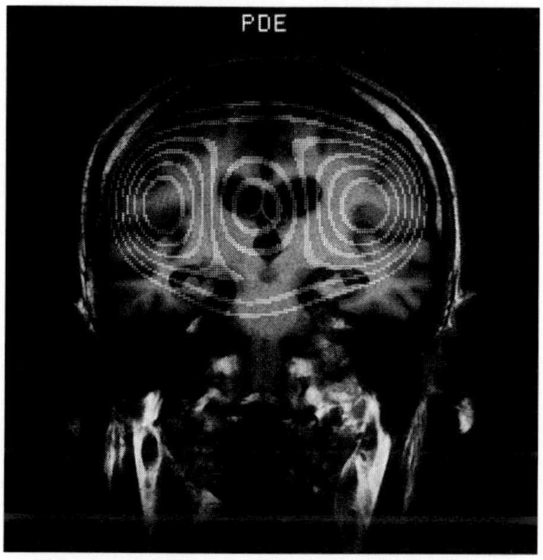

Fig. 57-4-7 Coronal PDE contour map superimposed on T_1-weighted image (500/15).

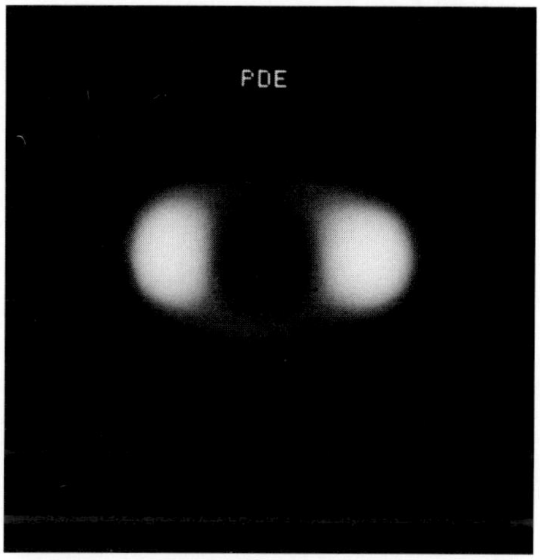

Fig. 57-4-8 Coronal PDE metabolite image.

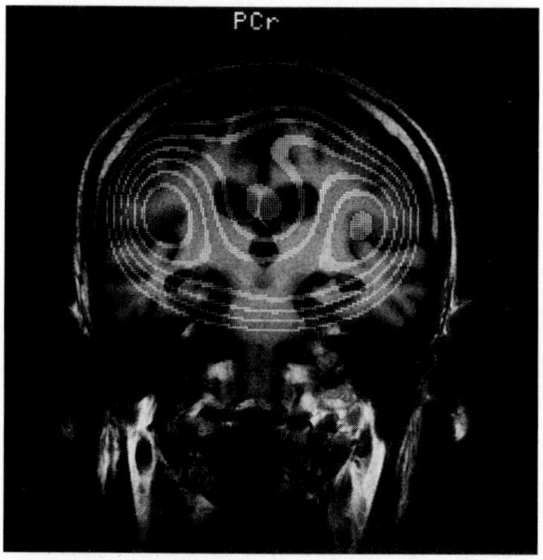

Fig. 57-4-9 Coronal PCr contour map superimposed on T_1-weighted image (500/15).

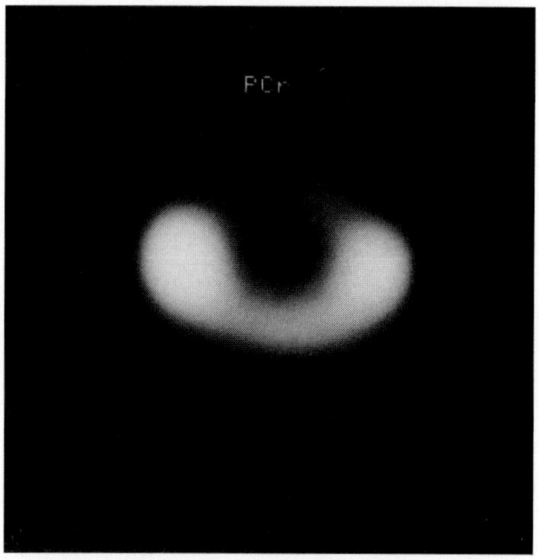

Fig. 57-4-10 Coronal PCr metabolite image.

CASE 57-5

CASE 57-5: **Probable Pick's disease**
Age at onset : 43 years.

^{1}H spectra in the temporal lobe in the late stage of Pick's disease, and ^{31}P spectra in the right and left frontal lobes taken from study 1-4.

^{1}H spectra in the temporal lobe in the late stage.

Figures 57-5-1 and 2 show ^{1}H spectra in the temporal lobe. ^{1}H spectra in the frontal lobe was not obtained, because the voxel size of $3\times3\times3cm^3$ was too large to place in the frontal lobe. The NAA/Cr ratio is reduced, and the Cho/Cr ratio is in the normal range in the right temporal lobe (Figure 57-5-1). The NAA/Cr ratio is decreased, and the Cho/Cr ratio is slightly increased in the left temporal lobe (Figure 57-5-2). The reduced NAA/Cr ratios suggest neuronal loss in the temporal lobe.

Changes in ^{31}P spectra from the first study to the fourth study.

The %PDE is increased in the early stage (Figures 57-5-3 and 4), increased further in the middle stage (Figures 57-5-7 and 8), and decreased at the late stage (Figures 57-5-9 and 10). The %PME in the left frontal lobe is increased in the middle stage (Figure 57-5-6), and the PME/PDE ratio is also markedly elevated at 0.50. The %PCr is increased in the early middle stage (Figures 57-5-5 and 6). The β-ATP is decreased, and is increased according to the progression of the disease. These findings suggest that alterations in phospholipids and high-energy metabolism are due to the progress of the disease.

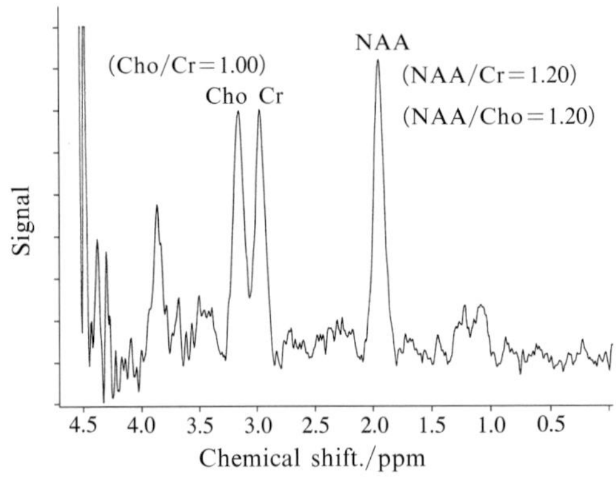

Fig. 57-5-1 ^{1}H spectrum of right mesial temporal lobe. PRESS (1,500/135)

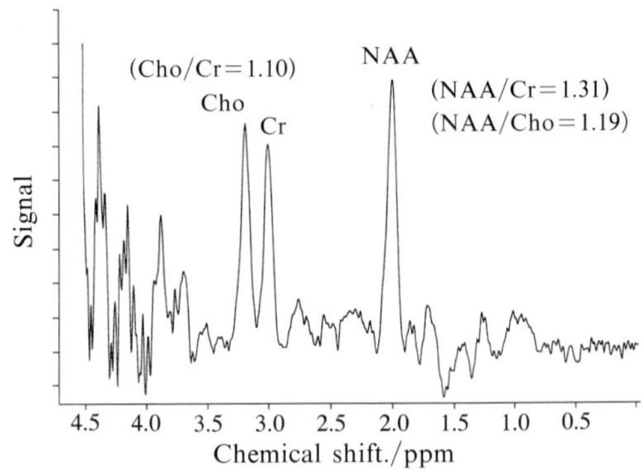

Fig. 57-5-2 ^{1}H spectrum of left mesial temporal lobe. PRESS (1,500/135)

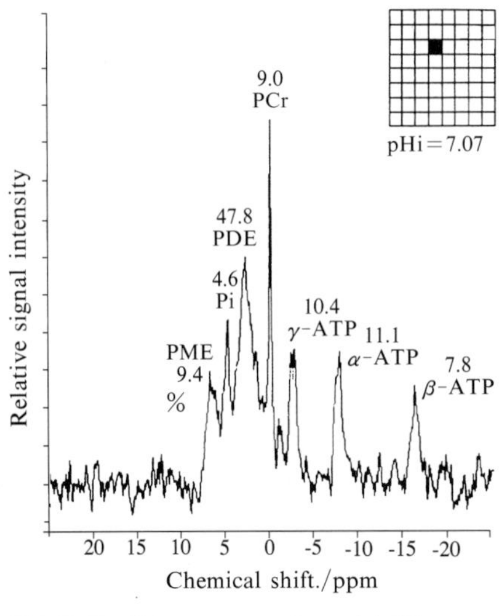

Fig. 57-5-3 ^{31}P spectrum of voxel 1 (first examination.) Early stage.

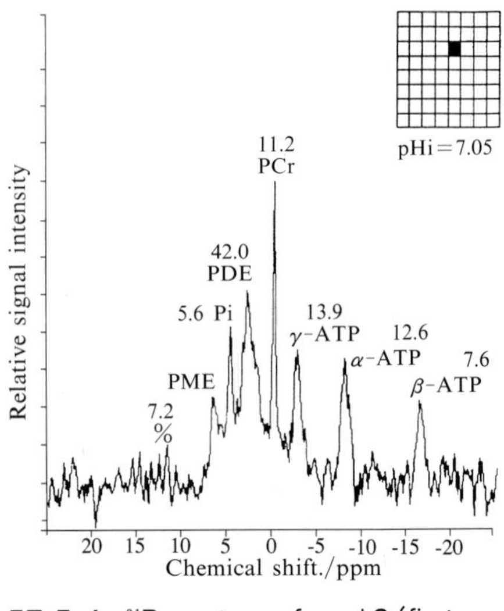

Fig. 57-5-4 ^{31}P spectrum of voxel 2 (first examination.) Early stage.

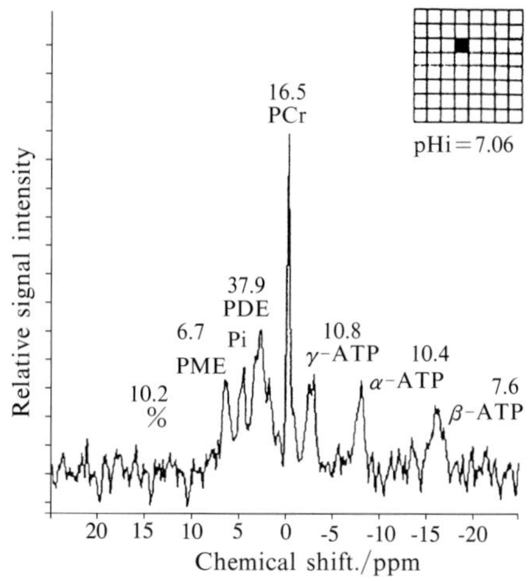

Fig. 57-5-5 ^{31}P spectrum of voxel 1. (Second examination: 4 months since the first examination.) Early middle stage.

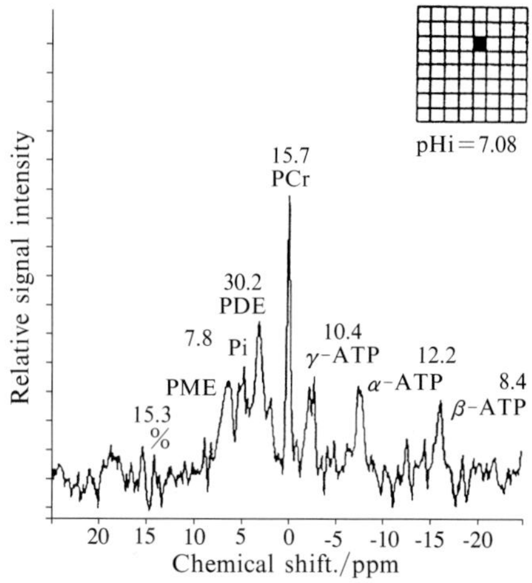

Fig. 57-5-6 ^{31}P spectrum of voxel 2. (Second examination: 4 months since the first examination.) Early middle stage.

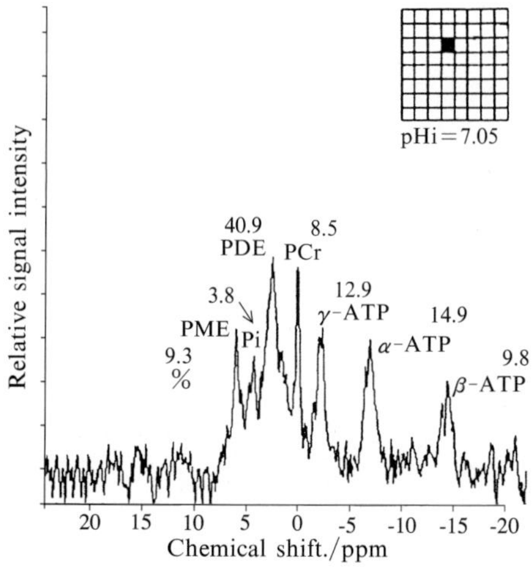

Fig. 57-5-7 ^{31}P spectrum of voxel 1. (Third examination: 10 months since the first examination.) Middle stage.

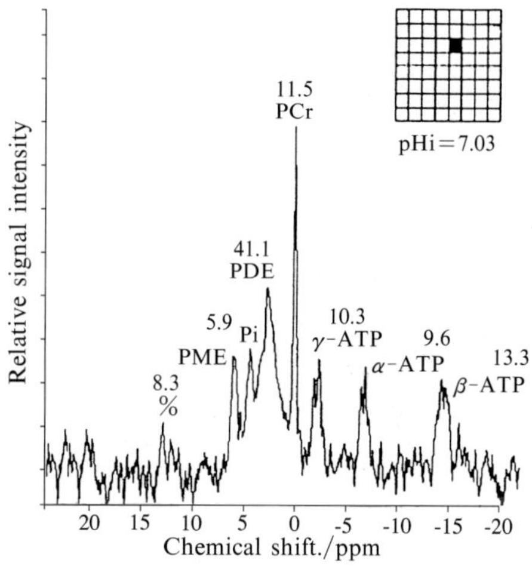

Fig. 57-5-8 ^{31}P spectrum of voxel 2. (Third examination: 10 months since the first examination.) Middle stage.

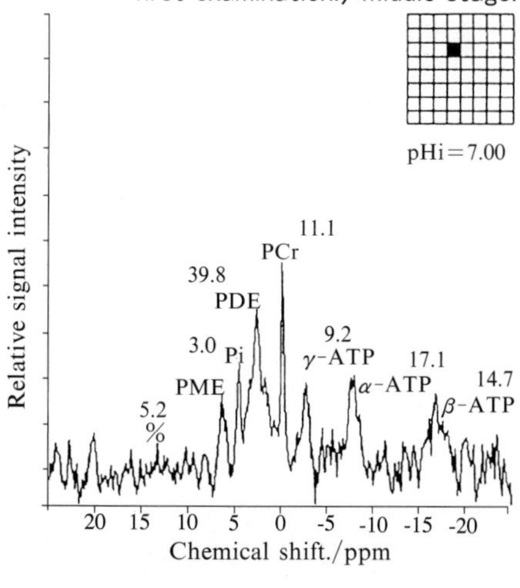

Fig. 57-5-9 ^{31}P spectrum of voxel 1. (Fourth examination: 2 years since the first examination.) Late stage.

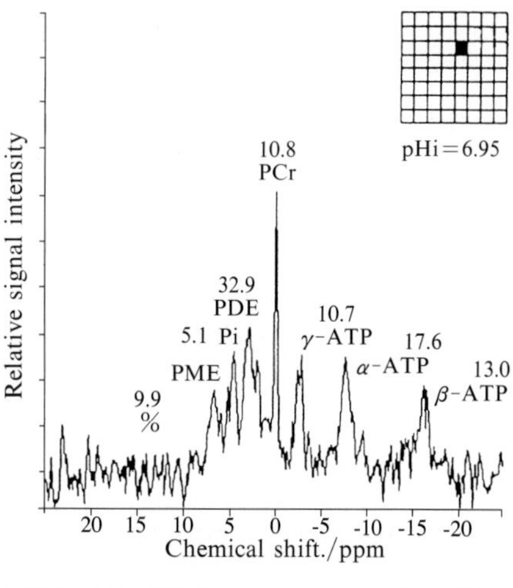

Fig. 57-5-10 ^{31}P spectrum of voxel 2. (Fourth examination: 2 years since the first examination.) Late stage.

CASE 58

CASE 58: A 66-year-old female

Multi-infarct dementia

Age at onset : 65 years.

The patient had mild dysarthria, left hemiprar-esis, tonic-clonic convulsion, and mild intellectual deterioration, but preserved her social competence. The T_2-weighted image in Figure 58-1 shows periventricular high signal intensity (PVH), multiple cerebral infarction, iron deposition in the basal ganglia, and enlargement of the ventricular system and cerebral sulci. In the ^{31}P metabolite image in Figure 58-2, the signal intensiy is reduced in the frontal lobe, indicating metabolic dysfunction due to vascular damage. The signal intensity is decreased in the left frontal lobe and the left mesial temporal lobe in the total ATP contour map and metabolite image, indicating a disturbance in high-energy phosphate metabolism (Figures 58-3 and 4). In the PME contour map and metabolite image in Figures 58-5 and 6, signal intensities are reduced in the frontal lobe and right temporal lobe. In the Pi contour map and metabolite image in Figures 58-7 and 8, signal intensities are also reduced in the frontal lobe and left temporal lobe. The PDE contour map and metabolite image in Figures 58-9 and 10 show reductions in signal intensity in the basal ganglia regions, the right frontal lobe and left mesial temporal lobe. Alterations in PDE and PME signal intensities suggest an abnormality of phospholipids.

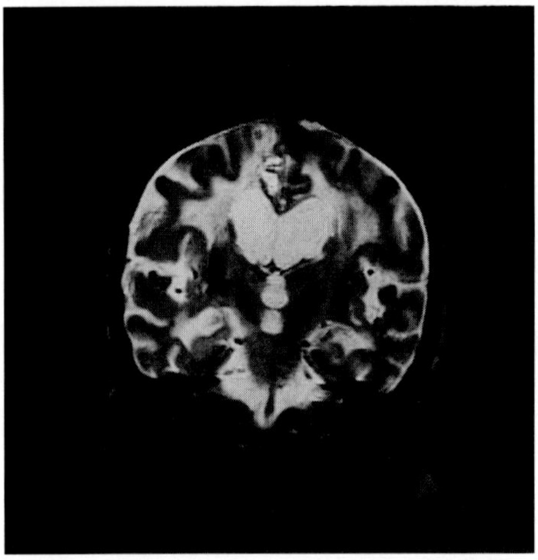

Fig. 58-1 Coronal T_2-weighted image (2,200/90).

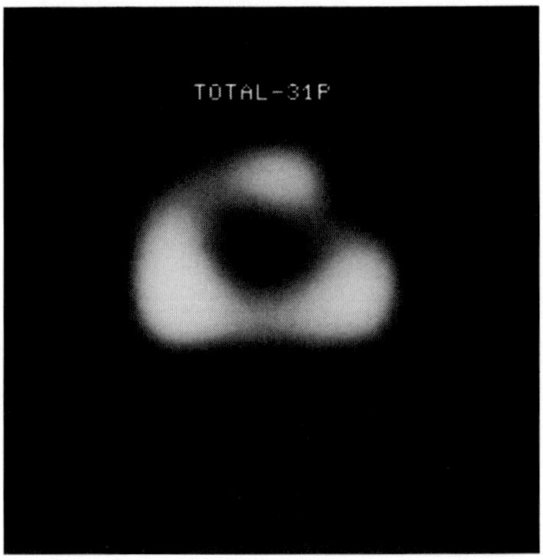

Fig. 58-2 Coronal ^{31}P metabolite image.

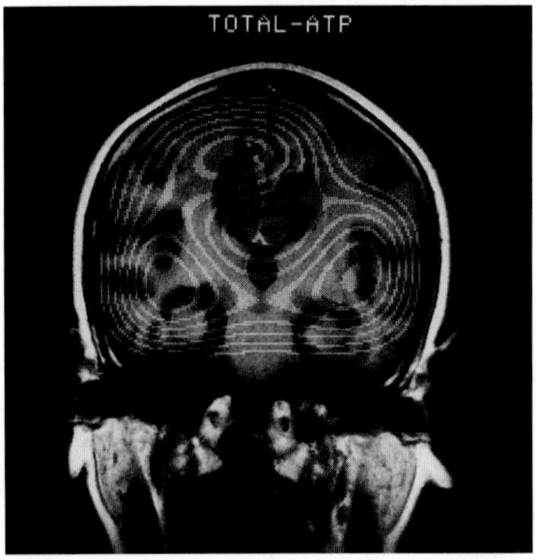

Fig. 58-3 Coronal total ATP contour map superimposed on T_1-weighted image (500/15).

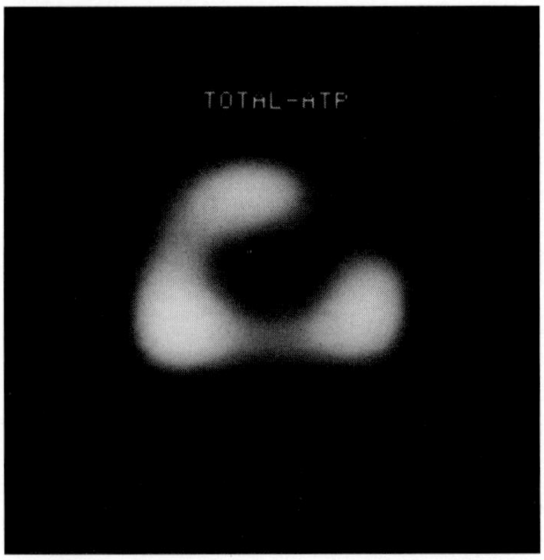

Fig. 58-4 Coronal total ATP metabolite image.

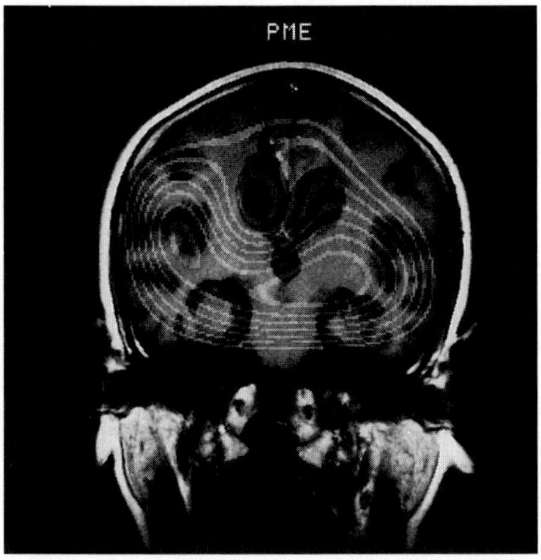

Fig. 58-5 Coronal PME contour map superimposed on T_1-weighted image (500/15).

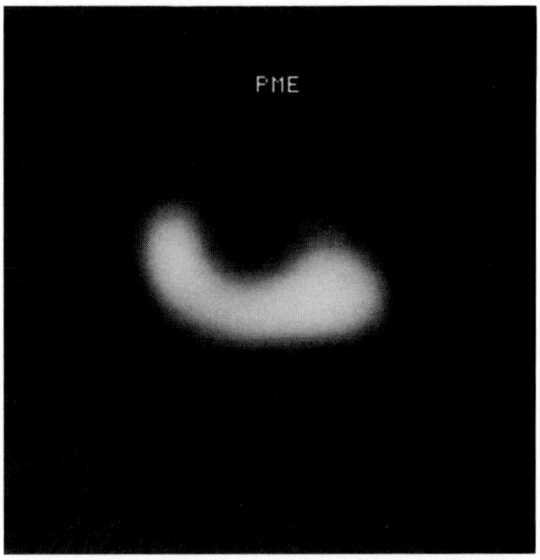

Fig. 58-6 Coronal PME metabolite image.

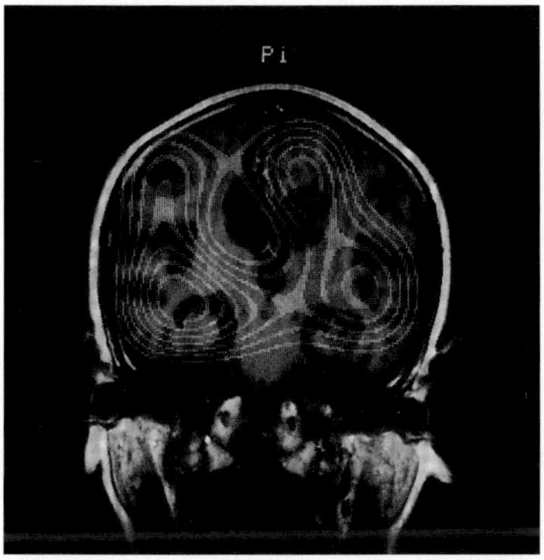

Fig. 58-7 Coronal Pi contour map superimposed on T_1-weighted image (500/15).

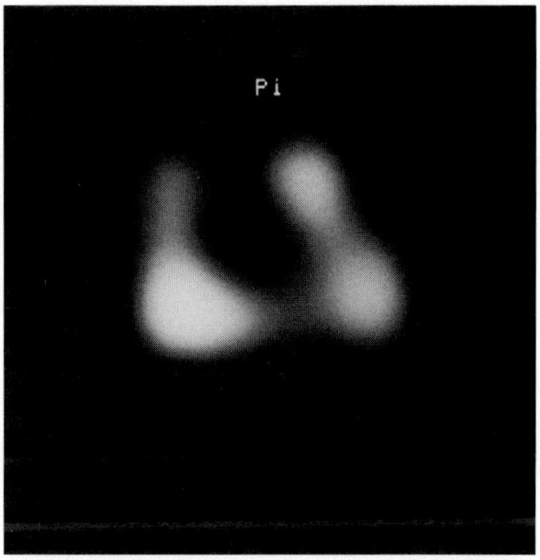

Fig. 58-8 Coronal Pi metabolite image.

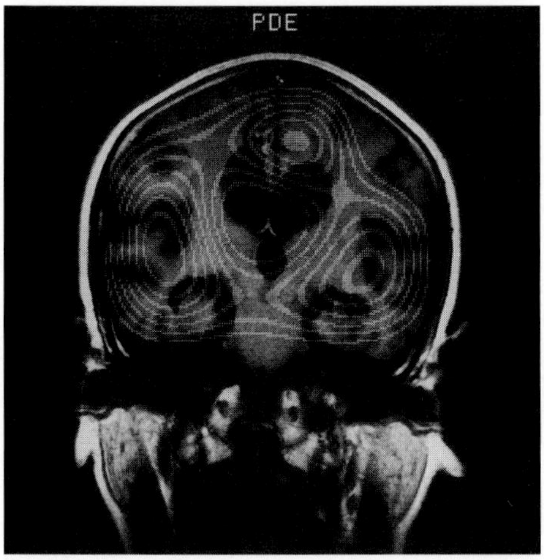

Fig. 58-9 Coronal PDE contour map superimposed on T_1-weighted image (500/15).

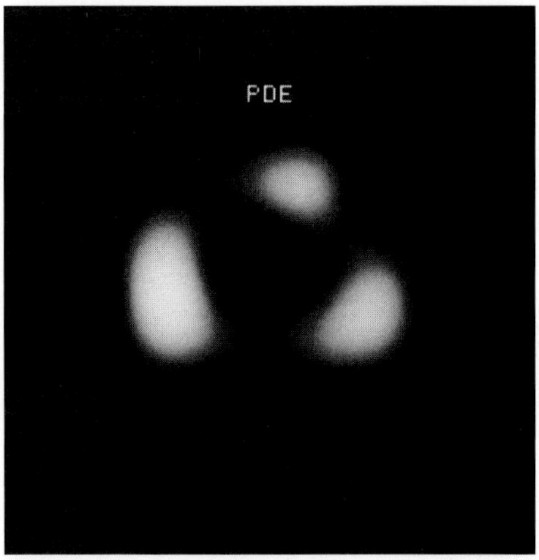

Fig. 58-10 Coronal PDE metabolite image.

CASE 59

CASE 59: An 86-year-old male

Multi-infarct dementia

Age at onset : 86 years.

Although personality was preserved, the patient exhibited emotional changes such as lability and psychotic episodes with paranoid delusions. The T_2-weighted image in Figure 59-1 shows periventricular high signal intensity (PVH) and multiple infarction in the basal ganglia region and the frontal lobe, and marked cerebral atrophy. In the ^{31}P metabolite image in Figure 59-2, signal intensities are reduced in the left basal ganglia region and mesial temporal lobe, suggesting metabolic changes due to vascular damage. In the total ATP contour map and metabolite image in Figures 59-3 and 4, signal intensities are decreased in the right temporal lobe and left basal ganglia region, suggesting dysfunction in high-energy phosphate metabolism. The PME signal intensity is reduced in the left temporal lobe and frontal lobe in the contour map and metabolite image (Figures 59-5 and 6). The PDE images in Figures 59-7 and 8 show reductions in the signal intensites in the bilateral basal ganglia regions and mesial temporal lobes, indicating disturbances in phospholipids. In the PCr contour map and metabolite image in Figures 59-9 and 10, the signal intensity is markedly elevated in the right basal ganglia region.

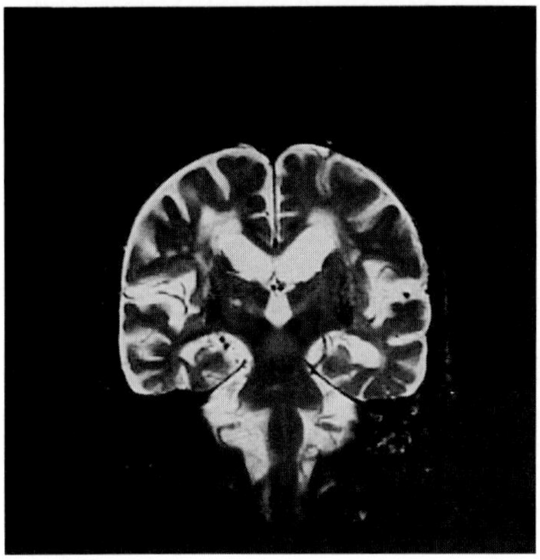

Fig. 59-1 Coronal T_2-weighted image (2,200/90).

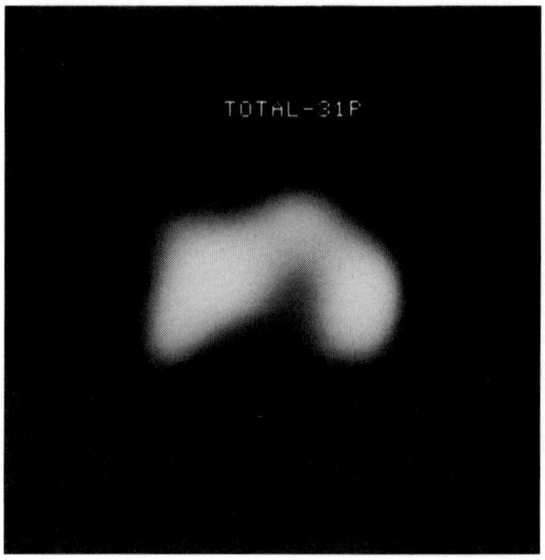

Fig. 59-2 Coronal ^{31}P metabolite image.

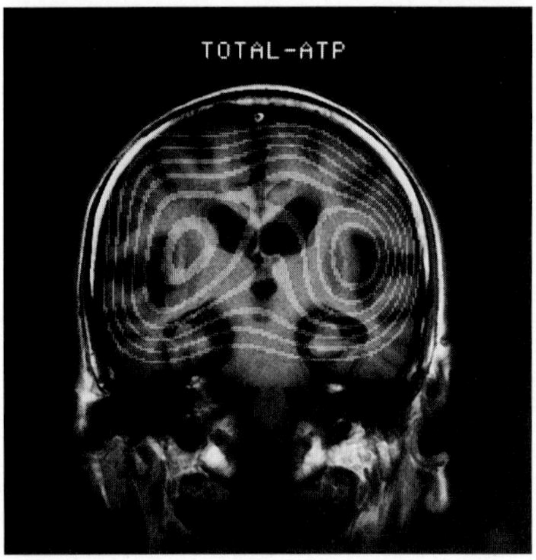

Fig. 59-3 Coronal total ATP contour map superimposed on T_1-weighted image (500/15).

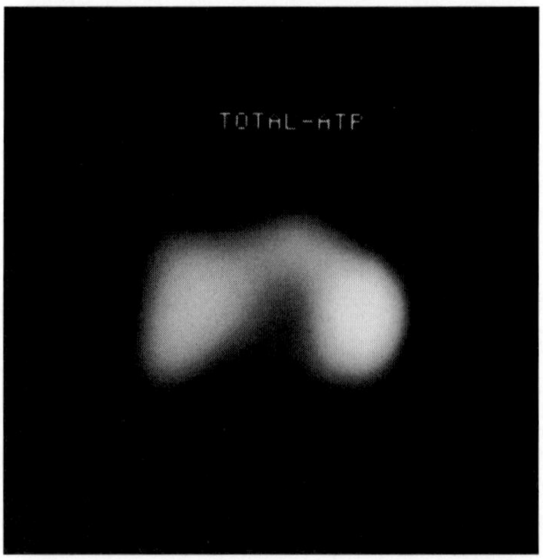

Fig. 59-4 Coronal total ATP metabolite image.

R 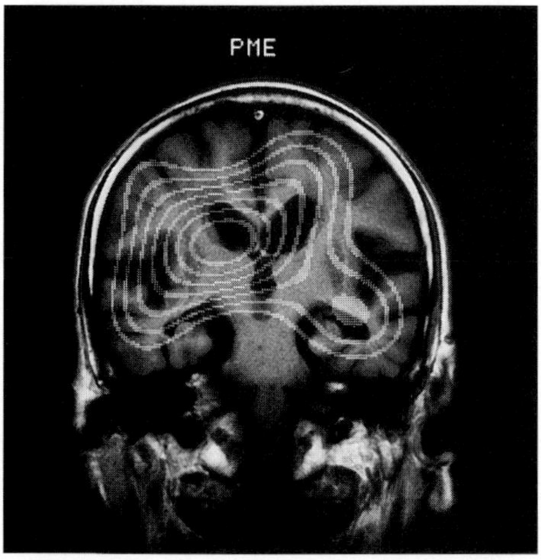 L

Fig. 59-5 Coronal PME contour map superimposed on T_1-weighted image (500/15).

R 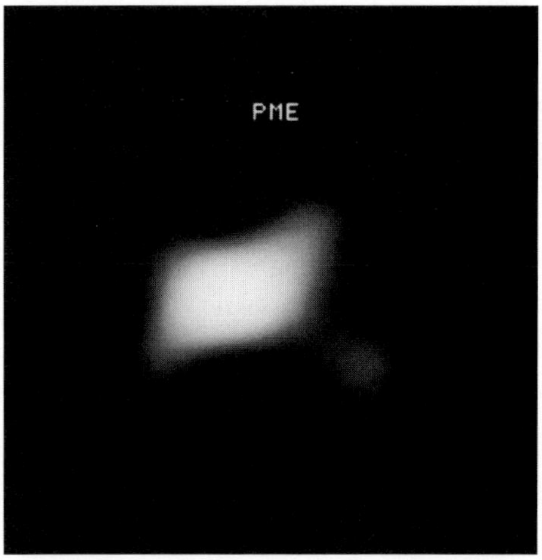 L

Fig. 59-6 Coronal PME metabolite image.

R 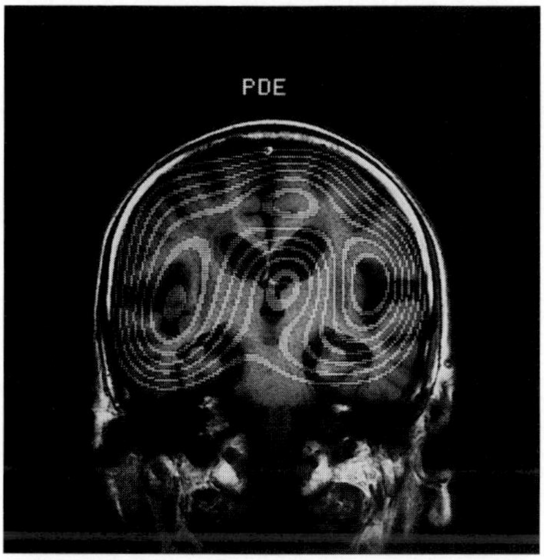 L

Fig. 59-7 Coronal PDE contour map superimposed on T_1-weighted image (500/15).

R 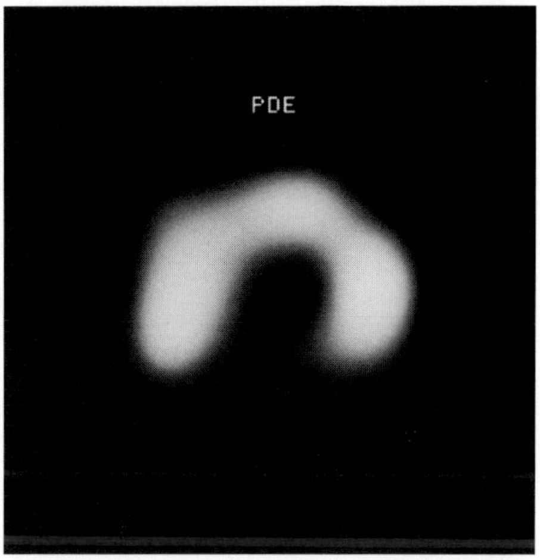 L

Fig. 59-8 Coronal PDE metabolite image.

R 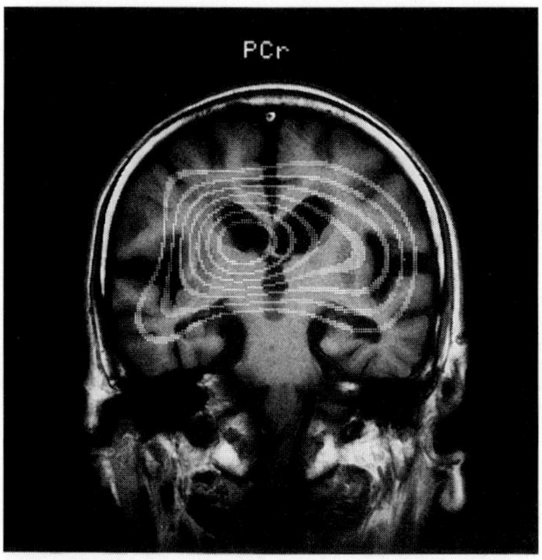 L

Fig. 59-9 Coronal PCr contour map superimposed on T_1-weighted image (500/15).

R 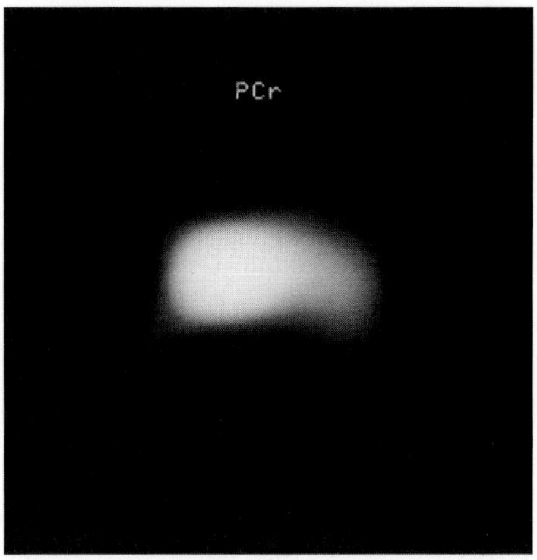 L

Fig. 59-10 Coronal PCr metabolite image.

CASE 60

CASE 60: A 70-year-old male

Binswanger's disease

Age at onset : 66 years.

The patient had gate disturbance and pseudobulbar palsy, and dementia with global intellectual impairment and loss of spontaneity. In the T_2-weighted image in Figure 60-1, multiple areas of high signal intensites are observed in the white matter, and enlargement of the lateral and third ventricles and atrophy of the hippocampus are noted. The ^{31}P metabolite image in Figure 60-2 shows decreases in the signal intensity in the frontal lobe, left basal ganglia region and right mesial temporal lobe. The total ATP contour map and metabolite image in Figures 60-3 and 4 show reductions in the signal intensities from the frontal lobe to the right temporal lobe, indicating a decreased high-energy phosphate metabolism. The PME contour map and metabolite image in Figures 60-5 and 6 show reduced signal intensites in the left temporal lobe. The PDE metabolite image in Figure 60-7 shows elevated signal intensites in the right frontal lobe and the left temporal lobe. The ^{31}P spectrum of the right frontal region (voxel 1 shown in Figure 60-9) shows increases in the % PDE and %PCr, and a decrease in the β-ATP. The pHi is increased. In the ^{31}P spectrum of the left frontal lobe (voxel 2) the %Pi and pHi are increased, also indicating dysfunction in high-energy phosphate metabolism (Figure 60-10).

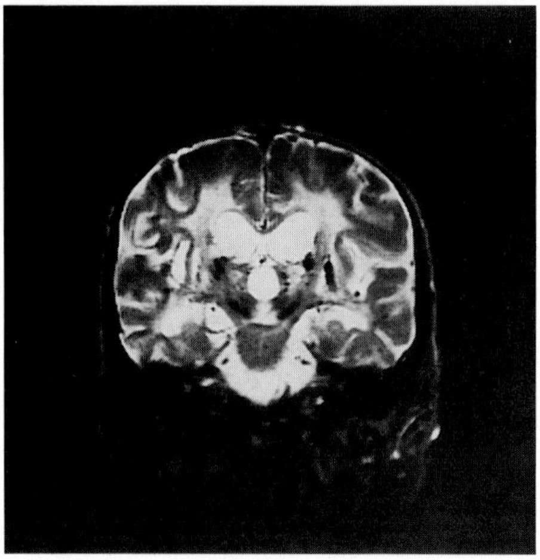

Fig. 60-1 Coronal T_2-weighted image (2,200/90).

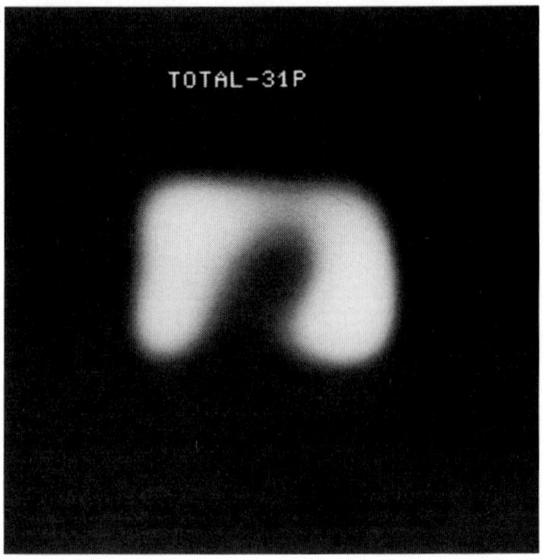

Fig. 60-2 Coronal ^{31}P metabolite image.

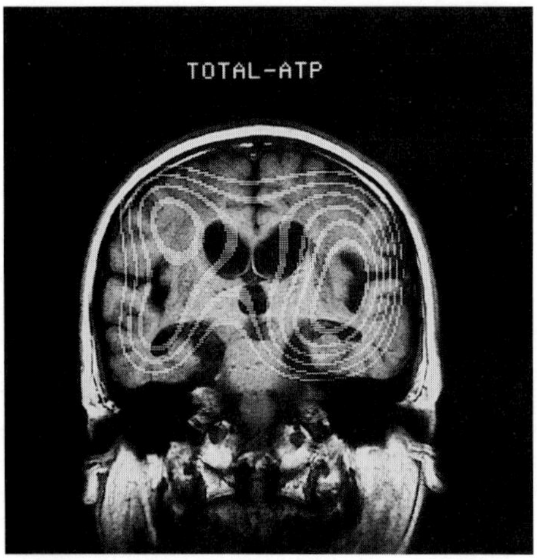

Fig. 60-3 Coronal total ATP contour map superimposed on T_1-weighted image (500/15).

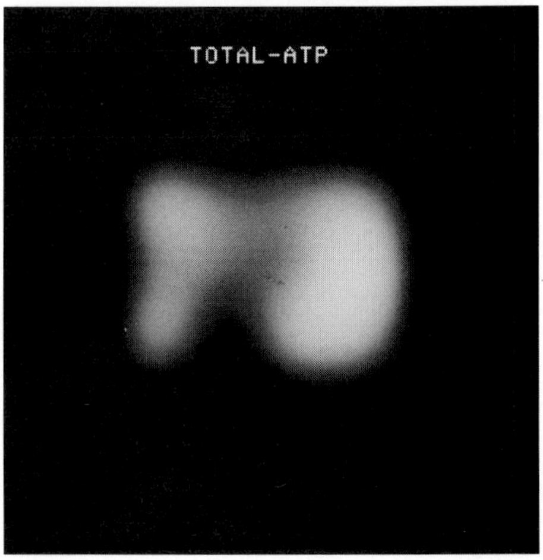

Fig. 60-4 Coronal total ATP metabolite image.

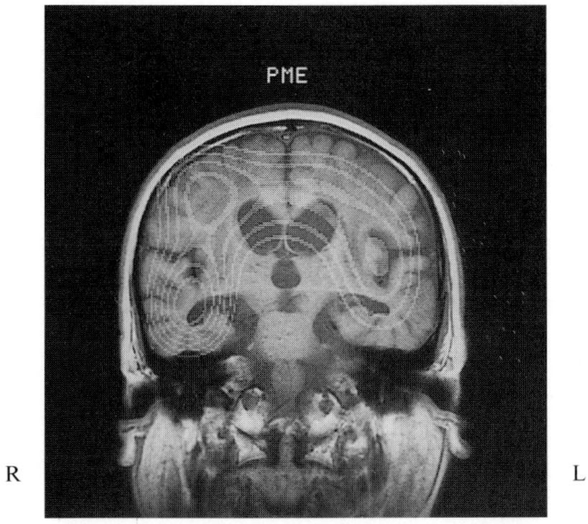

Fig. 60-5 Coronal PME contour map superimposed on T_1-weighted image (500/15).

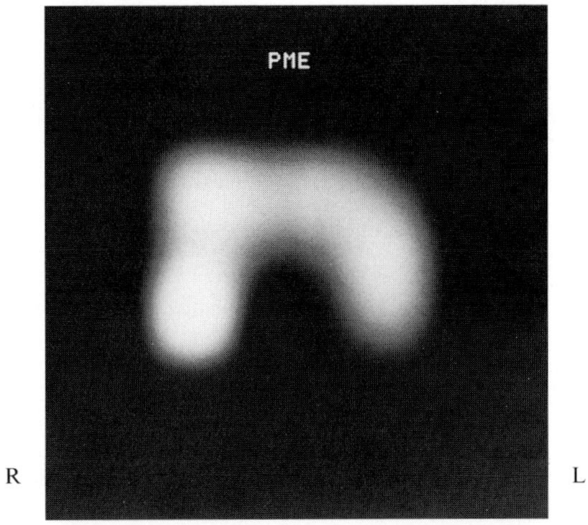

Fig. 60-6 Coronal PME metabolite image.

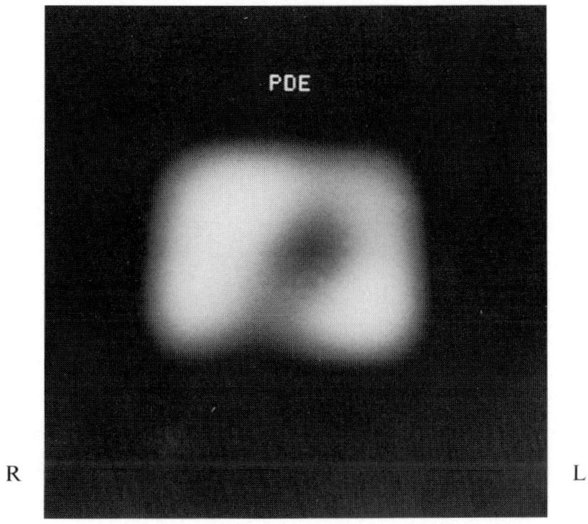

Fig. 60-7 Coronal PDE metabolite image.

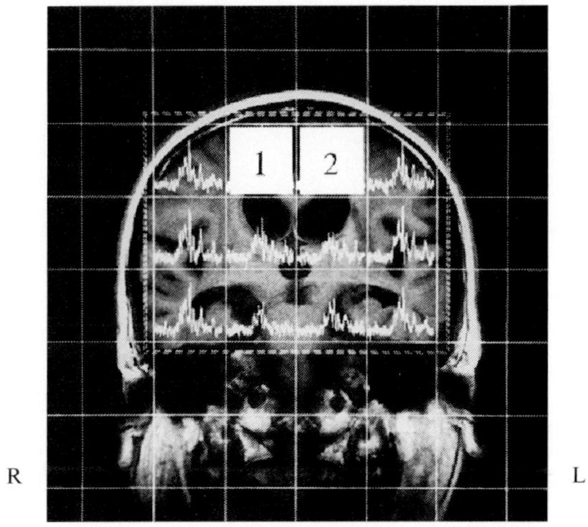

Fig. 60-8 T_1-weighted image showing the position of $3 \times 3 \times 4 cm^3$ voxels 1 and 2.

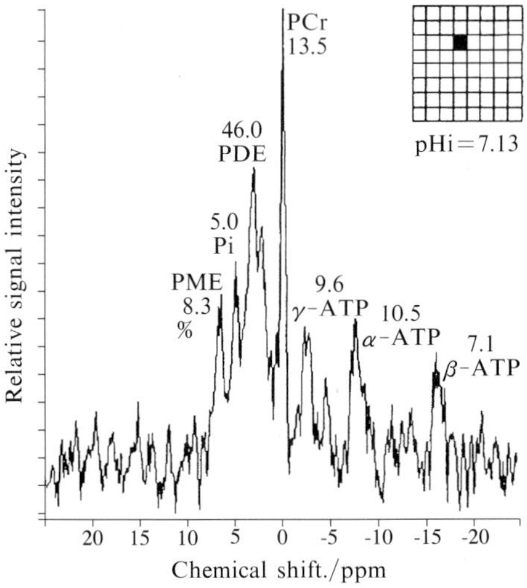

Fig. 60-9 ^{31}P spectrum of right frontal lobe (voxel 1).

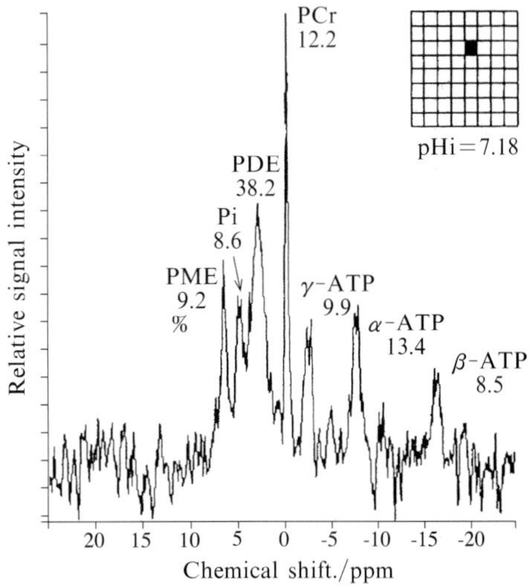

Fig. 60-10 ^{31}P spectrum of left frontal lobe (voxel 2).

Chapter 10 Other Neurological Disorders

Toshiro Fujimoto and Yasuhiko Utatsu

10.1 CHARACTERISTICS OF THE SPECTRUM

10.1.1 Multiple sclerosis (MS)

(1) ***^{31}P MRS***

Mooyaart et al.[1] reported decreased levels of PDE in patients with progressive multiple sclerosis. Minderhoud et al.[2] demonstrated increased PCr levels in multiple sclerosis, reflecting a reduced metabolic state of the brain. In Case 61, ^{31}P and total ATP signals are reduced not only in the lesions of MS but also in the right temporal lobe areas. This indicates that tissue damage and metabolic disturbance are present around as well as in the plaque. The PCr level remains unchanged, but the Pi level is increased in the area including the plaque, probably reflecting reduced high-energy phosphate metabolism. PDE levels tend to reduce. The PME level was elevated, presumably reflecting demyelination, inflammatory degradation of myelin, and an increased turnover in membrane phospholipid metabolism.

(2) ***^{1}H MRS***

Arnold et al.[3,4] found a decreased NAA/Cr ratio in the affected tissue with multiple sclerosis, suggesting damage marked pathologically by gliosis and axonal loss. Miller et al.[5] and Matthews et al.[6] reported that plaque with severe inflammatory changes has a decreased NAA/Cr ratio (Grossman et al.[7]). No correlation was found between decreased NAA and gadopentetate dimeglumine (Gd-DTPA) enhancement. Arnold et al.[4] and Davie et al.[8] suggested that reduction in the NAA/Cr ratio was partially reversible, and that axonal loss is not the only mechanism of reduction in the NAA/Cr ratio. Moreover, the presence of similar metabolic abnormalities has been suggested in the white matter surrounding the lesions that is imaged normally on MRI (Roser et al.[9]). Constans et al.[10] reported that the reduction of NAA/Cr ratio in normal appearing white matter may be due to a dissociation between osmotic or glial perturbation and demyelination or inflammation.

An increased ratio of Cho/Cr in some active plaque was also reported.[4,5,6,8] The increase in Cho is considered to be due to demyelination, inflammatory degradation of myelin, and elevated turnover of membrane components. Lactate resonance was also observed in some acute plaque, suggesting possible reduced oxygen delivery in those lesions.[5] Narayana et al.[11] found signals in the lipid region that were undetectable two weeks later, reflecting the dynamic stages of the evolution of the demyelinative process. Larsson et al.[12] suggested that lipids were detected as early as Day 10 in the acute plaque but appeared more distinct after 2 or 3 months, and that the production of free lipids is not a primary pathologic event in plaque formation. Bruhn et al.[13] and Koopmans et al.[14] reported an increase in inositol peak in multiple sclerosis lesions, reflecting the breakdown of myelin membrane phospholipids.

10.1.2 Leukodystrophy

(1) ***^{31}P MRS***

Reduced ^{31}P signals indicate a metabolic dysfunction in areas corresponding to diffusely increased signals involving the white matter of the frontal lobes in T_2-weighted images of MRI. In these areas, ATP and PCr signals are reduced, suggesting a disturbance in high-energy phosphate metabolism. The PDE level is also reduced, reflecting abnormal membrane phospholipids probably due to demyelination.

(2) ^{1}*H MRS*

Confort-Gouny et al.[15] reported a decrease in NAA and Cr resonances, and an increase in the Cho resonance in X-linked adrenoleukodystrophy. The increased level of Cho was accompanied by a lipid signal caused by the accumulation of very long chain fatty acids. In the last stage of the disease, all metabolite signals were reduced because of disturbances in the cerebral metabolism and the destruction of brain cells. Tzika et al.[16] showed an accumulation of lactate in some patients with X-linked childhood adrenoleukodystrophy, indicating a blood perfusion deficit rather than a specific metabolic defect at the mitochondrial level.

10.1.3 Huntington's disease

(1) ^{31}*P MRS*

Pettegrew et al.[17] reported increases in phosphomonoesters and phosphodiesters using perchlolic acid extracts of postmortem brain samples with Huntington's disease, suggesting abnormalities of phospholipid metabolism. Our *in vivo* spectra shows that the increase in PME level in the basal ganglia is consistent with the *in vitro* increases in PME. However, the decrease in the PDE level in the basal ganglia is not consistent with the *in vitro* results. In the basal ganglia region, our ^{31}P-CSI study of Huntington's disease shows decreases in PME and PDE levels, presumably reflecting phospholipids abnormalities, and reduction of ATP, indicating a reduction in high-energy phosphate metabolism. Positron emission tomography (PET) demonstrated decreased glucose and oxygen metabolism in the basal ganglia,[18,19] and the results of ^{31}P MRS were consistent with those of PET. The spectrum obtained from a voxel and the CSI gave different information. The CSI study illustrates differences in distribution of relative signal intensities in the whole brain, but the spectrum from the voxel only gives information from the local region.

(2) ^{1}*H MRS*

Dunlop et al.[20] found that concentration of NAA in the putamen was decreased in the perchloric acid extracts of postmortem brain tissue obtained from patients with Huntington's disease, and noted that the course of the disease may be monitored by NAA determination. Decreases in glutamate and gamma-aminobutyric acid (GABA) levels were reported in postmortem brain samples of Huntington's disease.[21,22] Using *in vivo* ^{1}H MRS, Jenkins et al.[23] demonstrated a decreased level of NAA and an increased level of Cho in the basal ganglia, suggesting neuronal loss and gliosis, and elevated lactate peaks in some patients, reflecting disturbance of energy metabolism. Davie et al.[24] and Taylor-Robinson et al.[25] reported increases in glutamine and glutamate (Glx) levels in the basal ganglia. The loss of neurons in Huntington's disease was considered to be a secondary phenomenon due to the excitotoxic effects of increased glutamate in the basal ganglia.[24]

References

1) Mooyaart, E. L.; Kamman, R. L.; Minderhoud, J. M. et al. ^{31}P NMR spectroscopy in patients with multiple sclerosis (MS): A correlation with clinical data. *In: Book of Abstracts: Eighth Annual Meeting and Exhibition of the Society of Magnetic Resonance in Medicine, Vol. 1. Amsterdam, The Netherlands: SMRM*; 1989: 456.

2) Minderhoud, J. M.; Mooyaart, E. L.; Kamman, R. L. et al. In vivo phosphorus magnetic resonance spectroscopy in multiple sclerosis. *Arch. Neurol*. 49: 161-165; 1992.

3) Arnold, D. L.; Matthews, P. M.; Francis, G. et al. Proton MR spectroscopy in the evaluation multiple sclerosis in humans in vivo: Assessment of the load of disease. *In: Book of Abstracts: Eighth Annual Meeting and Exhibition of the Society of Magnetic Resonance in Medicine, Vol. 1. Amsterdam, The Netherlands: SMRM*; 1989: 455.

4) Arnold, D. L.; Matthews, P. M.; Francis, G. S. et al. Proton magnetic resonance spectroscopic imaging for metabolic characterization of demyelinating plaques. *Ann. Neurol.* 31: 235–241; 1992.

5) Miller, D. H.; Austin, S. J.; Connelly, A. et al. Proton magnetic resonance spectroscopy of an acute and chronic lesion in multiple sclerosis. *Lancet* 337: 58–59; 1991.

6) Matthews, P. M.; Francis, G.; Antel, J. et al. Proton magnetic resonance spectroscopy for metabolic characterization of plaques in multiple sclerosis. *Neurology* 41: 1251–1256; 1991.

7) Grossman, R. I.; Lenkinski, R. E.; Ramer, K. N. et al. MR proton spectroscopy in multiple sclerosis. *AJNR Am. J. Neuroradiol.* 13: 1535–1543; 1992.

8) Davie, C. A.; Hawkins, C. P.; Barker, G. J. et al. Serial proton magnetic resonance spectroscopy in acute multiple sclerosis lesions. *Brain* 117: 49–58; 1994.

9) Roser, W.; Hagberg, G.; Mader, I. et al. Proton MRS of gadolinium-enhancing MS plaques and metabolic changes in normal-appearing white matter. *Magn. Reson. Med.* 33: 811–817; 1995.

10) Constans, J. M.; Fernandez, J.; Viader, F. et al. Automated single voxel ^{1}H MR spectroscopy in multiple sclerosis: Study of normal appearing white matter and study of differently aged lesions. *In: Proceedings : Fourth Scientific Meeting and Exhibition of the International Society for Magnetic Resonance in Medicine, Vol. 2. New York, USA: ISMRM*; 1996: 943.

11) Narayana, P. A.; Wolinsky, J. S.; Fenstermacher, M. J. Proton magnetic resonance spectroscopy in multiple sclerosis. *In: Book of Abstracts: Eighth Annual Meeting and Exhibition of the Society of Magnetic Resonance in Medicine, Vol. 1. Amsterdam, The Netherlands: SMRM*; 1989: 457.

12) Larsson, H. B. W.; Christiansen, P.; Jensen, M. et al. Localized *in vivo* proton spectroscopy in the brain of patients with multiple sclerosis. *Magn. Reson. Med.* 22: 23–31; 1991.

13) Bruhn, H.; Frahm, J.; Merboldt, K. D. et al. Multiple sclerosis in children: Cerebral metabolic alterations monitored by localized proton magnetic resonance spectroscopy in vivo. *Ann. Neurol.* 32: 140–150; 1992.

14) Koopmans, R. A.; Li, D. K. B.; Zhu, G. et al. Magnetic resonance spectroscopy of multiple sclerosis: in-vivo detection of myelin breakdown products. *Lancet* 341: 631–632; 1993.

15) Confort-Gouny, S.; Vion-Dury, J.; Chabrol, B. et al. Localized proton MR spectroscopy in X-linked adrenoleukodystrophy. *In: Proceedings: Twelfth Annual Scientific Meeting of the Society of Magnetic Resonance in Medicine, Vol. 3. New York, USA: SMRM*; 1993: 1565.

16) Tzika, A. A.; Ball, W. S.; Vigneron, D. B. et al. Childhood adrenoleukodystrophy: Assessment with proton MR spectroscopy. *Radiology* 189: 467–480; 1993.

17) Pettegrew, J. W.; Kopp, S. J.; Minshew, N. J. et al. ^{31}P nuclear magnetic resonance studies of phosphoglyceride metabolism in developing and degenerating brain: Preliminary observations. *J. Neuropathol. Exp. Neurol.* 46: 419–430; 1987.

18) Kuwert, T.; Lange, H. W.; Langen, K-J. et al. Cortical and subcortical glucose consumption measured by PET in patients with Huntington's disease. *Brain* 113: 1405–1423; 1990.

19) Martin, W. R. W.; Clark, C.; Ammann, W. et al. Cortical glucose metabolism in Huntington's disease. *Neurology* 42: 223–229; 1992.

20) Dunlop, D. S.; Mc Hale, D. M.; Lajtha, A. Decreased brain *N*-acetylaspartate in Huntington's disease. *Brain Research* 580: 44–48; 1992.

21) Ellison, D. W.; Beal, M. F.; Mazurek, M. F. et al. Amino acid neurotransmitter abnormalities in Huntington's disease and the quinolinic acid animal model of Huntington's disease. *Brain* 110: 1657–1673; 1987.

22) Perry, T. L.; Hansen, S. What excitotoxin kills striatal neurons in Huntington's disease ? Clues from neurochemical studies. *Neurology* 40: 20–24; 1990.

23) Jenkins, B. G.; Koroshetz, W. J.; Beal, M. F. et al. Evidence for impairment of energy metabolism in vivo in Huntington's disease using localized ^{1}H NMR spectroscopy. *Neurology* 43: 2689–2695; 1993.

24) Davie, C. A.; Barker, G. J.; Davies, S. E. C. et al. Proton magnetic resonance spectroscopy in Huntington's disease. *In: Proceedings: Second Meeting of the Society of Magnetic Resonance, Vol. 2. San Francisco, USA: SMR*; 1994: 577.

25) Taylor-Robinson, S. D.; Weeks, R. A.; Marcus, C. et al. ^{1}H MR spectroscopy demonstrated an increased Glx peak in the striatum of patients with Huntington's disease. *In: Proceedings: Second Meeting of the Society of Magnetic Resonance, Vol. 2. San Francisco, USA: SMR*; 1994: 578.

10.2 CASES (61-64)

CASE 61

Case 61: A 51-year-old female
Multiple sclerosis

The patient demonstrated numbness of bilateral hands and feet, dizziness, insomnia, diminished interest, and occasional repetition of speech and incoherent behavior. The T_2-weighted image in Figure 61-1 shows plaque in the right frontal lobe, the adjacent region of the left lateral ventricle, and the adjacent region of the left inferior horn of the lateral ventricle. The ^{31}P metabolite image in Figure 61-2 is almost normal. In the ATP metabolite image in Figure 61-3, signal intensities are reduced in the right frontal lobe corresponding to the plaque area, suggesting disturbance of high-energy phosphate metabolism. The PME image shows decreased signal intensity in the left frontal lobe corresponding to the area including the plaque (Figure 61-4). In Figure 61-6, the ^{1}H spectrum obtained from a voxel (Figure 61-5) containing the plaque area demonstrates the increased Cho/Cr ratio, the reduced NAA/Cho ratio, and the mildly reduced NAA/Cr ratio. In Figure 61-8, the ^{31}P spectrum from the plaque area in the right frontal lobe (A) (Figure 61-7) shows the mild reduction of %PDE. The pHi is normal. ^{31}P and ^{1}H spectra in almost the same plaque lesion suggest abnormality in membrane phospholipids. In Figure 61-9, a ^{31}P spectrum of an area including the plaque (B) shows a mild reduction in the %PDE and the %PME, and the mild elevation of %Pi. The pHi is normal. The ^{31}P spectrum in Figure 61-10 (C) presents increased levels in %Pi and %PME.

R 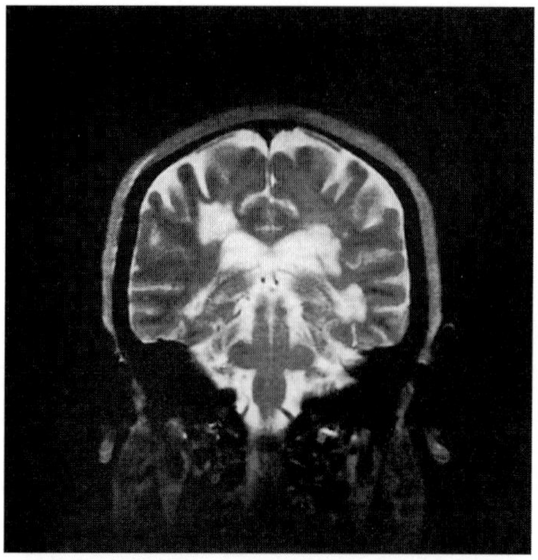 L

Fig. 61-1 Coronal T_2-weighted image (2,200/90).

R 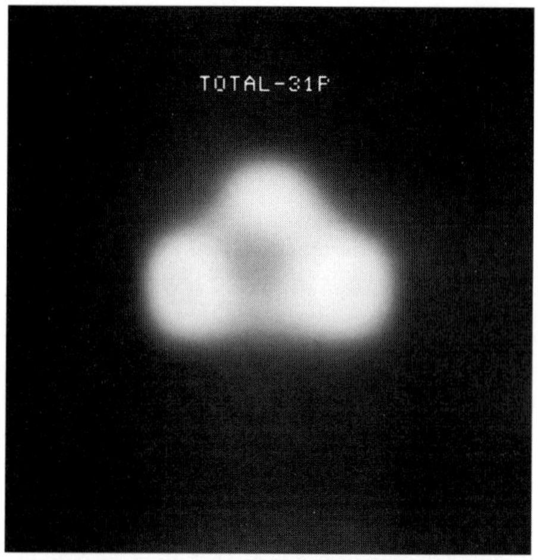 L

Fig. 61-2 Coronal ^{31}P metabolite image.

R 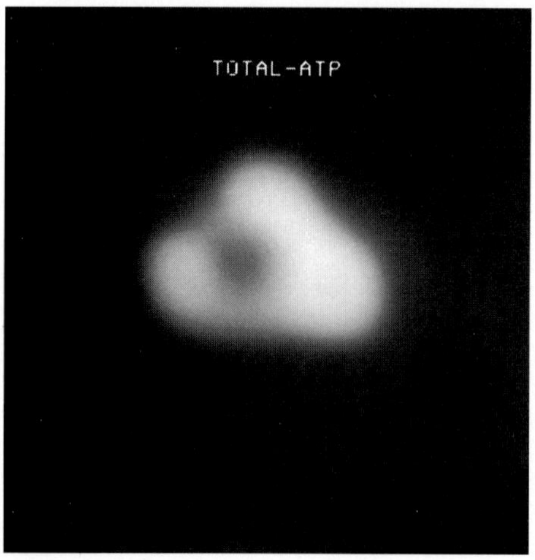 L

Fig. 61-3 Coronal total ATP metabolite image.

R 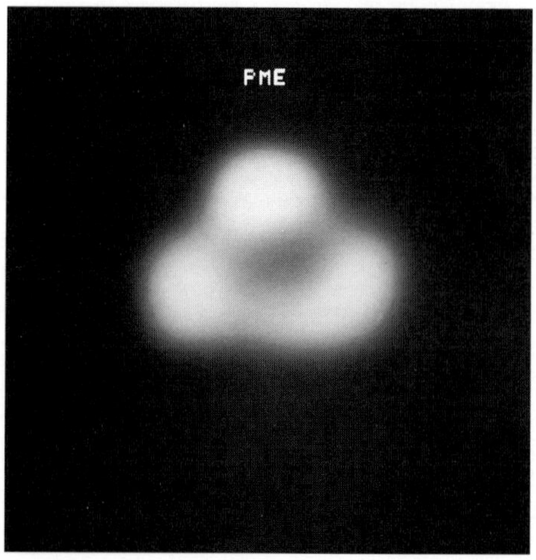 L

Fig. 61-4 Coronal PME metabolite image.

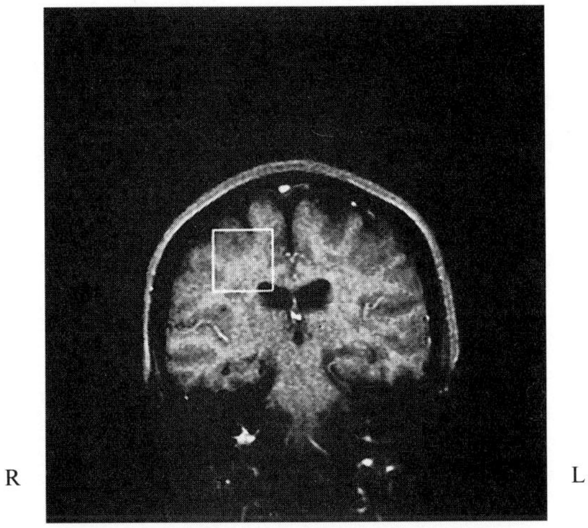

Fig. 61-5 T_1-weighted image showing the position of $3 \times 3 \times 3$ cm^3 voxel.

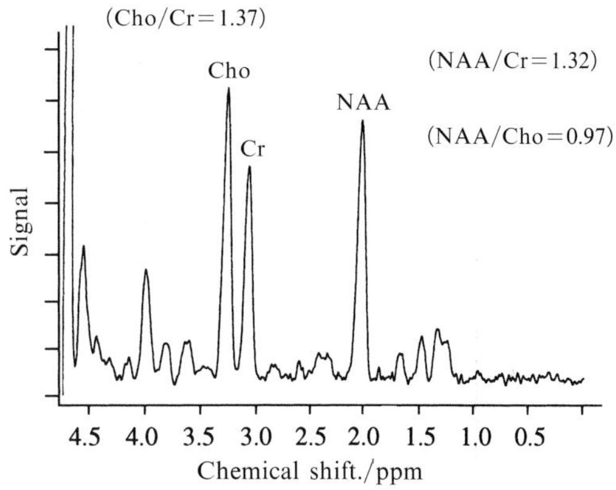

Fig. 61-6 ^1H spectrum in the area affected by plaque. PRESS (1,500/135).

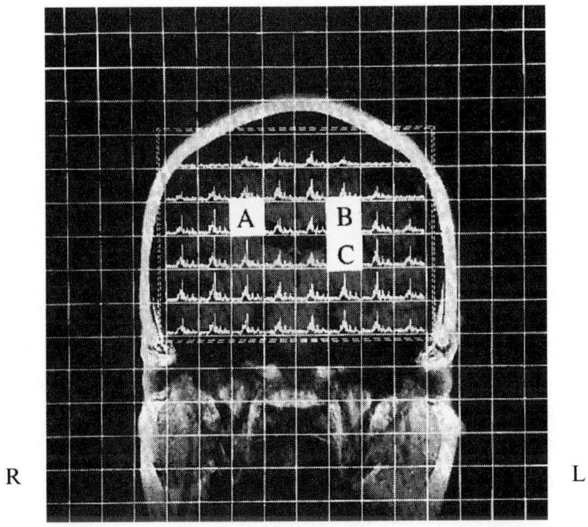

Fig. 61-7 T_1-weighted image showing the position of $1.5 \times 1.5 \times 4$ cm^3 voxels A, B and C.

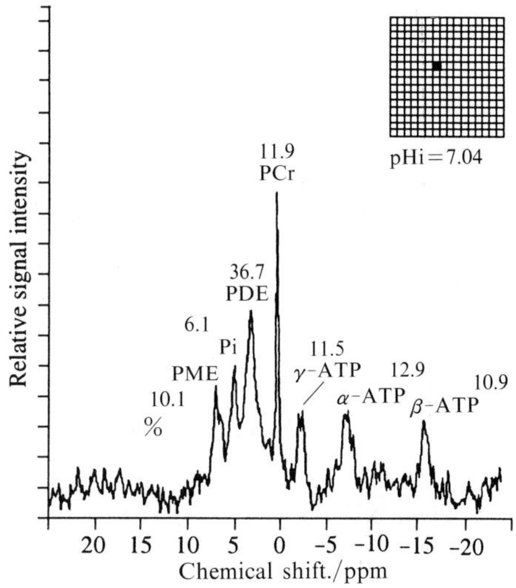

Fig. 61-8 ^{31}P spectrum of voxel A.

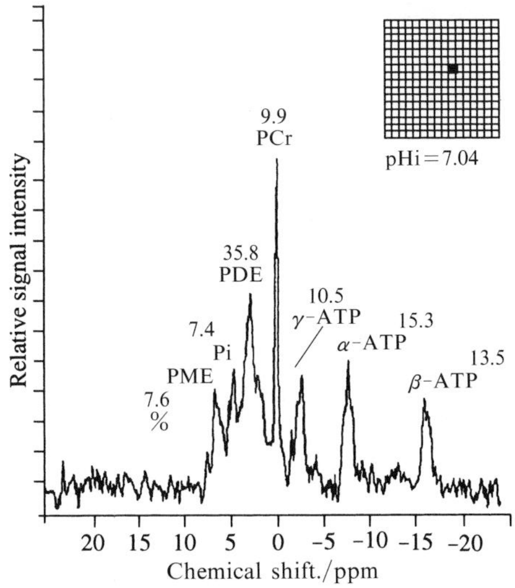

Fig. 61-9 ^{31}P spectrum of voxel B.

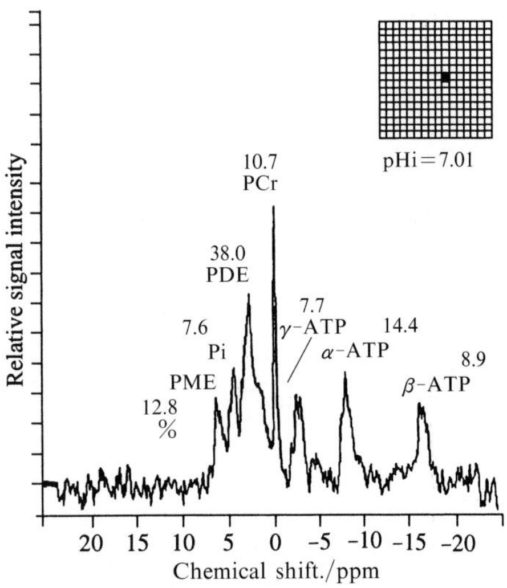

Fig. 61-10 ^{31}P spectrum of voxel C.

CASE 62

Case 62: A 66-year-old male

Leukodystrophy

The patient had exhibited tonic-clonic seizures and progressive dementia since 10 years of age. The T_2-weighted image of MRI in Figure 62-1 shows diffusely increased signal intensities in the white matter of the frontal lobes. In Figure 62-2, the signal intensity in the ^{31}P metabolite image is diffusely reduced in the frontal lobe, reflecting impairment of the cerebral metabolism in this region. Figure 62-3 illustrates a voxel for ^{1}H spectroscopy placed in the left frontal lobe, and the ^{1}H spectrum in Figure 62-4 shows a slight increase of the Cho level. In the Pi metabolite image in Figure 62-5, in spite of an irregular pattern, increased signal intensities in the frontal lobe and the left temporal lobe are observed. Signal intensities are reduced in the frontal lobe in both the PDE and PCr metabolite images in Figures 62-6 and 7, respectively. Figure 62-8 illustrates voxels A and B from which ^{31}P spectra were obtained and contains high signal intensity areas in the T_2-weighted image. In the ^{31}P spectrum in Figure 62-9 acquired from voxel A, the S/N ratio is reduced, and the %PME is increased, but the %PDE is slightly reduced. The pHi is normal. Figure 62-10 shows a ^{31}P spectrum from voxel B. The %PME is also increased, but the %PDE is reduced. The pHi is normal. ^{31}P and ^{1}H spectra suggest disturbances in membrane phospholipids and high-energy phosphate metabolism in the white matter, concoponding to high signal intensity areas of the T_2-weighted image.

R 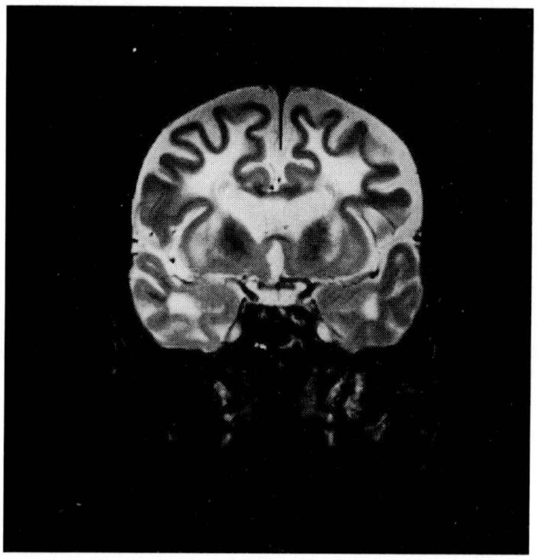 L

Fig. 62-1 Coronal T_2-weighted image (2,200/90).

R 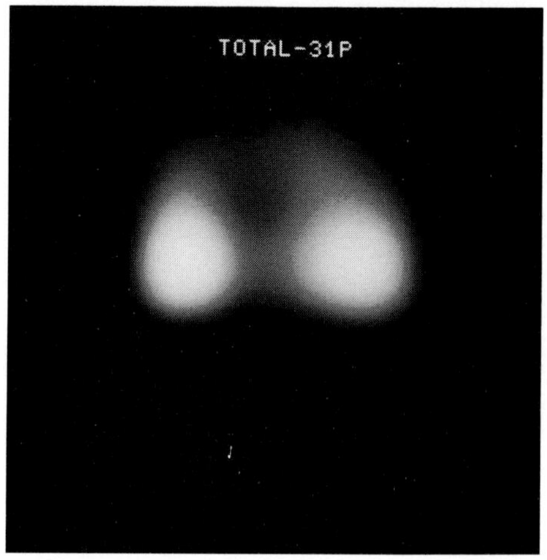 L

Fig. 62-2 Coronal ^{31}P metabolite image.

L 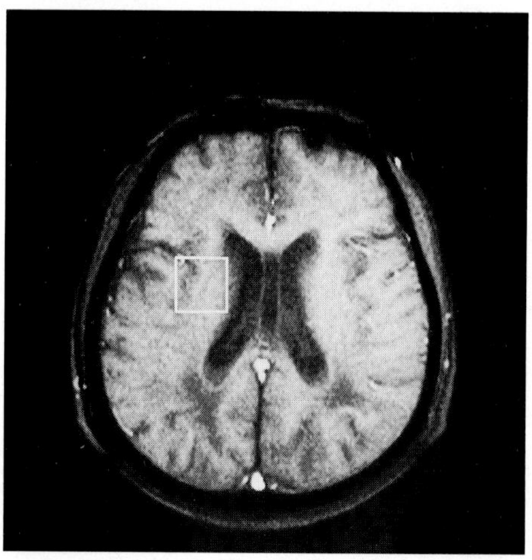 R

Fig. 62-3 T_1-weighted image showing the position of 3×3×3 cm^3 voxel.

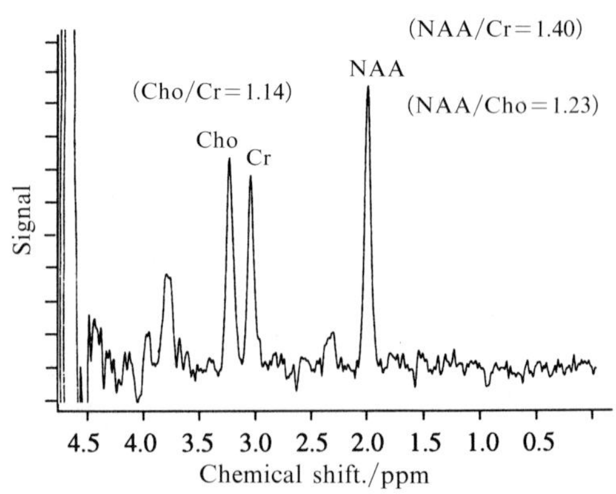

Fig. 62-4 ^{1}H spectrum in left frontal lobe. PRESS (1,500/135).

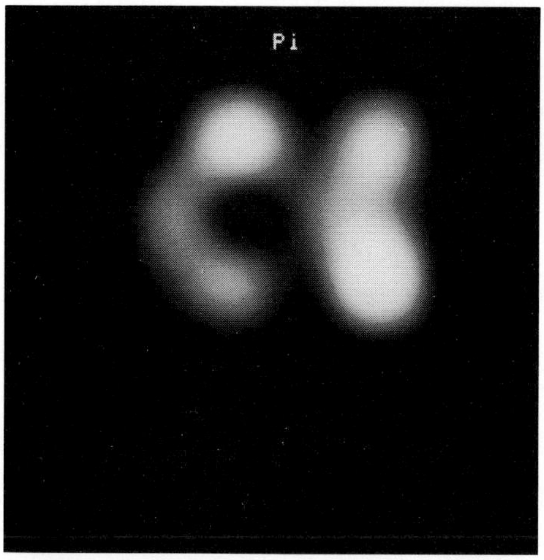

Fig. 62-5 Coronal Pi metabolite image.

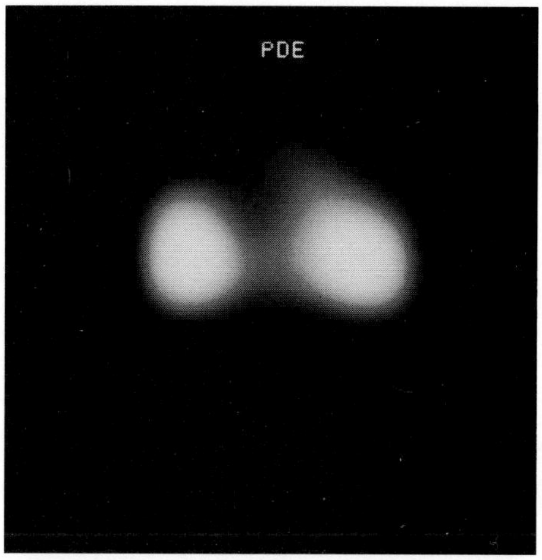

Fig. 62-6 Coronal PDE metabolite image.

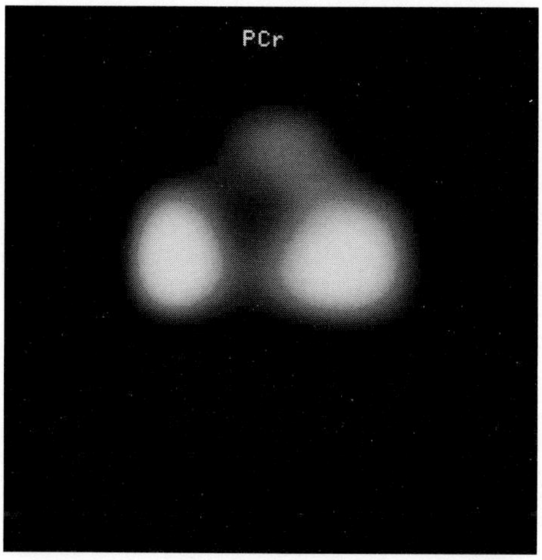

Fig. 62-7 Coronal PCr metabolite image.

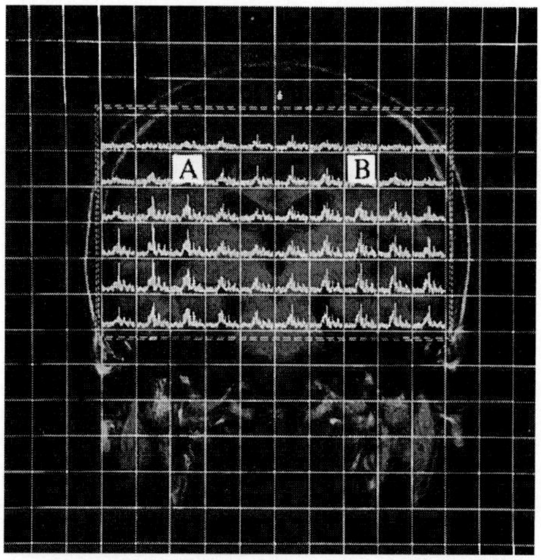

Fig. 62-8 T_1-weighted image showing the position of $1.5 \times 1.5 \times 4$ cm^3 voxels A and B.

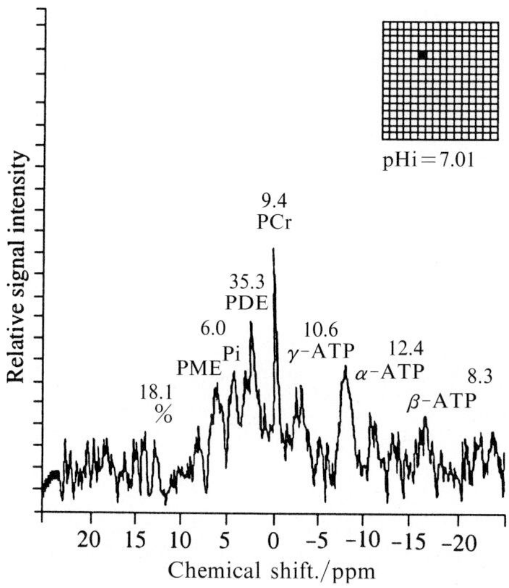

Fig. 62-9 ^{31}P spectrum of voxel A.

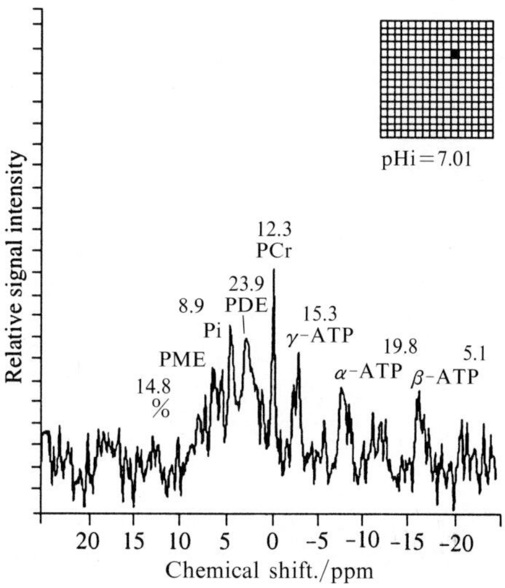

Fig. 62-10 ^{31}P spectrum of voxel B.

CASE 63

Case 63: A 46-year-old male

Huntington's disease

Age at onset was 42 years. The patient presented choreiform movements and dementia with schizophrenia-like disorder. The MRI in Figure 63-1 shows brain atrophy with enlargement of the lateral ventricle, third ventricle and cerebral sulci. The ^{31}P contour map in Figure 63-2 is almost symmetrical, and signal intensities are reduced bilaterally in the basal ganglia regions. Figures 63-3 and 4 show total ATP images in which signal intensities are reduced bilaterally in the basal ganglia regions, and the left temporal lobe, suggesting hypometabolism in these regions. In the PDE images in Figures 63-5 and 6, signal intensities are reduced bilaterally in the basal ganglia regions, indicating a disturbance in phospholipids. Figure 63-9, shows a spectrum obtained from voxel A (Figure 63-7) containing the right basal ganglia, and the %PDE is significantly decreased, and the %PME, the %Pi and %β-ATP are elevated, and %PCr is in the normal range. The pHi is high. In Figure 63-10, signals from the left basal ganglia (voxel B) are generally reduced, and the S/N ratio is reduced. The %PME and %PCr are increased, but the %Pi, the %PDE and the %β-ATP are in the normal range. The pHi is normal.

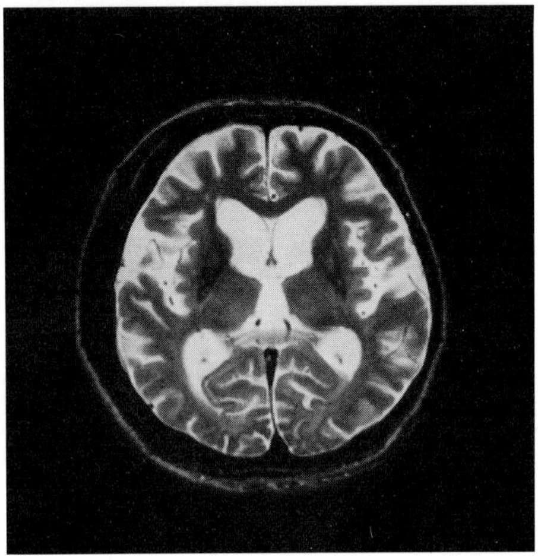

Fig. 63-1 Axial T_2-weighted image (2,200/90).

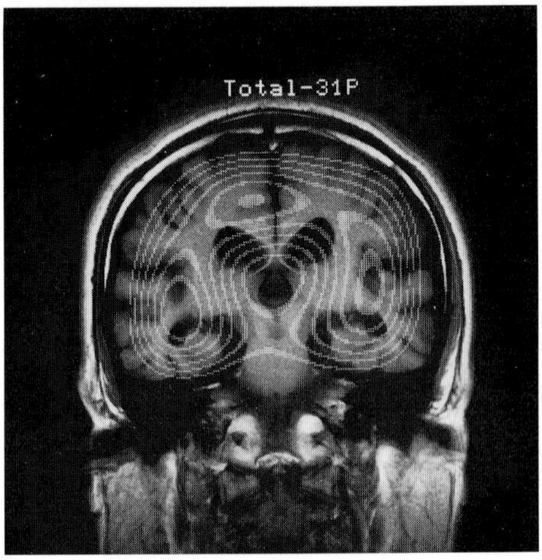

Fig. 63-2 Coronal ^{31}P contour map superimposed on T_1-weighted image.

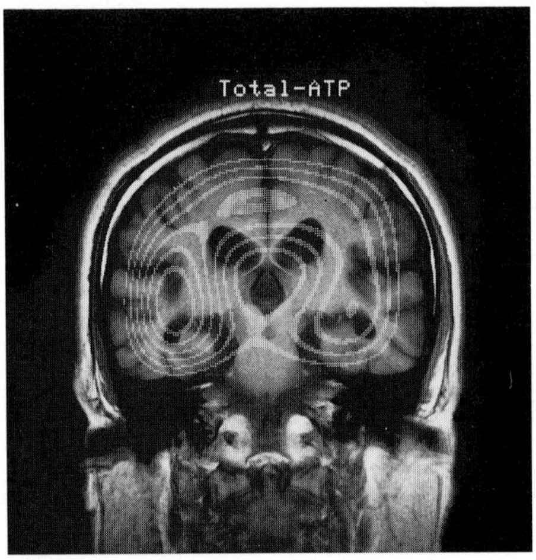

Fig. 63-3 Coronal total ATP contour map superimposed on T_1-weighted image.

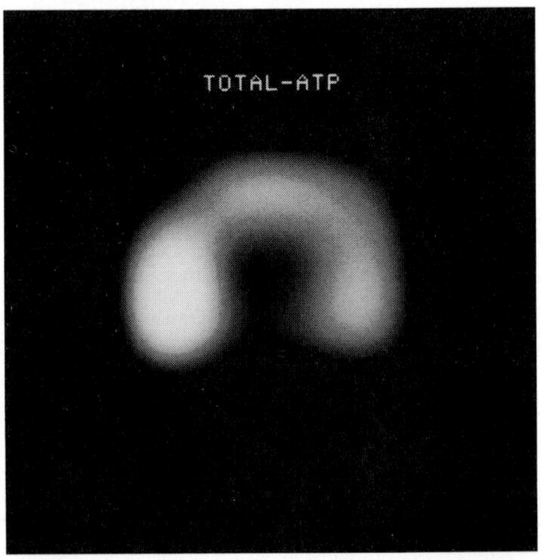

Fig. 63-4 Coronal total ATP metabolite image.

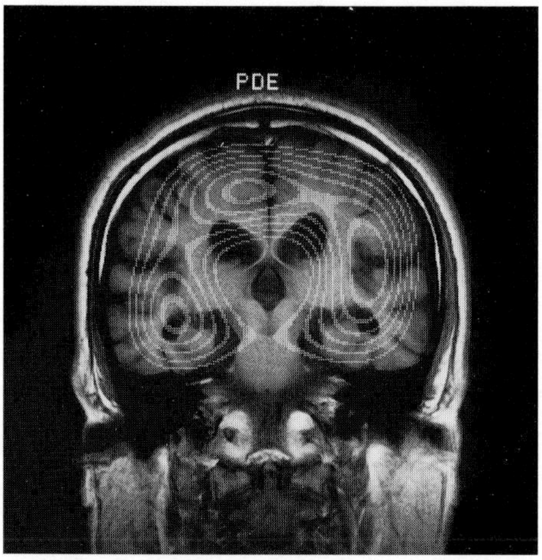

Fig. 63-5 Coronal PDE contour map superimposed on T_1-weighted image.

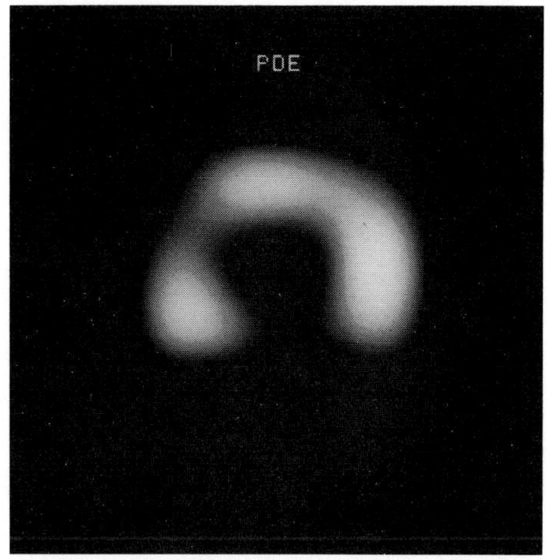

Fig. 63-6 Coronal PDE metabolite image.

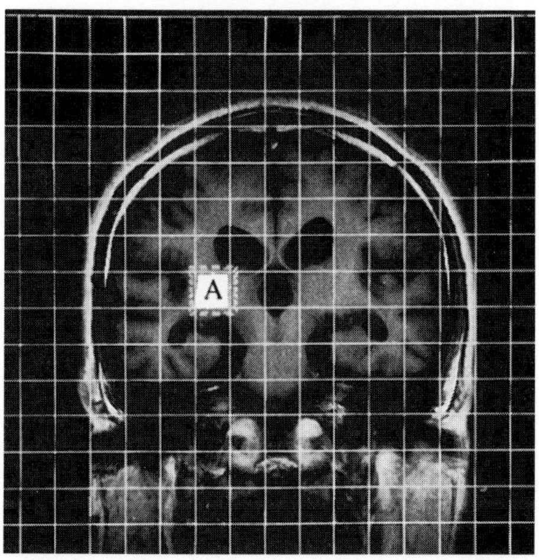

Fig. 63-7 T_1-weighted image showing the position of 1.5×1.5×4 cm^3 voxel A.

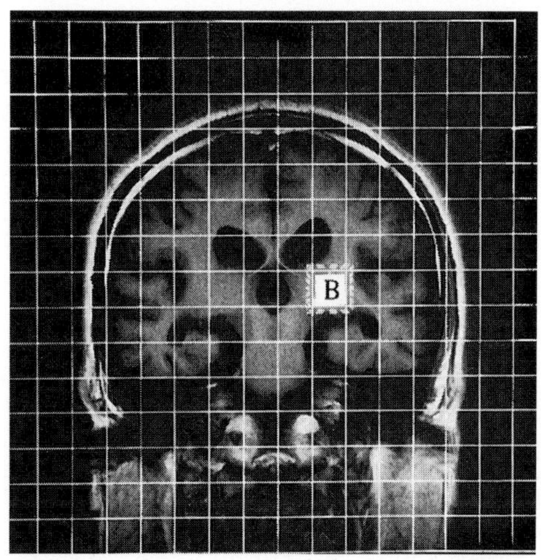

Fig. 63-8 T_1-weighted image showing the position of 1.5×1.5×4 cm^3 voxel B.

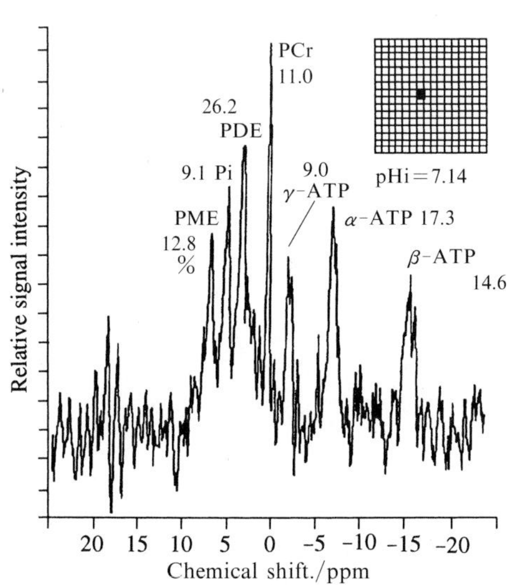

Fig. 63-9 ^{31}P spectrum of voxel A.

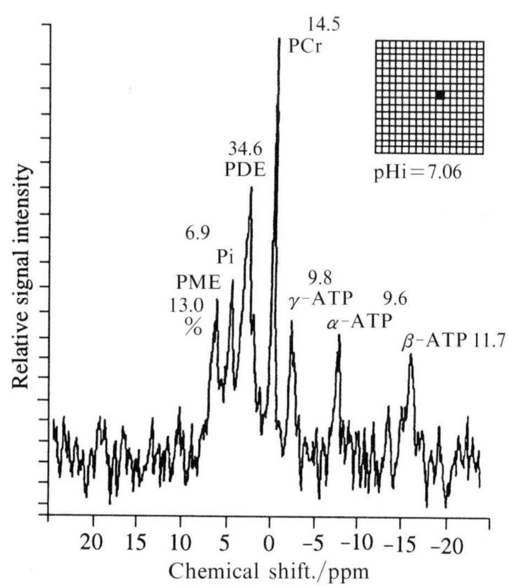

Fig. 63-10 ^{31}P spectrum of voxel B.

CASE 64

Case 64: A 40-year-old male

Huntington's disease

The patient was treated for schizophrenia at age 24. However, choreiform movements appeared at 36 years, and dementia has progressed since. The X-CT image in Figure 64-1 shows brain atrophy with enlargements of lateral and third ventricles and cerebral sulci. Figure 64-2 illustrates the voxels placed in the basal ganglia regions from which ^{1}H spectra were obtained. In Figure 64-3, an increased Cho/Cr ratio and a decreased NAA/Cr ratio are shown in the right basal ganglia. In Figure 64-4, an increased Cho/Cr ratio and a decreased NAA/Cr ratio are observed in the left basal ganglia. These findings suggest abnormality in membrane phospholipid metabolism and neuronal loss in the basal ganglia. The ^{31}P metabolite image shows a reduction in ^{31}P signal intensities in the basal ganglia regions, indicating dysfunction of metabolism (Figure 64-5). The PME metabolite image illustrates decreased signal intensities not only in the basal ganglia, but also in the right frontal regions (Figure 64-6). In Figures 64-7 and 8, a reduction in ATP signal intensities is observed in the basal ganglia, suggesting a reduction in high-energy phosphate metabolism. The PDE signal intensities are decreased in the basal ganglia regions and the right temporal lobe (Figures 64-9 and 10). Reduced PDE and PME signal intensities in the bilateral basal ganglia regions indicate abnormality in membrane phospholipids. ^{31}P and ^{1}H spectra demonstrate abnormality in the basal ganglia in Huntington's disease.

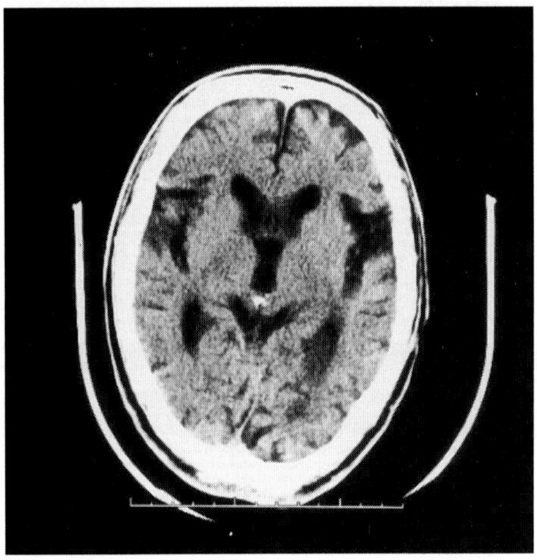

Fig. 64-1 Axial X-CT image.

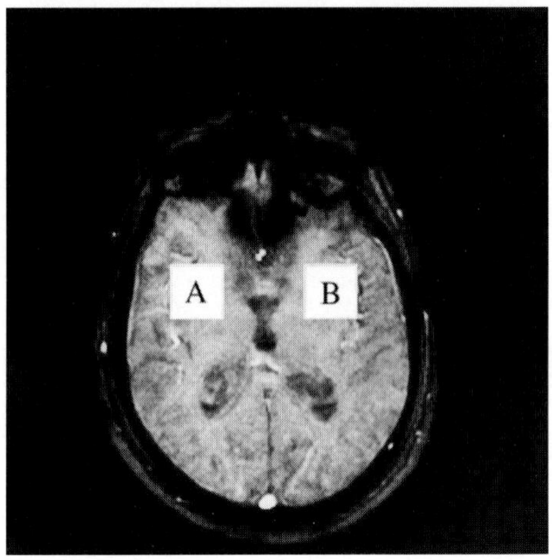

Fig. 64-2 T_1-weighted image showing the position $3 \times 3 \times 3 cm^3$ voxels A and B.

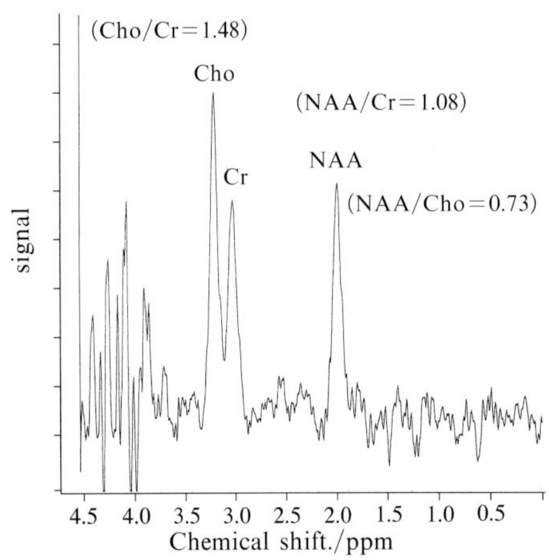

Fig. 64-3 ^{1}H spectrum of right basal ganglia (voxel B). PRESS (1,500/135)

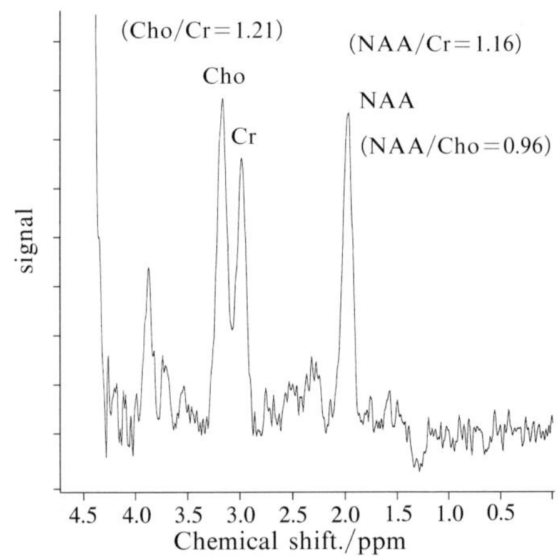

Fig. 64-4 ^{1}H spectrum of left basal ganglia (voxel A) PRESS (1,500/135)

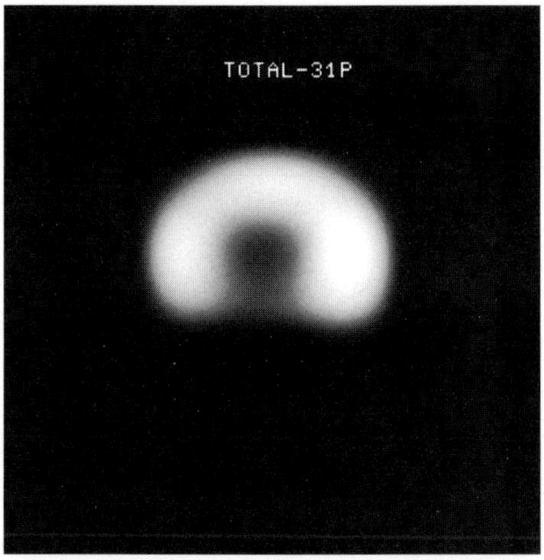

Fig. 64-5 Coronal ^{31}P metabolite image.

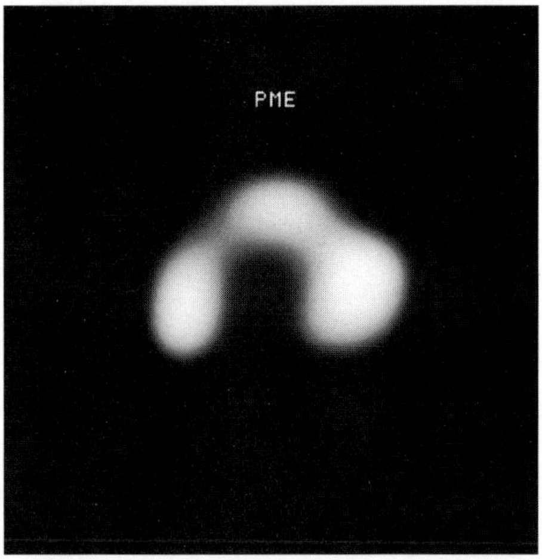

Fig. 64-6 Coronal PME metabolite image.

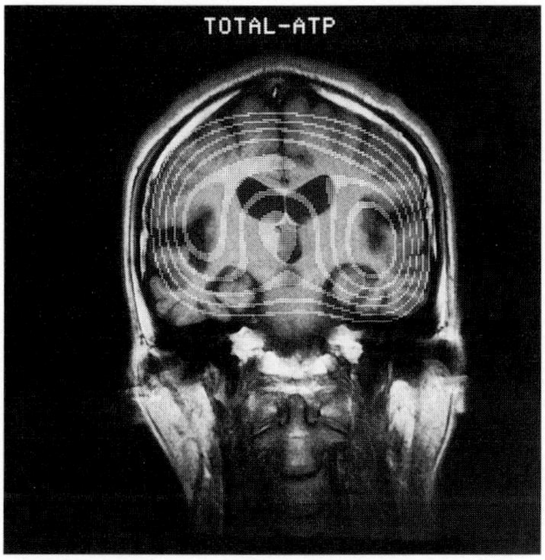

Fig. 64-7 Coronal total ATP contour map superimposed on T_1-weighted image (500/15).

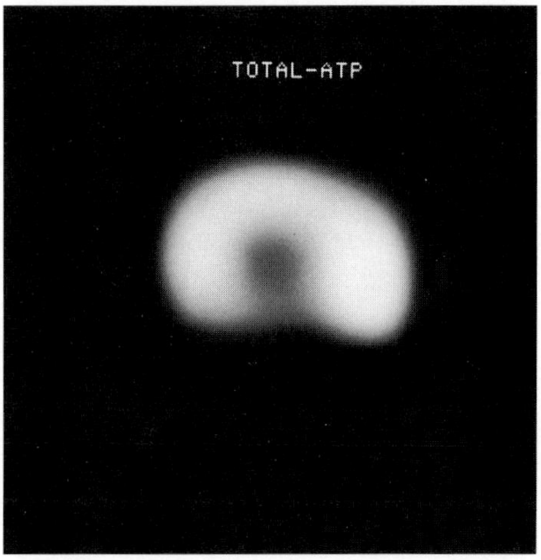

Fig. 64-8 Coronal total ATP metabolite image.

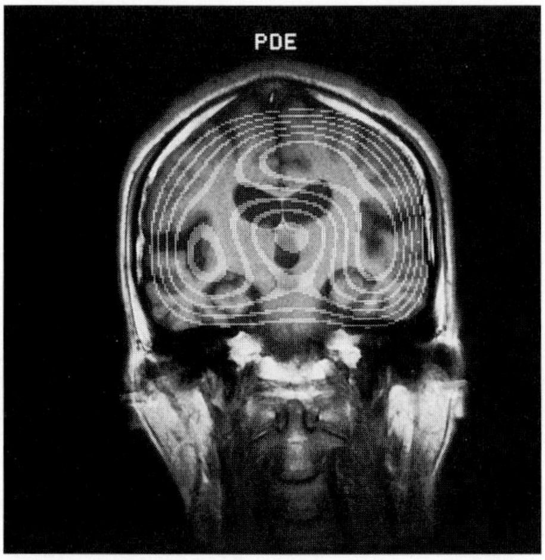

Fig. 64-9 Coronal PDE contour map superimposed on T_1-weighted image (500/15).

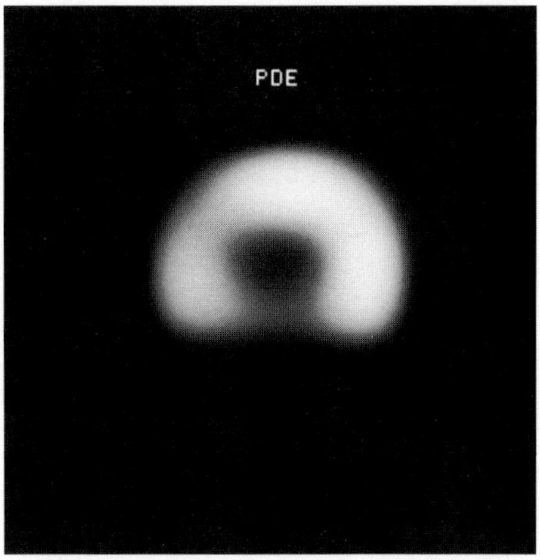

Fig. 64-10 Coronal PDE metabolite image.

Chapter 11 Epilepsy

Toshiro Fujimoto and Katsumi Nakamura

11.1 CHARACTERISTICS OF THE SPECTRUM

^{31}P MRS and ^{1}H MRS are used clinically and are known to be useful in biochemical and pathophysiological investigations of epilepsy. ^{31}P MRS allows detection of changes in high-energy phosphate metabolism of the brain and membrane phospholipids in patients with epilepsy. ^{1}H MRS provides not only information on neurons, phospholipids, neurotransmitters, and lactate, but also lateralizes the epileptogenic focus in focal epilepsy. With improvements in high-resolution NMR, many *in vivo* studies of epilepsy in animal models have been conducted using ^{31}P NMR, and the primary target of interest in these studies has detected changes in energy metabolism. Petroff et al.[1] studied the brain in status epilepticus in rabbits using ^{31}P NMR and reported that the PCr level decreased to 2/3 of the control and that the intracellular pH decreased. Using NMR spectroscopy of ^{1}H, ^{31}P and ^{23}Na, Schnall et al.[2] showed a decrease in PCr concentration and increases in Pi and lactate concentrations with no changes in ATP level, as well as an intracellular shift of the Na^{+} ion pool during generalized seizure induced by biccuculine. It has been shown recently, however, that more information could be obtained by technical improvements in MRS.[3–5] ^{1}H MRS (the single voxel method in which the echo time (TE) can be shortened), provides information on GABA, glutamine, glutamate and *myo*-inositol, and chemical shift imaging (CSI), which gives spatial information, are rapidly improving. High expectations are attached to their application in epilepsy.

(1) ^{31}*P MRS*

In localization-related epilepsies, changes in metabolism of high-energy phosphates and phospholipids can be represented directly as ^{31}P spectrum, metabolite image, and contour map by ^{31}P chemical shift imaging. Niiro et al.[6] demonstrated decreased signal intensity on PCr images and increased signal intensity on Pi images on the side of epileptic focus in patients with frequent spike discharge who were probably in the ictal period. In patients with apparent organic lesions, Nakamura et al.[7,8] showed decreases in signal intensities of PCr, ATP and Pi in the lesional hemisphere, compared to those in the contralateral hemisphere. Fujimoto et al.[9] reported alterations in PDE and PME in the focal lesions of the localization-related epilepsies in interictal period. However, in temporal lobe epilepsy in the interictal period, determination of the epileptogenic focus by ^{31}P MRS is difficult and controversial. Hugg et al.[10] and Laxer et al.[11] showed increases in pHi and Pi in the area including the epileptogenic focus in patients who had temporal lobe epilepsy with no ictal event occuring during the study.[10–12] On the other hand, Chu et al.[13,14] and Kuzniecky et al.[15] reported that no changes were observed in pHi, and that decreases were observed in the PCr/Pi ratio in patients who had temporal lobe epilepsy with no seizures during examination. Asakura et al.[16] and Nakamura et al.[17] observed that Pi levels increased in peri-ictal patients. According to our experience, the increased Pi level and increase in pHi did not always lateralize epileptogenic focus, and the PCr level is decreased occasionally in patients with temporal lobe epilepsy in the intrerictal period.[5,18] In addition, changes in the PDE and PME levels were noted,[5,7] and the PME level was decreased[10,12] or slightly increased[18] in areas containing the epileptogenic foci in patients with temporal lobe epilepsy. The discrepancy among these findings suggests that the ^{31}P MR spectra of epilepsy is complex, due to changes of various levels in energy metabolism in regions including the epileptogenic focus; and the state of high-energy phosphate metabolism of the brain depends on patients with ictal or peri-ictal or interictal states, which is difficult to decide in some cases. In addition, there is a large individual variation with respect to the location of the epileptogenic focus, type of attacks, and the effects of antiepileptic drugs, and also, changes in metabolism may be simultaneously detected not only in the epileptogenic focus but in its surrounding areas, using a voxel size as large as 36 cc. However, the fact that information concerning the metabolism of high-energy phosphates and the phospholipids can be obtained directly is an advantage.

(2) ^{1}*H MRS*

Since Matthews et al.,[19] Hugg et al.,[20] and Cendes et al.[21]reported reductions in NAA level on the side of the epileptogenic focus compared with the opposite side, in which many researchers[22–30] have confirmed the usefulness of ^{1}H MRS for lateralization of temporal lobe epilepsy. Ende et al.[31] reported that NAA is a sensitive marker of hippocampal disorders, and Laxer et al.[32] showed that memory function can be evaluated by measurement of NAA in hippocampal neurons in patients with temporal lobe epilepsy. Fujimoto et al.,[18] Ende et al.,[33] and Vermathen et al.[34] demonstrated that the NAA level is reduced not only in the temporal lobe including the epileptogenic focus, but also in the contralateral temporal lobe. Hugg et al.[35] observed that NAA levels recovered in unresected hippocampus in patients with bilateral temporal lobe epilepsy following surgical elimination of seizures, and suggested that early medical or surgical treatment in epilepsy may prevent secondary dysfunction due to chronic seizures. In schizophrenia-like epileptic psychosis, the NAA level is reduced in the left mesial temporal lobe, and attention is being directed to the relationship between the lateralization of the epileptogenic focus and psychotic symptoms (Fujimoto et al.,[36,37] and Maier et al.[38]).

Petroff et al.[39–42] and Rothman et al.[43] showed a decrease in the level of gamma-aminobutyric acid (GABA) in the occipital lobe of epilepsy patients, which is a major inhibitory neurotransmitter in the human cerebral cortex, and increased GABA levels after treatment of vigabatrin, which increases the GABA concentrations in the cerebral cortex by 2–3 fold through inhibiting GABA-transaminase. Petroff et al.[44] and Savic et al.[45] observed an increase in the level of glutamate, the major excitatory neurotrnasmitter, in the epileptic human brain. Novotny et al.[46] also reported elevated glutamate levels in the brain of pediatric epilepsies. ^{1}H MRS is expected to play a major role in monitoring GABA and glutamate in the brain of patients with epilepsy.

References

1) Petroff, O. A. C.; Prichard, J. W.; Behar, K. L. et al. In vivo phosphorus nuclear magnetic resonance spectroscopy in status epilepticus. *Ann. Neurol.* 16: 169–177; 1984.

2) Schnall, M. D.; Yoshizaki, K.; Chance, B. et al. Triple nuclear NMR studies of cerebral metabolism during generalized seizure. *Magn. Reson. Med.* 6: 15–23; 1988.

3) Prichard, J. W. Nuclear magnetic resonance spectroscopy of seizure states. *Epilepsia* 35 (Suppl. 6): S14–S20; 1994.

4) Kuzniecky, R. I.; Jackson, G. D. Magnetic resonance in epilepsy. New York: Raven Press, 1995.

5) Fujimoto, T.; Asakura, T.; Nakamura, K. Epilepsy and MRS. In: H. Akimoto, T. Yamauchi (Eds). Advances in Epileptology No. 3. Iwasaki Gakujutu Shuppansha, 1996: pp. 327–357. [Japanese]

6) Niiro, M.; Asakura, T.; Nakamura, K. et al. ^{31}P chemical shift imaging of epileptic brains. *Progress in CT* 12: 493–503; 1990. [Japanese]

7) Nakamura, K.; Yatsushiro, K.; Asakura, T. et al. A study of epileptic brains with ^{31}P-Chemical shift imaging. *Neurosciences* 18 (Suppl.): 159-162; 1992. [Japanese]

8) Nakamura, K.; Asakura, T.; Yatsushiro, K. A localized metabolic study of epileptic brains with ^{31}P-chemical shift imaging. *Jap. J. Psych. Neurol.* 46: 467-469; 1992.

9) Fujimoto, T.; Nakamura, K.; Haruzono, A. et al. Changes in ^{31}Phosphorus metabolism in localization-related epilepsies. *Epilepsia* 36 (Suppl. 3): S146; 1995.

10) Hugg, J. W.; Laxer, K. D.; Matson, G. B. et al. Lateralization of human focal epilepsy by ^{31}P magnetic resonance spectroscopic imaging. *Neurology* 42: 2011-2018; 1992.

11) Laxer, K. D.; Hubesch, B.; Sappey-Marinier, D. et al. Increased pH and inorganic phosphate in temporal seizure foci demonstrated by [^{31}P] MRS. *Epilepsia* 33: 618-623; 1992.

12) Garcia, P. A.; Laxer, K. D.; Ng, T. Application of spectroscopic imaging in epilepsy. *Magn. Reson. Imaging* 13: 1181-1185; 1995.

13) Chu, W-J.; Hetherington, H. P.; Kuzniecky, R. I. et al. Is the intracellular pH different from normal in the epileptic focus of epilepsy patients? *In: Proceedings: Third Scientific Meeting and Exhibition of the Society of Magnetic Resonance, Vol. 1. Nice, France: SMR*; 1995: 142.

14) Chu, W. -J.; Hetherington, H. P.; Vaughan, J. T. et al. High resolution in vivo ^{31}P spectroscopy of temporal lobe epilepsy on 4.1 tesla whole body NMR. *In: Proceedings: Fourth Scientific Meeting and Exhibition of the International Society for Magnetic Resonance in Medicine, Vol. 1. New York, USA: ISMRM*; 1996: 133.

15) Kuzniecky, R.; Elgavish, G. A.; Hetherington, H. P. et al. In vivo ^{31}P nuclear magnetic resonance spectroscopy of human temporal lobe epilepsy. *Neurology* 42: 1586-1590; 1992.

16) Asakura, T.; Nakamura, K.; Terada, K. et al. New method of presurgical evaluation of epilepsy surgery with ^{31}P-chemical shift imaging. *Epilepsia* 34 (Suppl. 2): 169; 1993.

17) Nakamura, K.; Asakura, T.; Niiro, M. et al. [^{31}P] MRS/Chemical shift imaging study as presurgical evaluation of partial epilepsy. *Epilepsia* 36 (Suppl. 3): S146; 1995.

18) Fujimoto, T.; Matsumoto, T.; Haruzono, A. et al. Study of temporal lobe epilepsy using ^{1}H and ^{31}P MRS. *In: Proceedings: Fourth Scientific Meeting and Exhibition of the International Society for Magnetic Resonance in Medicine, Vol. 2. New York, USA: ISMRM*; 1996: 959.

19) Matthews, P. M.; Andermann, F.; Arnold, D. L. A proton magnetic resonance spectroscopy study of focal epilepsy in humans. *Neurology* 40: 985-989; 1990.

20) Hugg, J. W.; Laxer, K. D.; Matson, G. B. et al. Neuron loss localizes human temporal lobe epilepsy by in vivo proton magnetic resonance spectroscopic imaging. *Ann. Neurol.* 34: 788-794; 1993.

21) Cendes, F.; Andermann, F.; Preul, M. C. et al. Lateralization of temporal lobe epilepsy based on regional metabolic abnormalities in proton magnetic resonance spectroscopic images. *Ann. Neurol.* 35: 211-216; 1994.

22) Connelly, A.; Jackson, G. D.; Duncan, J. S. et al. Magnetic resonance spectroscopy in temporal lobe epilepsy. *Neurology* 44: 1411-1417; 1994.

23) Ng, T. C.; Comair, Y. G.; Xue, M. et al. Temporal lobe epilepsy: Presurgical localization with proton chemical shift imaging. *Radiology* 193: 465-472; 1994.

24) Breiter, S. N.; Arroyo, S.; Mathews, V. P. et al. Proton MR spectroscopy in patients with seizure disorders. *AJNR Am. J. Neuroradiol.* 15: 373-384; 1994.

25) Garcia, P. A.; Laxer, K. D.; van der Grond, J. et al. Proton magnetic resonance spectroscopic imaging in patients with frontal lobe epilepsy. *Ann. Neurol.* 37: 279-281; 1995.

26) Cendes, F.; Andermann, F.; Dubeau, F. et al. Proton magnetic resonance spectroscopic images and MRI volumetric studies for lateralization of temporal lobe epilepsy. *Magn. Reson. Imaging* 13: 1187-1191; 1995.

27) Hetherington, H. P.; Kuzniecky, R. I.; Pan, J. W. et al. Application of high field spectroscopic imaging in the evaluation of temporal lobe epilepsy. *Magn. Reson. Imaging* 13: 1175-1180; 1995.

28) Hetherington, H.; Kuzniecky, R.; Pan, J. et al. Proton nuclear magnetic resonance spectroscopic imaging of human temporal lobe epilepsy at 4.1T. *Ann. Neurol.* 38: 396-404; 1995.

29) Gadian, D. G. *N*-acetylaspartate and epilepsy. *Magn. Reson. Imaging* 13: 1193-1195; 1995.

30) Cross, J. H.; Connelly, A.; Jackson, G. D. et al. Proton magnetic resonance spectroscopy in children with temporal lobe epilepsy. *Ann. Neurol.* 39: 107-113; 1996.

31) Ende, G.; Knowlton, R.; Laxer, K. D. et al. NAA is a more sensitive marker of hippocampal disease than atrophy: Evidence that NAA is a neuronal marker. *In: Proceedings: Fourth Scientific Meeting and Exhibition of the International Society for Magnetic Resonance in Medicine, Vol. 1. New York, USA: ISMRM*; 1996: 137.

32) Laxer, K. D.; Ende, G.; Walker, J. A. et al. NAA as a measure of hippocampal function in temporal lobe

epilepsy. *In: Proceedings: Fourth Scientific Meeting and Exhibition of the International Society for Magnetic Resonance in Medicine, Vol. 1. New York, USA: ISMRM*; 1996: 136.

33) Ende, G.; Laxer, K. D.; Knowlton, R. et al. Quantitative ^{1}H SI shows bilateral metabolite changes in unilateral TLE patients with and without hippocampal atrophy. *In: Proceedings: Third Scientific Meeting and Exhibition of the Society of Magnetic Resonance, Vol. 1. Nice, France: SMR*; 1995: 144.

34) Vermathen, P.; Ende, G.; Laxer, K. D. et al. Hippocampal NAA is not reduced in neocortical epilepsy: Contrast with medial temporal lobe epilepsy. *In: Proceedings: Fourth Scientific Meeting and Exhibition of the International Society for Magnetic Resonance in Medicine, Vol. 1. New York, USA: ISMRM*; 1996: 138.

35) Hugg, J. W.; Hetherington, H. P.; Butterworth, E. J. et al. High resolution ^{1}H MRSI at 4.1T localizes temporal lobe epilepsy and detects recovery after surgery. *In : Proceedings: Fourth Scientific Meeting and Exhibition of the International Society for Magnetic Resonance in Medicine, Vol. 1. New York, USA: ISMRM*; 1996: 134.

36) Fujimoto, T.; Yamada, K.; Nakano, T. et al. Proton magnetic resonance spectroscopy in patients with epileptic psychotic syndrome. *Jap. J. Psych. Neurol*. 48: 360–363; 1994.

37) Fujimoto, T.; Yamada, K.; Nakano, T. et al. Proton spectroscopy using MRS with 2T in patients with epileptic psychoses. *In: Proceedings: Twelfth Annual Scientific Meeting of the Society of Magnetic Resonance in Medicine, Vol. 3. New York, USA: SMRM*; 1993: 1541.

38) Maier, M.; Mellers, J.; Ron, M. A. et al. Association between hippocampal NAA and psychosis: ^{1}H MRS study of schizophrenia and epilepsy. *In: Proceedings: Third Scientific Meeting and Exhibition of the Society of Magnetic Resonance, Vol. 1. Nice, France: SMR*; 1995: 143.

39) Petroff, O. A. C.; Rothman, D. L.; Behar, K. L. et al. Gabapentin increases brain GABA levels in patients with epilepsy. *In: Proceedings: Third Scientific Meeting and Exhibition of the Society of Magnetic Resonance, Vol. 1. Nice, France: SMR*; 1995: 140.

40) Petroff, O. A. C.; Rothman, D. L.; Behar, K. L. et al. Initial observations on effect of vigabatrin on in vivo ^{1}H spectroscopic measurements of γ-aminobutyric acid, glutamate, and glutamine in human brain. *Epilepsia* 36: 457–464; 1995.

41) Petroff, O. A. C.; Rothman, D. L.; Behar, K. L. et al. Low brain GABA is associated with poor seizure control in patients with complex partial epilepsy. *In: Proceedings: Fourth Scientific Meeting and Exhibition of the International Society for Magnetic Resonance in Medicine, Vol. 1. New York, USA: ISMRM*; 1996: 131.

42) Petroff, O. A. C.; Rothman, D. L.; Behar, K. L. et al. Estimates of the rate of GABA synthesis in patients with epilepsy. *In: Proceedings: Fourth Scientific Meeting and Exhibition of the International Society for Magnetic Resonance in Medicine, Vol. 2. New York, USA: ISMRM*; 1996: 962.

43) Rothman, D. L.; Behar, K. L.; Mattson, R. H. et al. Homocarnosine levels are elevated in epileptic patients taking vigabatrin: a novel measure of cortical pH. *In: Proceedings: Fourth Scientific Meeting and Exhibition of the International Society for Magnetic Resonance in Medicine, Vol. 1. New York, USA: ISMRM*; 1996: 130.

44) Petroff, O. A. C.; Pleban, L. A.; Spencer, D. D. Symbiosis between in vivo and in vitro NMR spectroscopy: The creatine, *N*-acetylaspartate, glutamate, and GABA content of the epileptic human brain. *Magn. Reson. Imaging* 13: 1197–1211; 1995.

45) Savic, I.; Ke, Y.; Thomas, M. A. et al. Localized ^{1}H MR spectroscopy in partial epilepsy. *In: Proceedings: Fourth Scientific Meeting and Exhibition of the International Society for Magnetic Resonance in Medicine, Vol. 2. New York, USA: ISMRM*; 1996: 956.

46) Novotny, E. J.; Rothman, D. L. Altered amino acid levels in pediatric epilepsies. *In: Proceedings : Fourth Scientific Meeting and Exhibition of the International Society for Magnetic Resonance in Medicine, Vol. 1. New York, USA: ISMRM*; 1996: 132.

11.2 CASES (65-75)

CASE 65

Case 65: A 26-year-old male
Symptomatic epilepsy. Partial seizures.
Seizure onset at 15 years of age.

The patient with a history of cerebral palsy had partial seizures with auditory hallucinations and delusional moods occasionally evolving into secondary generalized seizures, and right hemiplegia. The T_2-weighted image in Figure 65-1 shows a diffuse high signal intensity region and atrophy in the left cerebral hemisphere. The ^{31}P contour map illustrates a decreased signal intensity in the left temporal lesion, indicating decreased concentrations of metabolites (Figure 65-2). The total ATP contour map and metabolite image show decreased signal intensities in the left temporal lesion (Figures 65-3 and 4). The PME and PDE contour maps in Figures 65-5 and 6 demonstrate decreases in the signal intensity in the lesion of the left temporal lobe. The signal intensity in the PCr/Pi contour map is decreased in the left hemisphere (Figure 65-7), suggesting reduced high-energy phosphate metabolism in the left temporal lobe. In the ^{31}P spectrum of the right temporal lobe (voxel 3), the %PME is increased, the %Pi is decreased, and %PDE, %β-ATP and pHi are in the normal ranges (Figure 65-9). Most signals other than PCr are reduced in the ^{31}P spectrum of the left temporal lesion (voxel 6) in Figure 65-10, indicating reduced concentrations of membrane phospholipids and ATP.

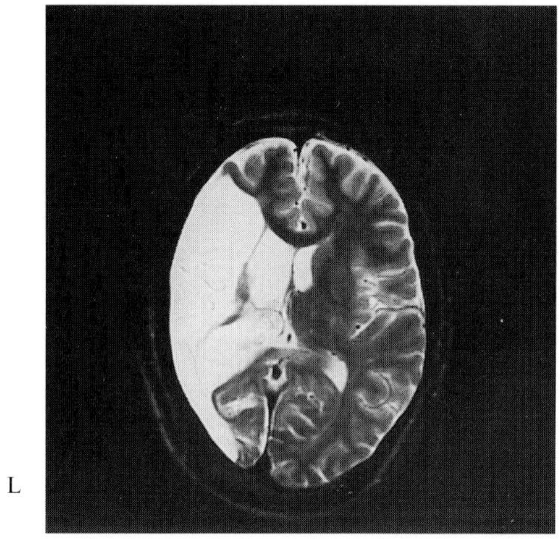

Fig. 65-1 Axial T_2-weighted image (2,200/90).

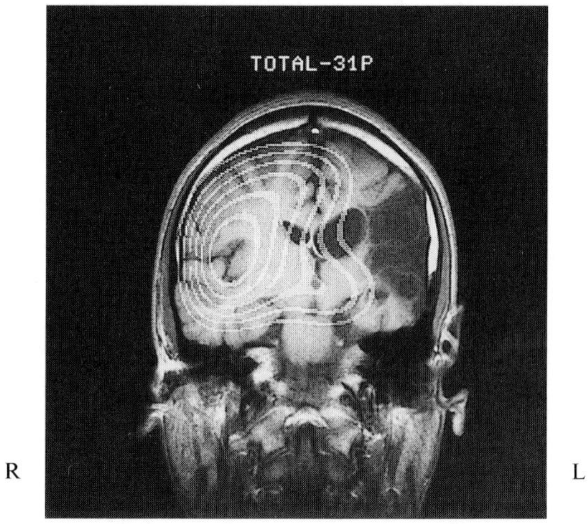

Fig. 65-2 Coronal ^{31}P contour map superimposed on T_1-weighted image (500/15).

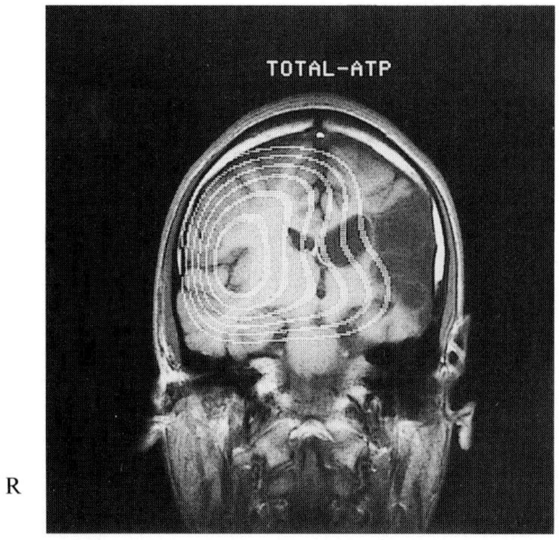

Fig. 65-3 Coronal total ATP contour map superimposed on T_1-weighted image (500/15).

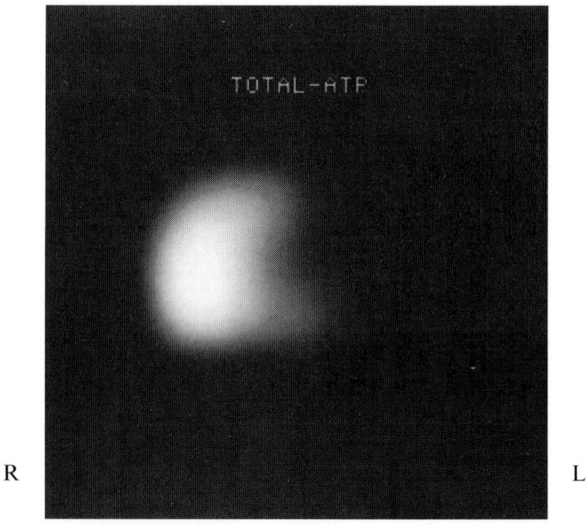

Fig. 65-4 Coronal total ATP metabolite image.

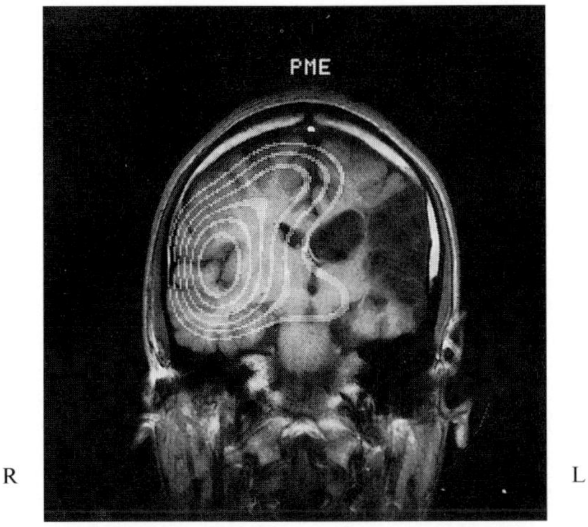

Fig. 65-5 Coronal PME contour map superimposed on T_1-weighted image (500/15).

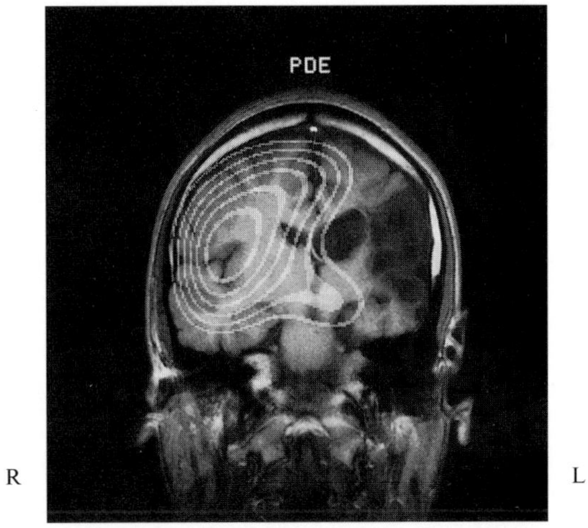

Fig. 65-6 Coronal PDE contour map superimposed on T_1-weighted image (500/15).

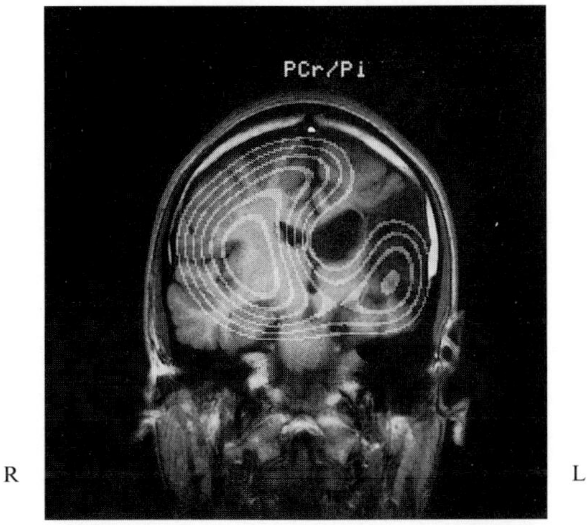

Fig. 65-7 Coronal PCr/Pi contour map superimposed on T_1-weighted image (500/15).

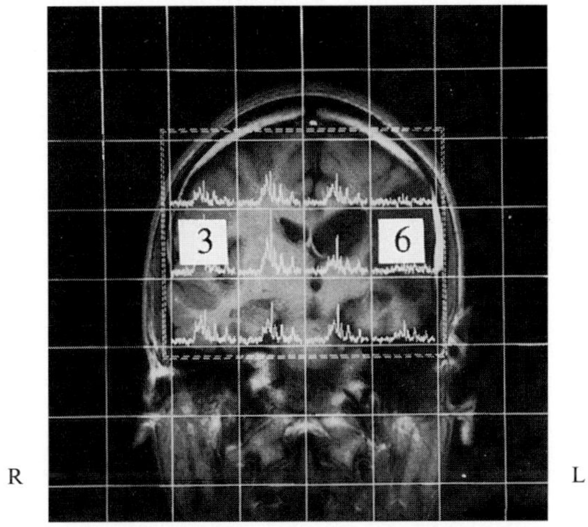

Fig. 65-8 T_1-weighted image showing the position of 3×3×4 cm³ voxels 3 and 6.

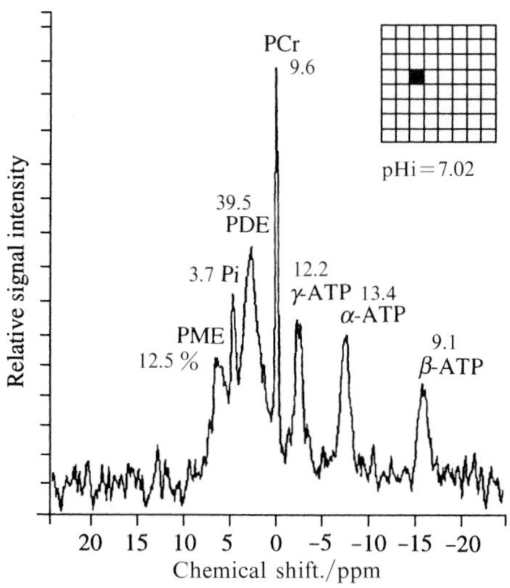

Fig. 65-9 ³¹P spectrum of voxel 3.

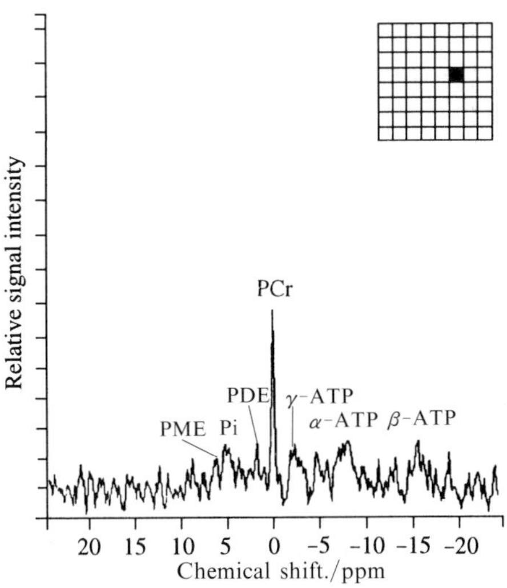

Fig. 65-10 ³¹P spectrum of voxel 6.

CASE 66

Case 66: A 51-year-old male

Symptomatic epilepsy. Complex partial seizure. Seizure onset at 22 years of age.

The patient presented complex partial seizure with automatism occasionally evolving into secondary generalized seizures and left hemianopsia following a head injury caused by a traffic accident at age 22 years. The T_2-weighted image in Figure 66-1 shows a high signal intensity region in the right occipital lobe and atrophy of bilateral occipital lobes. The signal intensity is almost symmetric in the ^{31}P contour map in Figure 66-2. The ATP metabolite image shows a decreased signal intensity in the right occipital region (Figure 66-3). The PME metabolite image shows increased signal intensities in the right occipital lesion (Figure 66-4). The Pi signal intensity of the contour map in Figure 66-5 is slightly decreased in the lesion and increased in the left mesial temporal lobe, compared to the contralateral areas. The signal intensity of PDE in the occipital lesion is elevated in the left mesial temporal lobe (Figure 66-6). The PCr/Pi ratio shows a complex pattern and is higher in the right occipital lesion than in the area opposite (Figure 66-7). Changes in signal intensities of Pi, PDE and PCr/Pi demonstrate metabolic abnormalities not only in the right occipital lobe but also in the left mesial temporal lobe. The %PME is increased in the right occipital lobe (voxel B), suggesting alterations in membrane phospholipids (Figure 66-10).

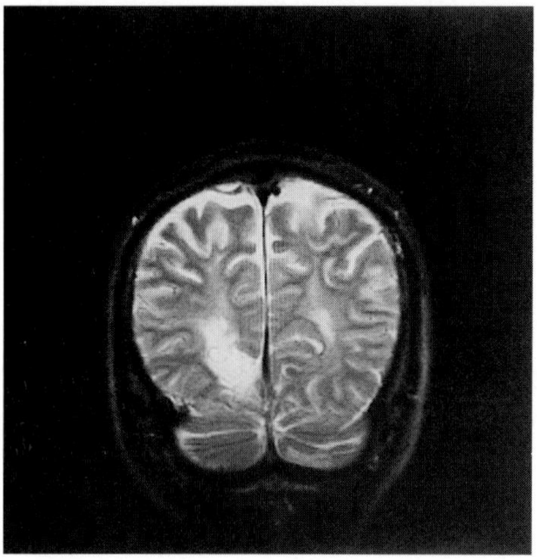

Fig. 66-1 Coronal T_2-weighted image (2,200/90).

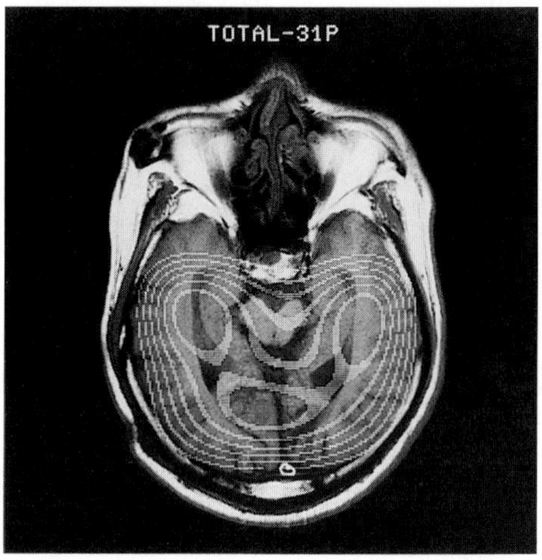

Fig. 66-2 Axial ^{31}P contour map superimposed on T_1-weighted image (500/15).

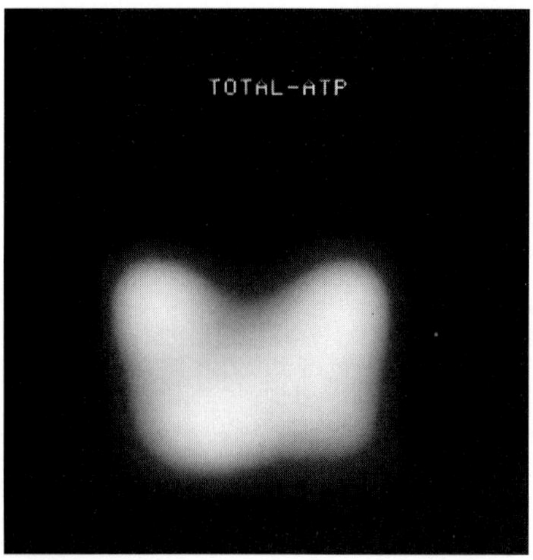

Fig. 66-3 Axial total ATP metabolite image.

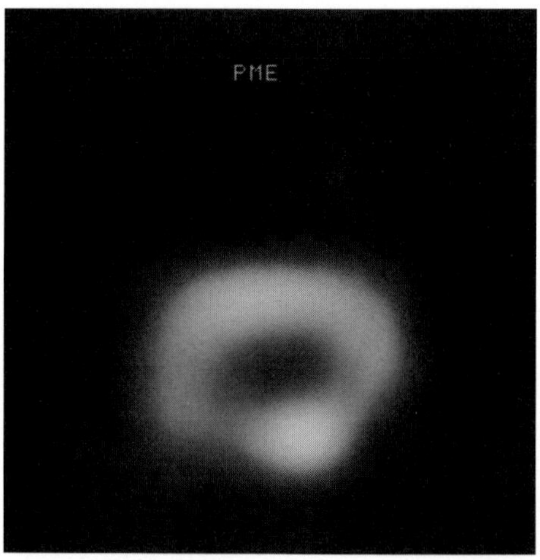

Fig. 66-4 Axial PME metabolite image.

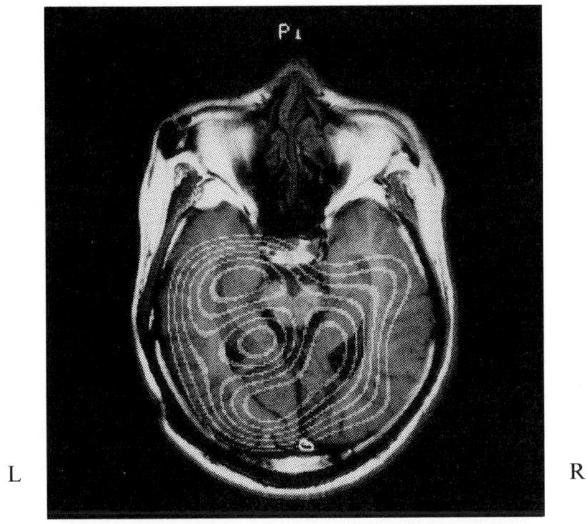

Fig. 66-5 Axial Pi contour map superimposed on T_1-weighted image (500/15).

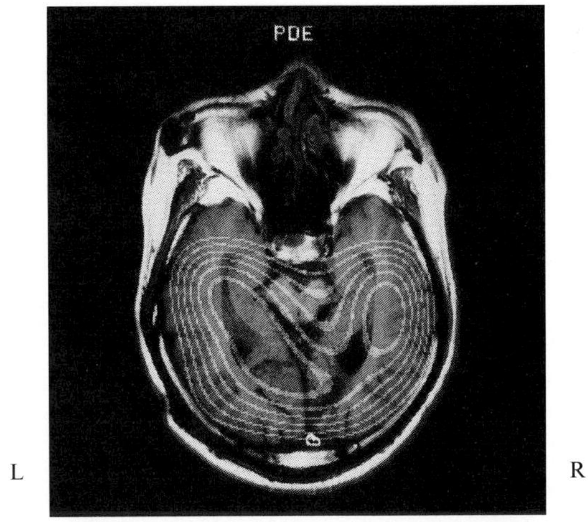

Fig. 66-6 Axial PDE contour map superimposed on T_1-weighted image (500/15).

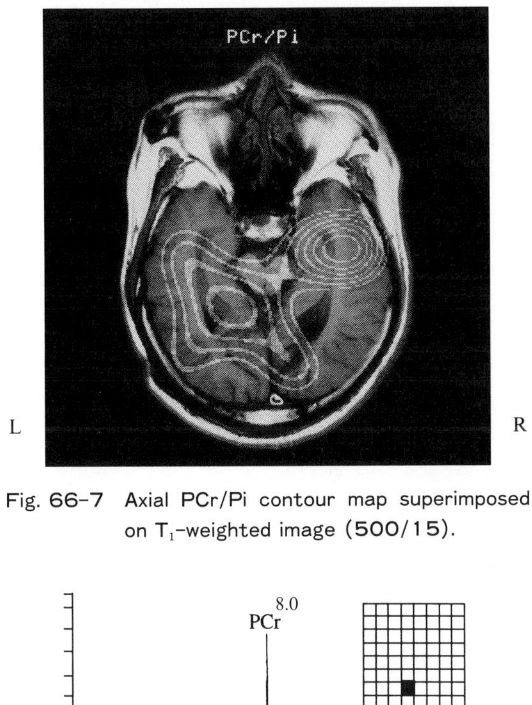

Fig. 66-7 Axial PCr/Pi contour map superimposed on T_1-weighted image (500/15).

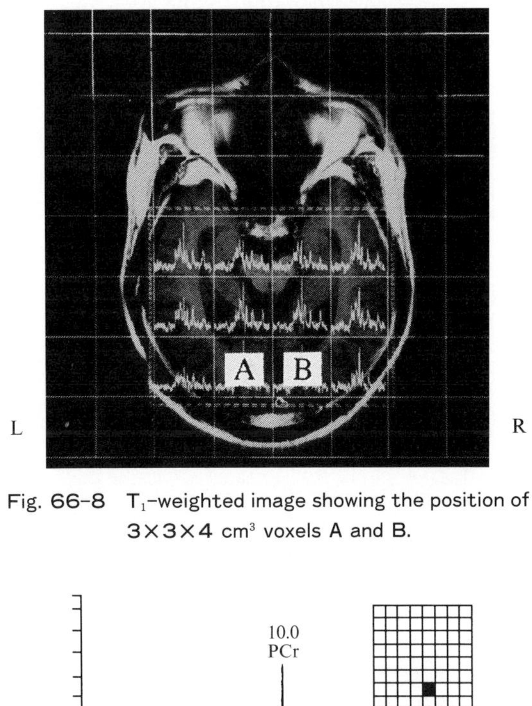

Fig. 66-8 T_1-weighted image showing the position of $3 \times 3 \times 4$ cm^3 voxels A and B.

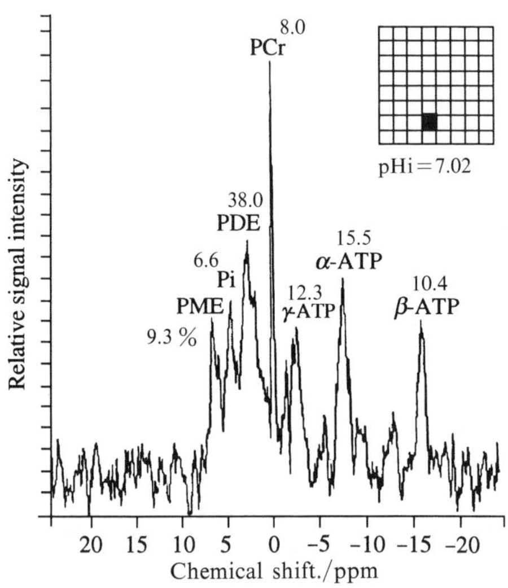

Fig. 66-9 ^{31}P spectrum of left occipital lobe (voxel A).

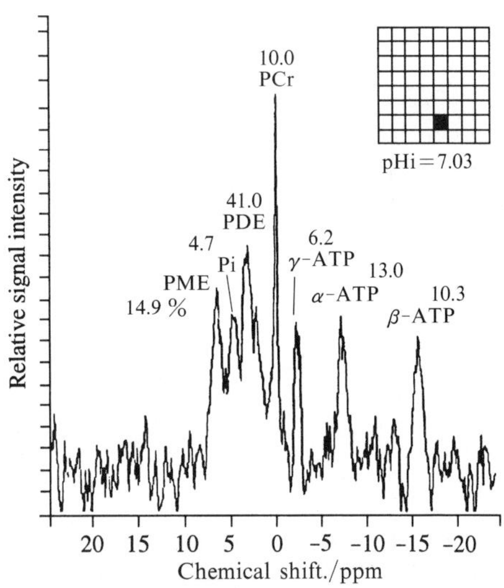

Fig. 66-10 ^{31}P spectrum of right occipital lobe (voxel B).

CASE 67

Case 67: A 25-year-old male
Symptomatic epilepsy. Partial seizures.
Seizure onset at 20 days after birth.

The patient with a history of cerebral palsy presented mental retardation and partial seizures with auditory hallucination of the right ear and autonomic signs occasionally evolving into secondary generalized seizures. The T_2-weighted image in Figure 67-1 shows high signal intensity regions and atrophy in the left temporal and frontal lobes with an enlargement of the left lateral ventricle. The ^{31}P contour map in Figure 67-2 shows reduced signal intensities in the left temporal and frontal lobes corresponding to the high intensity area in the T_2-weighted image. The total ATP contour map in Figure 67-3 shows a decreased signal intensity in the lesion of the left temporal lobe. The signal intensity of PME is also reduced in the left temporal lesion (Figure 67-4). The Pi metabolite image and the PDE contour map in Figures 67-5 and 6 also illustrate reduced signal intensities in the lesion of left temporal lobe. A reduced signal intesity in the PCr/Pi metabolite image in Figure 67-7 reflects decreased high-energy phosphate metabolism in the lesion of the left temporal lobe. In the ^{31}P spectrum in the right temporal lobe (voxel 3), the %PCr is elevated (Figure 67-9). In Figure 67-10, the S/N ratio of the ^{31}P spectrum in the left temporal lesion (voxel 6) is generally poor, and the %Pi and the %β-ATP are decreased, suggesting dysfunction in the high-energy phosphate metabolism in the lesion.

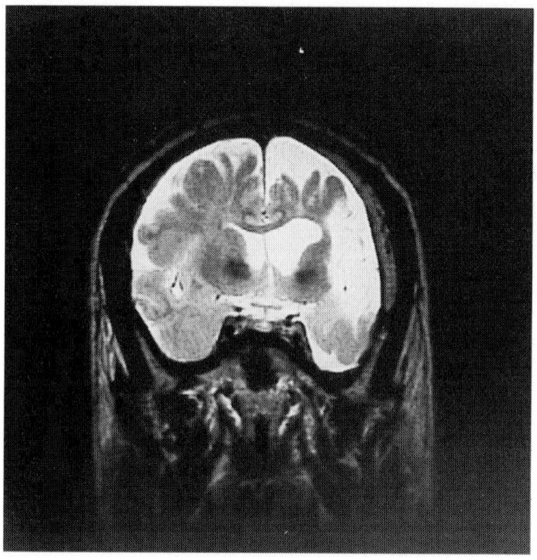

Fig. 67-1 Coronal T_2-weighted image (2,200/90).

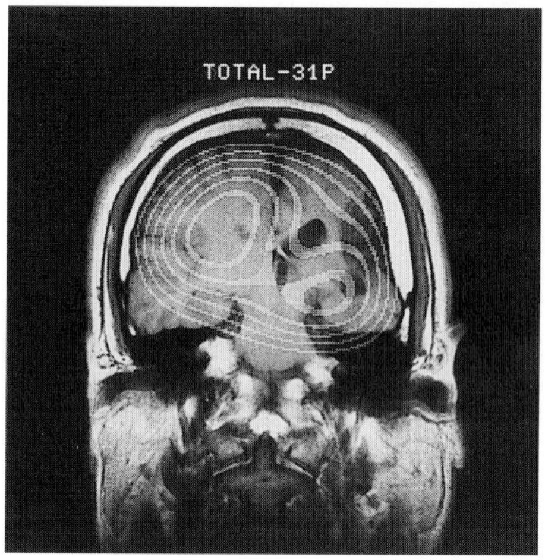

Fig. 67-2 Coronal ^{31}P contour map superimposed on T_1-weighted image (500/15).

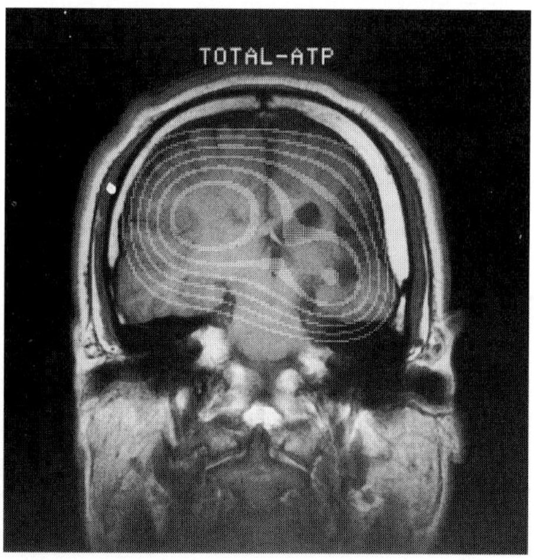

Fig. 67-3 Coronal total ATP contour map superimposed on T_1-weighted image (500/15).

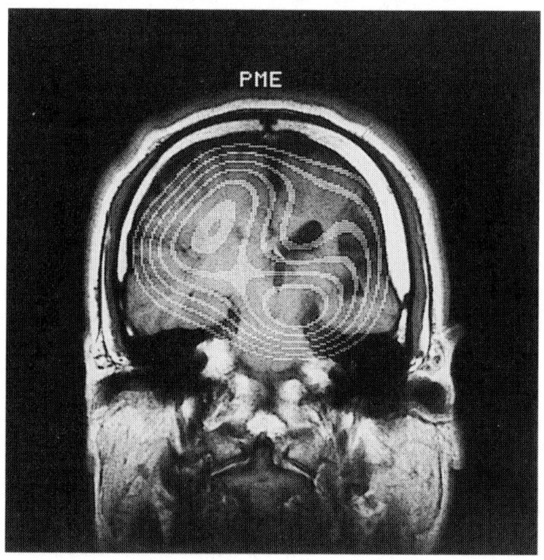

Fig. 67-4 Coronal PME contour map superimposed on T_1-weighted image (500/15).

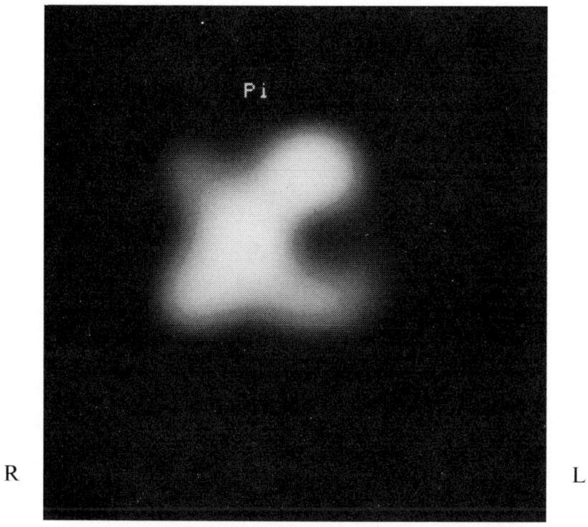

Fig. 67-5 Coronal Pi metabolite image.

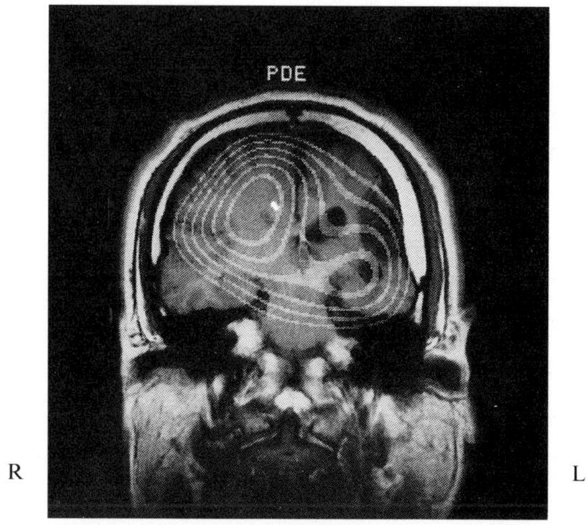

Fig. 67-6 Coronal PDE contour map superimposed on T_1-weighted image (500/15).

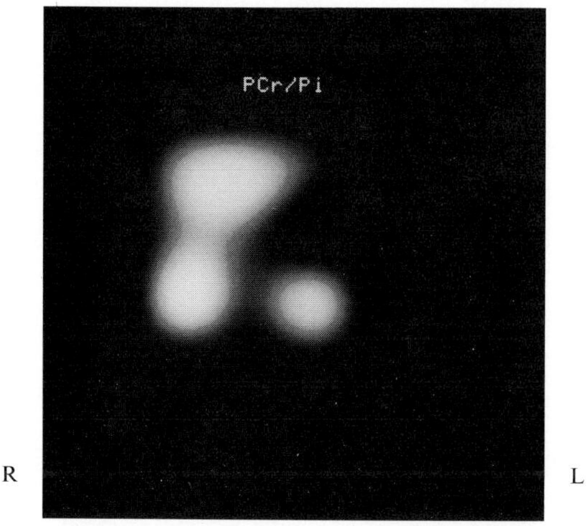

Fig. 67-7 Coronal PCr/Pi metabolite image.

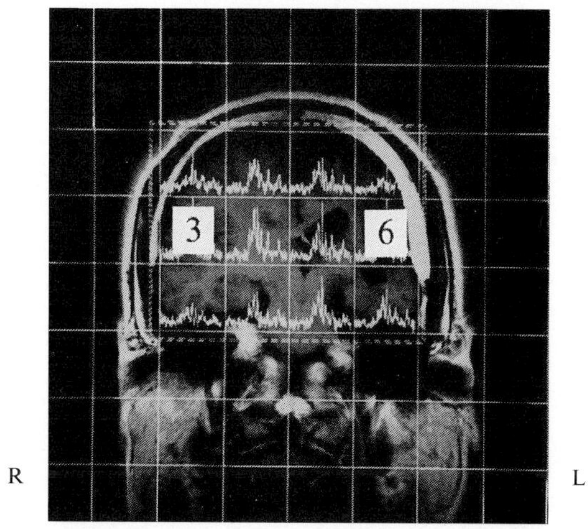

Fig. 67-8 T_1-weighted image showing the position of 3×3×4 cm^3 voxels 3 and 6.

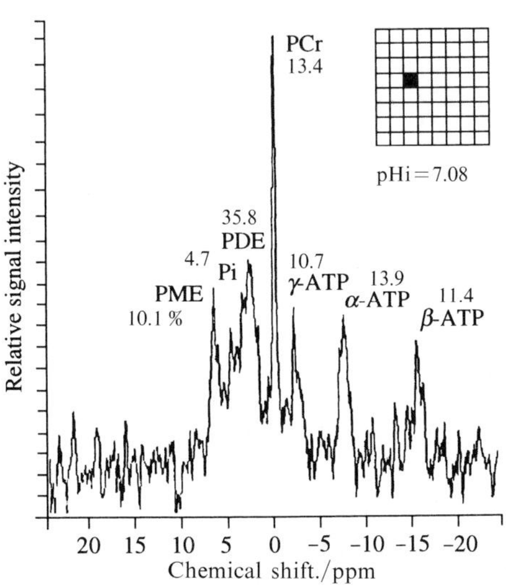

Fig. 67-9 ^{31}P spectrum of right temporal lobe (voxel 3).

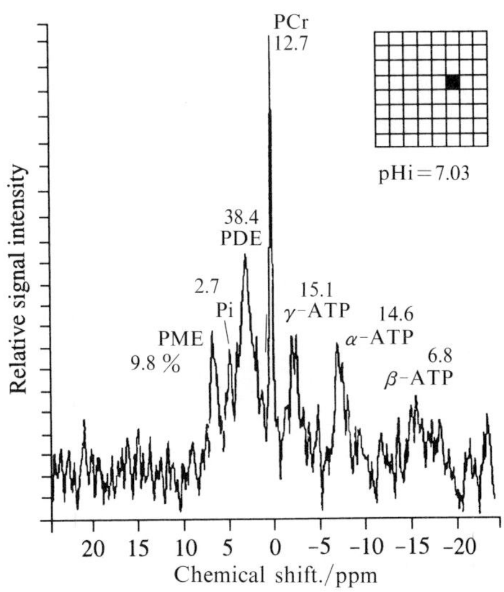

Fig. 67-10 ^{31}P spectrum of left temporal lobe (voxel 6).

CASE 68

Case 68: A 40-year-old male
Symptomatic epilepsy. Partial seizures.
Seizure onset at 11 years of age.

The patient presented partial seizures with imbalance and twisting movements of the bilateral upper limbs. The T_2-weighted image in Figure 68-1 shows high signal intensity regions and atrophy in the right temporal lobe. In the ^{31}P metabolite image in Figure 68-2 shows reduced signal intensities in the right temporal lobe corresponding to the high intensity area in the T_2-weighted image, suggesting a reduced metabolism. The total ATP contour map in Figure 68-3 shows a decreased signal intensity in the lesion of the right temporal lobe. The signal intensity of PME is also reduced in the right temporal lesion (Figure 68-4). The Pi contour map and the PDE metabolite image in Figures 68-5 and 6 also illustrate reduced signal intensities in the lesion. The PCr/Pi contour map in Figure 68-7 shows decreased signal intensity in the lesion and increased signal intensity in the left temporo-occipital and right temporo-frontal lobes. In the ^{31}P spectrum in the left temporal lobe (voxel A) shown in Figure 68-8, the %PME has a tendency to decrease (Figure 68-9). In Figure 68-10, the ^{31}P spectrum obtained from the voxel B including the right temporal lesion shows decreased %PME and increased %α-ATP. The reduced %PME suggests disturbance of the phospholipids in the lesion.

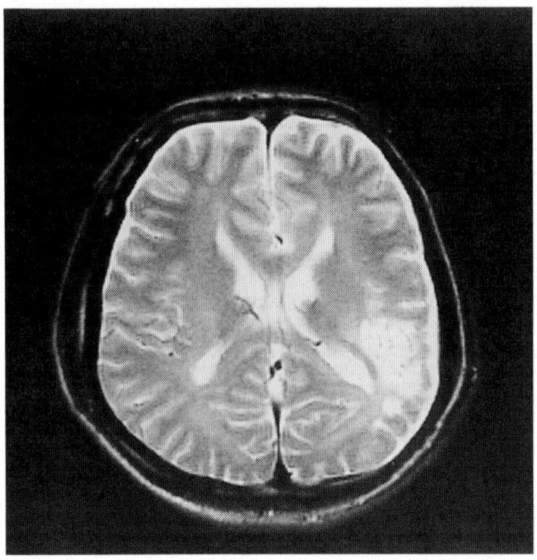

Fig. 68-1 Axial T_2-weighted image (2,200/90).

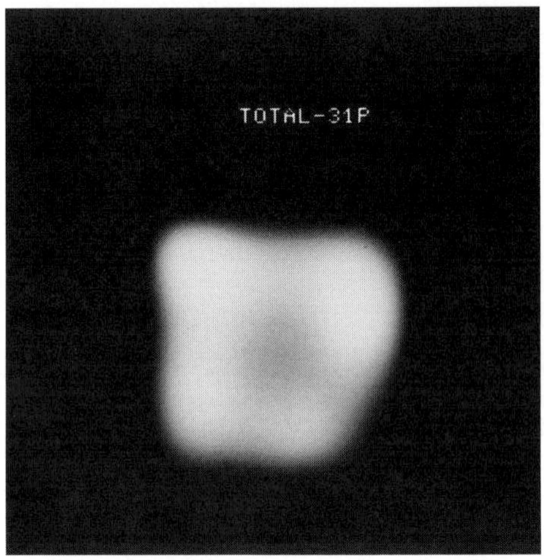

Fig. 68-2 Axial ^{31}P metabolite image.

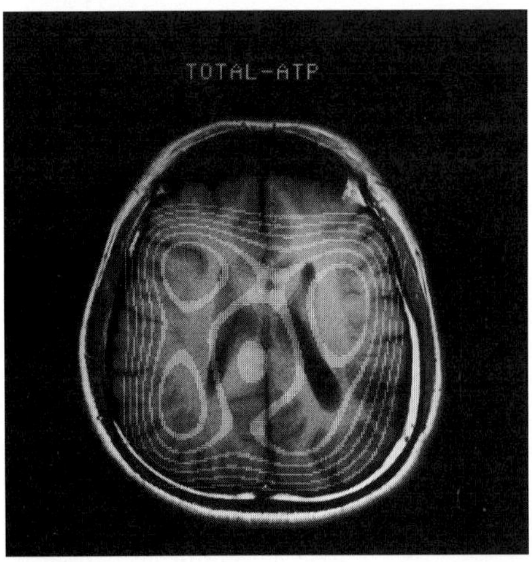

Fig. 68-3 Axial total ATP contour map superimposed on T_1-weighted image (500/15).

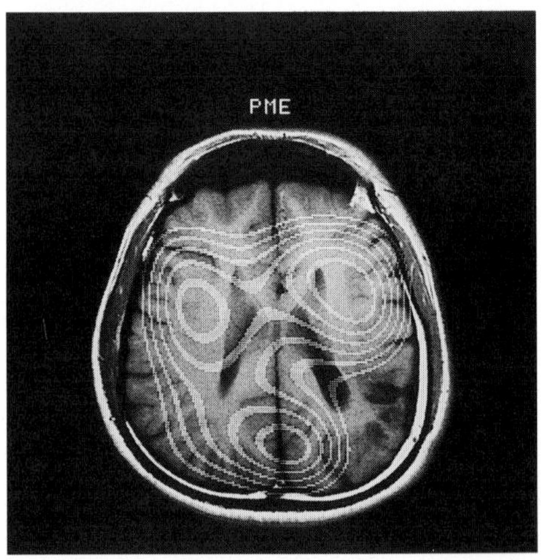

Fig. 68-4 Axial PME contour map superimposed on T_1-weighted image (500/15).

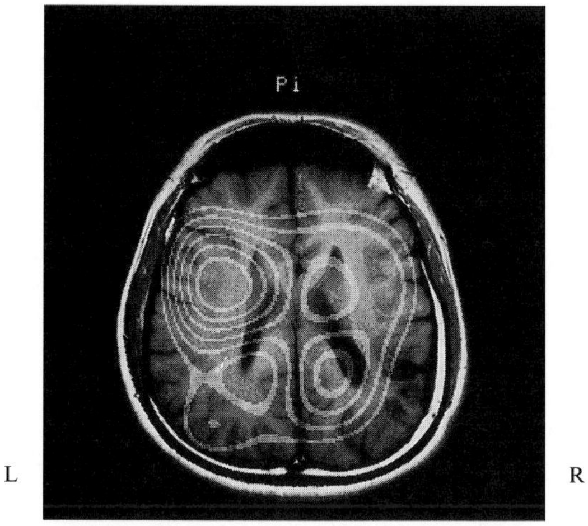

Fig. 68-5 Axial Pi contour map superimposed on T_1-weighted image (500/15).

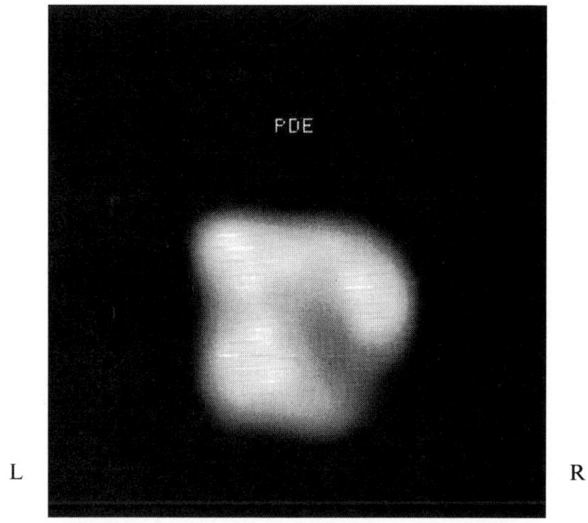

Fig. 68-6 Axial PDE metabolite image (500/15).

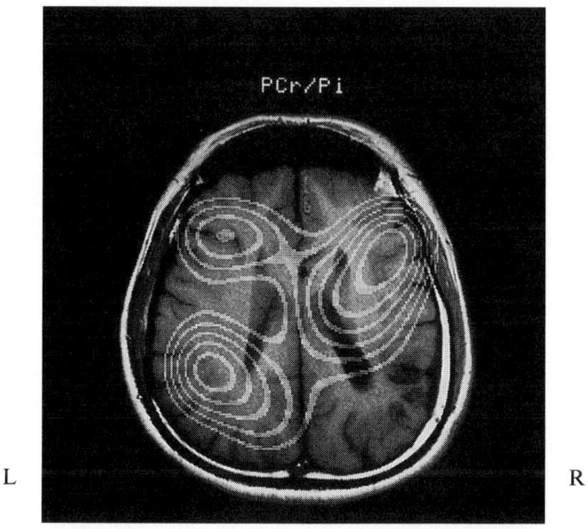

Fig. 68-7 Axial PCr/Pi contour map superimposed on T_1-weighted image (500/15).

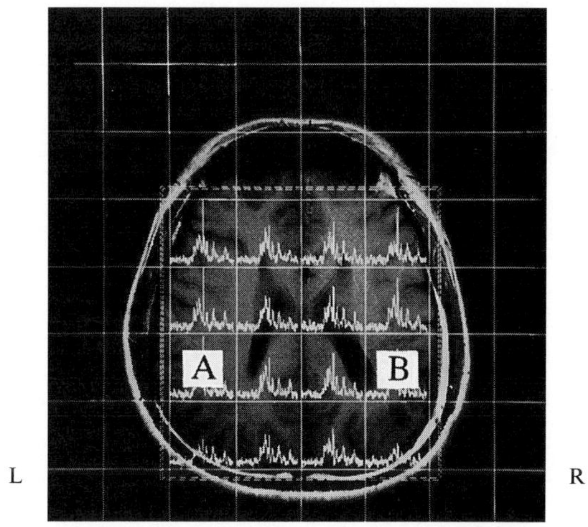

Fig. 68-8 T_1-weighted image showing the position of $3 \times 3 \times 4$ cm^3 voxels A and B.

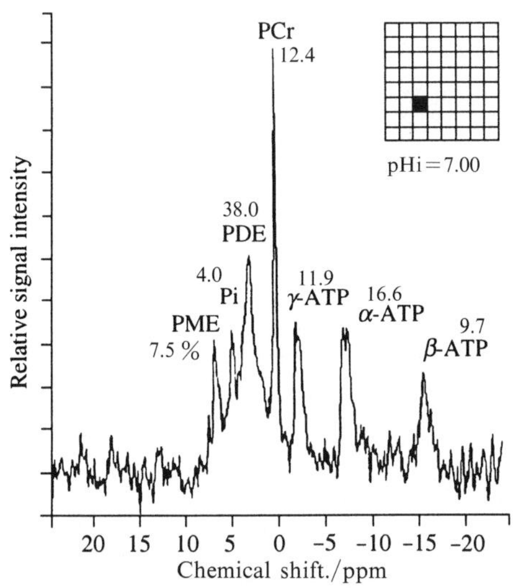

Fig. 68-9 ^{31}P spectrum of left temporal lobe (voxel A).

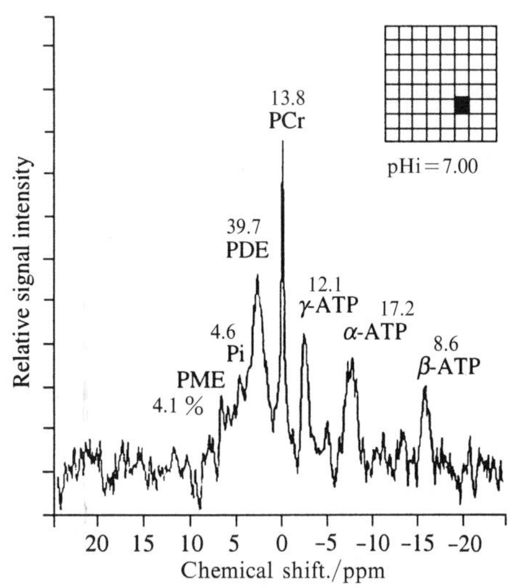

Fig. 68-10 ^{31}P spectrum of right temporal lobe (voxel B).

CASE 69

Case 69: A 44-year-old male
Symptomatic epilepsy. Partial seizure.
Seizure onset at 40 days from birth.

The patient with a history of cerebral palsy presented right hemiparesis, mental retardation, and partial seizures with impaired consciousness occasionally evolving into secondary generalized seizures. The T_2-weighted image in Figure 69-1 shows high signal intensity regions and atrophy in the left portion of the thalamus adjacent to the third ventricle and the frontal horn. The ^{31}P contour map in Figure 69-2 shows reduced signal intensities in the lesion corresponding to the high intensity area in the T_2-weighted image, suggesting a reduced concentration of metabolites. The total ATP metabolite image in Figure 69-3 shows decreased signal intensity in the lesion. The signal intensity of Pi is also reduced in the lesion (Figure 69-4). The PDE and the PCr contour maps in Figures 69-5 and 6 also illustrate reduced signal intensities in the lesion. The PCr/Pi contour map in Figure 69-7 shows decreased signal intensities in the lesion and in the left temporal lobe. In the ^{31}P spectrum in voxel 4 which is contralateral to the lesion shown in Figure 69-8, the %PDE is reduced, and the %α-ATP is elevated (Figure 69-9). In Figure 69-10, the ^{31}P spectrum obtained from voxel 5 in Figure 69-8 including the lesion shows a decreased %PDE. These findings suggest metabolic changes such as high-energy phosphate and phospholipids in the brain.

R 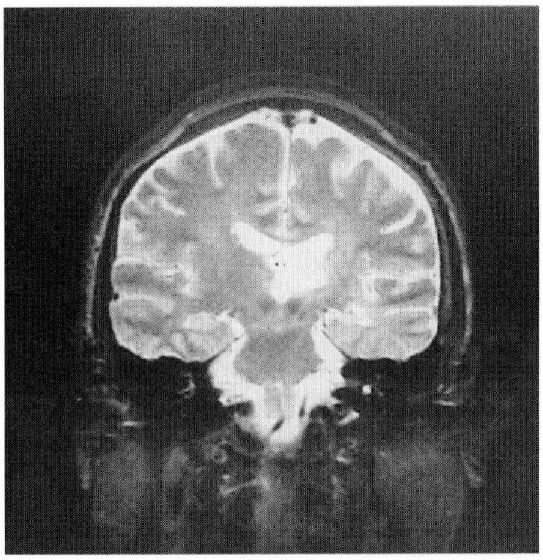 L

Fig. 69-1 Coronal T_2-weighted image (2,200/90).

R 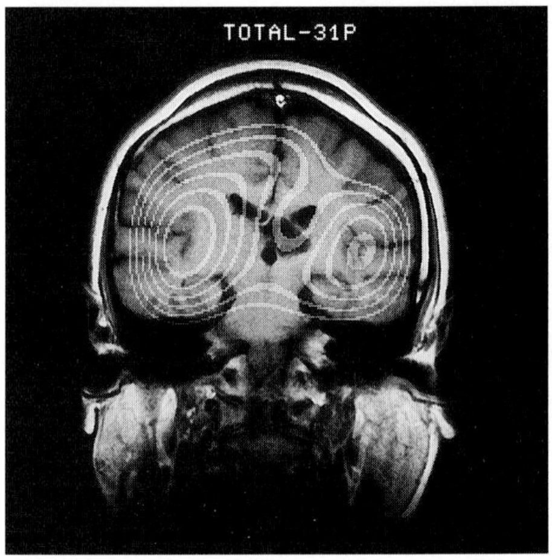 L

Fig. 69-2 Coronal ^{31}P contour map superimposed on T_1-weighted image (500/15).

R 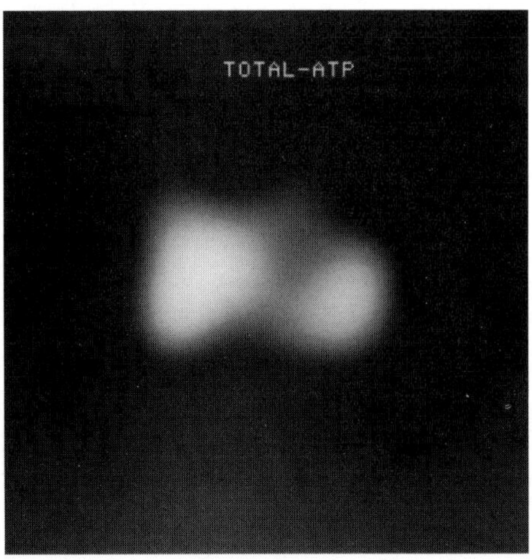 L

Fig. 69-3 Coronal total ATP metabolite image.

R 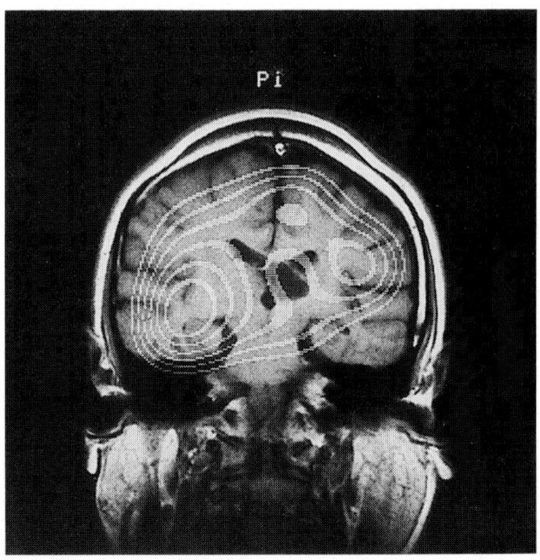 L

Fig. 69-4 Coronal Pi contour map superimposed on T_1-weighted image (500/15).

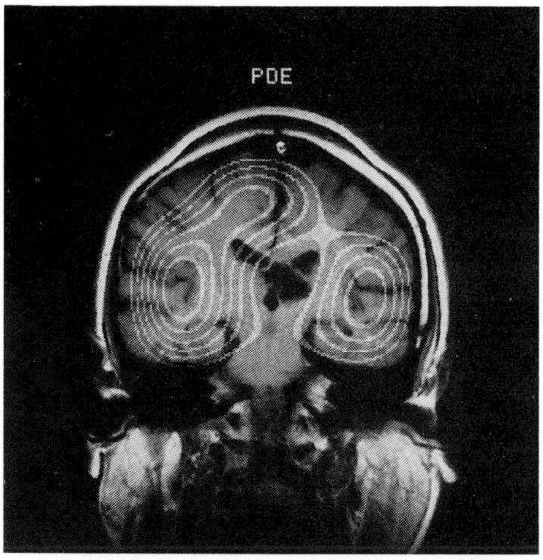

Fig. 69-5 Coronal PDE contour map superimposed on T_1-weighted image (500/15).

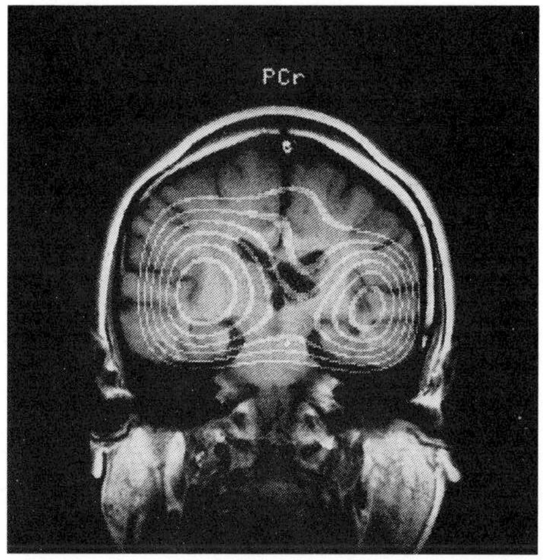

Fig. 69-6 Coronal PCr contour map superimposed on T_1-weighted image (500/15).

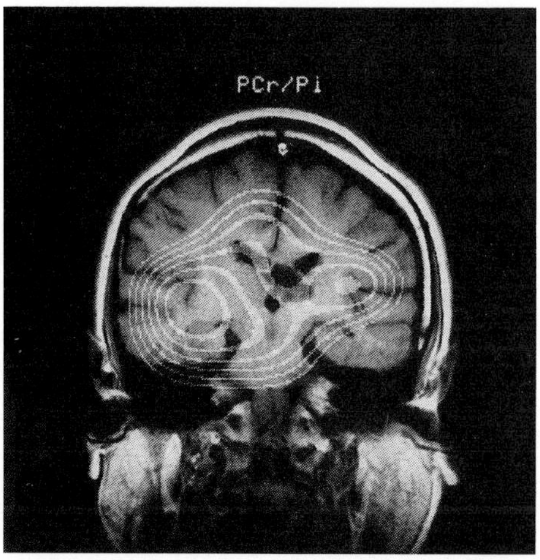

Fig. 69-7 Coronal PCr/Pi contour map superimposed on T_1-weighted image (500/15).

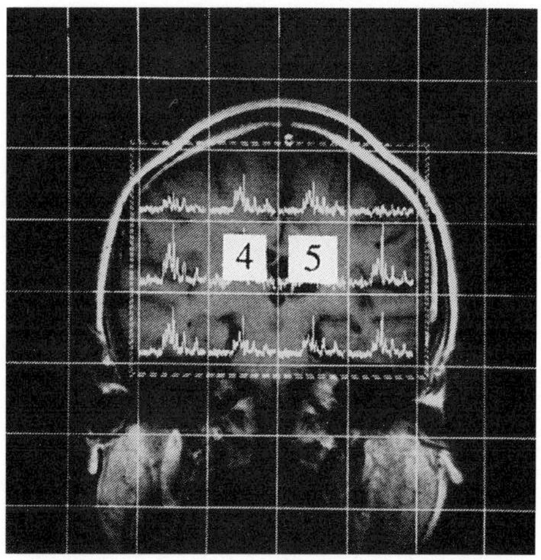

Fig. 69-8 T_1-weighted image showing the position of $3 \times 3 \times 4$ cm^3 voxels 4 and 5.

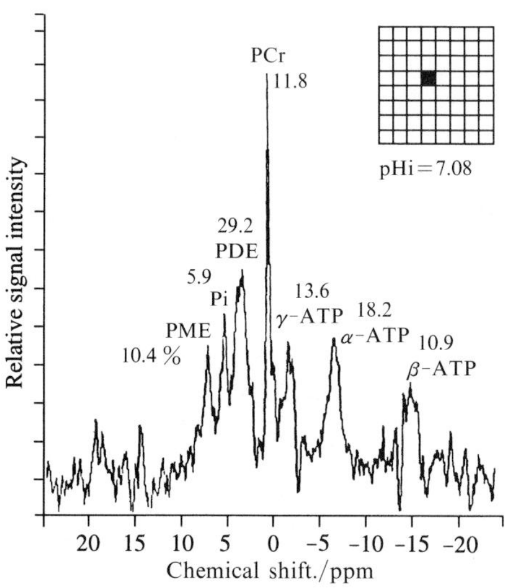

Fig. 69-9 ^{31}P spectrum of voxel 4.

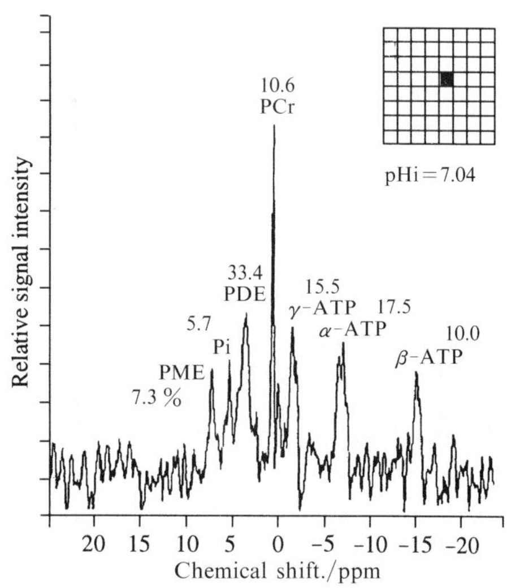

Fig. 69-10 ^{31}P spectrum of voxel 5.

CASE 70

Case 70: A 37-year-old male

Symptomatic epilepsy. Complex partial seizure with cavernous angioma.

Seizure onset at 26 years of age.

The patient presented unconsciousness and automatism seizure with twisting movement of the right upper limb and oral movement. He had been operated on for left cavernous angioma. The T_2-weighted image in Figure 70-1 shows a cavernous angioma in the left temporal lobe. The SPECT image in Figure 70-2 indicates reduced blood flow in the left temporal lobe. The ^{31}P, total ATP, and PME metabolite images show almost symmetrical signal intensities (Figures 70-3,4 and 5). Signal intensities are reduced around the left basal ganglia region in the PCr/Pi contour map in Figure 70-6. The Pi contour map and metabolite image in Figures 70-7 and 8 show increased signal intensities in the left temporal lobe, probably due to hypometabolism in this region. The signal intensities are symmetrical in the PCr metabolite image and contour map in Figures 70-9 and 10.

R 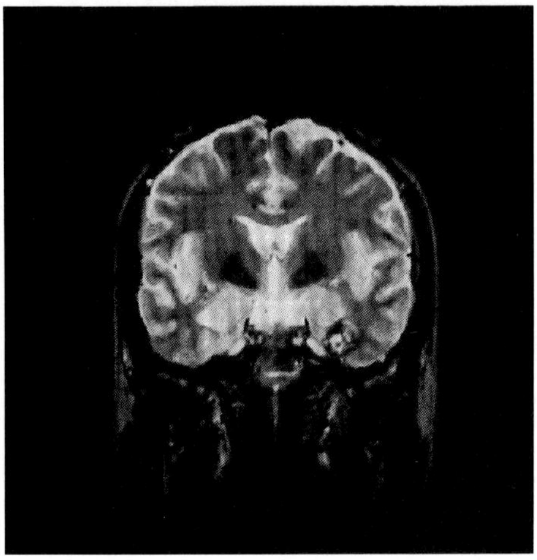 L

Fig. 70-1 Coronal T_2-weighted image (2,200/90).

L 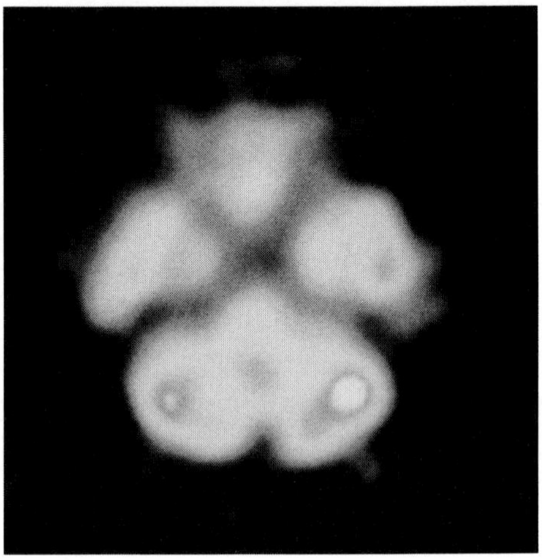 R

Fig. 70-2 SPECT.

R 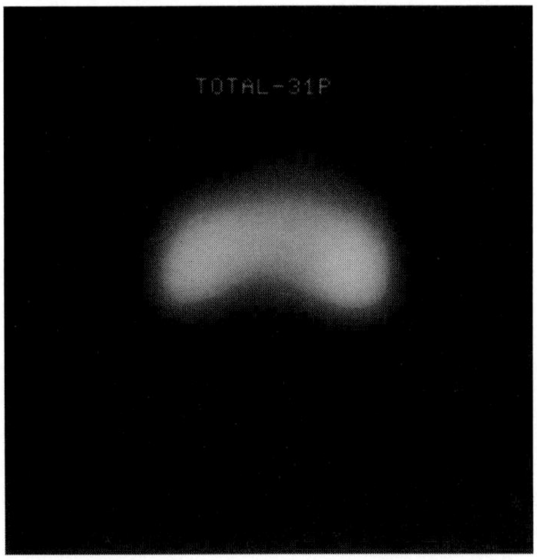 L

Fig. 70-3 Coronal ^{31}P metabolite image.

R 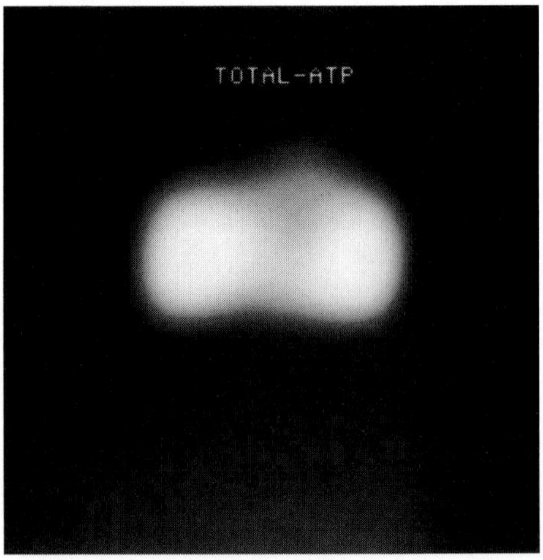 L

Fig. 70-4 Coronal total ATP metabolite image.

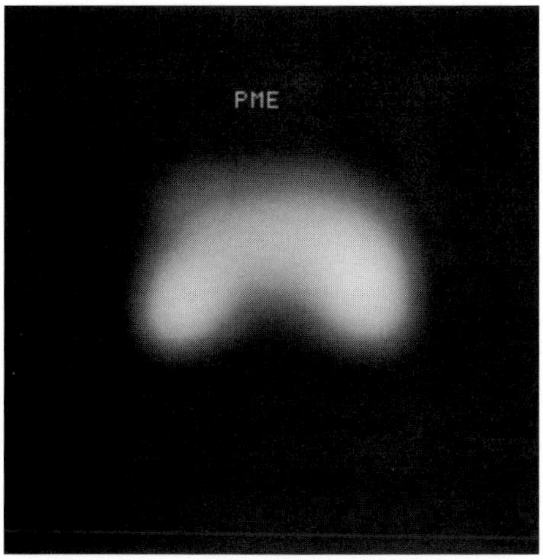

Fig. 70-5 Coronal PME metabolite image.

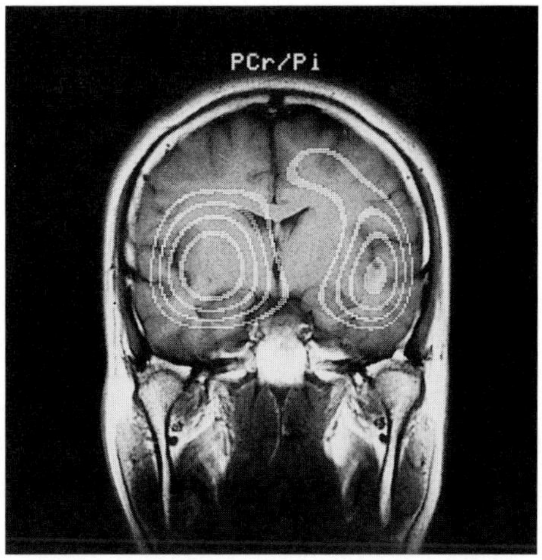

Fig. 70-6 Coronal PCr/Pi contour map superimposed on T_1-weighted image (500/15).

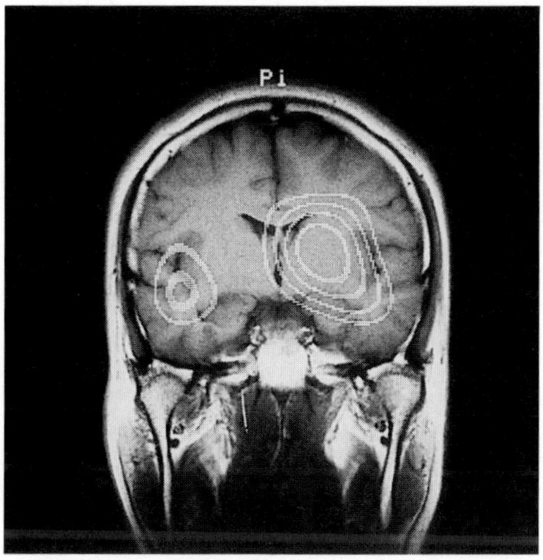

Fig. 70-7 Coronal Pi contour map superimposed on T_1-weighted image (500/15).

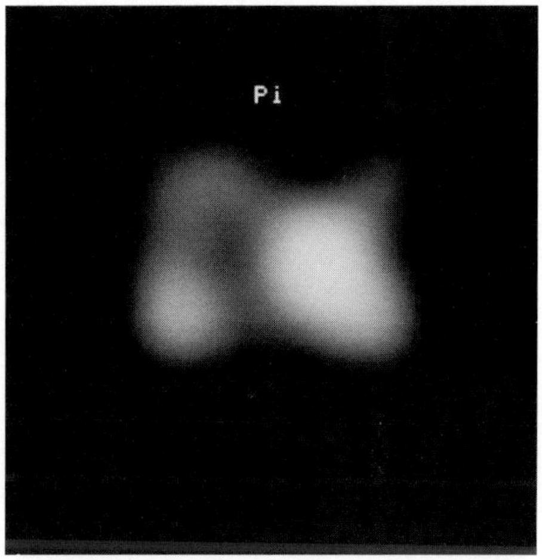

Fig. 70-8 Coronal Pi metabolite image.

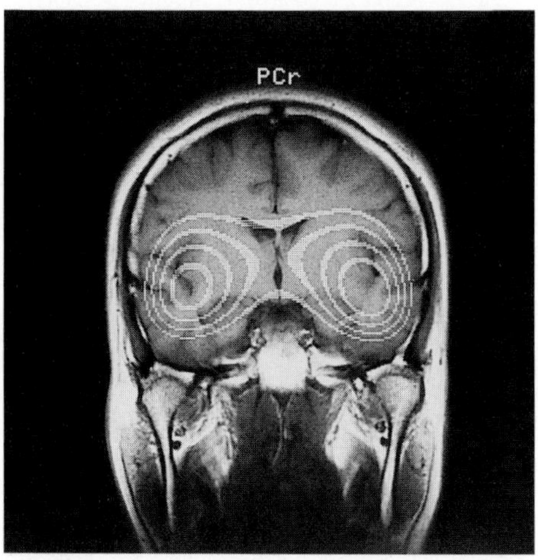

Fig. 70-9 Coronal PCr contour map superimposed on T_1-weighted image (500/15).

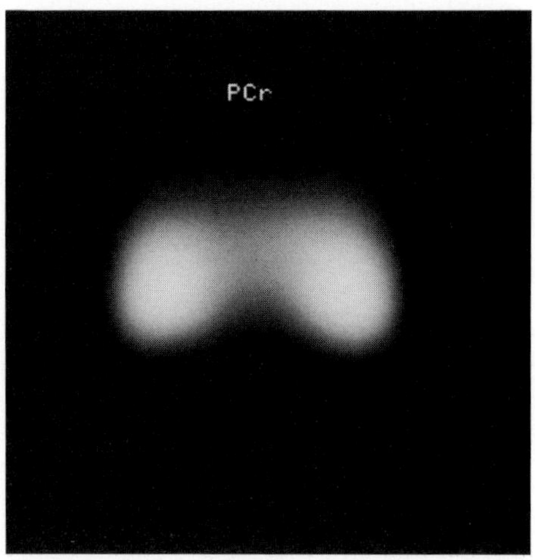

Fig. 70-10 Coronal PCr metabolite image.

CASE 71

Case 71: A 12-year-old female
Absence (before and after corpus callosotomy).
Seizure onset at 5 months after birth.

The first seizure occurred as a generalized seizure. Bilateral chronic subdural hematoma was detected by CT scan, and surgery (burr hole irrigation) was performed. Thereafter, seizures were uncontrolled with anticonvulsant, and seizures occured 2–3 times a day. Callosotomy was conducted. No particular abnormality is noted in the T_2-weighted images in Figures 71–1 and 2. Figure 71–3 is a preoperative sagittal image. In Figure 71–4, a postoperative sagittal image shows that the anterior two-thirds of the corpus callosum is separated. In the ^{31}P metabolite image after corpus callosotomy in Figure 71–6, ^{31}P signal intensity is more evenly distributed, compared to before surgery as in Figure 71–5. The total ATP metabolite image before operation (Figure 71–7) shows a higher decrease in signal intensity in the left temporal lobe than after surgery in Figure 71–8, which shows a tendency to almost symmetrical signal distribution. In the PME metabolite image before surgery in Figure 71–9, the PME signal intensity shows irregular distribution, compared to that after surgery in Figure 71-10. These metabolite images may suggest that the ^{31}P metabolites distribute more evenly due to corpus callosotomy, but further investigation is necessary to determine the effects of corpus callosotomy in epilepsy.

L 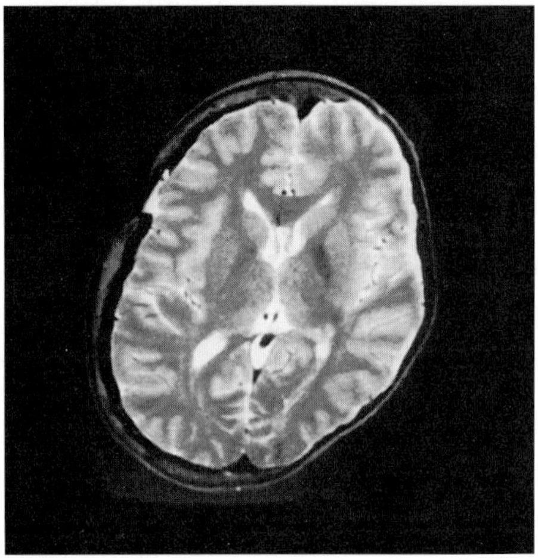 R

Fig. 71–1 Axial T_2-weighted image (2,200/90).

L 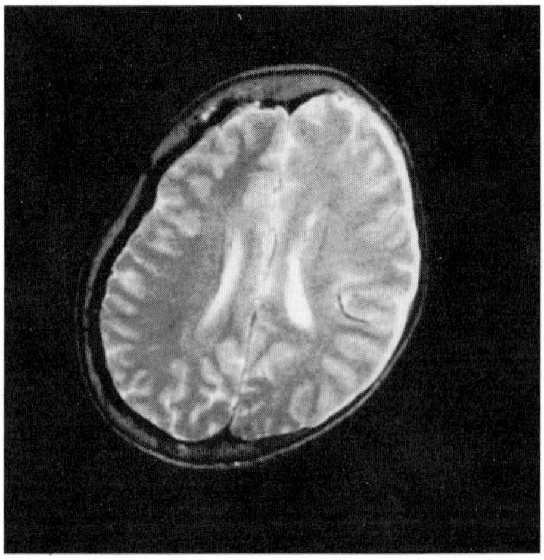 R

Fig. 71–2 Axial T_2-weighted image (2,200/90).

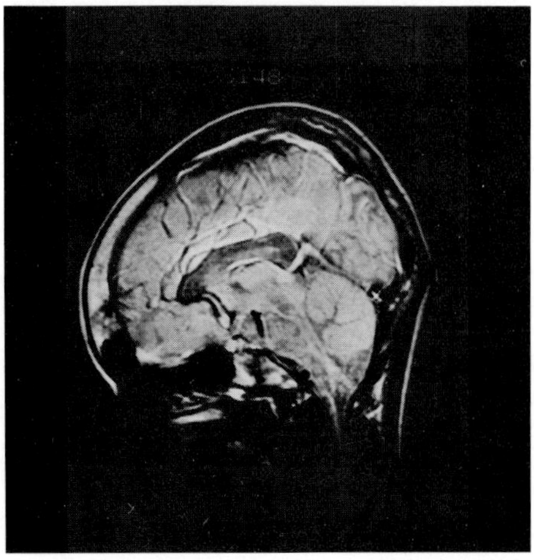

Fig. 71–3 Sagittal image before corpus callosotomy.

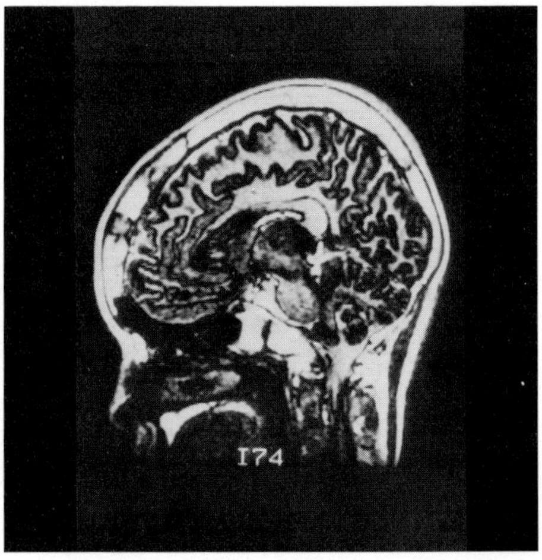

Fig. 71–4 Sagittal image after corpus callosotomy.

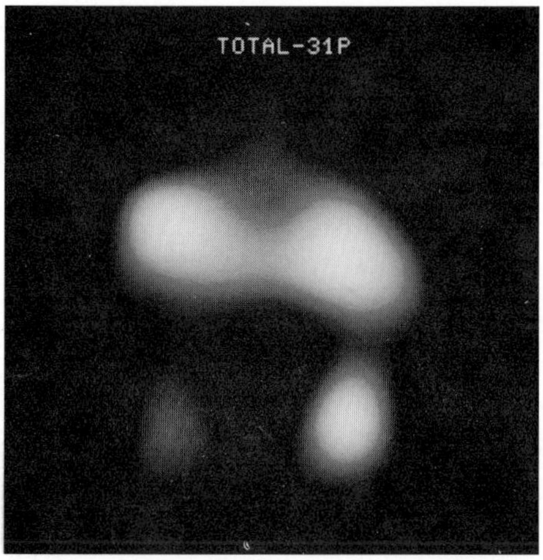

Fig. 71-5 Coronal ^{31}P metabolite image before corpus callosotomy.

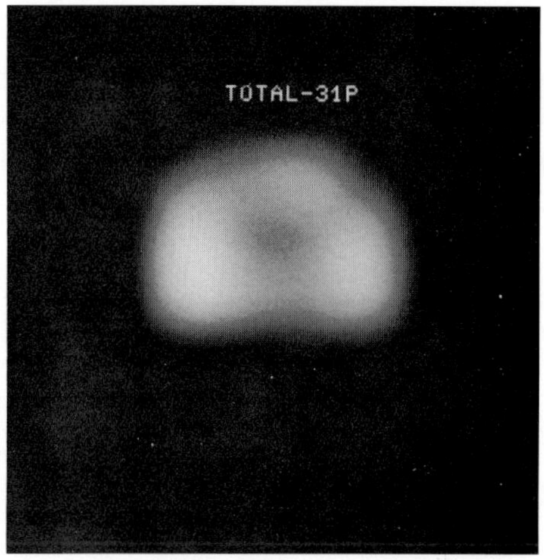

Fig. 71-6 Coronal ^{31}P metabolite image after corpus callosotomy.

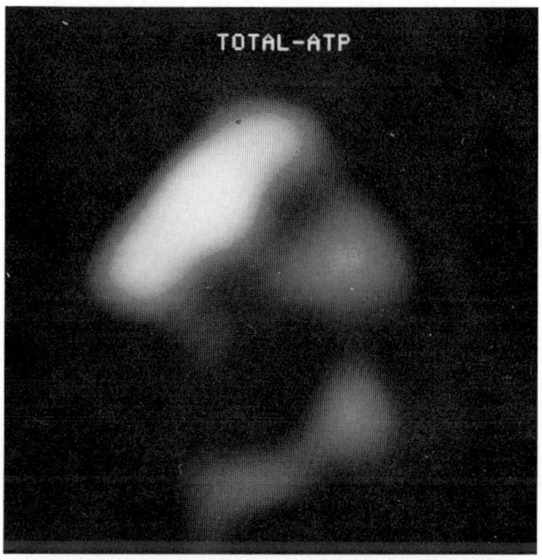

Fig. 71-7 Coronal total ATP metabolite image before corpus callosotomy.

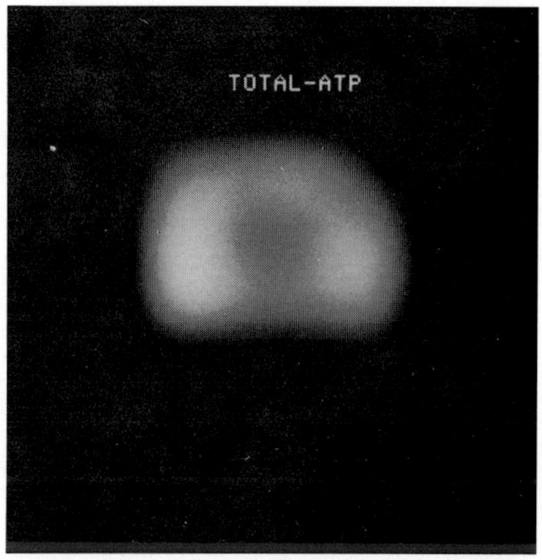

Fig. 71-8 Coronal total ATP metabolite image after corpus callosotomy.

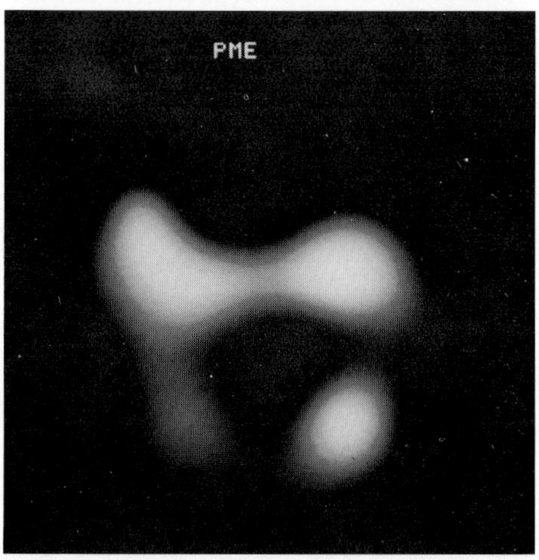

Fig. 71-9 Coronal PME metabolite image before corpus callosotomy.

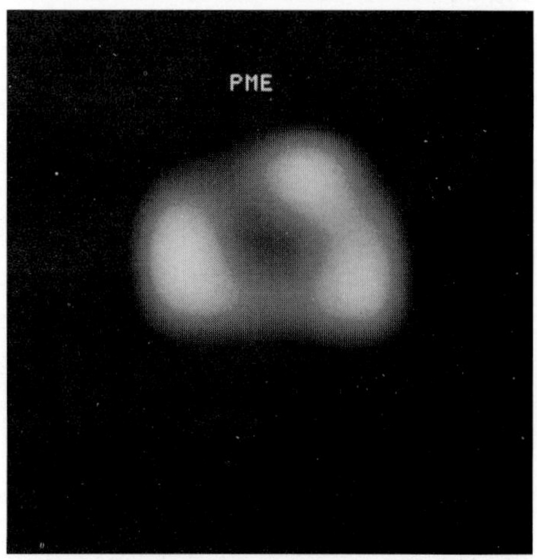

Fig. 71-10 Coronal PME metabolite image after corpus callosotomy.

CASE 72

Case 72: A 25-year-old male

Symptomatic temporal lobe epilepsy. Complex partial seizures (focus on the left temporal lobe on EEG)

Seizure onset at 2 years of age.

The patient had been suffering from complex partial seizures which occured a few times a week. It is suspected that he had a seizure during this MRS examination. The T_2-weighted image in Figure 72-1 shows atrophy of the left temporal lobe and hippocampus. The signal intensity in the ^{31}P metabolite image in Figure 72-2 shows a slight increase in the left temporal lobe. In the total ATP metabolite image, signal intensity is also mildly elevated in the left temporal lobe (Figure 72-3). The PCr metabolite image shows an increased signal intensity in the left temporal lobe. The PME contour map and metabolite image in Figures 72-5 and 6 demonstrate increased signal intensity in the left mesial temporal lobe. The distribution of signal intensities is nearly symmetrical in the PDE contour map and metabolite image in Figures 72-7 and 8. The signal intensity is increased in the left mesial temporal lobe in the PME/PDE contour map in Figure 72-9, suggesting alterations of phospholipids in the region including the epileptogenic focus. The PCr/Pi contour map in Figure 72-10 also illustrates an elevated signal intensity in the left temporal lobe, indicating an increased high-energy phosphate metabolism due to the seizures.

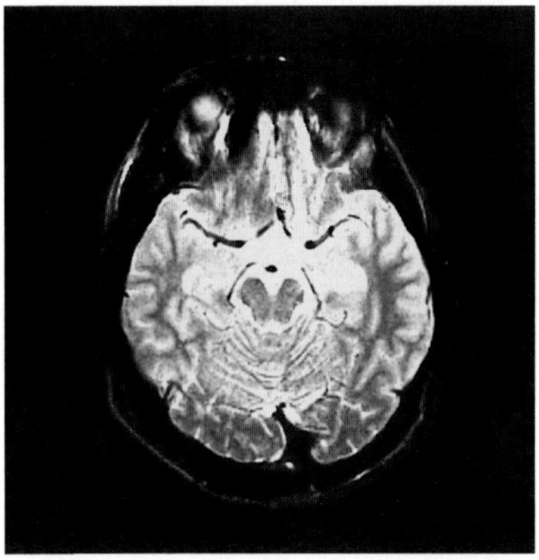

Fig. 72-1 Axial T_2-weighted image (2,200/90).

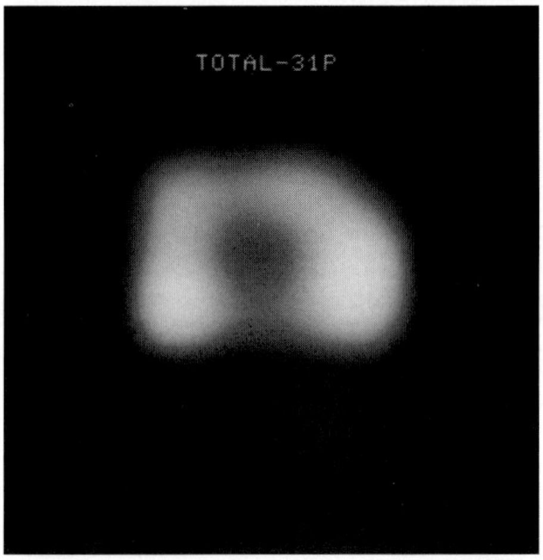

Fig. 72-2 Coronal ^{31}P metabolite image.

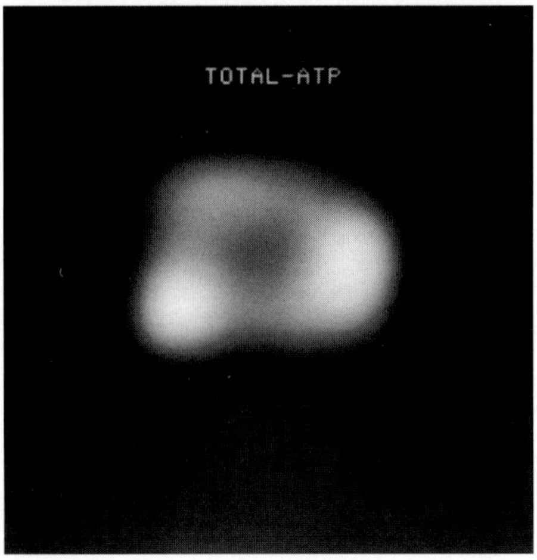

Fig. 72-3 Coronal total ATP metabolite image.

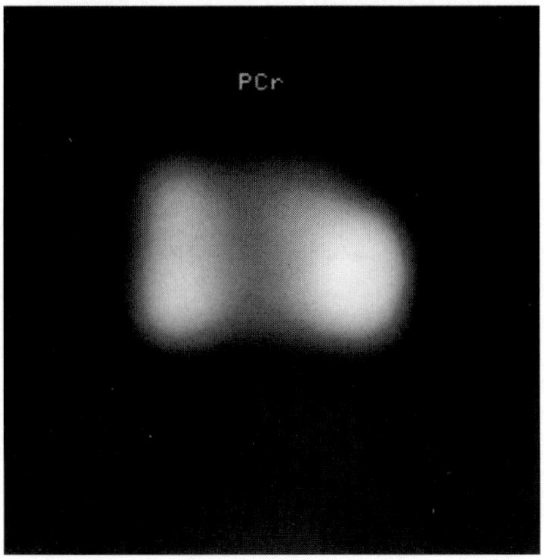

Fig. 72-4 Coronal PCr metabolite image.

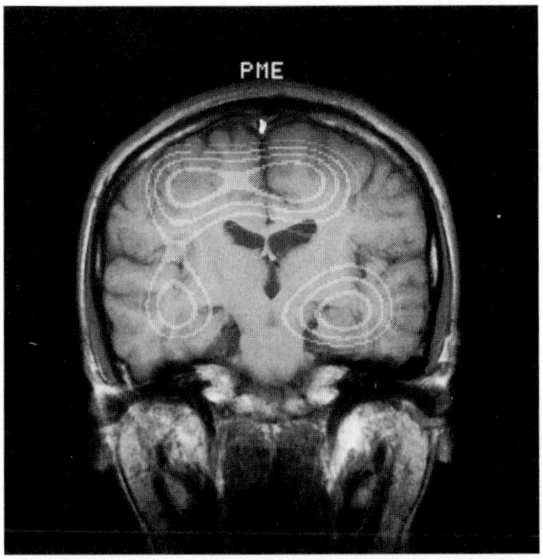

Fig. 72-5 Coronal PME contour map superimposed on T_1-weighted image (500/15).

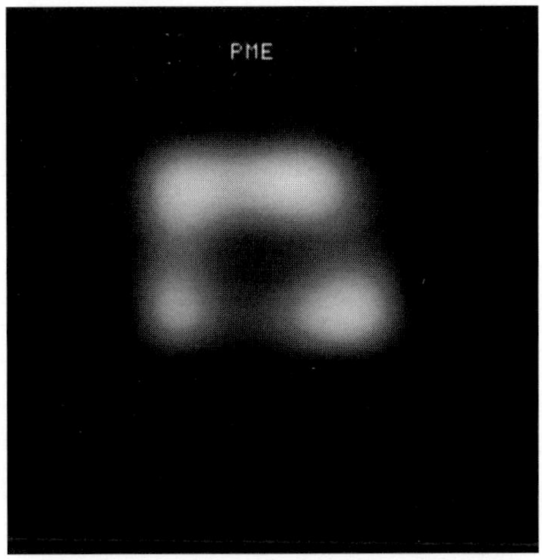

Fig. 72-6 Coronal PME metabolite image.

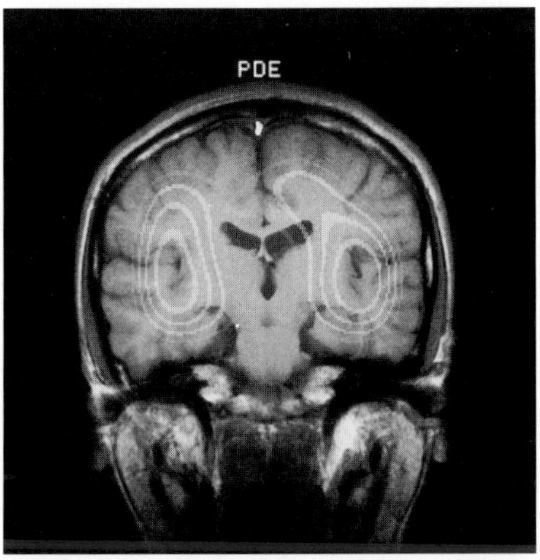

Fig. 72-7 Coronal PDE contour map superimposed on T_1-weighted image (500/15).

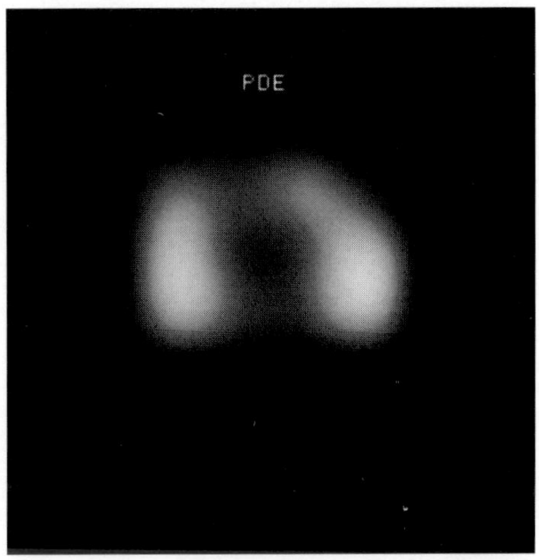

Fig. 72-8 Coronal PDE metabolite image.

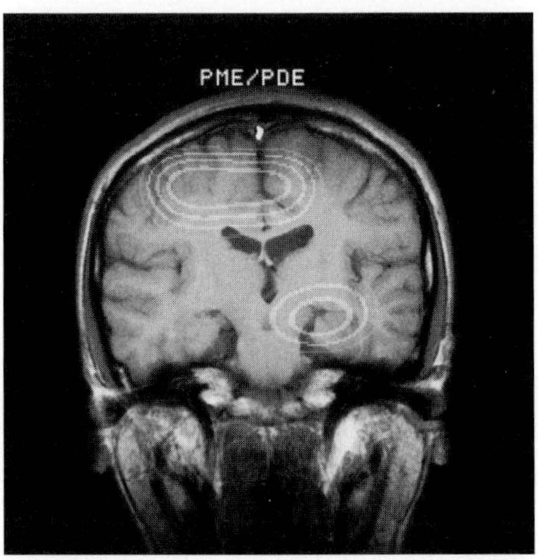

Fig. 72-9 Coronal PME/PDE contour map superimposed on T_1-weighted image (500/15).

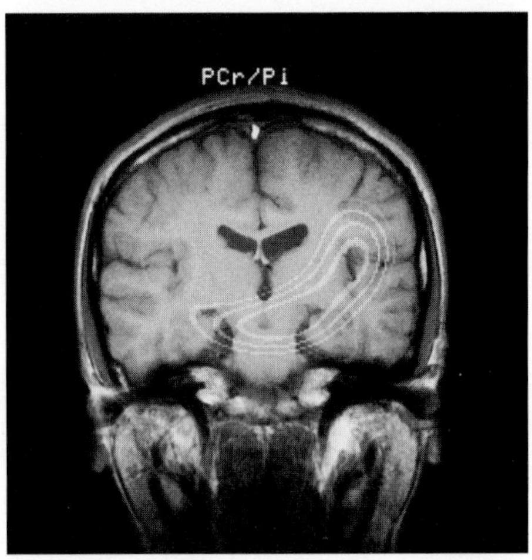

Fig. 72-10 Coronal PCr/Pi contour map superimposed on T_1-weighted image (500/15).

CASE 73

Case 73: A 32-year-old male

Symptomatic temporal lobe epilepsy. Complex partial seizures (focus on the left temporal lobe on EEG)

Seizure onset at 1 year of age.

The patient presented mental retardation and complex partial seizures with automatism such as lip smacking and walking, and psychic phenomenon such as fear of a murderous presence. The proton density-weighted image in Figure 73-1 shows a hippocampal sclerosis on the left. The ^{31}P contour map in Figure 73-2 shows almost symmetrical signal intensities in the left and right hemispheres. The β-ATP contour map and metabolite image in Figures 73-3 and 4 show a decreased signal intensity in the left mesial temporal lobe. The contour map of PCr/Pi ratio shows a decrease in the left mesial temporal lobe (Figure 73-5). In the ^{31}P spectrum in the right mesial temporal lobe (voxel 11), the %Pi, %α-ATP and pHi are increased (Figure 73-7). In Figure 73-8, ^{31}P spectrum in the left mesial temporal lobe (voxel 13) shows increased %Pi suggesting hypometabolism. In the ^{1}H spectrum of the right mesial temporal lobe in Figure 73-9, the NAA/Cr ratio decreased. The NAA/Cr ratio in the left temporal lobe is also reduced and has decreased more than that of the right. This confirms the left temporal epileptogenic focus.

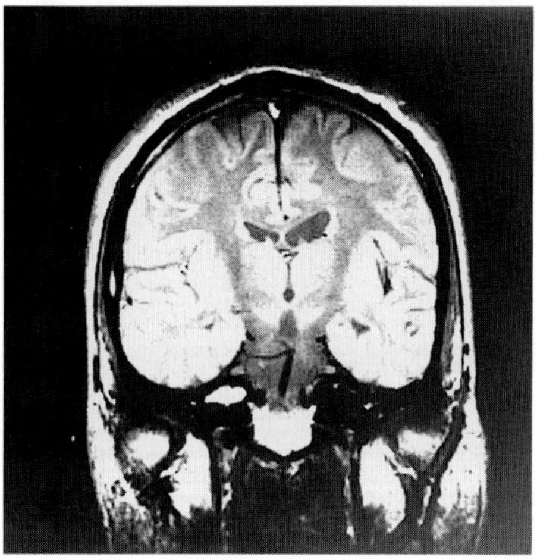

Fig. 73-1 Coronal proton density-weighted image (2,200/15).

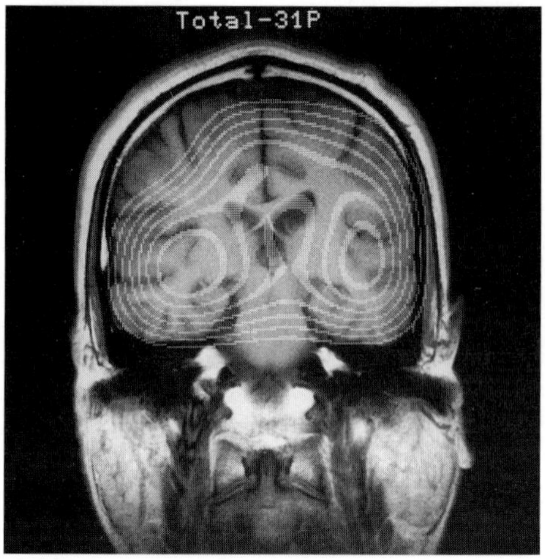

Fig. 73-2 Coronal ^{31}P contour map superimposed on T_1-weighted image (500/15).

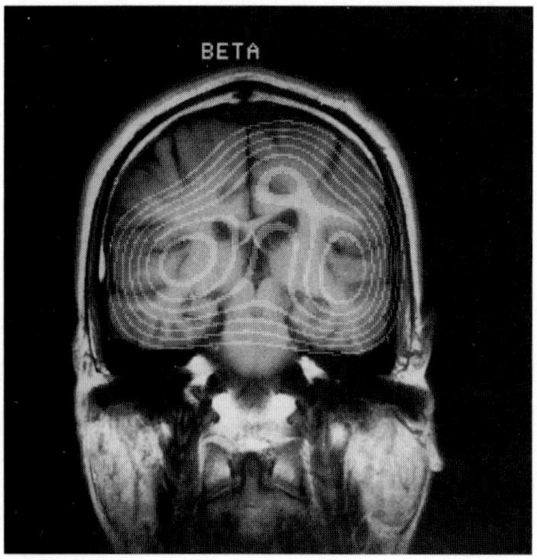

Fig. 73-3 Coronal β-ATP contour map superimposed on T_1-weighted image (500/15).

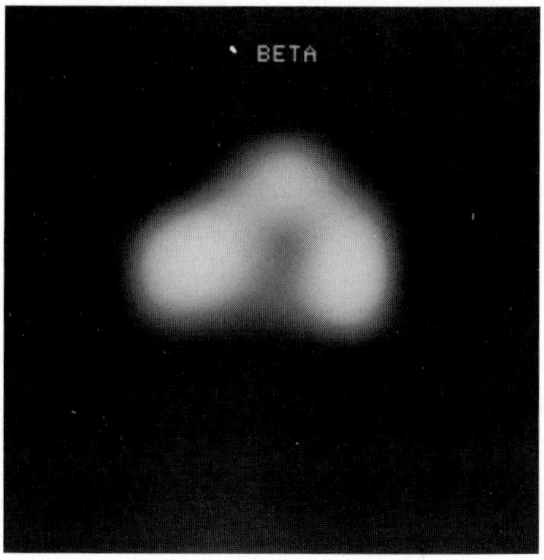

Fig. 73-4 Coronal β-ATP metabolite image.

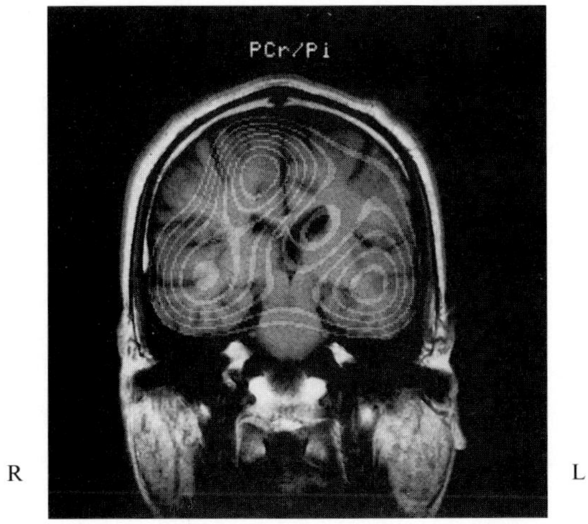

Fig. 73-5 Coronal PCr/Pi contour map superimposed on T_1-weighted image (500/15).

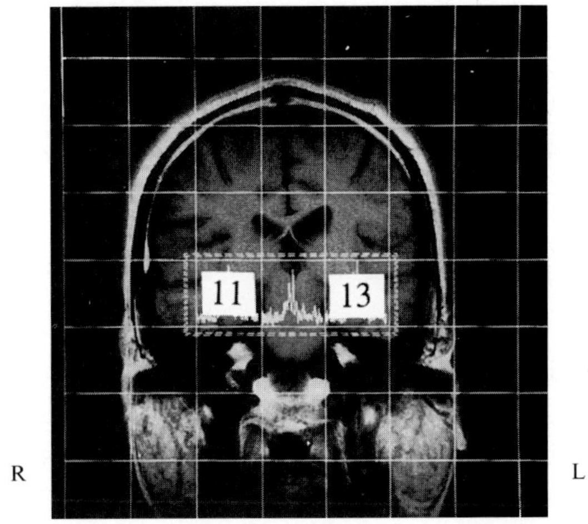

Fig. 73-6 T_1-weighted image showing the position of 3×3×4 cm³ voxels 11 and 13.

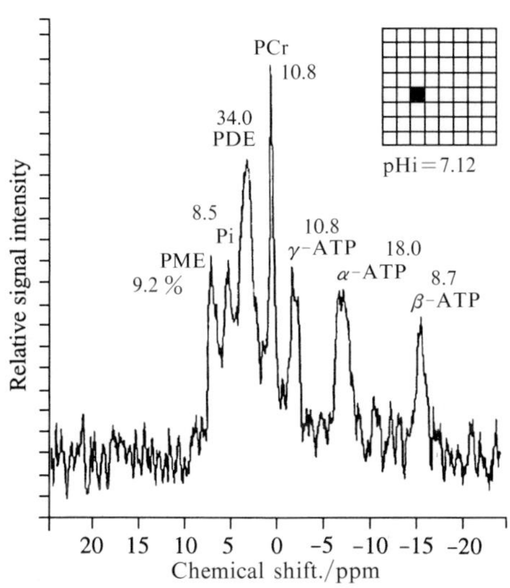

Fig. 73-7 ³¹P spectrum of right mesial temporal lobe (voxel 11).

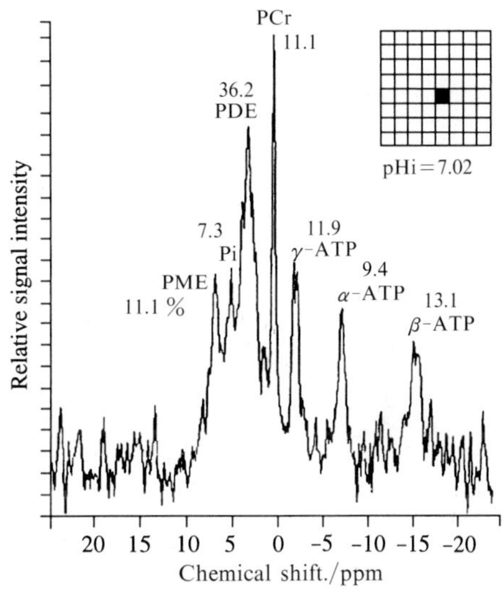

Fig. 73-8 ³¹P spectrum of left mesial temporal lobe (voxel 13).

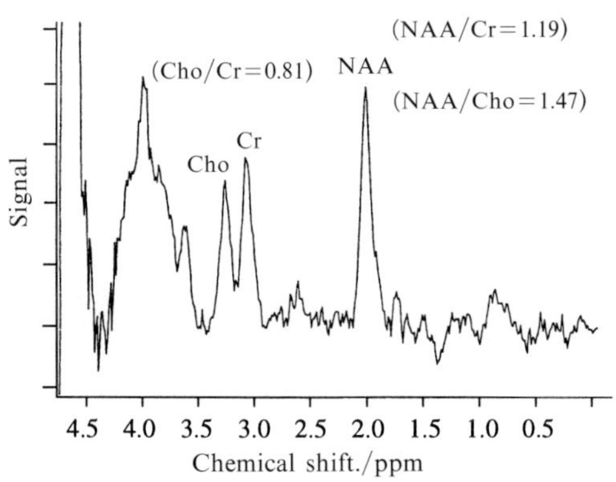

Fig. 73-9 ¹H spectrum of right mesial temporal lobe (STEAM : 2,000/60) Voxel size : 2.5×2.5×2.5 cm³.

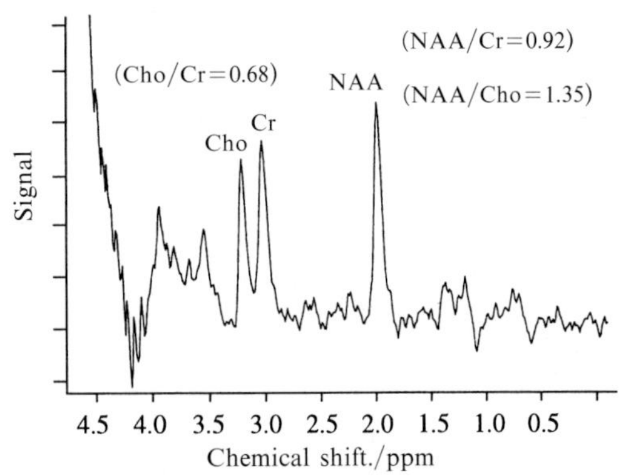

Fig. 73-10 ¹H spectrum of left mesial temporal lobe (STEAM : 2,000/60) Voxel size : 2.5× 2.5×2.5 cm³.

CASE 74

Case 74: A 41-year-old male

Symptomatic temporal lobe epilepsy. Complex partial seizures (focus on the left temporal lobe on EEG)

Seizure onset at 13 years of age.

The patient presented complex partial seizures with psychic phenomenon such as memory recall, jamais vu, sadness, and aphasia, occasionally evolving into secondary generalized seizures. The T_2-weighted image in Figure 74-1 shows mild cerebral atrophy. The total ATP contour map in Figure 74-2 shows a reduced signal intensity in the left temporal lobe. The Pi contour map in Figure 74-3 shows a decreased signal intensity in the left mesial temporal lobe. The PCr/Pi ratio is elevated in the left mesial temporal lobe (Figure 74-4). In the ^{31}P spectrum in the right mesial temporal lobe (voxel A), the %PME is decreased, %α-ATP is increased (Figure 74-7). In Figure 74-8, ^{31}P spectrum in the left mesial temporal lobe (voxel B) shows increased %PME and decreased %β-ATP, compared to the right, suggesting disturbances in membrane phospholipids and high-energy metabolism in the epileptogenic region. In the ^1H spectrum of the right mesial temporal lobe in Figure 74- 9, the NAA/Cr ratio and Cho/Cr ratio are in the normal ranges. However, the NAA/Cr ratio is reduced in the left mesial temporal lobe, reflecting neuronal loss in the epileptogenic region (Figure 74-10).

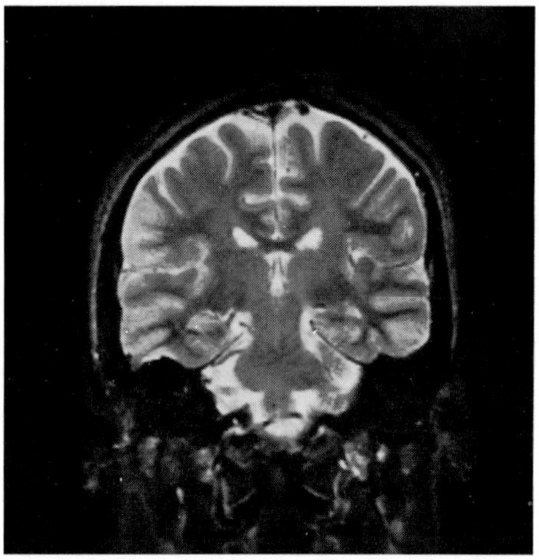

Fig. 74-1 Coronal T_2-weighted image (2,200/90).

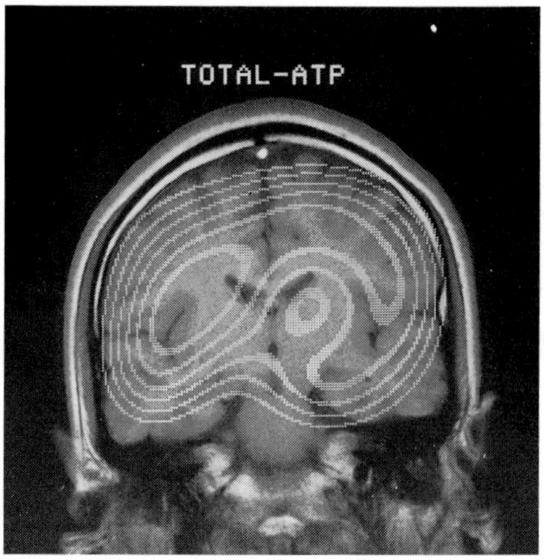

Fig. 74-2 Coronal total ATP contour map superimposed on T_1-weighted image (500/15).

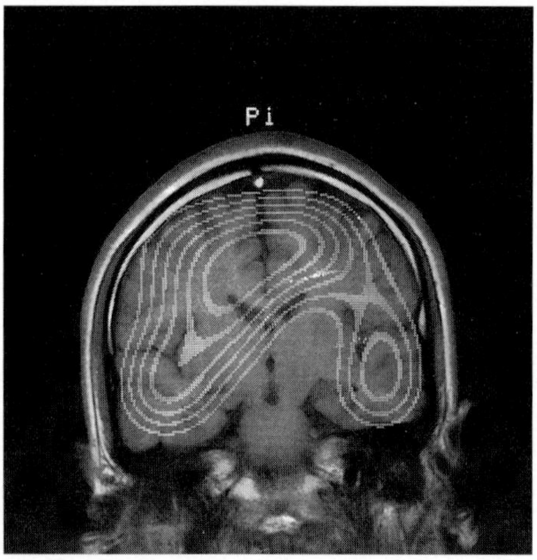

Fig. 74-3 Coronal Pi contour map superimposed on T_1-weighted image (500/15).

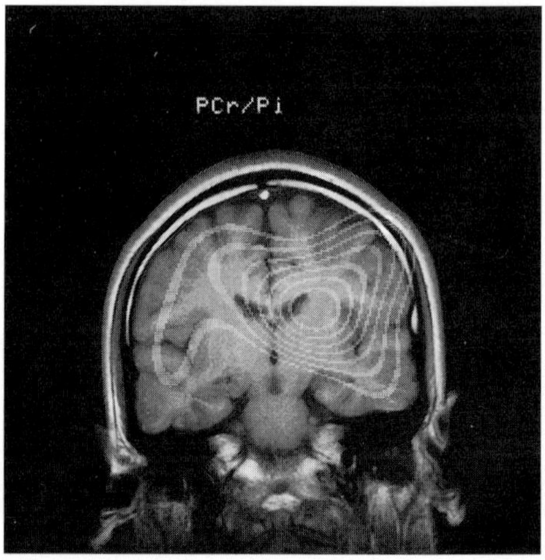

Fig. 74-4 Coronal PCr/Pi contour map superimposed on T_1-weighted image (500/15).

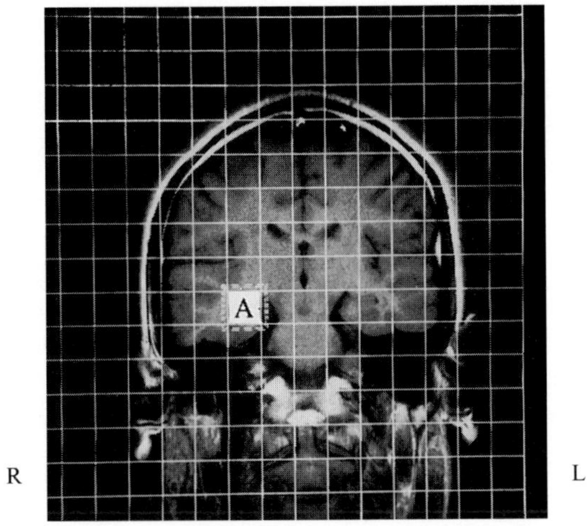

Fig. 74-5 T_1-weighted image showing the position of $1.5 \times 1.5 \times 4$ cm^3 voxel A.

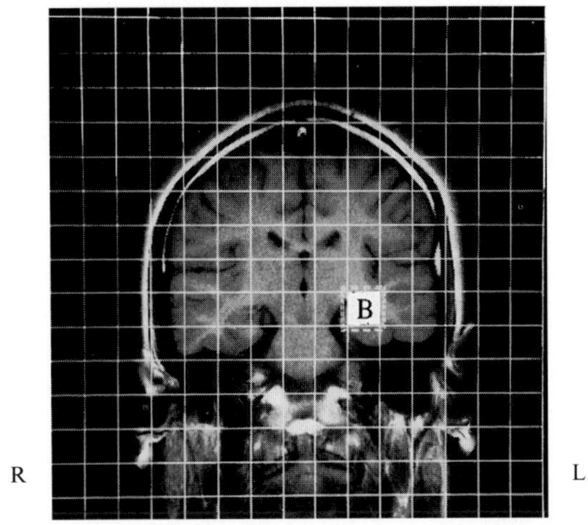

Fig. 74-6 T_1-weighted image showing the position of $1.5 \times 1.5 \times 4$ cm^3 voxel B.

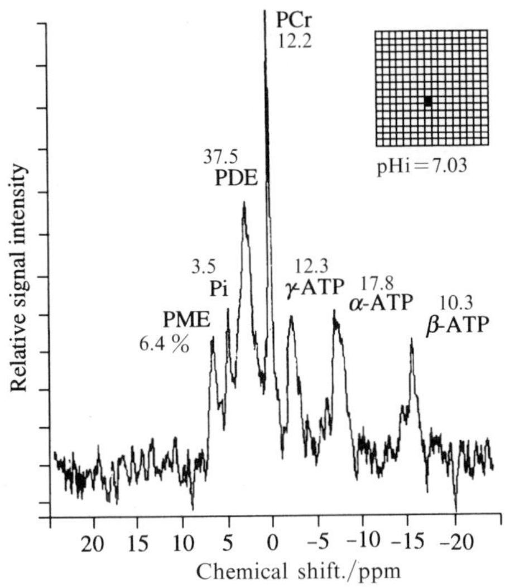

Fig. 74-7 ^{31}P spectrum of right mesial temporal lobe (voxel A).

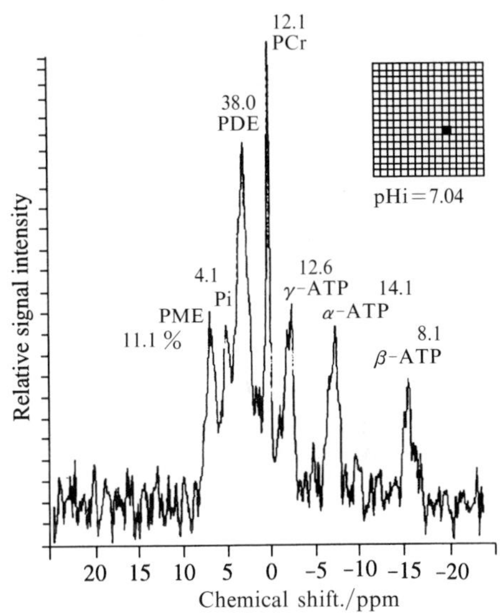

Fig. 74-8 ^{31}P spectrum of left mesial temporal lobe (voxel B).

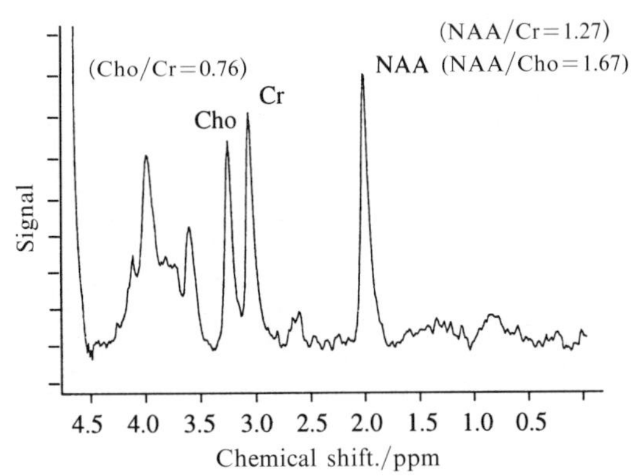

Fig. 74-9 ^{1}H spectrum of right mesial temporal lobe (STEAM: 2,000/60) Voxel size: $2.5 \times 2.5 \times 2.5$ cm^3.

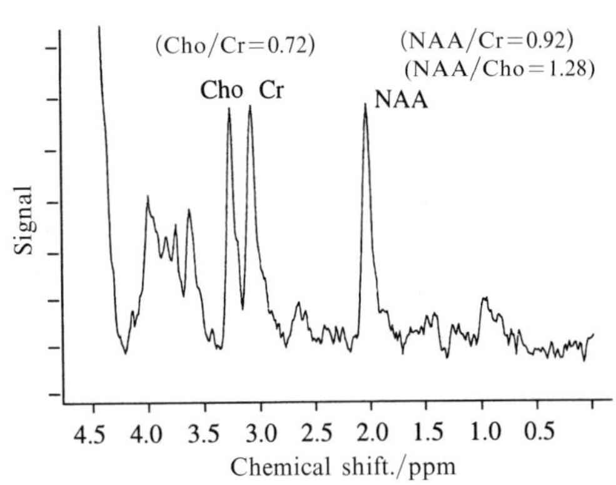

Fig. 74-10 ^{1}H spectrum of left mesial temporal lobe (STEAM: 2,000/60) Voxel size: $2.5 \times 2.5 \times 2.5$ cm^3.

CASE 75

Case 75: A female (First ^{31}P MRS study at 12 years of age; second study at 13 years of age)

Generalized seizures

Seizure onset at 12 years of age.

The first generalized convulsion occurred at 12 years of age, and the first ^{31}P MRS study was performed before treatment. The patient was treated with antiepileptic drugs which gave good control. The second study of the MRS was conducted after one year. Results of ^{31}P chemical shift imaging were compared before and after treatments. The ^{31}P contour map before treatment shows a decreased signal intensity in the right temporal lobe (Figure 75-1). However, the ^{31}P signal intensity is almost symmetrical in the contour map after treatment (Figure 75-2). The reduced signal intensity of the total ATP before treatment is elevated after treatement (Figures 75-3 and 4). After treatment, the PME signal intensity is increased in the left temporal lobe, compared to before (Figures 75-5 and 6). In the Pi metabolite images, a reduced signal intensity in the right temporal lobe before treatment is elevated after treatment (Figures 75-7 and 8). In the PCr metabolite image, the signal intensity before treatment is decreased, but is increased after treatment in the right temporal lobe (Figures 75-9 and 10).

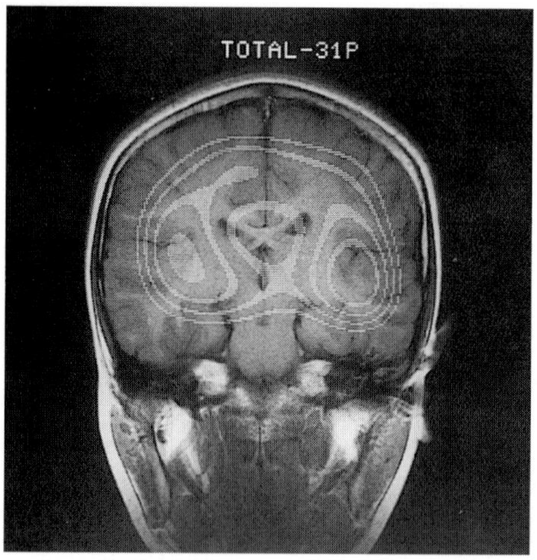

Fig. 75-1 Coronal ^{31}P contour map superimposed on T_1-weighted image (500/15) (before treatment).

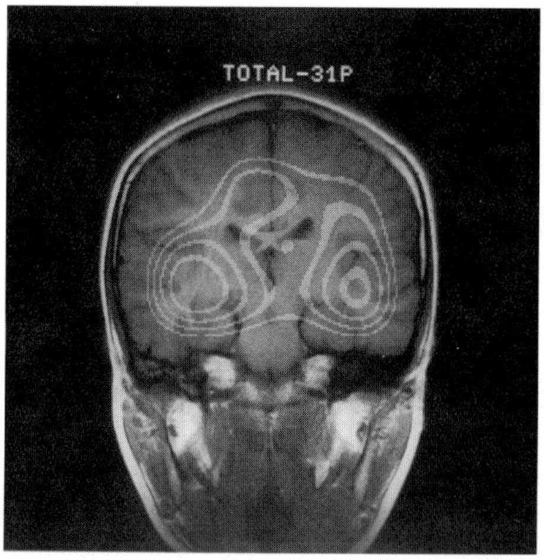

Fig. 75-2 Coronal ^{31}P contour map superimposed on T_1-weighted image (500/15) under antiepileptic drug treatment. (1 year since first examination.)

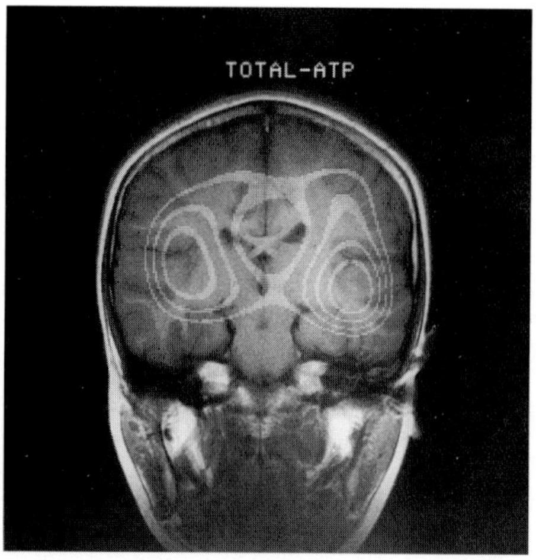

Fig. 75-3 Coronal total ATP contour map superimposed on T_1-weighted image (500/15) (before treatment).

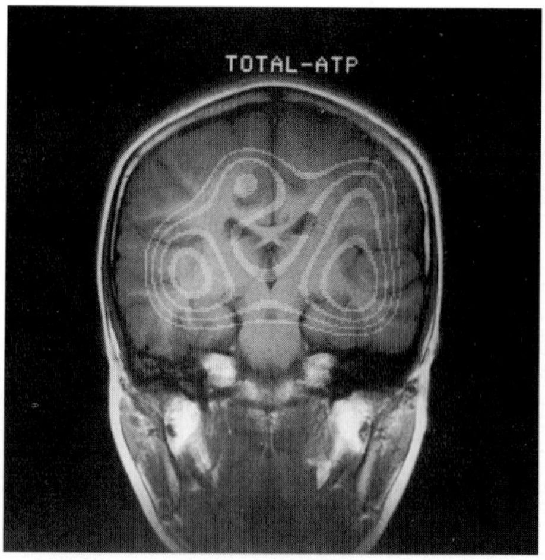

Fig. 75-4 Coronal total ATP contour map superimposed on T_1-weighted image (500/15) under antiepileptic drug treatment. (1 year since first examination.)

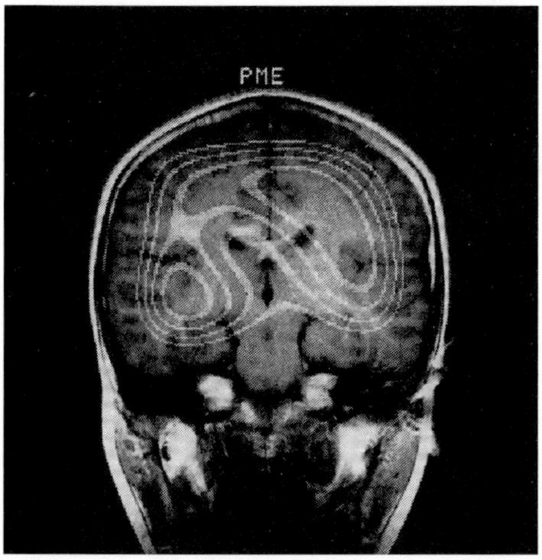

Fig. 75-5 Coronal PME contour map superimposed on T_1-weighted image (500/15) (before treatment).

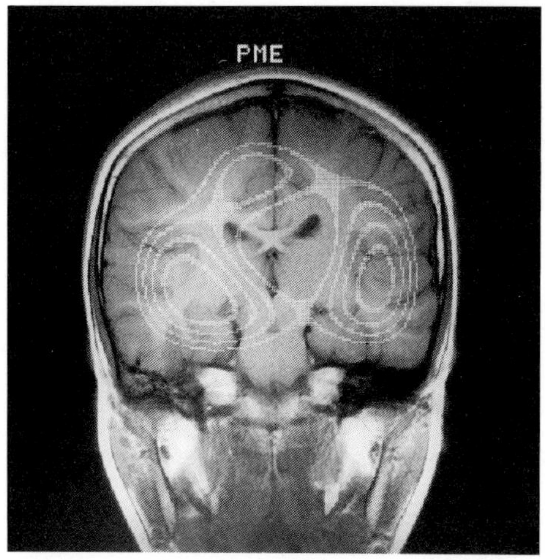

Fig. 75-6 Coronal PME contour map superimposed on T_1-weighted image (500/15) under antiepileptic drug treatment. (1 year since first examination.)

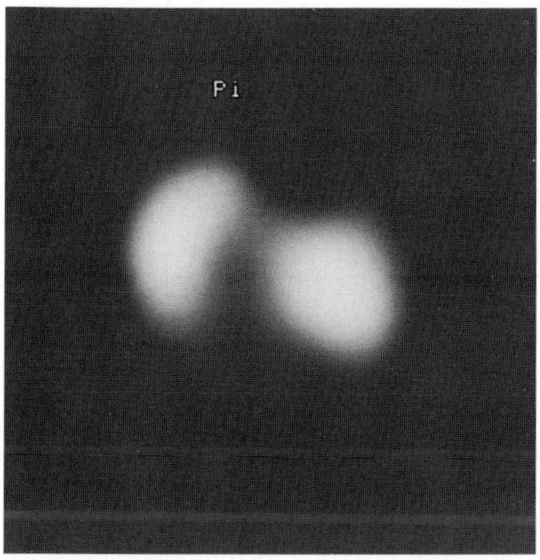

Fig. 75-7 Coronal Pi metabolite image (before treatment).

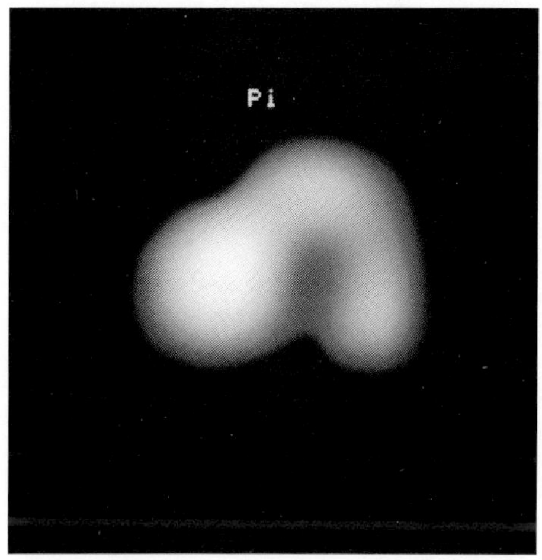

Fig. 75-8 Coronal Pi metabolite image under antiepileptic drug treatment. (1 year since first examination.)

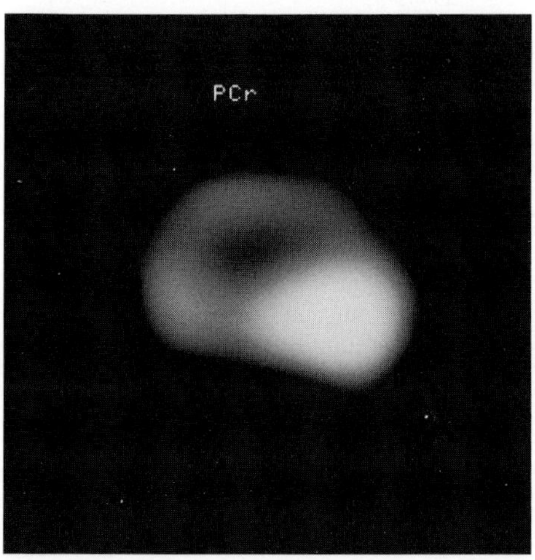

Fig. 75-9 Coronal PCr metabolite image (before treatment).

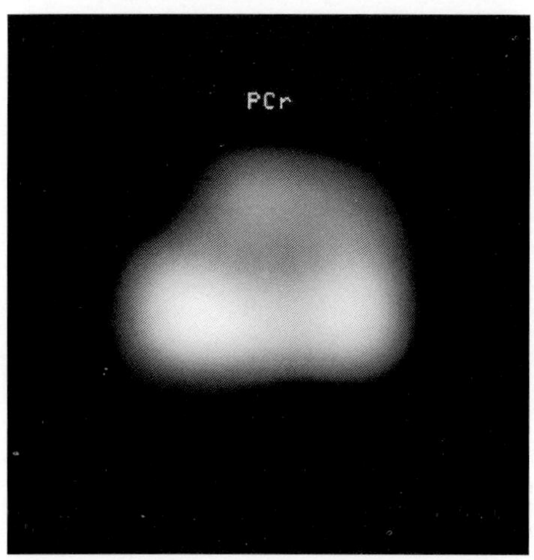

Fig. 75-10 Coronal PCr metabolite image under antiepileptic drug treatment. (1 year since first examination.)

Chapter 12 Psychiatric Disorders

Toshiro Fujimoto

12.1 CHARACTERISTICS OF THE SPECTRUM

Studies on the neurobiological pathology of psychiatric brain disorders, which at present are poorly understood, are becoming clearer with the application of MRS which provides noninvasive information of localized metabolic changes in the brain.[1–3] Investigations of pathophysiological mechanisms by MRS are expected to lead to an understanding of the causes of psychiatric disorders, the monitoring of drug effects and the development of new therapies.

12.1.1 Schizophrenia

(1) ***^{31}P MRS***

The first study of schizophrenia using ^{31}P MRS was conducted by Pettegrew et al.,[4] and ^{31}P MRS with the surface coil method was applied. An increase in PDE level, a decrease in PME level, an increase in ATP level, and a decrease in Pi level in the dorsal prefrontal cortex of drug naïve, first episode schizophrenic patients[5,6] were observed. Changes in PDE and PME reflect abnormalities of phospholipids, and alterations in ATP and PCr reflect impairment in the metabolism of high-energy phosphates. Fujimoto et al.[7,8] investigated many regions of the schizophrenic brain using the ^{31}P chemical shift imaging (CSI) technique, which is as reliable as the single voxel method. The evaluation of the ^{31}P spectra of patients with schizophrenia by CSI demonstrated localized abnormalities in PDE, PME, PCr and ATP in disorganized type of schizophrenia (DSM-III-R diagnostic criteria) under neuroleptic treatment. These changes varied according to the region of the brain and indicated the complexity of metabolic changes in the brain of schizophrenics. The PDE level was reduced in the basal ganglia but was increased in the left medial frontal and temporal lobes. The PME level was increased in the basal ganglia, and the PCr level was reduced in the medial frontal lobes. The ATP level was reduced in the left temporal lobe but was increased in the right basal ganglia region.

Regarding the ^{31}P spectra of the prefrontal cortex in drug naïve patients with schizophrenia, Stanley et al.[9] observed decreases in PME levels and an increase in PDE levels and the intracellular free magnesium level, but no abnormalities in high-energy phosphate levels, by employing the surface coil method with fast rotating gradient spectroscopy (FROG). Using the FROG method, Williamson et al.[10,11] noted a decrease in PME, an increase in PDE, and free magnesium in the left prefrontal region of patients, and reported a negative correlation between PDE levels and the duration of illness. According to the report of Kato et al.[12,13] using the surface coil method, the PME levels were decreased in bilateral frontal lobes, but β-ATP levels and PCr levels were increased in the left frontal lobe, and the PCr levels had a positive correlation with scores on the Scale for Assessment of Negative Symptoms (SANS). However, the PDE levels did not show significant changes in the frontal lobes. Employing the CSI, Deicken[14] showed higher levels of PDE in both right and left frontal lobes and decreased levels of PCr and Pi in medicated schizophrenic patients.

Deicken et al.[15] demonstrated higher right versus left temporal PCr/ATP, PCr/Pi, and PCr as well as lower right versus left temporal ATP, indicating the asymmetry of high-energy phosphate metabolism in the temporal lobe of patients with schizophrenia. In the basal ganglia, Deicken et al.[16] reported that the β-ATP levels were reduced in patients, and impairment of high-energy phosphate metabolism of the brain was suspected. Using the CSI, Arias-Mendoza et al.[17] showed that the concentration of PCr was lower in schizophrenic patients, indicating an impairment in brain bioenergetics, and they also showed that PCr levels were increased in some patients during CoQ_{10} treatment. Dogomori et al.[18] with the CSI, found that schizophrenic patients with neuroleptic malignant syndrome showed increases in PME levels in bilateral basal ganglia regions and PDE levels in the bilateral temporal lobes. In contrast, a decrease in the ATP level in the bilateral temporal lobes was observed, compared with normal controls and other schizophrenic patients.

Bachert-Baumann et al.[19] suggested that irradiation of proton improves the spectral resolution due to the NOE (nuclear Overhauser effect). Potwarka et al.[20] investigated the prefrontal lobe of schizophrenic patients, using the CSI with proton decoupling method by which the PDE signals were assigned to glycerophosphocholine (GPC), glycerophosphoethanolamine (GPE), and membrane phospholipids (MP). The increased resonance of PDE in schizophrenic patients was not due to the peak of GPC or GPE, but mainly due to membrane phospholipids. This finding is important for interpreting of the increase in PDE resonance in schizophrenic patients.

(2) ^{1}***H MRS***

Moore et al.[21] found that %NAA levels in the left temporal and frontal lobes in schizophrenic patients were decreased, using stimulated echo acquisition mode (STEAM) spectroscopy. Yurgelun-Todd et al.[22–24] with the modified STEAM sequence reported a decrease in the NAA/Cr ratio in both right and left temporal lobes of patients, and Nasrallah et al. [25,26] using the STEAM noted decreased NAA intensities in the right hippocumpus/amygdala region of patients. Other researchers have confirmed reduced NAA levels in the temporal lobe in patients with schizophrenia.[27–29] Bertolino et al.,[30] Buckley et al.[31] and Choe et al.[32] reported that the NAA level is reduced also in the frontal lobe. Bertolino et al.[33] suggested that NAA levels in the temporal lobe and the dorsolateral prefrontal lobe were reduced in drug naïve patients with schizophrenia, and that decreased NAA levels are independent of neuroleptic treatment. In patients with first-episode schizophrenia, Renshaw et al.[28] using a STEAM pulse sequence reported a decrease in the NAA level in the temporal lobe, and and Paul et al.,[34] also noted the same in the frontal lobe of patients.

Fujimoto et al.[35] using a spin-echo pulse sequence found that the NAA level is also reduced in the basal ganglia in patients receiving neuroleptic treatment. The decreased level in the NAA resonance in these reports is interpreted as neuronal loss or dysfunction in schizophrenia. Increased ratios of Cho/Cr were observed in the left basal ganglia of patients, suggesting that the anabolic activities of the membrane phospholipid metabolism may be increased, since the PME level was also increased in the left basal ganglia on ^{31}P MRS.[31] Thomas et al.[36] employing the STEAM sequence reported that the peak of Glx (GABA, glutamine, and glutamate) was reduced in schizophrenic children. Choe et al.[37,38] using a STEAM pulse sequence reported that (GABA and Glu)/Cr ratios in the prefrontal lobe of adult patients with chronic schizophrenia were increased, and that this increased level was associated with neuroleptic treatment. Changes in Glx levels reflect alterations in the neurotransmitters of GABA and Glu, and is considered to be an important subject of future research in ^{1}H MRS. Komoroski et al.[39] demonstrated that in *in vitro* studies using high-resolution ^{1}H NMR presented small differences between schizophrenics and controls in metabolites such as

NAA, NAAG, Cho, Cr, GABA, glutamate and glutamine, and that NAA was significantly reduced in the thalamus. The small differences between schizophrenics and controls in metabolites in this *in vitro* study may be caused by the differences between the methods *in vitro* and *in vivo*.

12.1.2 Depression

(1) ^{31}*P MRS*

Reports of ^{31}P MRS in depression are inconsistent, but it was suggested that there are reductions of ATP and PCr and abnormalities of phospholipids in basal ganglia and frontal lobe regions (Fujimoto et al.[40]). The ATP and PCr levels were decreased in the basal ganglia region, and PME levels were increased in the left as shown in Case 80. In Case 81, the PCr level was also reduced in the bilateral basal ganglia regions, and the PME level was increased in the right. As for other reports, Moore et al.[41] reported that the β-ATP level was reduced and the ADP was also possibly reduced in the basal ganglia of unmedicated patients with depression. Christensen et al.[42] reported elevation of the sum of PDE and PME peaks in major depression. This finding was consistent with the increased level of the choline peak in ^{1}H MRS of depressive patients, and suggested the disturbance of adrenergic/cholinergic balance in the brain. Kato et al.[43] observed that the PCr level was reduced in the left hemisphere, indicating asymmetry of high-energy phosphate metabolism. In depression, the pathologic phases and medications are diverse, and the results of ^{31}P MRS are considered to reflect this diversity.

(2) ^{1}*H MRS*

Charles et al.[44] and Sharma et al.[45] found that the choline (Cho) levels of patients with depression were elevated and fell to sub-control levels after therapy. Renshaw et al.[46] reported that choline/creatine ratios in the basal ganglia were increased by 65% in unmedicated depressed patients. Kato et al.[47] also suggested elevation of the Cho peak in patients with bipolar disorders in the depressive state. Since the Cho peak may arise from glycerophosphocholine (GPC) and phosphocholine (PC), the increase in the Cho levels reflects increased PC caused by increased second messenger generation and/or a decrease rate of PC incorporation into membrane lipid, and elevated GPC due to the degenerative process.[48] Case 81 clearly shows elevation in both the Cho level in the ^{1}H spectrum and the PME level in the ^{31}P spectrum in the basal ganglia of depressed patients. Bruhn et al.[48] observed that manic-depressive patients treated with lithium did not change in Cho resonance despite an increase in the erythrocyte choline concentration after lithium administration, probably because small concentration changes in free choline of the order of 0.05mM are not reflected in the Cho peak.

12.1.3 Mania

(1) ^{31}*P MRS*

The MRS examination of patients with mania is difficult, because the patients exhibit hyperactivity or excitement during manic episodes. Spectra of Case 82 were obtained in the state of mild mania. Asymmetrical distributions of ATP and PCr which were relatively decreased in the left basal ganglia region were noted. Whether these findings indicate reduced metabolism or increased consumption of PCr and ATP cannot be determined solely by these spectra. The PDE level was reduced in the right basal ganglia region, when compared to the left. The PME level was increased in the left basal ganglia. These changes in PME and PDE also indicate abnormalities of phospholipids in mania.

12.1.4 Alcoholism

(1) ^{31}*P MRS*

Denays et al.[49] found that in the rat brain, the consumption of ATP and PCr was reduced, reflecting a reduction in the metabolism of the brain, in both the acute and chronic periods of alcohol intoxication. The PME/PDE ratio was also reduced, and the PDE/β-ATP ratio was increased, in the chronic period, and these changes were considered to indicate the breakdown of membrane phospholipids. These findings may explain the progression of brain atrophy due to alcoholism. Case 83, an alcoholic patient, showed decreased PDE signal intensities in the bilateral basal ganglia regions indicating abnormality of the phospholipids. In the total ATP and PCr images, signal intensities of the basal ganglia were relatively reduced suggesting dysfunction of high energy phosphate metabolism.

(2) ^{1}*H MRS*

Yamaguchi et al.[50] reported a decrease in NAA levels in the basal ganglia of alcoholic patients. The decrease in the NAA level in the basal ganglia is considered to indicate neuronal dysfunction or loss. Gibbs et al.[51] showed that ^{1}H spectra in the voxel centered in the superior vermis showed an increased Cho/NAA ratio and a decrease with time after abstinence. This increase in the Cho level is associated with changes in the lipid constituents of myelin or in the acetylcholine precursor, choline. On the other hand, Fujimoto et al.[52] did not observe reduction in NAA levels in the mesial temporal lobe in alcoholic patients. This suggests that biochemical changes differ between the temporal lobe and basal ganglia in alcoholic patients. Fujimoto et al.[53] showed that the NAA level is also reduced in the basal ganglia in patients with alcohol-induced persisting dementia. Behar et al.[54] reported that the GABA levels were reduced in the occipital lobe, and that the GABAergic mechanism was important in alcoholism. Mendelson et al.[55], and Kaufman et al.[56] showed that alcohol in the brain can be detected directly by ^{1}H MRS. Chiu et al.[57] reported that the ethanol concentration ratio in the brain was greater in heavy drinkers than in occasional drinkers. Chiu et al.[58] observed that the alcohol resonance including overlapping lipid resonance was increased, and assumed that this reflected increases in catabolism of phospholipids or alterations in mobility characteristic fatty acid side chains within the membrane. ^{1}H MRS is expected to advance research into the cause of, and treatment for, alcoholism.

References

1) Fujimoto, T.; Nakano, T.; Terada, K. et al. Study of dementia, epilepsy and shizophrenia using ^{31}P-CSI. *Japanese Journal of Clinical Medicine* 49: 233-237; 1991. [Japanese]
2) Nasrallah, H. A.; Pettegrew, J. W. In: NMR Spectroscopy in Psychiatric Brain Disorders. Washington, DC: American Psychiatric Press, Inc. 1995.
3) Maier, M. *In vivo* magnetic resonance spectroscopy: Applications in psychiatry. *Br. J. Psychiatry* 167: 299-306; 1995.
4) Pettegrew, J. W.; Panchalingam, K.; Keshevan, M. et al. Alterations in membrane phospholipid and high energy phosphate metabolism in the dorsal prefrontal cortex of schizophrenics. *In: Book of Abstracts: Eighth Annual Meeting and Exhibition of the Society of Magnetic Resonance in Medicine, Vol. 1. Amsterdam, The Netherlands: SMRM*; 1989: 463.
5) Pettegrew, J. W.; Keshavan, M. S.; Panchalingam, K. et al. Alterations in brain high-energy phosphate and membrane phospholipid metabolism in first-episode, drug-naive schizophrenics. *Arch. Gen. Psychiatry* 48: 563-568; 1991.
6) Pettegrew, J. W.; Minshew, N. J. Chapter 12. Molecular insights into schizophrenia. In: N. C. Andreasen (Ed). Schizophrenia: From Mind to Molecule. Washington, DC: American Psychiatric Press, Inc. 1994: pp. 221-243.
7) Fujimoto, T.; Nakano, T.; Takano, T. et al. Study of in vivo phosphorus 31 NMR spectra of chronic schizophrenics. *Japanese Journal of Clinical Psychiatry* 21: 1471-1480; 1992. [Japanese]
8) Fujimoto, T.; Nakano, T.; Takano, T. et al. Study of chronic schizophrenics using ^{31}P magnetic resonance chemical shift imaging. *Acta. Psychiatr. Scand*. 86: 455-462; 1992.
9) Stanley, J. A.; Williamson, P. C.; Drost, D. J. et al. An in vivo study of the prefrontal cortex of schizophrenic patients at different stages of illness via phosphorus magnetic resonance spectroscopy. *Arch. Gen. Psychiatry* 52: 399-406; 1995.
10) Williamson, P.; Drost, D.; Stanley, J. et al. Localized

phosphorus 31 magnetic resonance spectroscopy in chronic schizophrenic patients and normal controls. *Arch. Gen. Psychiatry* 48: 578; 1991.

11) Williamson, P. C.; Drost, D. J. Stanley, J. A. et al. ^{31}P–MRS in the study of schizophrenia. In: H. A. Nasrallah, J. W. Pettegrew (Eds). NMR Spectroscopy in Psychiatric Brain Disorders. Washington, DC: American Psychiatric Press, Inc. 1995: pp. 107–129.

12) Kato, T.; Shioiri, T.; Murashita, J. et al. Lateralized abnormality of high-energy phosphate and bilateral reduction of phosphomonoester measured by phosphorus-31 magnetic resonance spectroscopy of the frontal lobes in schizophrenia. *Psychiatry Res. Neuroimaging* 61: 151–160; 1995.

13) Kato, T.; Shioiri, T.; Murashita, J. et al. Phase-encoded ^{31}P–MRS of the frontal lobes in patients with schizophrenia. *In: Proceedings: Second Meeting of the Society of Magnetic Resonance, Vol. 2. San Francisco, California USA: SMR*; 1994: 602.

14) Deicken, R. F. Chapter 4, ^{31}P–MRS of the human brain in the study of schizophrenia. In: H. A. Nasrallah, J. W. Pettegrew (Eds). NMR Spectroscopy in Psychiatric Brain Disorders. Washington, DC: American Psychiatric Press, Inc. 1995: pp. 79–106.

15) Deicken, R. F.; Calabrese, G.; Merrin, E. L. et al. Asymmetry of temporal lobe phosphorous metabolism in schizophrenia: A ^{31}Phosphorous magnetic resonance spectroscopic imaging study. *Biol. Psychiatry* 38: 279–286; 1995.

16) Deicken, R. F.; Calabrese, G.; Merrin, E. L. et al. Basal ganglia phosphorous metabolism in chronic schizophrenia. *Am. J. Psychiatry* 152: 126–129; 1995.

17) Arias–Mendoza, F.; Elkashef, A.; Stoyanova, R. et al. Coenzyme Q_{10} effect on cognitive functions and bioenergetics in schizophrenia: an anatomically localized ^{31}P magnetic resonance study. *In: Proceedings: Fourth Scientific Meeting and Exhibition of the International Society for Magnetic Resonance in Medicine, Vol. 2. New York, USA: ISMRM*; 1996: 1003.

18) Dogomori, H.; Fujimoto, T.; Nakano, T. et al. Study of *in vivo* phoshorus 31 NMR spectra of neuroleptic malignant syndrome. *Japanese Journal of Clinical Psychiatry* 23: 1067–1076; 1994. [Japanese]

19) Bachert–Baumann, P.; Ermark, F.; Zabel, H. –J. et al. *In vivo* nuclear overhauser effect in ^{31}P–{^{1}H}double-resonance experiments in a 1.5–T whole-body MR system. *Magn. Reson. Med.* 15: 165–172; 1990.

20) Potwarka, J.; Drost, D. J.; Williamson, P. C. A study of schizophrenia using 2D ^{31}P chemical shift imaging with ^{1}H decoupling. *In: Proceedings: Fourth Scientific Meeting and Exhibition of the International Society for Magnetic Resonance in Medicine, Vol. 2. New York, USA: ISMRM*; 1996: 998.

21) Moore, C. M.; Redmond, O. M.; Buckley, P. et al. In vivo proton NMR spectroscopy (STEAM) in patients with schizophrenia. *In: Book of Abstracts: Eleventh Annual Scientific Meeting of the Society of Magnetic Resonance in Medicine, Vol. 1. Berlin, Germany: SMRM*; 1992: 1933.

22) Yurgelun–Todd, D. A.; Renshaw, P. F.; Waternaux, C. M. et al. ^{1}H spectroscopy of the temporal lobes in schizophrenic and bipolar patients. *In: Proceedings: Twelfth Annual Scientific Meeting of the Society of Magnetic Resonance in Medicine, Vol. 3. New York, USA: SMRM*; 1993: 1539.

23) Yurgelun–Todd, D. A.; Moore, C. M.; Bonello, C. M. et al. NAA/Cr ratio correlates inversely with gray matter in the left temporal lobe of schizophrenic patients. *In: Proceedings: Fourth Scientific Meeting and Exhibition of the International Society for Magnetic Resonance in Medicine, Vol. 2. New York, USA: ISMRM*; 1996: 999.

24) Yurgelun–Todd, D. A.; Renshaw, P. F.; Gruber, S. A. et al. Proton magnetic resonance spectroscopy of the temporal lobes in schizophrenics and normal controls. *Schizophr. Res.* 19: 55–59; 1996.

25) Nasrallah, H. A.; Skinner, T. E.; Schmalbrock, P. et al. Chapter 1, In vivo ^{1}H–NMR Spectroscopy of the limbic temporal lobe in patients with schizophrenia. In: H. A. Nasrallah, J. W. Pettegrew (Eds). NMR Spectroscopy in Psychiatric Brain Disorders. Washington, DC: American Psychiatric Press, Inc. 1995: pp. 1–20.

26) Nasrallah, H. A.; Skinner, T. E.; Schmalbrock, P. et al. Proton magnetic resonance spectroscopy (^{1}H MRS) of the hippocampal formation in schizophrenia: A pilot study. *Br. J. Psychiatry* 165: 481–485; 1994.

27) Komoroski, R. A.; Heimberg, C.; Lawson, W. et al. A localized, *in vivo* ^{1}H NMR spectroscopy study of schizophrenics. *In: Proceedings: Third Scientific Meeting and Exhibition of the Society of Magnetic Resonance, Vol. 3. Nice, France: SMR*; 1995: 1846.

28) Renshaw, P. F.; Yurgelun–Todd, D. A.; Tohen, M. et al. Temporal lobe proton magnetic resonance spectroscopy of patients with first-episode psychosis. *Am. J. Psychiatry* 152: 444–446; 1995.

29) Fukuzako, H.; Takeuchi, K.; Hokazono, Y. et al. Proton magnetic resonance spectroscopy of the left medial temporal and frontal lobes in chronic schizophrenia: preliminary report. *Psychiatry Res. Neuroimaging* 61: 193–200; 1995.

30) Bertolino, A.; Nawroz, S.; Mattay, V. S. et al. A specific anatomical pattern of neuronal impairment in schizophrenia as assessed by multislice ^{1}H–MRSI. *In: Proceedings: Third Scientific Meeting and Exhibition*

of the Society of Magnetic Resonance, Vol. 3. Nice, France: SMR; 1995: 1844.

31) Buckley, P. F.; Moore, C.; Long, H. et al. [1]H-Magnetic resonance spectroscopy of the left temporal and frontal lobes in schizophrenia: Clinical, neurodevelopmental, and cognitive correlates. *Biol. Psychiatry* 36: 792-800; 1994.

32) Choe, B. -Y.; Kim, K. -T.; Suh, T. -S. et al. Alterations of proton metabolites in drug-naive, chronic schizophrenia by MRS. *In: Proceedings: Second Meeting of the Society of Magnetic Resonance, Vol. 2. San Francisco, California USA: SMR*; 1994: 603.

33) Bertolino, A.; Callicott, J. H.; Elman, I. et al. Proton magnetic resonance spectroscopic imaging in drug naive patients with schizophrenia: Regionality of neuronal damage. *In: Proceedings: Fourth Scientific Meeting and Exhibition of the International Society for Magnetic Resonance in Medicine, Vol. 2. New York, USA: ISMRM*; 1996: 1002.

34) Paul, C. R.; Lenkinski, R. E.; Boyko, O. B. et al. Proton magnetic resonance spectroscopy of patients with first episode of schizophrenia. *In: Proceedings: Fourth Scientific Meeting and Exhibition of the International Society for Magnetic Resonance in Medicine, Vol. 2. New York, USA: ISMRM*; 1996: 1001.

35) Fujimoto, T.; Nakano, T.; Takano, T. et al. Proton magnetic resonance spectroscopy of basal ganglia in chronic schizophrenia. *Biol. Psychiatry* 40: 14-18; 1996.

36) Thomas, M. A.; Ke, Y.; Caplan, R. et al. Frontal lobe ^{1}H MR spectroscopy of children with schizophrenia. *In: Proceedings: Fourth Scientific Meeting and Exhibition of the International Society for Magnetic Resonance in Medicine, Vol. 2. New York, USA: ISMRM*; 1996: 1000.

37) Choe, B. -Y.; Suh, T. -S.; Shinn, K. -S. et al. Correlation between clinical evaluations and metabolic changes in chronic schizophrenia after neuroleptic treatment by *in vivo* ^{1}H MRS. *In: Proceedings: Fourth Scientific Meeting and Exhibition of the International Society for Magnetic Resonance in Medicine, Vol. 2. New York, USA: ISMRM*; 1996: 1004.

38) Choe, B. -Y.; Suh, T. -S.; Shinn, K. -S. et al. Evaluation of neuroleptic treatment in chronic schizophrenia by ^{1}H MRS. *In: Proceedings: Second Meeting of the Society of Magnetic Resonance, Vol. 2. San Francisco, California USA: SMR*; 1994: 604.

39) Komoroski, R. A.; Omori, M.; Pearce, J. et al. An *in vitro* ^{1}H NMR study of post-mortem brains of schizophrenics. *In: Proceedings: Third Scientific Meeting and Exhibition of the Society of Magnetic Resonance, Vol. 3. Nice, France: SMR*; 1995: 1845.

40) Fujimoto, T.; Matsumoto, T.; Uchida, T. et al. [31]P chemical shift imaging in bipolar disorder. *In: Proceedings: Fifth Scientific Meeting and Exhibition of the International Society for Magnetic Resonance in Medicine, Vol. 2. Vancouver, B. C., Canada: ISMRM*; 1997: 1168.

41) Moore, C. M.; Christensen, J. D.; Lafer, B. et al. Decreased adenosine triphosphate in the basal ganglia of depressed subjects: A phosphorus-31 magnetic resonance spectroscopy study. *In: Proceedings: Fourth Scientific Meeting and Exhibition of the International Society for Magnetic Resonance in Medicine, Vol. 2. New York, USA: ISMRM*; 1996: 996.

42) Christensen, J. D.; Renshaw, P. F.; Stoll, A. L. et al. [31]P spectroscopy of the basal ganglia in major depression. *In: Proceedings: Second Meeting of the Society of Magnetic Resonance, Vol. 2. San Francisco, California, USA: SMR*; 1994: 608.

43) Kato, T.; Shioiri, T.; Murashita, J. et al. Cerebral asymmetry of high energy phosphate metabolism in manic-depressive illness measured with ^{31}P one-dimensional chemical shift imaging. *In: Proceedings: Twelfth Annual Scientific Meeting of the Society of Magnetic Resonance in Medicine, Vol. 3. New York, USA: SMRM*; 1993: 1544.

44) Charles, H. C.; Lazeyras, F.; Krishnan, R. K. K. et al. Brain choline in depression: *In vivo* detection of potential pharmacodynamic effects of antidepressant therapy using hydrogen localized spectroscopy. *In: Book of Abstracts: Eleventh Annual Scientific Meeting of the Society of Magnetic Resonance in Medicine, Vol. 1. Berlin, Germany: SMRM*; 1992: 757.

45) Sharma, R.; Venkatasubramanian, P. N.; Bárány, M. et al. Proton magnetic resonance spectroscopy of the brain in schizophrenic and affective patients. *Schizophr. Res.* 8: 43-49; 1992.

46) Renshaw, P. F.; Stoll, A. L.; Rothschild, A. et al. Proton MRS studies of the basal ganglia in major depression: Side and treatment effects. *In: Proceedings: Twelfth Annual Scientific Meeting of the Society of Magnetic Resonance in Medicine, Vol. 1. New York, USA: SMRM*; 1993: 433.

47) Kato, T.; Hamakawa, H.; Shioiri, T. et al. Proton MRS of the basal ganglia in patients with bipolar disorder. *In: Proceedings: Second Meeting of the Society of Magnetic Resonance, Vol. 2. San Francisco, California USA: SMR*; 1994: 605.

48) Bruhn, H.; Stoppe, G.; Staedt, J. et al. Quantitative proton MRS *in vivo* shows cerebral *myo*-inositol and cholines to be unchanged in manic-depressive patients

treated with lithium. *In: Proceedings: Twelfth Annual Scientific Meeting of the Society of Magnetic Resonance in Medicine, Vol. 3. New York, USA: SMRM*; 1993: 1543.

49) Denays, R.; Chao, S. L.; Mathur-Devrē, R. et al. Metabolic changes in the rat brain after acute and chronic ethanol intoxication: A ^{31}P NMR spectroscopy study. *Magn. Reson. Med.* 29: 719-723; 1993.

50) Yamaguchi, H.; Uchida, T.; Fujimoto, T. et al. ^{1}H MRS findings of brains in patients with alcoholism. *Japanese Journal of Psychiatric Research on Alcohol* 3: 49-54; 1996. [Japanese]

51) Gibbs, S. J.; Riddle, W. R.; Welch, L. W. et al. Recovery of brain function in newly abstinent alcoholics: Correlation with proton single voxel spectroscopy. *In: Proceedings: Third Scientific Meeting and Exhibition of the Society of Magnetic Resonance, Vol. 1. Nice, France: SMR*; 1995: 61.

52) Fujimoto, T.; Uchida, T.; Yamaguchi, H. et al. ^{1}H MRS study of temporal lobe in alcoholic patients. *In: Abstracts of the X World Congress of Psychiatry, Vol. 2. Madrid;* 1996: 130.

53) Fujimoto, T.; Uchida, T.; Yamaguchi, H. et al. Localized ^{1}H MRS in alcoholic dementia. *In: Proceedings: Fourth Scientific Meeting and Exhibition of the International Society for Magnetic Resonance in Medicine, Vol. 2. New York, USA: ISMRM*; 1996: 952.

54) Behar, K.; Rothman, D.; Petersen, K. et al. Cortical GABA levels are reduced in localized ^{1}H NMR spectra of alcoholic and hepatic encephalopathy patients. *In: Proceedings: Fourth Scientific Meeting and Exhibition of the International Society for Magnetic Resonance in Medicine, Vol. 1. New York, USA: ISMRM*; 1996: 408.

55) Mendelson, J. H.; Woods, B. T.; Chiu, T. -M. et al. In vivo proton magnetic resonance spectroscopy of alcohol in human brain. *Alcohol* 7: 443-447; 1990.

56) Kaufman, M. J.; Chiu, T. -M.; Mendelson, J. H. et al. Brain alcohol detectability increase with repeated administration in humans: a proton spectroscopy study. *Magn. Reson. Med.* 35: 435-440; 1996.

57) Chiu, T. -M.; Mendelson, J. H.; Woods, B. T. et al. *In vivo* proton magnetic resonance spectroscopy detection of human alcohol tolerance. *Magn. Reson. Med.* 32: 511-516; 1994.

58) Chiu, T. -M.; Woods, B. T.; Teoh, S. K. et al. Proton spectroscopy of brain alcohol signals at short echo times in alcohol-tolerant and alcohol non-tolerant human subjects. *In: Book of Abstracts: Eleventh Annual Scientific Meeting of the Society of Magnetic Resonance in Medicine, Berlin, Germany: SMRM*; 1992: 1958.

12.2 CASES (76-85)

CASE 76

Case 76: A 34-year-old male
Schizophrenia (Disorganized type)
Age at onset : 28 years.

The patient presented a marked regression to primitive, uninhibited, and unorganized behavior, thought disorders, affective flatness, and poor contact with reality. The signal intensities in the ^{31}P contour map and metabolite image in Figures 76-1 and 2 are almost symmetrical. In Figures 76-3 and 4, signal intensites of β-ATP are slightly reduced in the left temporal lobe. In Figures 76-5 and 6, signal intensites of PDE are reduced in the basal ganglia regions, but increased in the left temporal lobe. Signal intensities in the PCr metabolite image are reduced in the medial frontal lobe (Figure 76-7), suggesting a decreased high-energy phosphate metabolism in this region. In the ^{31}P spectrum of voxel 1, obtained from the right medial frontal region, shown in Figure 76-9, the %PCr and %PME are reduced. In the^{31}P spectrum of voxel 2 from the left frontal region, the %PCr and %PME are reduced, and %PDE is elevated (Figure 76-10). The decreased %PME and increased % PDE may indicate disturbances in membrane phospholipids in the medial frontal lobe.

R 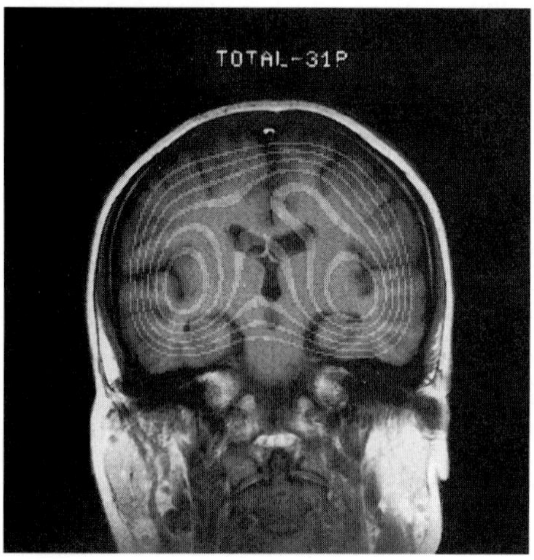 L

Fig. 76-1 Coronal ^{31}P contour map superimposed on T_1-weighted image (500/15).

R 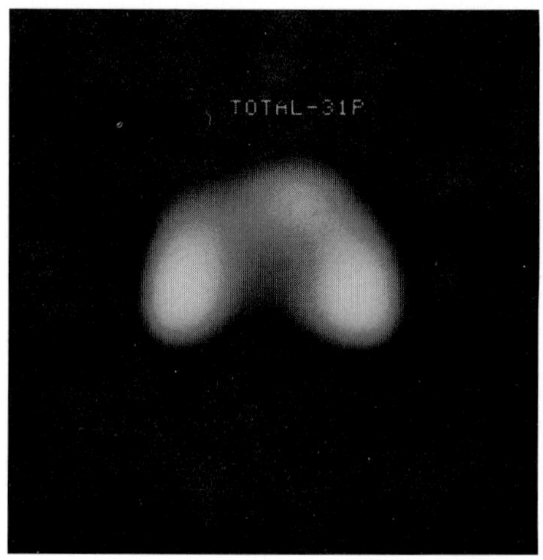 L

Fig. 76-2 Coronal ^{31}P metabolite image.

R 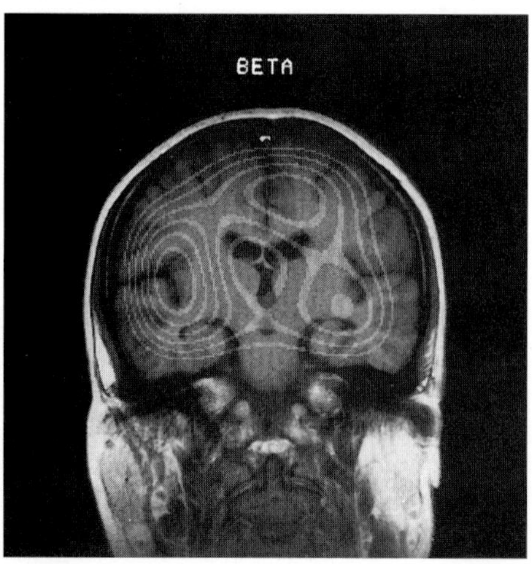 L

Fig. 76-3 Coronal β-ATP contour map superimposed on T_1-weighted image (500/15).

R 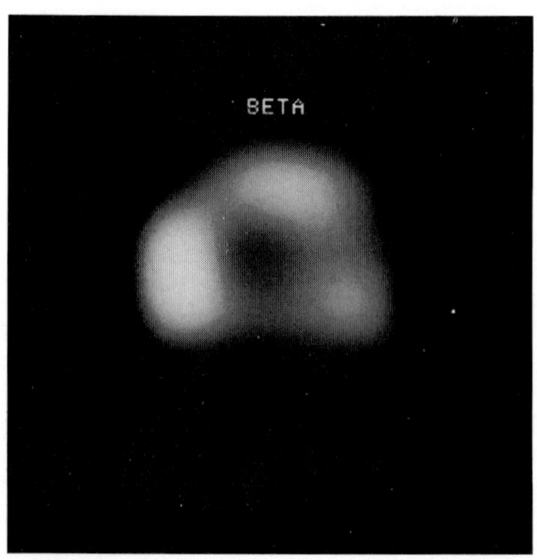 L

Fig. 76-4 Coronal β-ATP metabolite image.

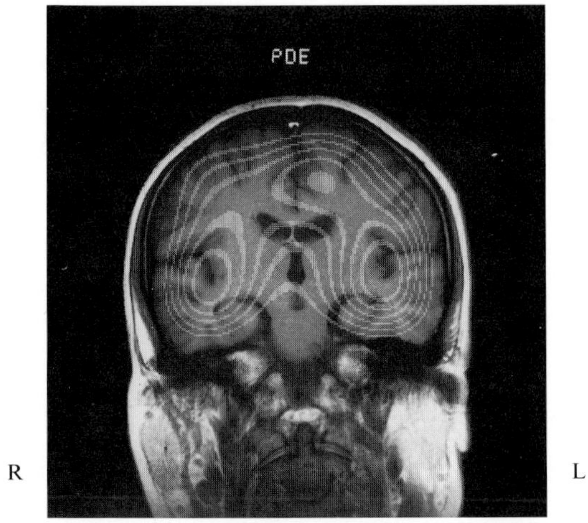

Fig. 76-5 Coronal PDE contour map superimposed on T_1-weighted image (500/15).

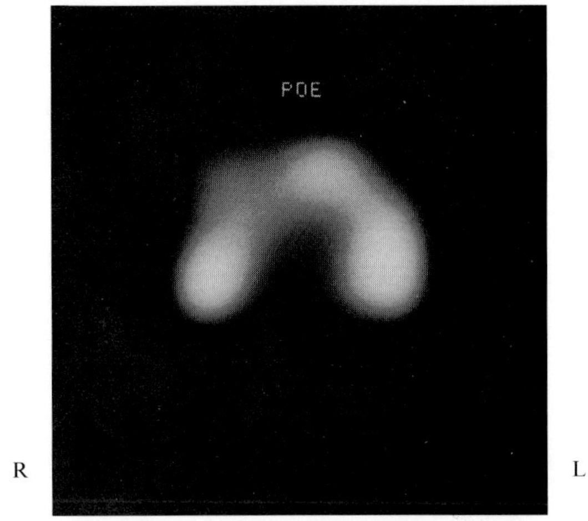

Fig. 76-6 Coronal PDE metabolite image.

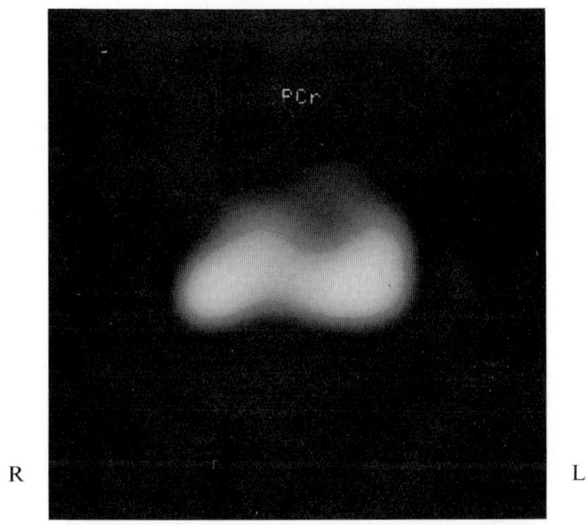

Fig. 76-7 Coronal PCr metabolite image.

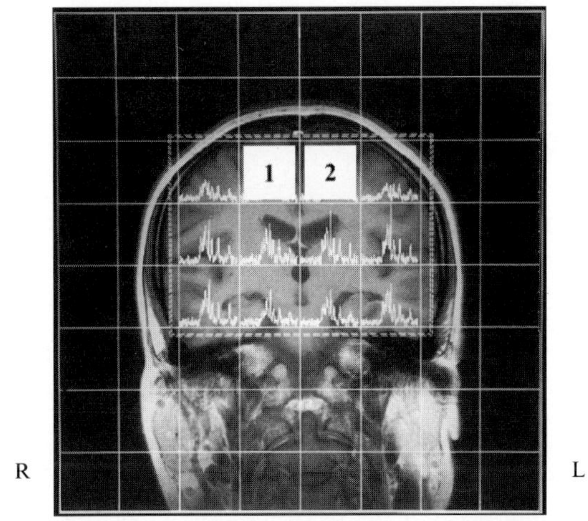

Fig. 76-8 T_1-weighted image showing the position of $3 \times 3 \times 4 cm^3$ voxels 1 and 2.

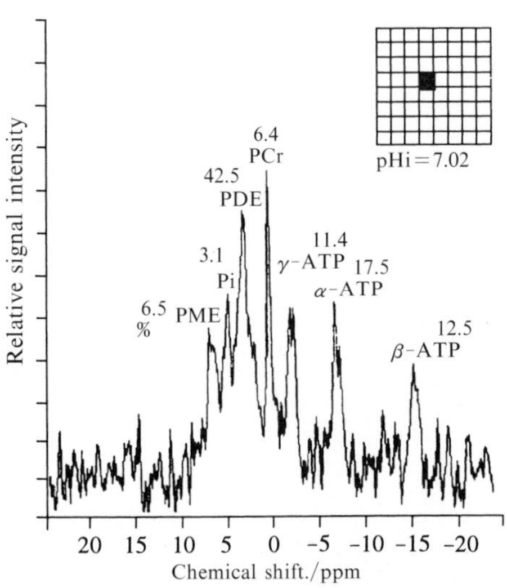

Fig. 76-9 ^{31}P spectrum of voxel 1. (Right medial frontal lobe.)

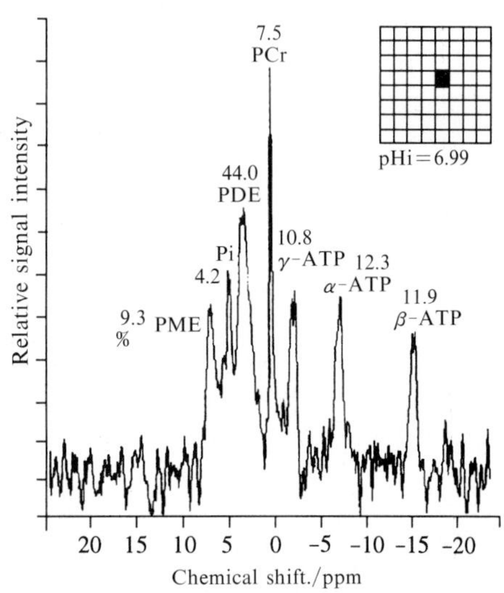

Fig. 76-10 ^{31}P spectrum of voxel 2. (Left medial frontal lobe.)

CASE 77

Case 77: A 35-year-old male
Schizophrenia (Disorganized type)
Age at onset : 32 years.

The patient presented blunted affect, disorganized behavior, alogia, anhedonia, ideas of persecution, and social/occupational dysfunction. The T_2-weighted image in Figure 77-1 shows slight enlargements of cerebral sulci and the lateral ventricle. In Figure 77-2, the distribution of ^{31}P signal intensities is almost symmetrical. In the PDE contour map and metabolite image in Figures 77-3 and 4, signal intensities are reduced in basal ganglia regions, but elevated in the left temporal lobe. The PCr metabolite image shows a decrease in signal intensities in the medial frontal region, suggesting a decrease in high-energy phosphate metabolism (Figure 77-5). In the ^{31}P spectrum in the right basal ganglia (voxel 4) shown in Figure 77-7, %PDE is reduced. In the ^{31}P spectrum of the left basal ganglia region (voxel 5), the %PME and %Pi are increased, and the %PDE is decreased (Figure 77- 8). In Figure 77-9, all peaks and pHi are also almost in the normal ranges in the right temporal lobe (voxel 3). In Figure 77-10, the %PDE and %PCr are increased, and %PME is decreased in the left temporal lobe (voxel 6). These findings suggest the dysfunction of membrane phospholipids in the basal ganglia regions and the left temporal lobe.

R 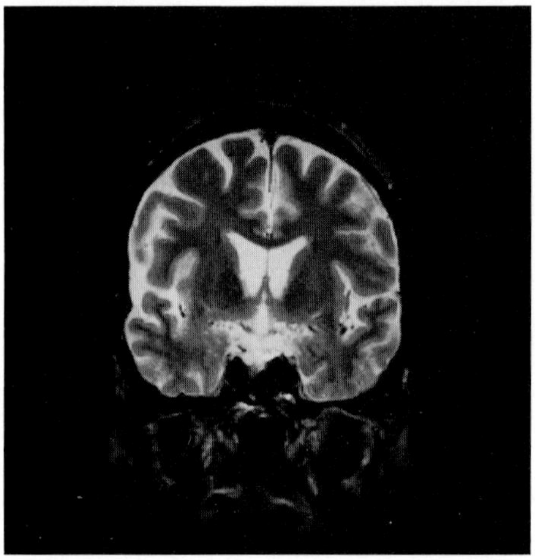 L

Fig. 77-1 Coronal T_2-weighted image (2,200/90).

R 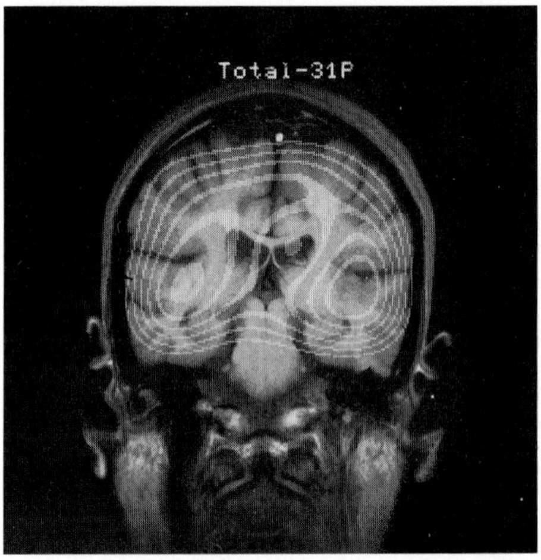 L

Fig. 77-2 Coronal ^{31}P contour map superimposed on T_1-weighted image (500/15).

R 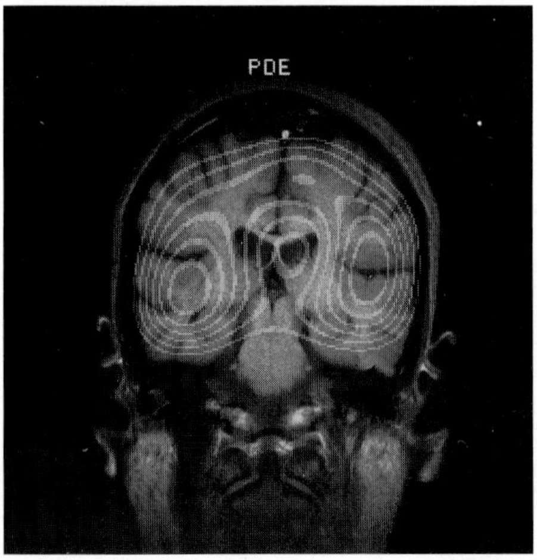 L

Fig. 77-3 Coronal PDE contour map superimposed on T_1-weighted image (500/15).

R 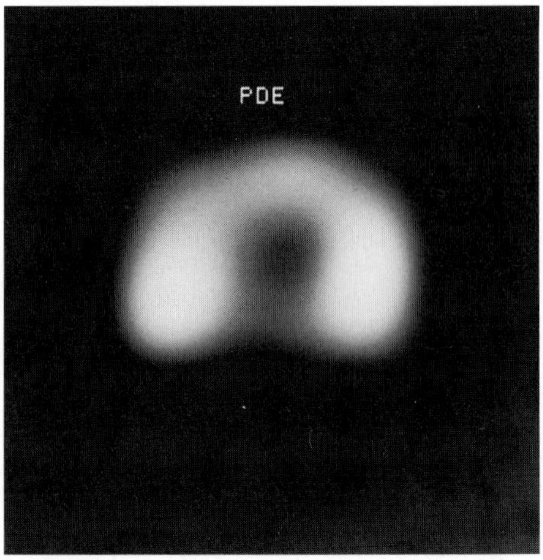 L

Fig. 77-4 Coronal PDE metabolite image.

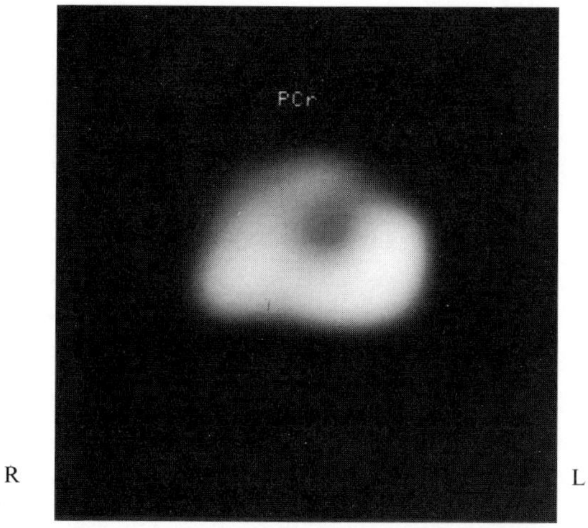

Fig. 77-5 Coronal PCr metabolite image.

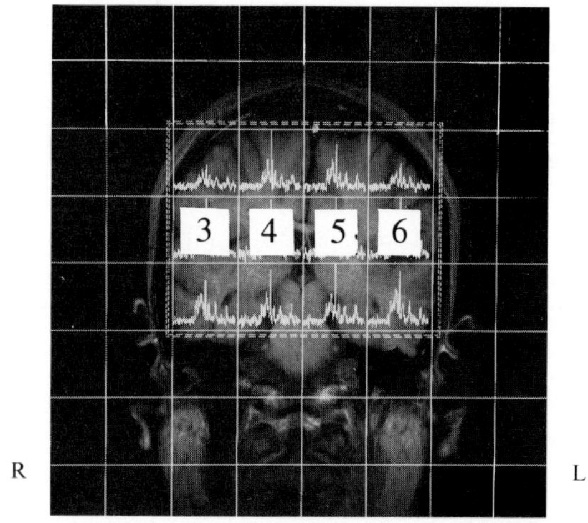

Fig. 77-6 T_1-weighted image showing the position of $3 \times 3 \times 4 cm^3$ voxels 4, 5, 3 and 6.

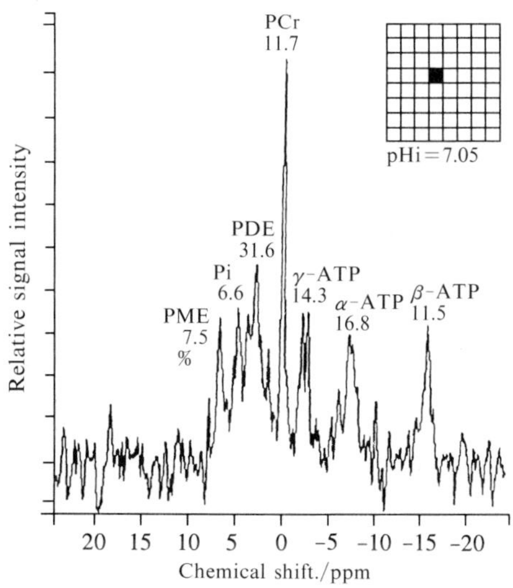

Fig. 77-7 ^{31}P spectrum of voxel 4. (Right basal ganglia.)

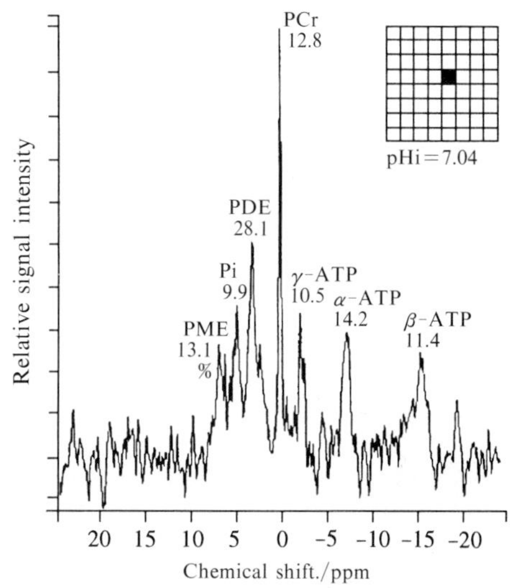

Fig. 77-8 ^{31}P spectrum of voxel 5. (Left basal ganglia.)

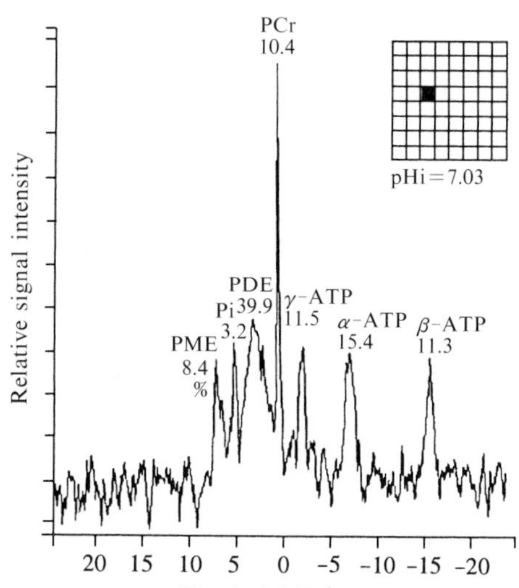

Fig. 77-9 ^{31}P spectrum of voxel 3. (Right temporal lobe.)

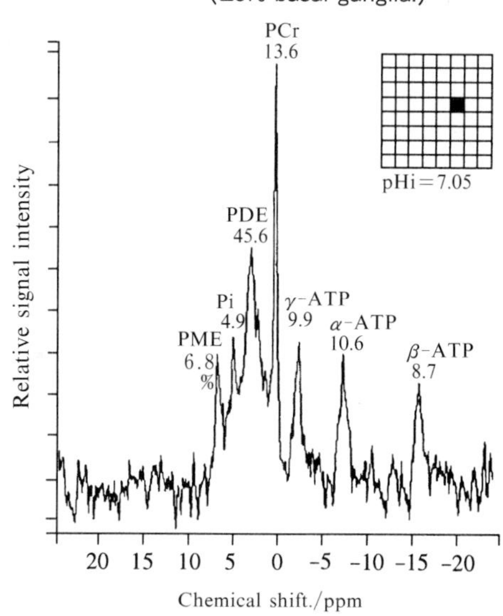

Fig. 77-10 ^{31}P spectrum of voxel 6. (Left temporal lobe.)

CASE 78

Case 78: A 43-year-old male
Schizophrenia (Disorganized type)
Age at onset : 27 years.

The patient presented disorganized speech and behavior, affective flattening, and dysfunction in interpersonal relations and self-care. In Figure 78-1, the T_2-weighted image shows slight brain atrophy. In the ^1H spectrum of Figure 78-3, the NAA/Cho and NAA/Cr ratios in the right basal ganglia are reduced, and the Cho/Cr ratio is slightly increased. In Figure 78-4, the NAA/Cho ratio is reduced, but the NAA/Cr and the Cho/Cr ratio are in the normal ranges in the left basal ganglia (Figure 78-4). Decreased NAA/Cr ratios suggest neuronal loss and dysfunction. The PDE metabolite image shows reduced signal intensities in areas including the basal ganglia (Figure 78-5). In Figure 78-7, the %PDE is decreased, and the %PME and pHi are increased in the area of the right basal ganglia (voxel 4). In Figure 78-8, the %PDE is decreased and the pHi is increased in the area of the left basal ganglia (voxel 5). In the ^{31}P spectrum in Figure 78-9, the %PDE is elevated in the right temporal region (voxel 7), indicating a disturbance of the membrane phospholipids metabolism. In the ^{31}P spectrum of the left temporal lobe obtained from voxel 10, all peaks and pHi are in the normal ranges (Figure 78-10). The decreased %PDE and increased %PME in the ^{31}P spectrum and increased Cho/Cr ratio in the ^1H spectrum both suggest dysfunction of phospholipids metabolism in the right basal ganglia region.

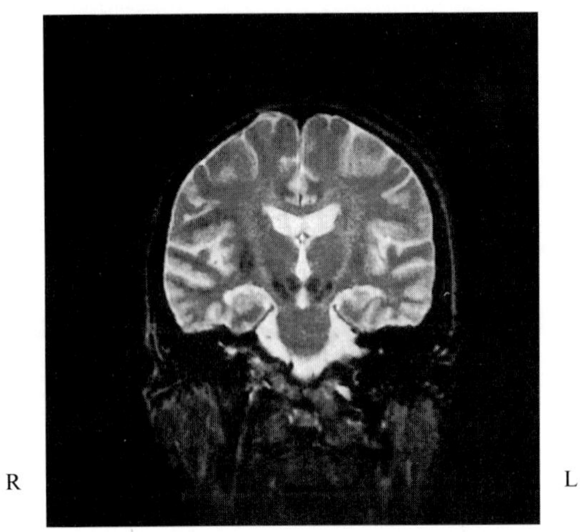

Fig. 78-1 Coronal T_2-weighted image (2,200/90).

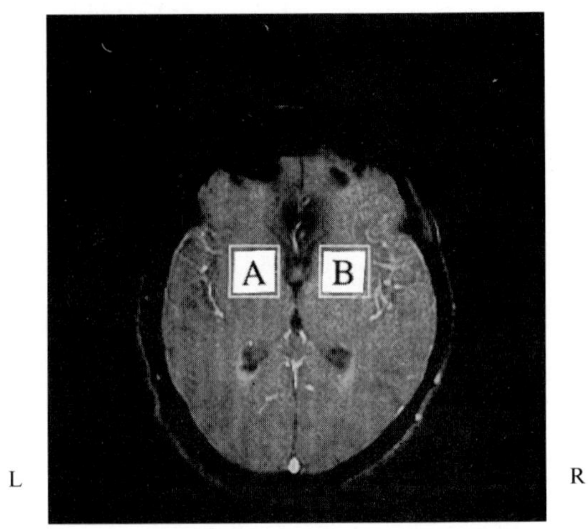

Fig. 78-2 T_1-weighted image showing the position of $3\times3\times3$ cm^3 voxels A and B.

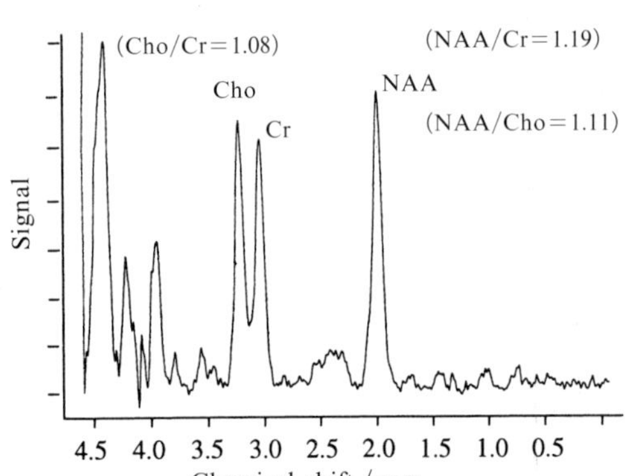

Fig. 78-3 ^1H spectrum of right basal ganglia (voxel B). PRESS (1,500/135).

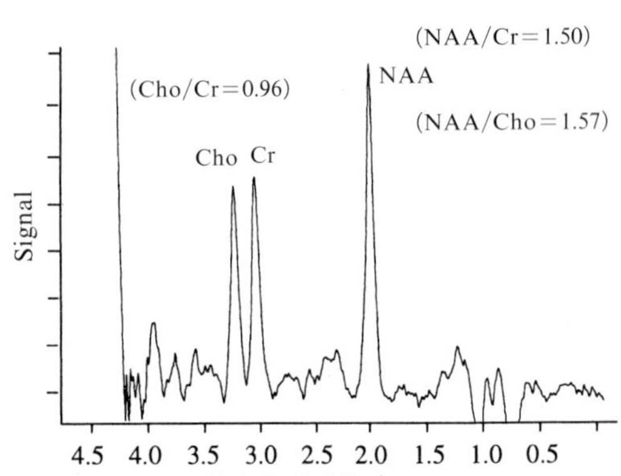

Fig. 78-4 ^1H spectrum of left basal ganglia (voxel A). PRESS (1,500/135).

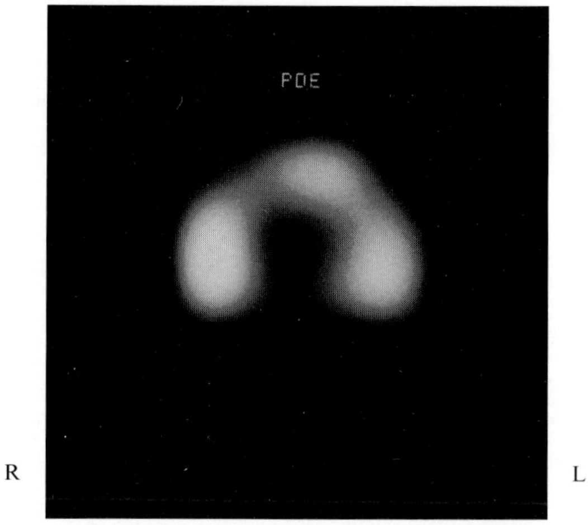

Fig. 78-5 Coronal PDE metabolite image.

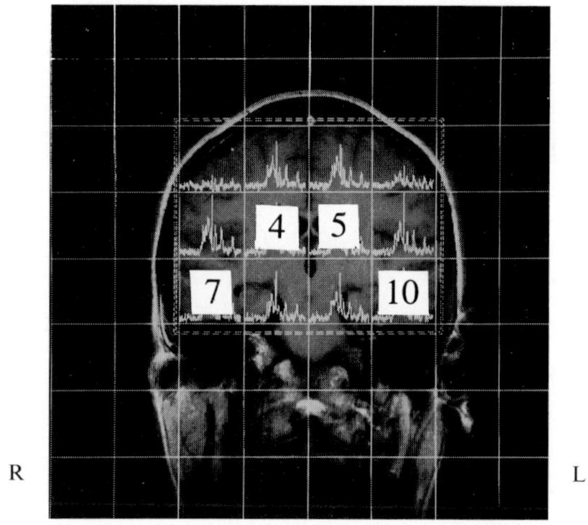

Fig. 78-6 T_1-weighted image showing the position of $3 \times 3 \times 4$ cm^3 voxels 4, 5, 7 and 10.

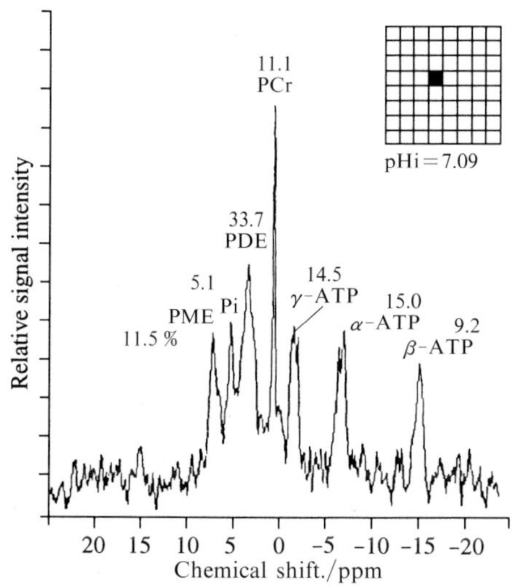

Fig. 78-7 ^{31}P spectrum of voxel 4. (Right basal ganglia.)

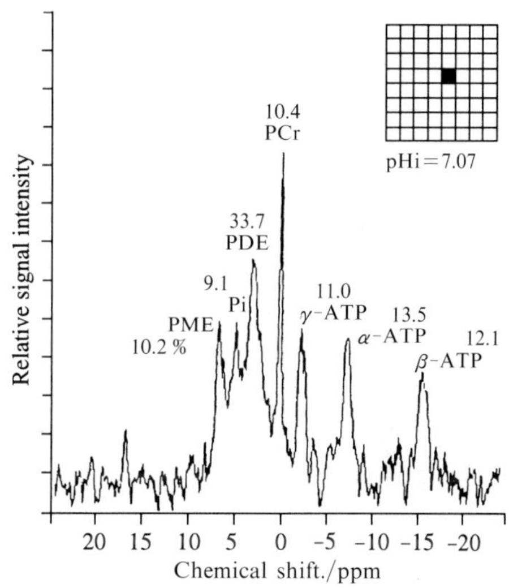

Fig. 78-8 ^{31}P spectrum of voxel 5. (Left basal ganglia.)

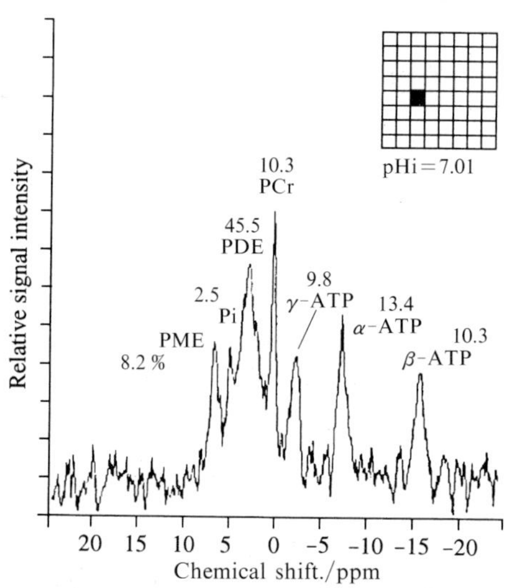

Fig. 78-9 ^{31}P spectrum of voxel 7. (Right temporal lobe.)

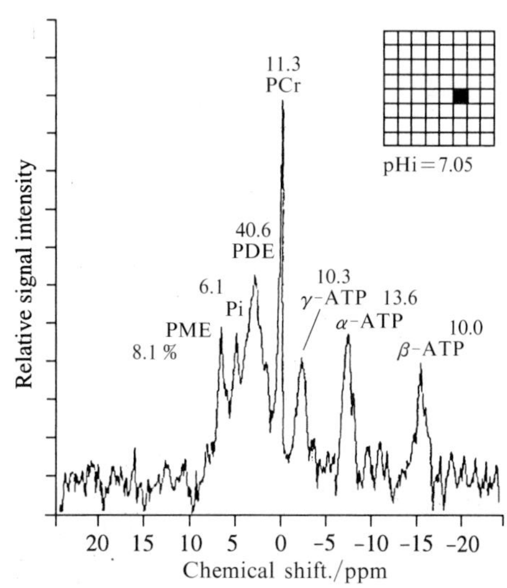

Fig. 78-10 ^{31}P spectrum of voxel 10. (Left temporal lobe.)

CASE 79

Case 79: A 47-year-old male
Schizophrenia (Catatonic type)
Age at onset, 27 years.

The patient was hospitalized due to excessive motor activity and disorganized behavior and speech. When MRS was performed after three weeks of hospitalization, his catatonic state had been reduced. The T_2-weighted image in Figure 79-1 shows slight brain atrophy. In the ^1H spectrum of the right mesial temporal lobe, the NAA/Cho ratio and the NAA/Cr ratio are reduced, and the Cho/Cr ratio is slightly increased (Figure 79-3). In Figure 79-4, the NAA/Cho ratio and the NAA/Cr ratio are reduced, and the Cho/Cr ratio is elevated in the left mesial temporal lobe. The decreased NAA/Cr ratio and increased Cho/Cr ratio suggests neuronal loss and membrane dysfunction, respectively. In the ^{31}P spectrum of an area including the right basal ganglia (voxel 4) shown in Figure 79-6, the %PDE is reduced, and the %PME and %PCr are increased (Figure 79-6). In Figure 79-7, the %PDE is decreased and the PME is increased in the left basal ganglia region (voxel 5). In the ^{31}P spectrum in Figure 79-9, the %β-ATP is reduced in the right mesial temporal region (voxel 11). In the ^{31}P spectrum of the left mesial temporal lobe obtained from voxel 13, the %β-ATP is increased (Figure 79-10). The decreased %PDE and increased %PME in the ^{31}P spectrum and increased Cho/Cr ratio in the ^1H spectrum together suggest dysfunction of the phospholipid metabolism in the basal ganglia region.

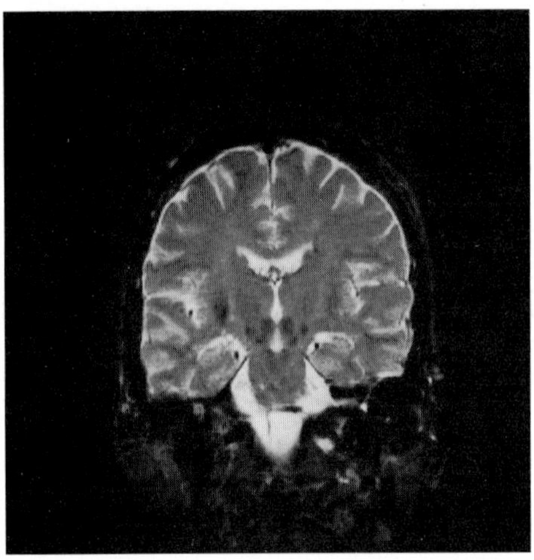

Fig. 79-1 Coronal T_2-weighted image (2,200/90).

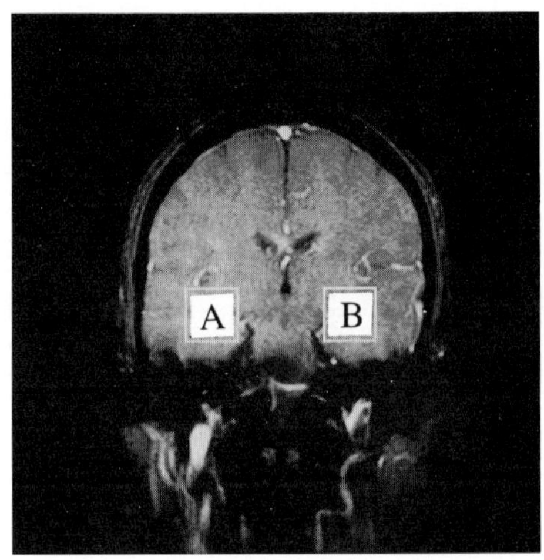

Fig. 79-2 T_1-weighted image showing the position of $3 \times 3 \times 3$ cm^3 voxels A and B.

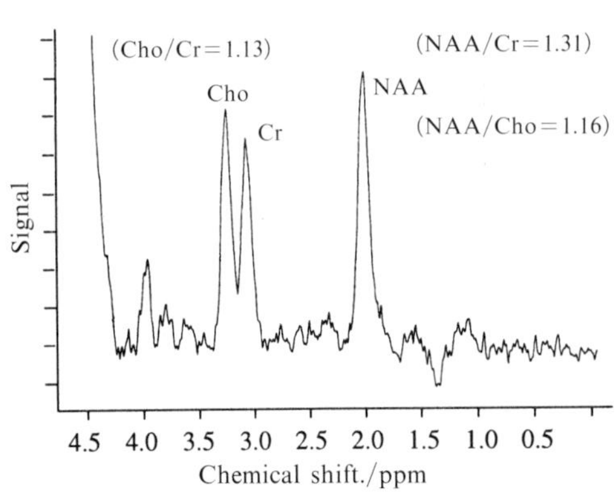

Fig. 79-3 ^1H spectrum of right mesial temporal lobe (voxel A). PRESS (1,500/135).

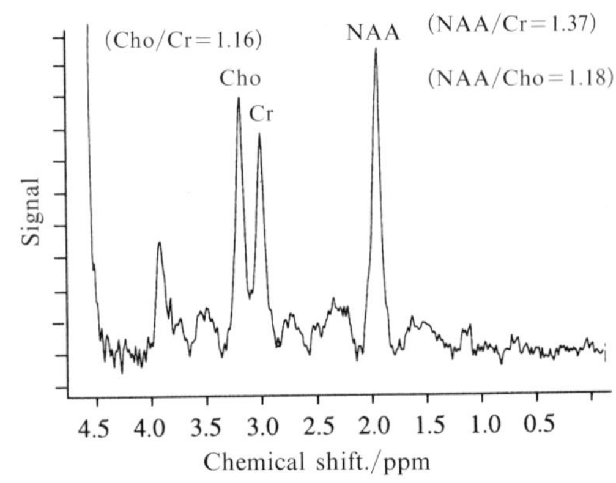

Fig. 79-4 ^1H spectrum of left mesial temporal lobe (voxel B). PRESS (1,500/135).

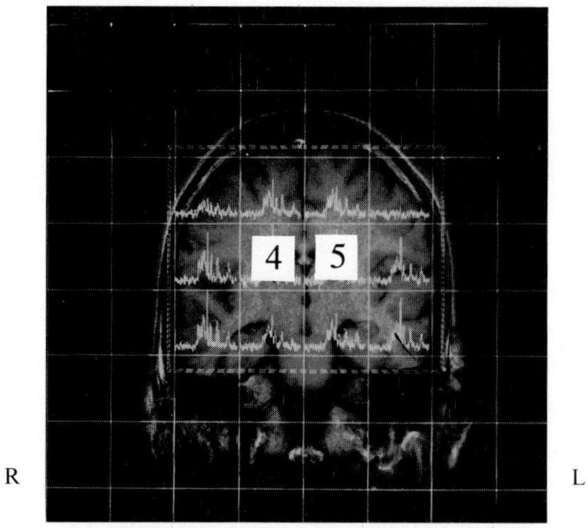

Fig. 79-5 T_1-weighted image showing the position of $3 \times 3 \times 4$ cm^3 voxels 4 and 5.

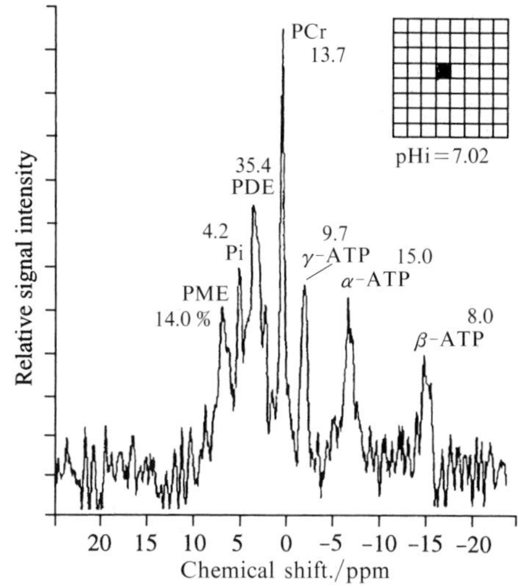

Fig. 79-6 ^{31}P spectrum of voxel 4. (Right basal ganglia.)

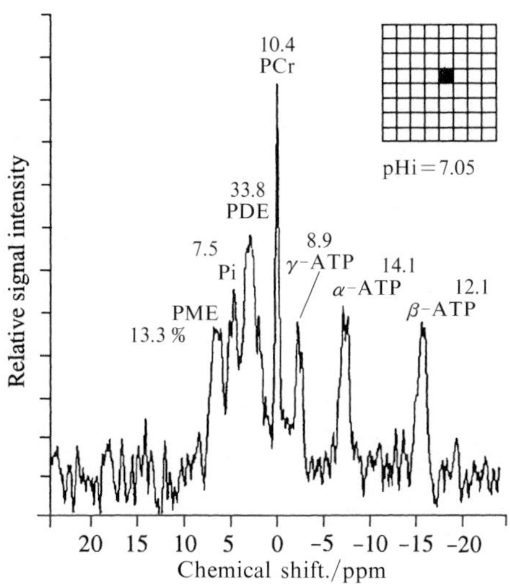

Fig. 79-7 ^{31}P spectrum of voxel 5. (Left basal ganglia.)

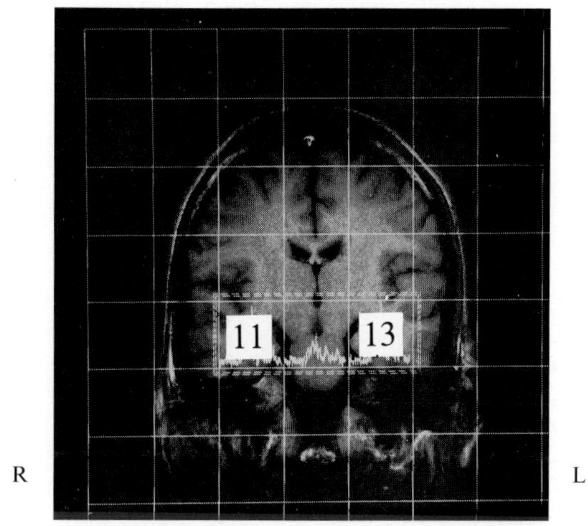

Fig. 79-8 T_1-weighted image showing the position of $3 \times 3 \times 4$ cm^3 voxels 11 and 13.

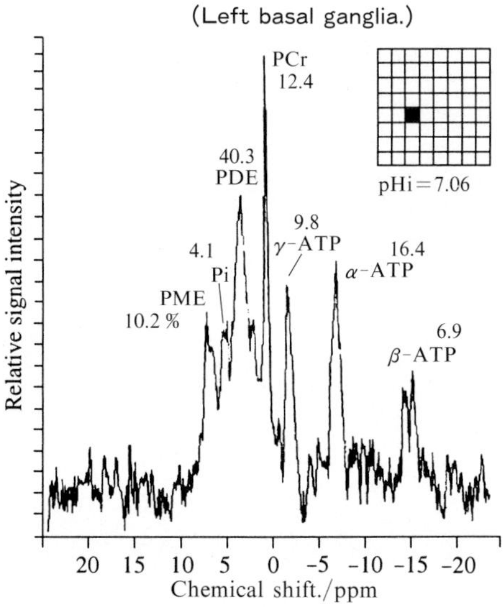

Fig. 79-9 ^{31}P spectrum of voxel 11. (Right mesial temporal lobe.)

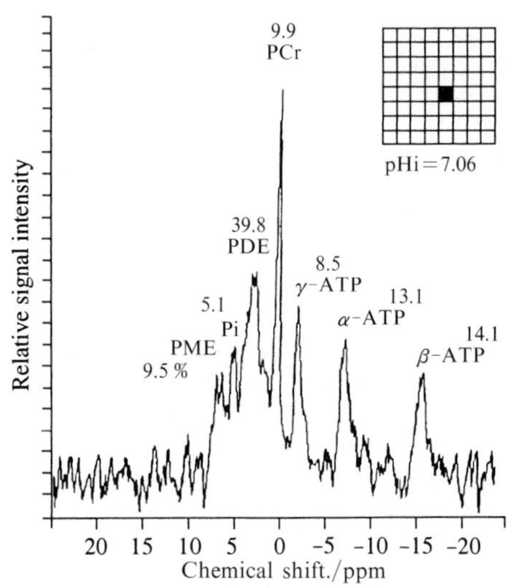

Fig. 79-10 ^{31}P spectrum of voxel 13. (Left mesial temporal lobe.)

CASE 80

Case 80: A 42-year-old male

Bipolar 1 Disorder, Most Recent Episode Depressed (DSM-IV 296. 52)

Age at onset : 39 years.

The patient had two previous manic episodes. At the MRS examination his mental state showed mild depression with diminished interest, insomnia, and psychomotor agitation. In the ^{31}P contour map and metabolite image in Figures 80-1 and 2, signal intensities are slightly reduced in the left temporal lobe. In the total ATP contour map in Figure 80-3, the signal intensity is decreased in the frontal and left basal ganglia, suggesting dysfunction of the high-energy phosphate metabolism. The total ATP metabolite image also shows decreased signal intensities in the medial frontal lobe and basal ganglia region (Figure 80-4). In the PME contour map and metabolite image in Figures 80-5 and 6, the signal intensities are reduced in the right basal ganglia region but increased in the left. The PDE contour map and metabolite image show elevated signal intensities in the medial frontal lobe (Figures 80-7 and 8). Increased signal intensities of PDE and PME indicate alterations in membrane phospholipids. In the PCr contour map and metabolite image in Figures 80-9 and 10, signal intensities are reduced in the medial frontal lobe and basal ganglia region, suggesting decreased high-energy phosphate metabolism. The pHi levels are in the normal ranges in all voxels.

R 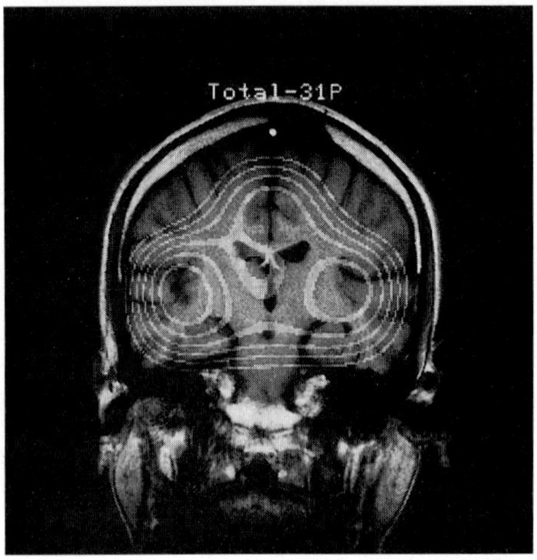 L

Fig. 80-1 Coronal ^{31}P contour map superimposed on T_1-weighted image (500/15).

R 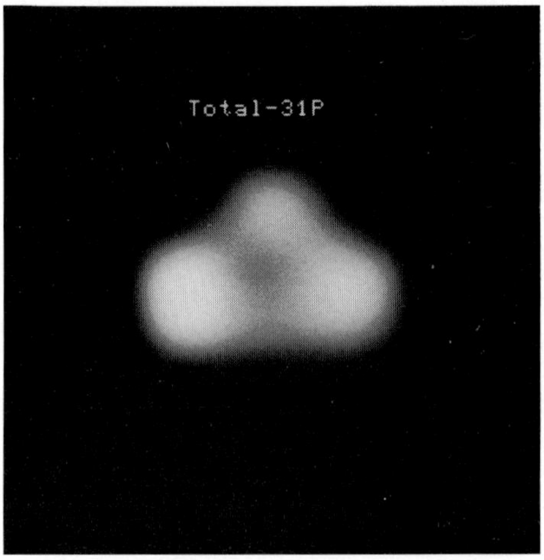 L

Fig. 80-2 Coronal ^{31}P metabolite image.

R 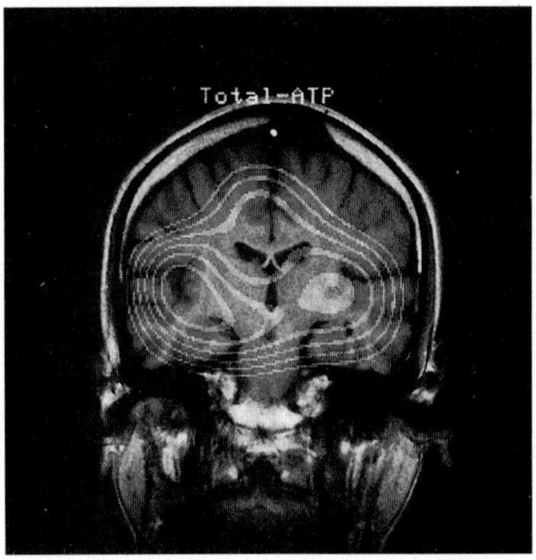 L

Fig. 80-3 Coronal total ATP contour map superimposed on T_1-weighted image (500/15).

R 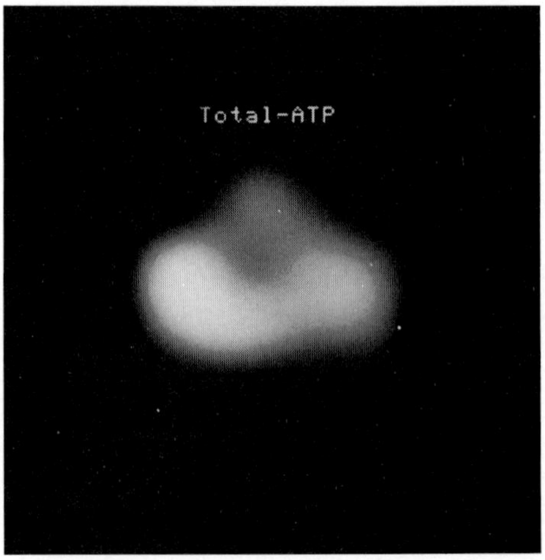 L

Fig. 80-4 Coronal total ATP metabolite image.

R 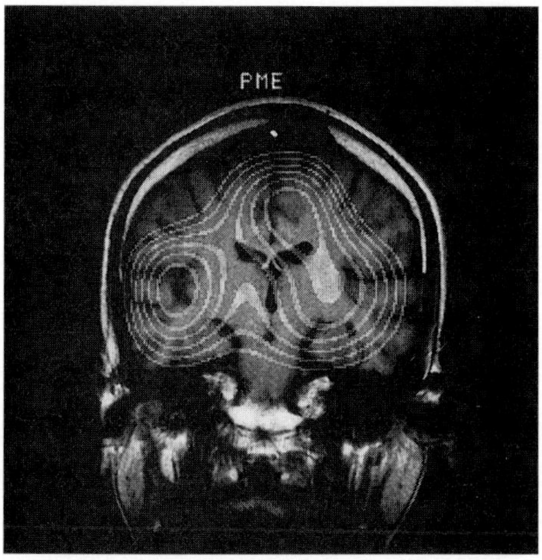 L

Fig. 80-5 Coronal PME contour map superimposed on T_1-weighted image (500/15).

R 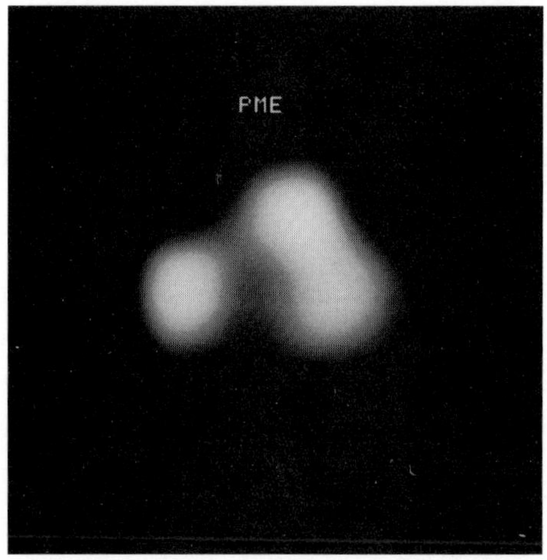 L

Fig. 80-6 Coronal PME metabolite image.

R 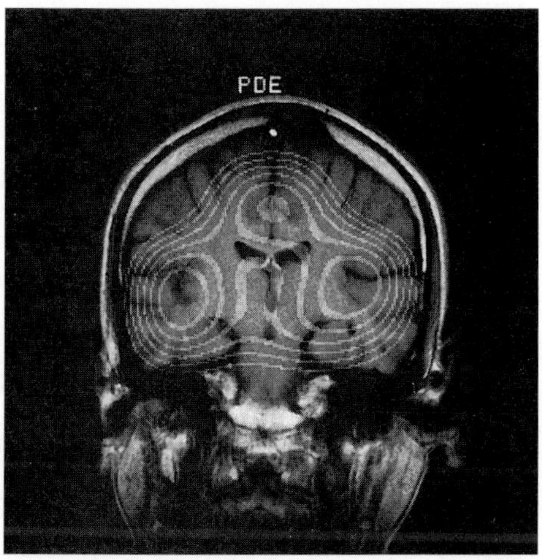 L

Fig. 80-7 Coronal PDE contour map superimposed on T_1-weighted image (500/15).

R 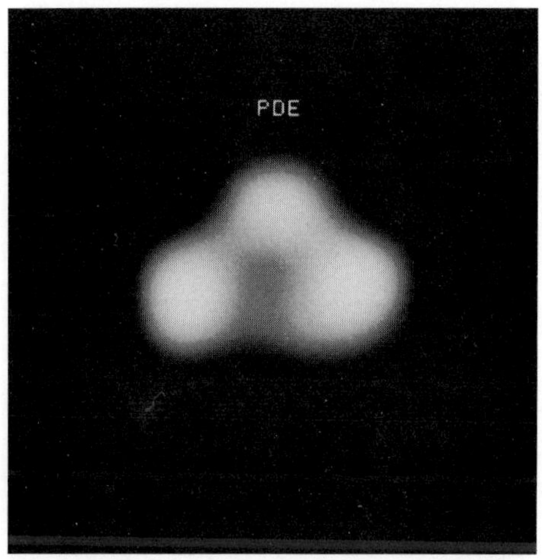 L

Fig. 80-8 Coronal PDE metabolite image.

R 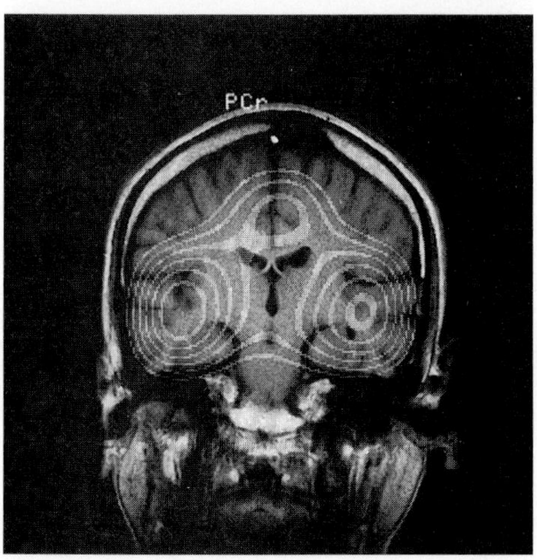 L

Fig. 80-9 Coronal PCr contour map superimposed on T_1-weighted image (500/15).

R 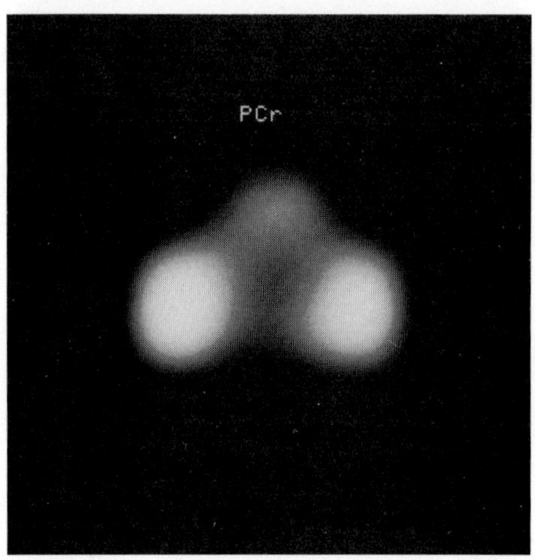 L

Fig. 80-10 Coronal PCr metabolite image.

CASE 81

Case 81: A 68-year-old male

Bipolar 1 Disorder, Most Recent Episode Depressed

Age at onset : 67 years.

The patient had one previous manic episode. At the MRS examination his mental state showed mild depression with insomnia, loss of energy, feelings of worthlessness, and guilt. The T_2-weighted image in Figure 81-1 shows slight brain atrophy. In the ^1H spectrum of the right basal ganglia (voxel B shown in Figure 81-2), the Cho/Cr ratio is increased, and the NAA/Cho ratio and NAA/Cr ratio are reduced (Figure 81-3). In the ^1H spectrum of the left basal ganglia (voxel A), the Cho/Cr ratio is also increased, the NAA/Cho ratio is decreased, but the NAA/Cr ratio is in the normal range (Figure 81-4). The elevated Cho/Cr ratio suggest alterations in membrane phospholipid metabolism and the decreased NAA/Cr ratios suggest neuronal loss and dysfunction. In Figure 81-5, signal intensity of ^{31}P are slightly decreased in the left basal ganglia region. In Figure 81-6, the PDE signal intensity is reduced in the left basal ganglia region. In the PCr contour map and metabolite image in Figures 81-7 and 8, signal intensities are reduced in the medial frontal lobe and basal ganglia regions, suggesting dysfunction in the high-energy phosphate metabolism. In the ^{31}P spectrum obtained from the voxel shown in Figure 81-10, the %PME of the right basal ganglia is increased, and the %Pi is decreased. Both ^{31}P and ^1H spectra demonstrate an alteration in phospholipids in the basal ganglia region.

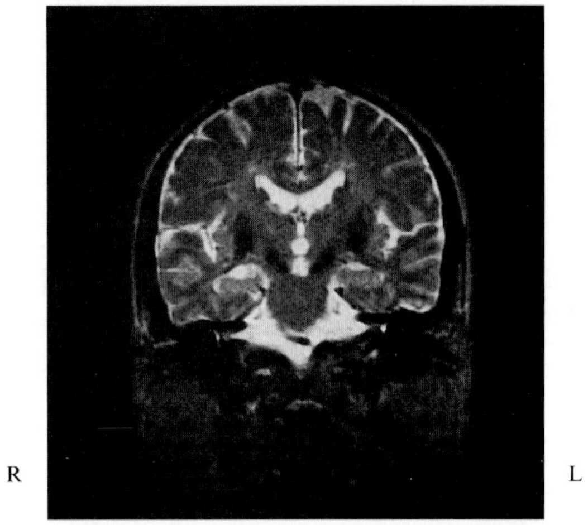

Fig. 81-1 Coronal T_2-weighted image (2,200/90).

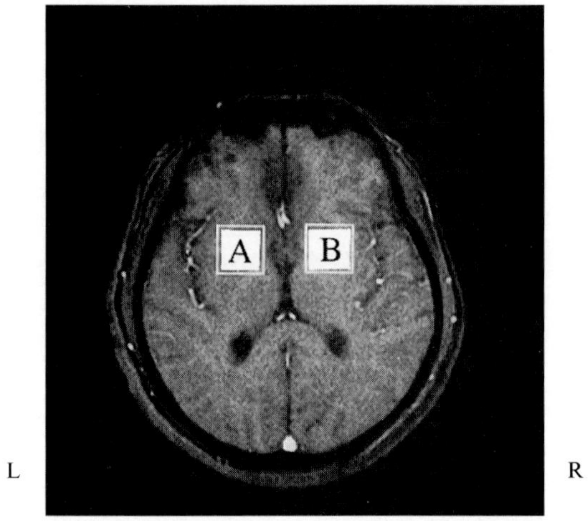

Fig. 81-2 T_1-weighted image showing the position of $3 \times 3 \times 3$ cm^3 voxels A and B.

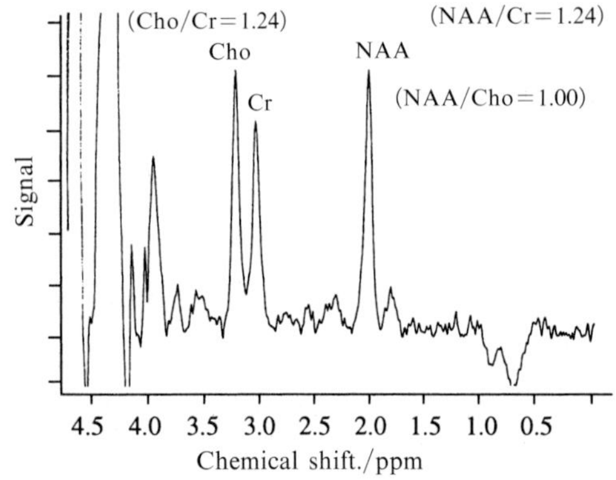

Fig. 81-3 ^1H spectrum of right basal ganglia (voxel B). PRESS (1,500/135).

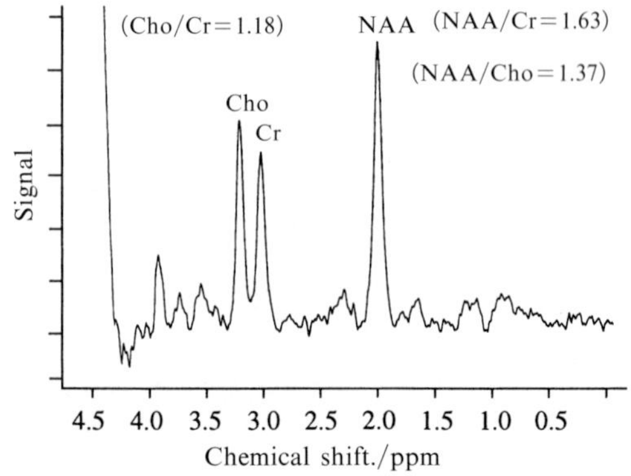

Fig. 81-4 ^1H spectrum of left basal ganglia (voxel A). PRESS (1,500/135).

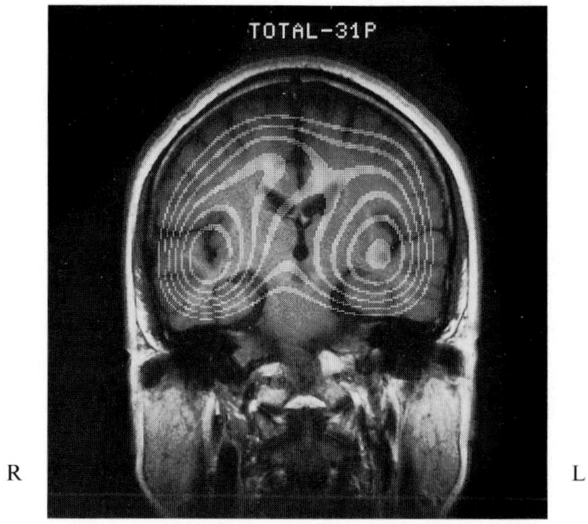

Fig. 81-5 Coronal ^{31}P contour map superimposed on T_1-weighted image (500/15).

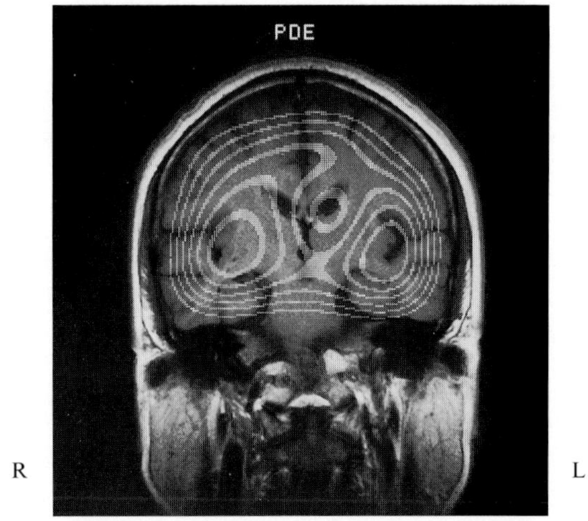

Fig. 81-6 Coronal PDE contour map superimposed on T_1-weighted image (500/15).

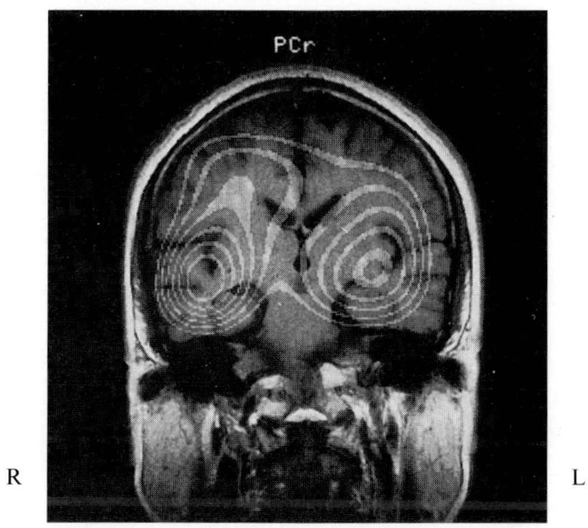

Fig. 81-7 Coronal PCr contour map superimposed on T_1-weighted image (500/15).

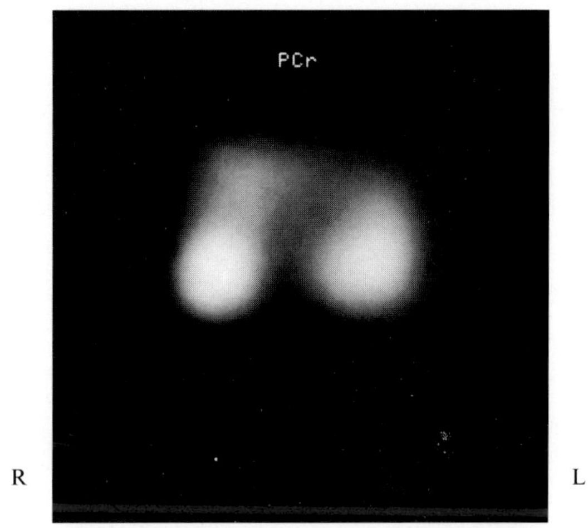

Fig. 81-8 Coronal PCr metabolite image.

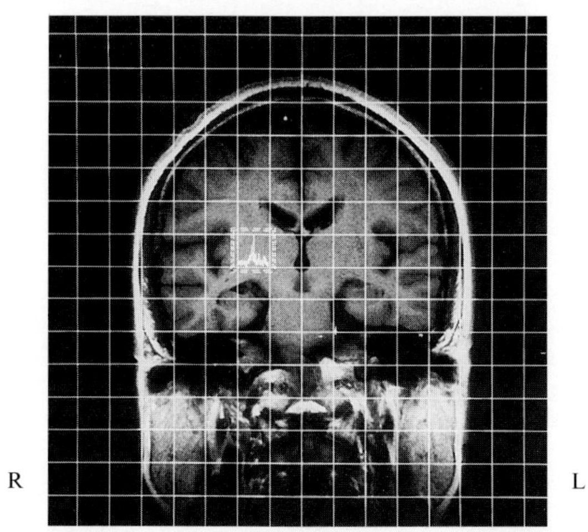

Fig. 81-9 T_1-weighted image showing the position of $1.5 \times 1.5 \times 4$ cm^3 voxel.

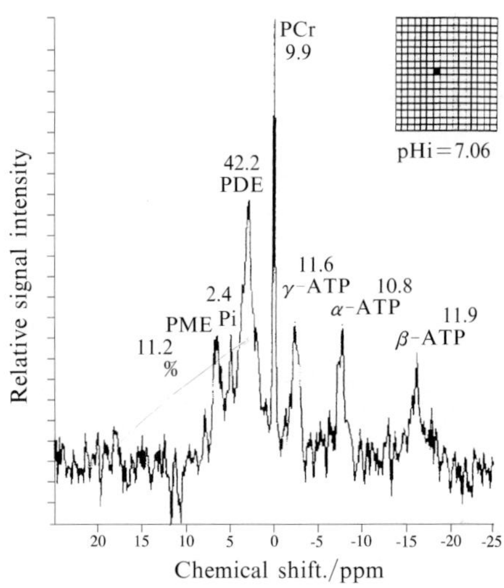

Fig. 81-10 ^{31}P spectrum of right basal ganglia.

CASE 82

Case 82: A 42-year-old male

Bipolar 1 Disorder, Most Recent Episode Manic

Age at onset : 29 years.

Although the patient presented a severe manic episode at admission, manic symptoms were subsiding. The MRS examination was performed at 72 days after admission, when his condition was relatively stabilized to a state of mild mania with inflated self-esteem and talkativeness. The T_2-weighted image in Figure 82-1 shows slight brain atrophy. The signal intensity in the ^{31}P contour map in Figure 82-2 is almost symmetrical. In the total ATP contour map in Figure 82-3, signal intensites are reduced in the left basal ganglia region. In the PME contour map signal intensities are reduced in the right medial frontal lobe and increased in the left basal ganglia region (Figure 82-4). In Figures 82-5 and 6, PDE signal intensities are reduced in the right basal ganglia region. PCr signals are decreased in the left temporal lobe and left basal ganglia region (Figure 82-7). In the ^{31}P spectrum of the right basal ganglia region obtained from voxel 4 shown in Figure 82-8, the %PCr is slightly increased (Figure 82-9). In the spectrum of the left basal ganglia (voxel 5), the %PME is increased, and %PCr and %γ-ATP are decreased (Figure 82-10). In the left basal ganglia region, the increased %PME suggests an alteration in phospholipids and the reduced PCr indicates dysfunction in the high-energy phosphate metabolism.

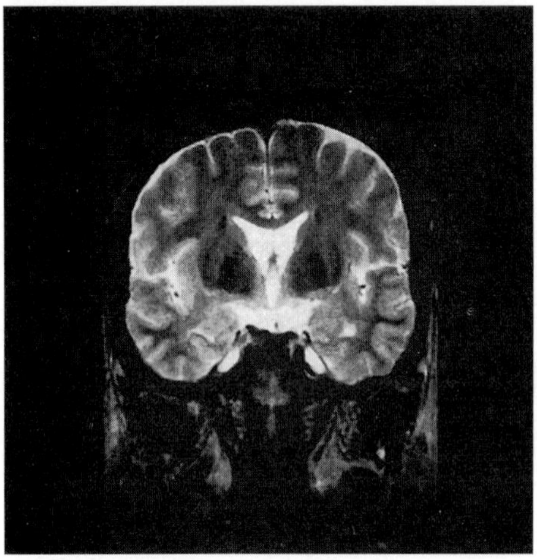

Fig. 82-1 Coronal T_2-weighted image (2,200/90).

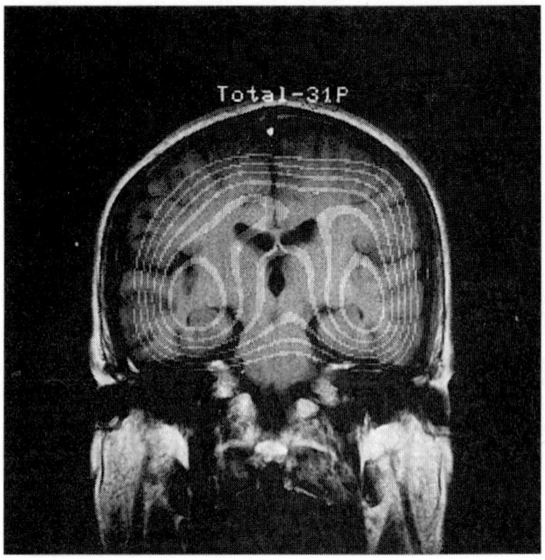

Fig. 82-2 Coronal ^{31}P contour map superimposed on T_1-weighted image (500/15).

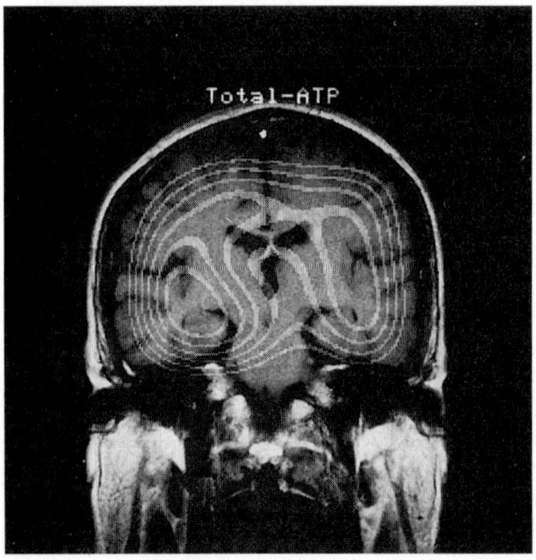

Fig. 82-3 Coronal total ATP contour map superimposed on T_1-weighted image (500/15).

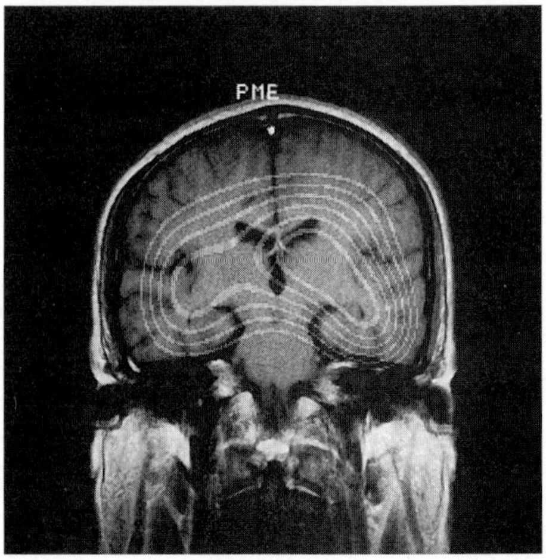

Fig. 82-4 Coronal PME contour map superimposed on T_1-weighted image (500/15).

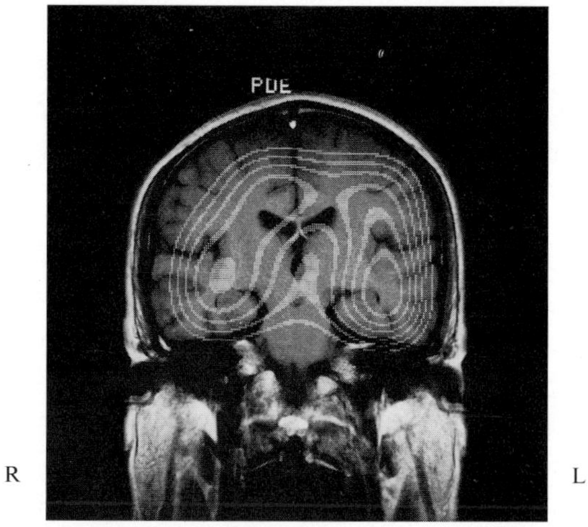

Fig. 82-5 Coronal PDE contour map superimposed on T_1-weighted image (500/15).

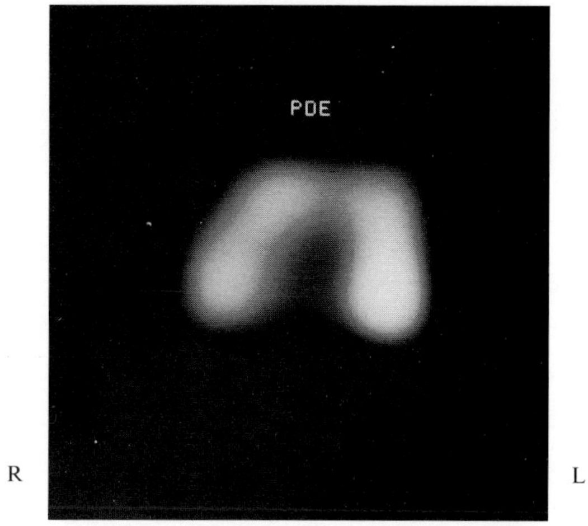

Fig. 82-6 Coronal PDE metabolite image.

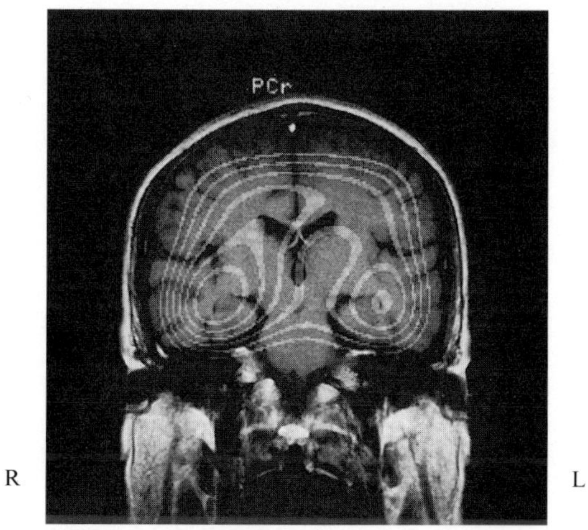

Fig. 82-7 Coronal PCr contour map superimposed on T_1-weighted image (500/15).

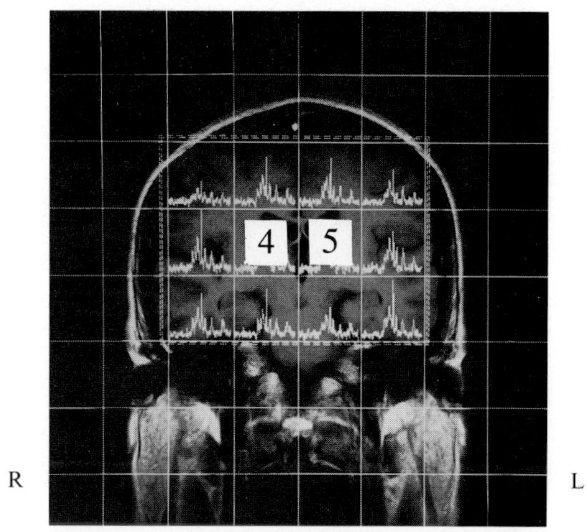

Fig. 82-8 T_1-weighted image showing the position of $3 \times 3 \times 4$ cm^3 voxels 4 and 5.

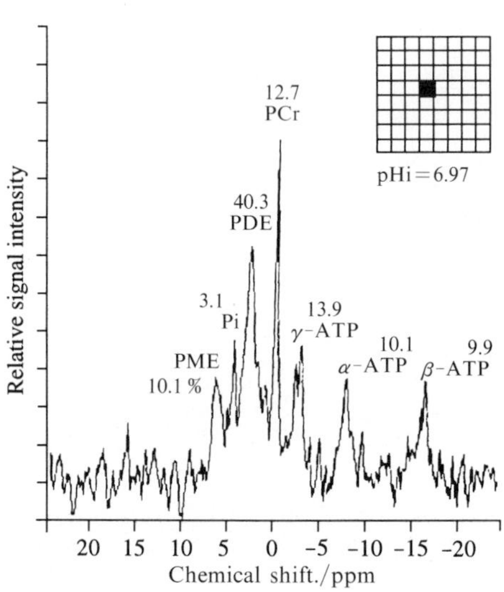

Fig. 82-9 ^{31}P spectrum of voxel 4. (Right basal ganglia.)

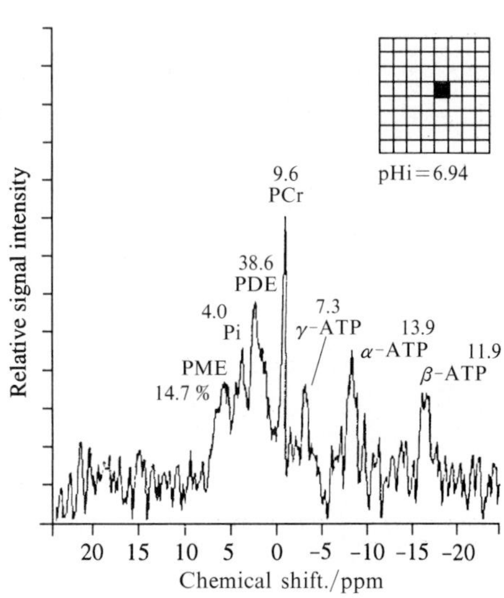

Fig. 82-10 ^{31}P spectrum of voxel 5. (Left basal ganglia.)

CASE 83

Case 83: A 48-year-old male

Alcohol Dependence

History of drinking : about 20 years.

The patient was admitted because of chronic alcoholism, diabetes mellitus, chronic liver disease, delusion of persecution, and impaired social functioning such as violence to his wife. The MRS study was performed at 17 days after hospitalization. The T_2-weighted image in Figure 83-1 shows moderate brain atrophy. In the ^{31}P contour map in Figure 83-2, signal intensities are reduced in the basal ganglia region. In the total ATP contour map and metabolite image in Figures 83-3 and 4, signal intensities are reduced in the basal ganglia region and the left temporal lobe, suggesting dysfunction in high-energy phosphate metabolism. The PME contour map and metabolite image show decreased signal intensities in the basal ganglia and right temporal regions (Figures 83-5 and 6). In the PDE contour map and metabolite image (Figures 83-7 and 8), signal intensities are reduced in the basal ganglia regions. In the PCr contour map and metabolite image in Figures 83-9 and 10, signal intensities are decreased in the bilateral basal ganglia regions. The spectra acquired from the basal ganglia region suggest disturbances in phospholipids and high-energy phosphate metabolism.

R 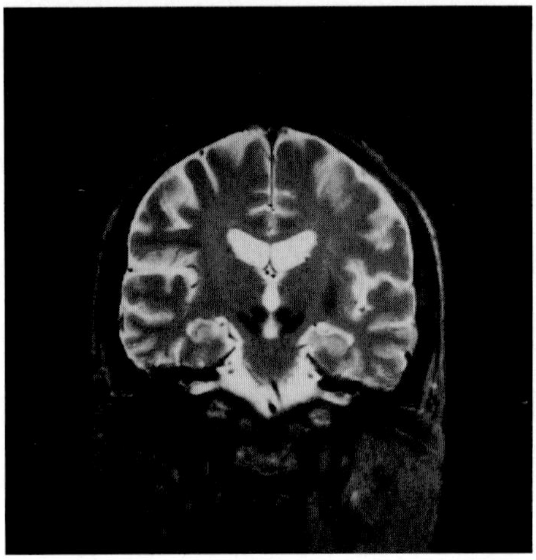 L

Fig. 83-1 Coronal T_2-weighted image (2,200/90).

R 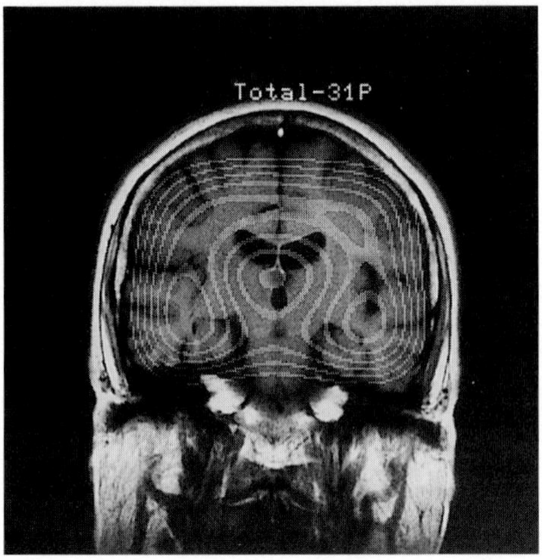 L

Fig. 83-2 Coronal ^{31}P contour map superimposed on T_1-weighted image (500/15).

R 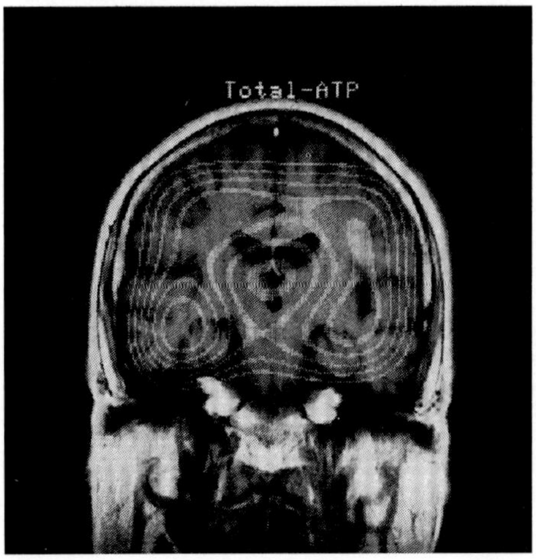 L

Fig. 83-3 Coronal total ATP contour map superimposed on T_1-weighted image (500/15).

R 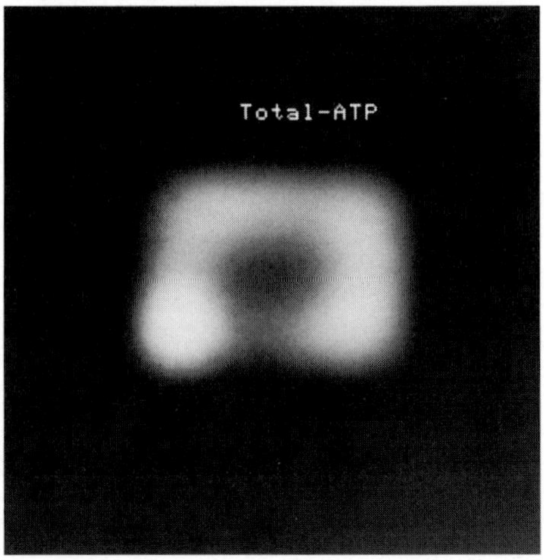 L

Fig. 83-4 Coronal total ATP metabolite image.

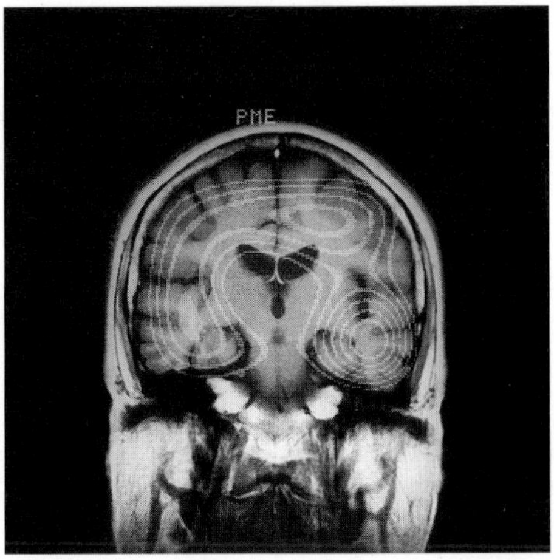

Fig. 83-5 Coronal PME contour map superimposed on T_1-weighted image (500/15).

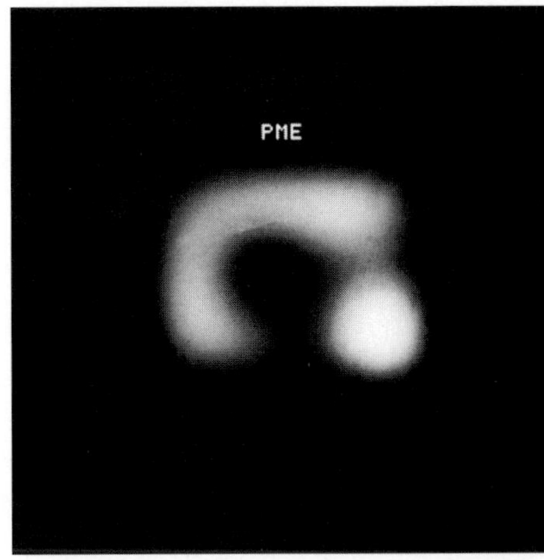

Fig. 83-6 Coronal PME metabolite image.

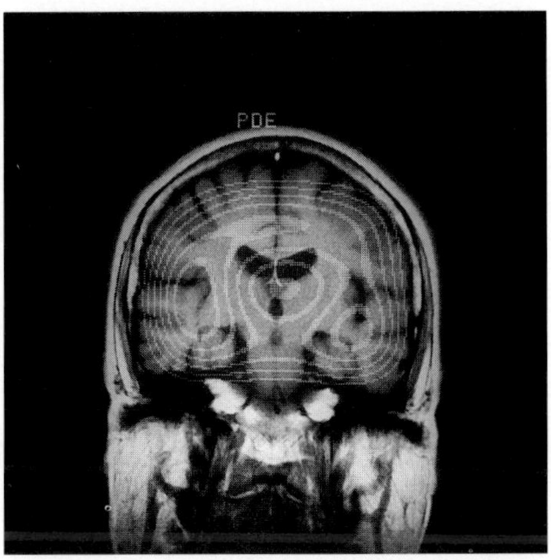

Fig. 83-7 Coronal PDE contour map superimposed on T_1-weighted image (500/15).

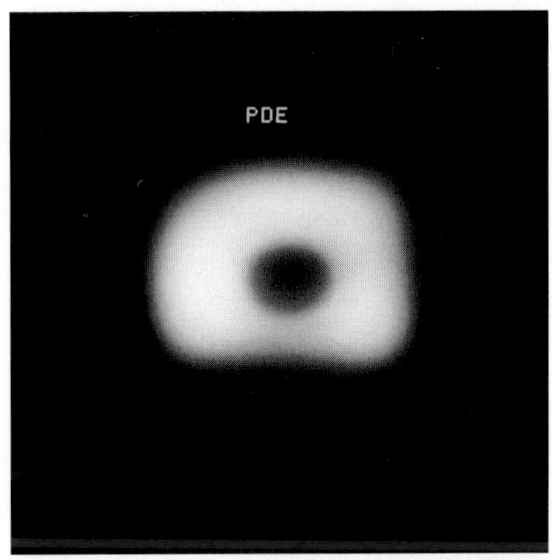

Fig. 83-8 Coronal PDE metabolite image.

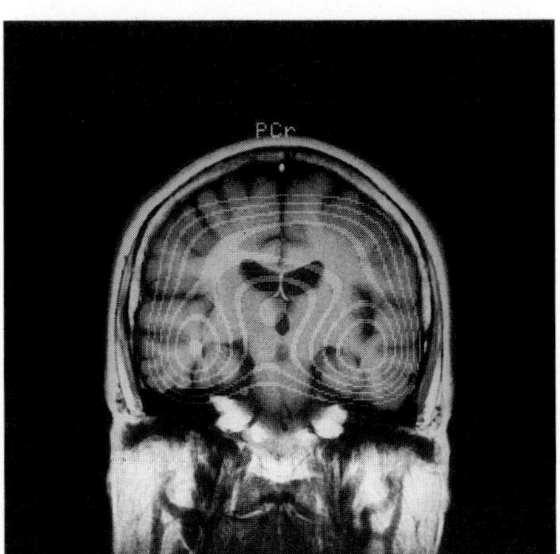

Fig. 83-9 Coronal PCr contour map superimposed on T_1-weighted image (500/15).

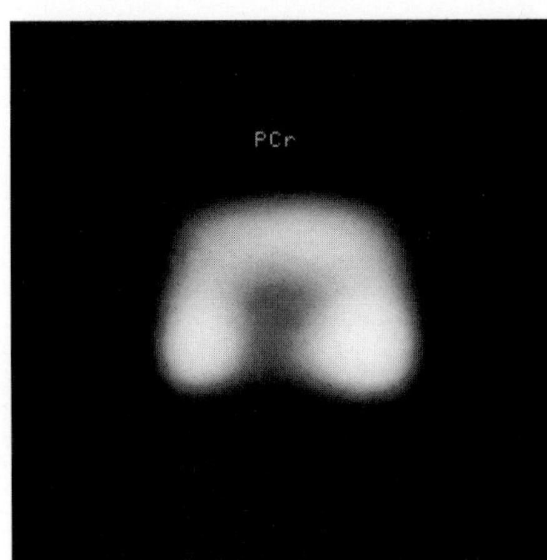

Fig. 83-10 Coronal PCr metabolite image.

CASE 84

Case 84: A 57-year-old male

Alcohol-induced mood disorder

History of drinking : about 20 years.

The patient had previously been hospitalized 4 times because of alcohol dependence, and had abstained from drinking for more than 60 months. However, he had a marked diminished interest in all activites which had persisted since the onset of withdrawal, and showed personality change. The T_2-weighted image in Figure 84-1 shows slight brain atrophy. In the ^1H spectrum obtained from the right basal ganglia region (voxel A shown in Figure 84-2), NAA/Cr ratio and the NAA/Cho ratio are reduced and the Cho/Cr ratio also has a tendency to decrease (Figure 84-3). In the ^1H spectrum of the left basal ganglia region (voxel B), NAA/Cr ratio is decreased and the NAA/Cho ratio is in the normal range, and the Cho/Cr ratio has a tendency to decrease (Figure 84-4). Decreased NAA/Cr ratios suggest neuronal loss and dysfunction in the basal ganglia region.

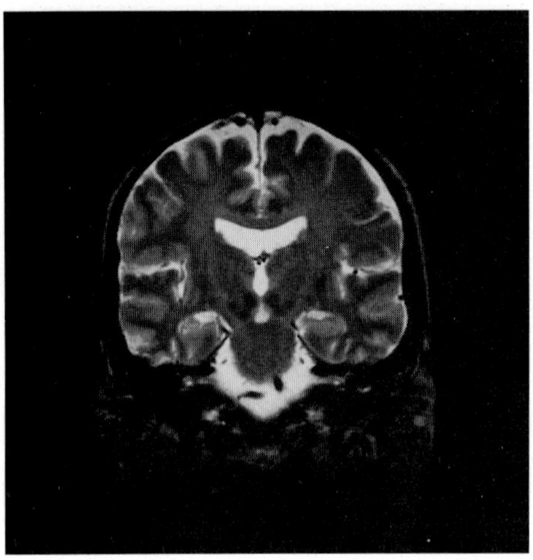

Fig. 84-1 Coronal T_2-weighted image (2,200/90).

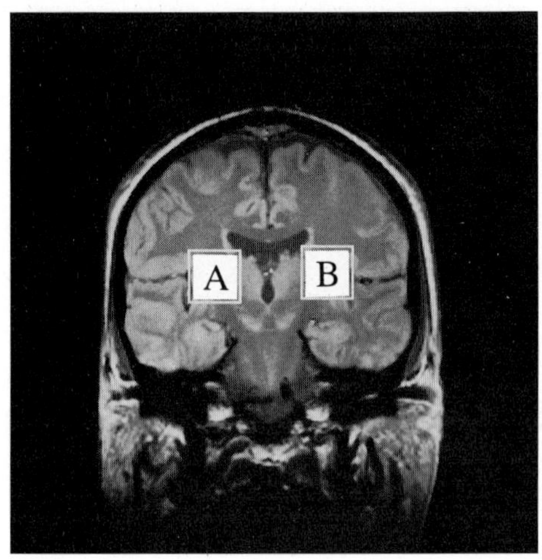

Fig. 84-2 T_1-weighted image showing the position of $2.5 \times 2.5 \times 2.5$ cm^3 voxels A and B.

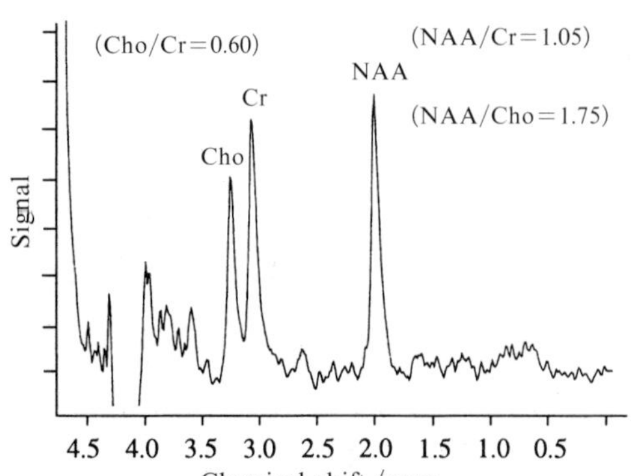

Fig. 84-3 ^1H spectrum of right basal ganglia (voxel A). STEAM (2,000/60).

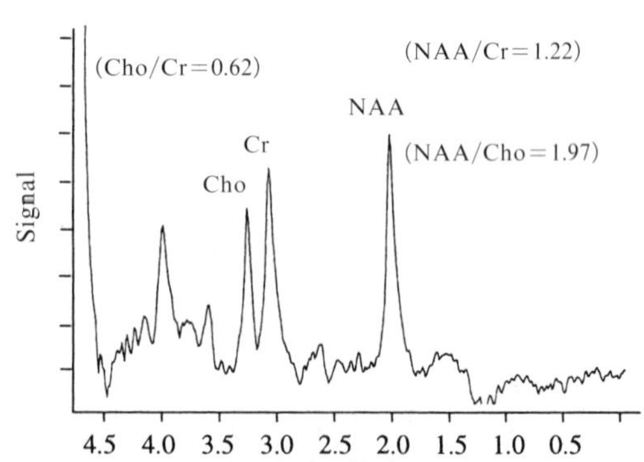

Fig. 84-4 ^1H spectrum of left basal ganglia (voxel B). STEAM (2,000/60).

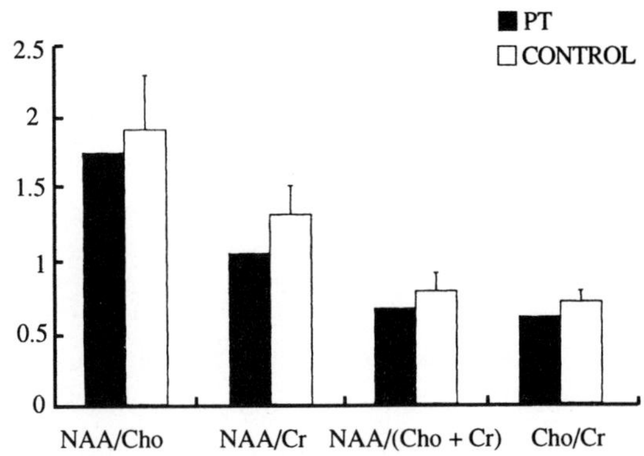

Fig. 84-5 Comparison of peak ratios in ^{1}H spectra of the right basal ganglia between patient and control group.

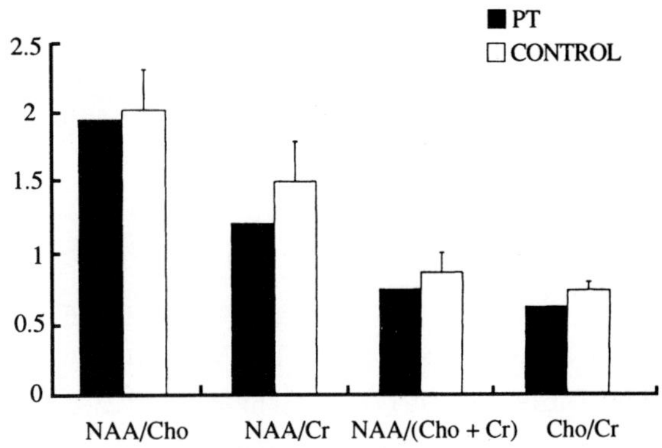

Fig. 84-6 Comparison of peak ratios in ^{1}H spectra of the left basal ganglia between patient and control group.

CASE 85

Case 85: A 48-year-old male

Alcohol Dependence

History of drinking : about 28 years.

The patient with a chronic excessive use of alcohol was admitted because of amnestic syndrome, anorexia, disturbance of liver function, and impaired social functioning. The MRS study was obtained 19 days after the beginning of abstinence. The T_2-weighted image in Figure 85-1 shows moderate brain atrophy. In the ^1H spectrum obtained from the right mesial temporal lobe (voxel B shown in Figure 85-2), the NAA/Cho ratio is reduced, but NAA/Cr ratio is in the normal range, and the Cho/Cr ratio is increased (Figure 85-3). In the ^1H spectrum of the left mesial temporal lobe (voxel A), NAA/Cr ratio and the NAA/Cho ratio are decreased, and the Cho/Cr ratio has a tendency to increase (Figure 85-4). Decreased NAA/Cr ratios suggest neuronal loss and dysfunction, and increased Cho/Cr ratios indicate alterations of the membrane phospholipid metabolism in the mesial temporal lobe.

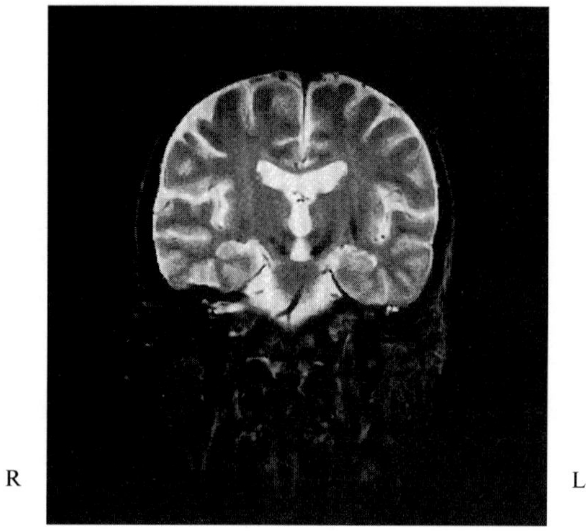

Fig. 85-1 Coronal T_2-weighted image (2,200/90).

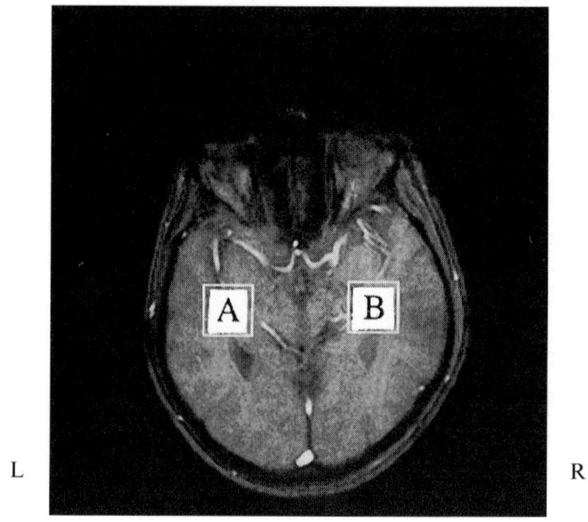

Fig. 85-2 T_1-weighted image showing the position of $2.5 \times 2.5 \times 2.5\ cm^3$ voxels A and B.

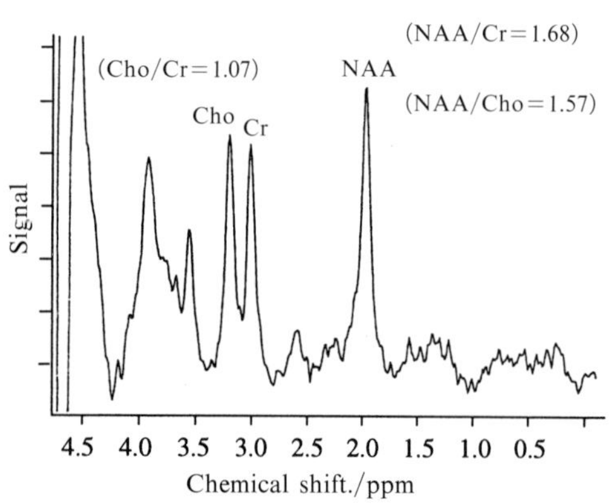

Fig. 85-3 ^1H spectrum of right mesial temporal lobe (voxel B). STEAM (2,000/60).

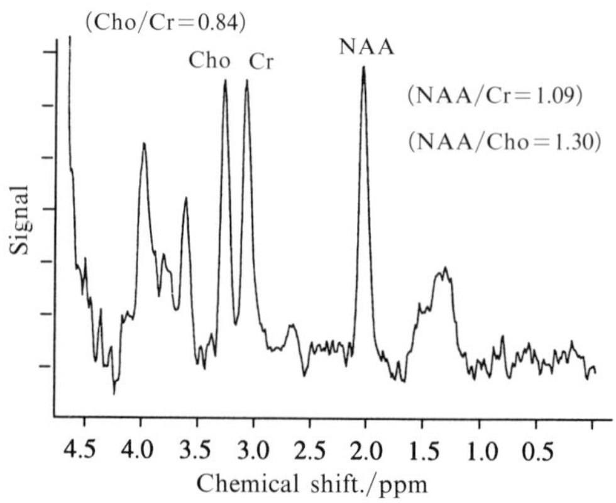

Fig. 85-4 ^1H spectrum of left mesial temporal lobe (voxel A). STEAM (2,000/60).

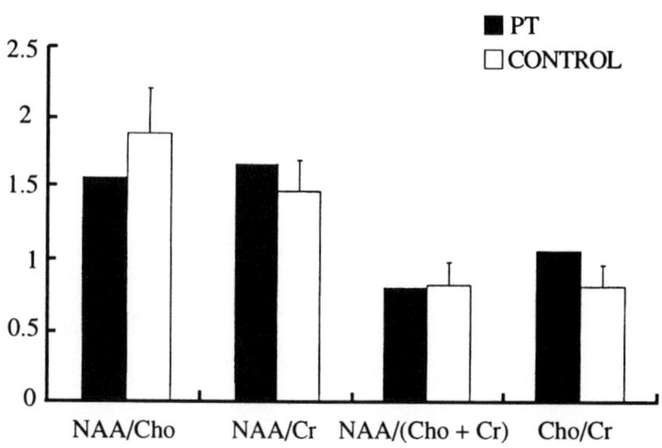

Fig. 85-5 Comparison of peak ratios in ^{1}H spectra of the right mesial temporal lobe between patient and control group.

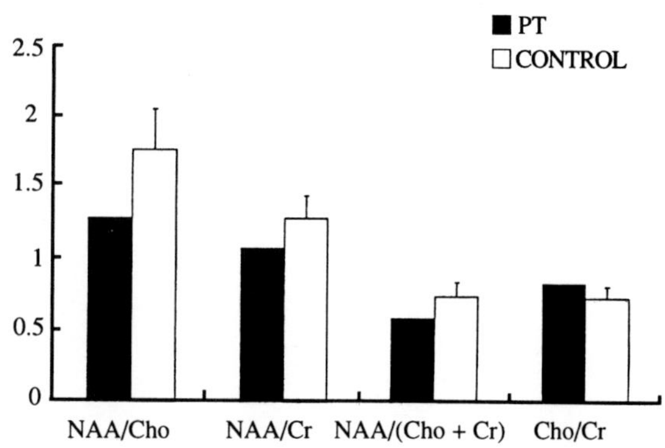

Fig. 85-6 Comparison of peak ratios in ^{1}H spectra of the left mesial temporal lobe between patient and control group.

Author Index

Subject Index